P9-CRE-949

May. 79.

Medical neurobiology

FROM THE LIBRARY OF
Fred Cornell, M.D., M.S.C., F.A.C.C.

Medical neurobiology

Neuroanatomical and neurophysiological
principles basic to clinical neuroscience

William D. Willis, Jr., M.D., Ph.D.

Chief, Comparative Neurobiology, Marine Biomedical Institute;
Professor of Anatomy and Physiology,
University of Texas Medical Branch,
Galveston, Texas

Robert G. Grossman, M.D.

Chief of Neurosurgery;
Professor of Surgery,
University of Texas Medical Branch,
Galveston, Texas

SECOND EDITION

with 638 illustrations

The C. V. Mosby Company

Saint Louis 1977

SECOND EDITION

Copyright © 1977 by The C. V. Mosby Company

All rights reserved. No part of this book may be reproduced in any manner without written permission of the publisher.

Previous edition copyrighted 1973

Printed in the United States of America

Distributed in Great Britain by Henry Kimpton, London

Library of Congress Cataloging in Publication Data

Willis, William D   1934-
   Medical neurobiology.

   Includes bibliographies and index.
   1. Neurobiology. I. Grossman, Robert G.,
joint author. II. Title. [DNLM: 1. Nervous
system—Anatomy and histology. 2. Nervous system—
Physiology. WL102 W735m]
QP356.W45 1977   612'.8   76-41192
ISBN 0-8016-5583-8

CB/CB/B 9 8 7 6 5 4 3 2 1

To

William D. Willis, M.D.

and

Ferenc Grossman, M.D.

Preface

The second edition of *Medical Neurobiology* has much the same organization as the first edition, with some notable exceptions. The main emphasis in the revision has been the addition of a considerable number of new illustrations (almost 200), mostly of neuroanatomical material, with the intent of making the book more useful in the neuroanatomical laboratory. To further this end, the Atlas (Appendix III) has been revised by including photographs of brain sections with better contrast between gray and white matter than in the previous edition and also a series of brain sections in the horizontal plane.

Chapter 1, on neurohistology and cellular neurophysiology, has been altered only slightly, by revision of the section on neurocytology and the addition of several figures. Chapter 2, on sensory receptors and their function, was improved by a more modern treatment of the cutaneous receptors and by several new illustrations. In Chapter 3, the consideration of the peripheral nervous system was not changed greatly, although there was some expansion of the discussion of neuromuscular transmission, including consideration of membrane recycling. Chapter 4, on the spinal cord, now includes material on motor unit properties and the motoneuron size principle. Major revisions are in Chapters 5 and 6, which deal with brain organization. The gross anatomy of the brain and the ventricular system and vascular supply of the brain are the subject matter of Chapter 5. Cross-sectional and microscopic anatomy of the brain and the cranial nerves now form the subject of a new Chapter 6. Chapter 7 has many new illustrations that help guide the student in tracing the sensory pathways, and the subject of pain is treated more extensively. Chapter 8 now contains sections on the reticular formation, the cerebellum, and the basal ganglia, so that the motor system can be studied as a whole. Again, many new illustrations should assist students in following motor pathways. Chapter 10, on the limbic system, has been restructured and better illustrated. Appendix I was expanded to include consideration of several additional techniques. Little was done to alter Chapters 9, 11, 12, or Appendix II. As mentioned above, the Atlas has been significantly improved.

We hope that the changes made in this edition will serve to make the text more valuable for teaching neuroanatomy and neurophysiology. We wish to thank those individuals who have contributed so much to the revision: Gail Silver, for most of the new figures; Drs. P. Coates, R. E. Coggeshall, J. D. Coulter, and M. Sarwar, for a number of illustrations; and Pat Williamson and Myrna Bratcher, for typing the manuscript.

William D. Willis, Jr.

Robert G. Grossman

Contents

The neuron and the nerve impulse

NEURON THEORY

One of the fundamental concepts of modern neurobiology is the neuron theory. Perhaps more than to any other single person we owe this concept to the

Spanish neurohistologist, Santiago Ramón y Cajal (1852-1934).

During Cajal's career there developed a controversy over the question of how nerve cells interconnect. One group favored the idea that there is protoplasmic continuity between various nervous elements. This idea was called the reticular theory, and it appeared to simplify the problem of nervous transmission (Fig. 1-1). Cajal led an opposing group who felt that histologic and other evidence proved that nerve cells are contiguous but not continuous. Cajal summarized this evidence in *Neuron Theory or Reticular Theory?* which was published after his death.

The evidence of Cajal and others that a nerve cell is an anatomical entity has been fully confirmed by modern histological techniques, including electron microscopy, and by neurophysiological methods.

Although Cajal did much to develop the neuron theory, it was His and Forel who originated it, Wal-

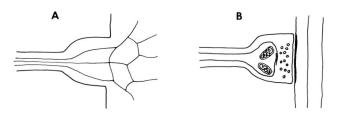

Fig. 1-1. Reticular theory versus neuron theory. The reticular theory was the concept that elements of the nervous system have protoplasmic interconnections. This idea was based on light microscopic observations. **A** shows neurofibrils forming a network that is continuous between two neural elements. The neuron theory, championed by Cajal, was the idea that neural elements are individual cells and that these cells come into contiguity at functional zones of contact, but that there is no cytoplasmic continuity between nerve cells. **B** shows such a contact point between neural elements. The neurofibrils remain within the confines of the cell membranes of the two nerve cells. Final proof of the structural arrangements present at such regions of contact between nerve cells came with the invention of the electron microscope.

deyer who coined the term neuron, and Sherrington who gave the name synapse to the region of functional connection between two neurons.

Neurons as a communications network

The properties of neurons and their interconnections form a major part of the subject matter of neurobiology. Neurons are cells that are specialized for receiving and transmitting information (Fig. 1-2). The nervous system obtains data from the environment, both external and internal, by means of receptor organs. The data are coded by the receptor organs in spatial and temporal patterns of nerve impulses. The information is conveyed to the central nervous system, where it is interpreted. The result may be a decision by the central nervous system to alter some ongoing activity or to initiate an action. The command to do either is relayed to effector organs, such as muscles or glands, by nerve impulses. Communication between neurons and other neurons or effector cells is accom-

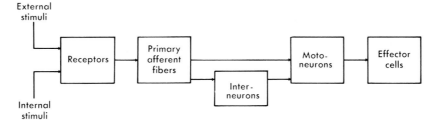

Fig. 1-2. Information flow in the nervous system. Stimuli, both from the external world and from within the body, activate receptor organs. The information gathered by receptor organs is transmitted to the central nervous system by way of primary afferent fibers. These synapse either directly on motoneurons or, more commonly, on interneurons. The interneurons may activate other interneurons, either in the spinal cord or in the brain. The patterns of interaction among these cells can be exceedingly complex. Eventually, however, the interneuron chains feed information to motoneurons. These command actions by effectors, which include muscle and gland cells.

Fig. 1-3. Basic events in the development of the nervous system. The neural tube is shown developing from the walls of the neural groove. The preceding stage was the neural plate. As the neural folds approximate each other, the neural crest buds off, forming, among other things, the dorsal root ganglia and the sympathetic paravertebral ganglia. Cells of the dorsal root ganglia include neuroblasts, which eventually form the pseudounipolar dorsal root ganglion cells, the precursors of Schwann cells, which ensheath the developing afferent fibers, and satellite cells, which surround the cell bodies of the ganglion cells. Dorsal root ganglion cells send processes centrally into dorsal roots and peripherally into spinal nerves. The sympathetic paravertebral ganglia also contain neuroblasts, which develop into sympathetic postganglionic neurons, and the precursors of Schwann and satellite cells. The cells of the neural tube form the ependymal layer adjacent to the lumen of the tube. The ependymal layer is also called the ventricular zone. In the telencephalon of a number of mammals studied, eventually a subependymal or a subventricular layer can be distinguished in which proliferation of cells may occur into adult life. The radially directed terminal processes of these cells form the marginal layer. Neuroblasts and neuroglial precursor cells are formed after mitosis and differentiation of some of the elements of the ependymal layer. Neuroblasts are actually postmitotic cells that migrate and differentiate; medulloblasts, or apolar spongioblasts, are interphase germinal cells that can undergo further division, with subsequent differentiation into the macroglia (astrocytes and oligodendrocytes). The new cells form the mantle layer just external to the ependymal layer. The mantle layer is also called the intermediate zone. As the neural elements mature, many send axons into the outer, or marginal, layer of the neural tube. Motoneurons send their axons into the developing ventral roots and from there into spinal nerves. The pattern of development of the spinal cord and of the neocortex is that the deepest layers develop first, and then new cells migrate outward to the surface. However, in the cerebellum the superficial layers develop first, and cells then migrate inward to form the deeper layers. Abbreviations: *EP*, ependymal layer; *Mant*, mantle layer; *Marg*, marginal layer; *SN*, spinal nerve; *Med*, medulloblast; *Ast*, astroblast; *Olig*, oligodendroblast; *Peri*, pericyte; *Micr*, microglial cell; *AN*, apolar neuroblast; *BN*, bipolar neuroblast; *UN*, unipolar neuroblast; *MN*, multipolar neuroblast; *Neur*, neuron; *Pseu N*, pseudounipolar neuron.

plished by a special process known as synaptic transmission.

A useful analogy can be made between these two basic communications processes in the nervous system—nerve impulses and synaptic transmission—and the two types of signals employed by computers. Some computers utilize signals that are either present or absent. These are called digital signals. Arithmetic can be done with digital information, using binary mathematics. Information is stored in a digital computer by memory elements, which can be put into either of two states, often described as "on" or "off." In many ways, the traffic of nerve impulses in the nervous system resembles the transfer of digital information in a computer. However, it is unlikely that anything resembling a binary memory exists in the nervous system.

Another type of computer uses continuously variable signals in its handling of information. This kind of signal is called an analog. An example of an analog

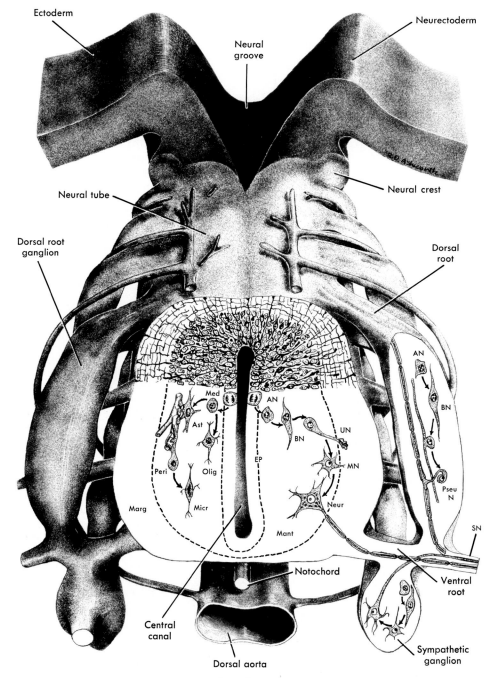

Fig. 1-3. For legend see opposite page.

signal is the electrocardiogram. The activity of the heart produces a continuously variable electrical signal, which is generally recorded on a strip of paper by a penwriter after suitable amplification. A signal of this kind can also be analyzed by an analog computer. Transmission between nerve cells in the nervous system resembles in some respects the processing of analog signals, because transmission of information across a synapse produces a continuously variable alteration in the excitability of the postsynaptic cell.

Because the nervous system uses both analog and digital types of signals, it acts more like a hybrid analog and digital computer than like either kind alone. The nervous system can "digitize" analog signals, such as sensory information, coding it in patterns of nerve impulses. At synapses, the information conveyed by nerve impulses is translated back into time-variant analog form during synaptic transmission.

Much of this and the next three chapters is devoted to a consideration of the mechanisms of nervous transmission, receptor organ function, and synaptic transmission. The nerve impulses are discussed in some detail later in this chapter. But first it is necessary to describe the development and structure of neurons and their supporting cells.

EMBRYOLOGY OF NEURONS AND NEUROGLIA

The nervous system of vertebrates develops from the outermost of the three germ layers, the ectoderm (Fig. 1-3). In the region of the primitive streak of the embryo, a portion of the ectoderm differentiates into the neural plate. A neural groove forms, and eventually the margins of the neural groove meet to produce the neural tube, which then separates from the surface ectoderm. Some ectodermal cells pinch off at the lateral borders of the neural tube adjacent to the surface. These cells form the neural crests.

The majority of neurons and their supporting cells, the neuroglia, originate from cells of the neural tube. These form the central nervous system. Ganglionic neurons of the peripheral nervous system and their supporting cells originate, at least in part, from the neural crests.

As the cells within the neural tube divide and differentiate, the wall of the tube develops a three-layered structure. The innermost layer, adjacent to the lumen of the neural tube, is the ependymal layer. It contains germinal cells and cells destined to become the adult ependymal cells. As the germinal cells divide, many of the daughter cells become situated in the zone around the ependymal layer, forming the mantle layer. As some of the cells differentiate into neurons they

develop processes, which extend superficially to form the marginal layer.

The germinal cells give rise to intermediate forms that later become either neurons or neuroglia. Early neurons are often called neuroblasts. These may at first lack processes (apolar neuroblasts), in which case they resemble the medulloblasts (apolar spongioblasts), which are cells that give rise to astrocytes and oligodendroglia. As a neuroblast matures, it typically develops two processes (bipolar neuroblast). Later, one of these regresses, leaving a single process that is destined to become the axon (unipolar neuroblast). Finally, a number of additional processes, which eventually become dendrites (multipolar neuroblasts), may develop. This sequence may vary considerably, depending on the particular type of neuron.

Medulloblasts (and also spongioblasts with processes) differentiate into precursor cells that later become astrocytes and oligodendroglia. The most important of the intermediate forms are the astroblast and the oligodendroblast.

The microglia are different from the other types of neuroglia in that they originate from mesoderm and enter the central nervous system with the vasculature. They may assume an inactive form as pericytes adjacent to blood vessels until there is damage to nervous tissue.

Neural crest cells migrate to positions lateral and anterior to the neural tube. The former develop into the ganglion cells and satellite cells of the dorsal root ganglia and cranial nerve ganglia. Those that become located anterior to the neural tube may differentiate into sympathetic ganglion cells or chromaffin cells, including those of the adrenal medulla. In addition, the neural crest seems to give rise to some of the Schwann cells, which are responsible for myelin formation in the peripheral nervous system. Other Schwann cells may originate from the neural tube.

MORPHOLOGY OF NEURONS AND NEUROGLIA
Size of neurons

If multinucleated cells, like those of skeletal muscle, are discounted, neurons include the largest cells of the body. However, there is a wide range of sizes of neurons. The diameter of the largest neurons in mammals, measuring the long axis of the cell body, is about 125 μm; that of the smallest is about 4 μm. Such measurements are a bit misleading, because the cell body of a neuron may represent only a fraction of the total extent of the neuron. For example, the surface area of the cell body of a cerebral cortical neuron may be only 10% of the total; the remaining

90% of the surface area is accounted for by the neuronal processes (the axon and the dendrites). The volume of mammalian neurons ranges up to 10^6 μm^3, and the net weight up to about 8×10^{-7} g.

The neurons of many invertebrates are much larger than those of vertebrates. For instance, the cell body of the identified neuron R2 in the sea slug *Aplysia* has a diameter approaching 1 mm. Even axons in the invertebrates may reach enormous size. The best known giant axon is that of the squid, which is described in further detail (p. 26) in connection with its use as a model preparation for the study of the action potential. Its diameter may also approach 1 mm.

Structural properties of neurons

There are many types of neurons. Drawings of some are shown in Fig. 1-4. Despite the diversity of neuronal types, they share the normal complement of organelles found in most cells. What distinguishes neurons from each other and from other cell types is the number, extent, and arrangement of neuronal processes. The most unique feature of neurons is the synapse (Figs. 1-5 and 1-8).

The cytoplasm of neurons is bounded by a unit membrane similar to that of other cells of the body. The unit membrane is a three-layered structure with an electron-dense layer on each side of an electron-translucent layer. The total thickness of the unit membrane is about 7.5 nm. It is thought that the electron-dense layers represent the location of bonds between protein and lipid, and the electron-translucent layer indicates the bimolecular leaflet of lipids in the membrane.

The nucleus of most neurons is large, spherical, and lightly staining (with hematoxylin and eosin) and contains a single large nucleolus (Figs. 1-5 and 1-6). A Barr body (sex chromatin) may be seen in nuclei of neurons in females. The nucleus of a neuron is surrounded by two membranes, the outer one being a part of the endoplasmic reticulum (Figs. 1-6 and 1-7). These membranes form the nuclear envelope. Although most of the chromatin material of the nucleus is dispersed, some appears in electron micrographs as dense strands within the karyoplasm.

The cytoplasm of neurons stained with a basic dye contains masses of a chromophilic material called Nissl substance (after Franz Nissl). This material corresponds to organized areas of granular endoplasmic reticulum in electron micrographs (Figs. 1-5 to 1-7). As in other cells, the granular endoplasmic reticulum of neurons is involved in protein synthesis. The highly developed granular endoplasmic reticulum of neurons reflects the fact that neurons are especially active in protein synthesis. Nissl bodies are distributed

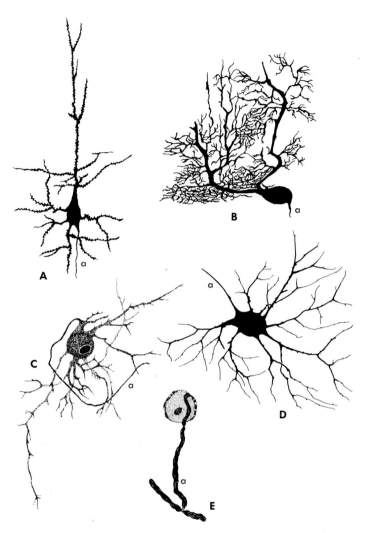

Fig. 1-4. Variety of forms of neurons. The neuron in **A** is characterized by a cell body that has a roughly pyramidal shape. This type of neuron, called a pyramidal cell, is typical of the cerebral cortex. Note the many spinous processes lining the surface of the dendrites. The axon is labelled *a* in this and the other drawings. The cell type in **B** was first described by the Czechoslovakian neuroanatomist Purkinje, and it has since been known as the Purkinje cell. Purkinje cells are characteristic of the cerebellar cortex. The cell body is pear shaped, with a rich dendritic plexus originating from one end and the axon from the other. The fine branches of the dendrites are covered with spines (not shown). The neurons in **C** and **D** are motor in function. **C** shows a sympathetic postganglionic neuron; **D** is an alpha motoneuron of the spinal cord. Both are multipolar neurons with radially arranged dendrites. The cell in **E** is sensory in function. It is a dorsal root ganglion cell. There are no dendrites. The axon branches into a central and a peripheral process. Because the axon is the result of fusion of two processes during embryonic development, these cells are described as pseudounipolar neurons rather than unipolar.

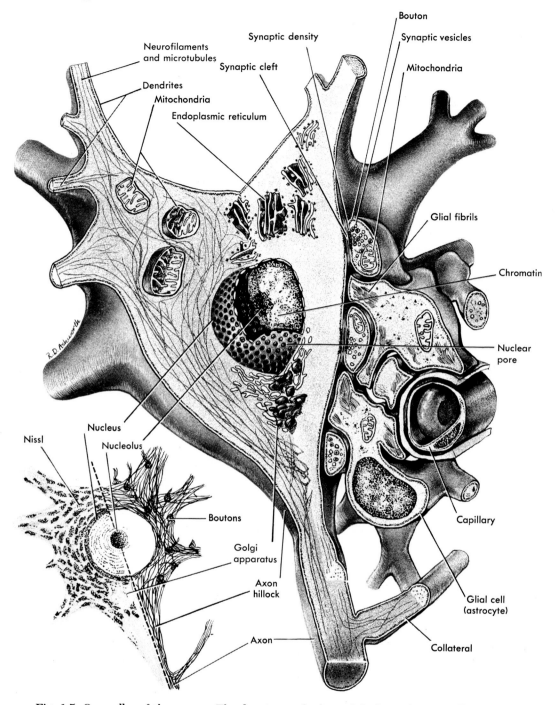

Fig. 1-5. Organelles of the neuron. The drawing to the lower left shows the organelles typical of a neuron as seen with the light microscope. The portion of the drawing to the left of the broken line represents structures seen with a Nissl stain. These include the nucleus and nucleolus, Nissl bodies in the cytoplasm of the cell body and proximal dendrites, and, as a negative image, the Golgi apparatus. The absence of Nissl bodies in the axon hillock and axon is also shown. To the right of the broken line are structures seen with a heavy-metal stain. These include neurofibrils. With the appropriate heavy-metal stain, the Golgi apparatus may be demonstrated (not shown). On the surface of the neuron, a number of synaptic endings are indicated as stained by the heavy metal. The large drawing shows structures visible at the electron microscopic level. The nucleus, nucleolus, chromatin, and nuclear pores are represented. In the cytoplasm are mitochondria, rough endoplasmic reticulum, the Golgi apparatus, neurofilaments, and microtubules. Along the surface membrane are such associated structures as synaptic endings, astrocytic processes, and a capillary containing a red blood corpuscle.

throughout the cell body of the neuron and may also be seen in the basal parts of the processes called dendrites, but they are not found in the axon hillock or in the axon (see p. 8 for a description of neuronal processes). The staining quality of Nissl bodies is altered in the pathological reaction of chromatolysis, described on p. 19.

The cell bodies and processes of neurons contain neurofibrils, best demonstrated at the light microscopic level by heavy metal stains (Fig. 1-5). The neurofibrils appear to correspond to groups of microtubules and neurofilaments seen with the electron microscope. Microtubules are elongated structures having a diameter of 20 to 26 nm. Their name reflects the observation that in cross section they have a circular profile, with a ring-shaped wall 6 nm thick surrounding an electron-lucent core. Microtubules have

been implicated in the movement of substances and organelles within neuronal cytoplasm. Of particular interest is the discovery that there is a substantial movement of cytoplasm from the region of the cell body down the axon and also in the reverse direction (axoplasmic flow and retrograde axoplasmic flow, p. 38). There is also a movement of cytoplasm within the cell body and along the dendrites. The movement can be halted by cytotoxic agents, such as colchicine and the *Vinca* alkaloids, which disrupt the microtubules. The neurofilaments are also elongated structures, with a diameter of 10 nm. It has been proposed that neuro-

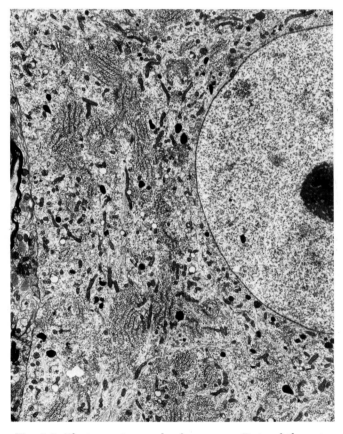

Fig. 1-6. Electron micrograph of a neuron. Parts of the cytoplasm and nucleus of a neuron are shown. The nucleus and nucleolus are at the right. Within the nucleoplasm is scattered chromatin material. The cytoplasm of the neuron contains clusters of rough endoplasmic reticulum (Nissl bodies), components of the Golgi apparatus, mitochondria, and neurofilaments. Along the plasma membrane to the left of the micrograph are associated structures, including synaptic endings, glial processes, and passing myelinated axons. (×4,550.) (Courtesy Dr. Murray Matthews.)

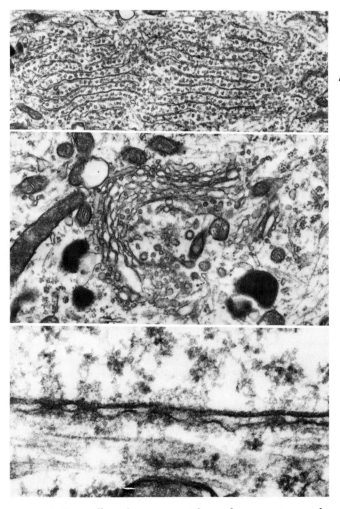

Fig. 1-7. Organelles of a neuron. Three electron micrographs of neuronal organelles are shown. **A** shows an area of rough endoplasmic reticulum (Nissl body). (×12,400.) At the center of **B** is a view of a Golgi apparatus. In addition, other structures are seen, including mitochondria, neurofilaments, and microtubules. (×15,250.) **C** shows the nuclear envelope. The nucleoplasm is at the top and the cytoplasm at the bottom. The two separate layers of the nuclear envelope are seen to join periodically, presumably at the sites of nuclear pores. (×53,800.) (Courtesy Dr. Murray Matthews.)

filaments may represent fragments or precursors of microtubules, but this is controversial. Other than this possibility, the function of neurofilaments is unknown, although they may play a role in maintaining the structural configuration of neuronal processes. Neuron cell bodies also contain the system of flattened cisternae and small vesicles known as the Golgi apparatus (Fig. 1-7). The first description of this organelle by Golgi was based on histological preparations of nervous tissue showing the apparatus in the Purkinje cells of the barn owl. As in other cells, the Golgi apparatus of neurons is considered to be involved in secretory activity. One secretion product of the neuron is the synaptic transmitter, which may be packaged in vesicles by the Golgi apparatus and then transported down the axon to synaptic endings. The Golgi apparatus may also be involved in the formation of lysosomes, according to the Golgi endoplasmic reticulum lysosome hypothesis (GERL).

Other organelles found in neurons include numerous mitochondria. These are found in all regions of the cytoplasm, both in the cell body region and in the processes. They are especially abundant in synaptic terminals. Some neurons have been found with cilia. Neuronal cilia are thought to be vestigial in most instances, although in retinal photoreceptors and in several kinds of hair cells the cilia have a sensory function. Neurons may also contain inclusions, such as pigment granules. The most common type of pigment in neurons is called lipofuscin, which tends to increase in quantity with advancing age. Lipofuscin pigment appears to be derived from lysosomes and may represent the undigested residue of material that cannot be catabolized by lysosomal enzymes. In the usual amounts found, lipofuscin seems to be harmless, but an excess accumulation of this or other residues is the basis for a number of storage diseases affecting neurons. Certain neurons in the substantia nigra (p. 191) and in the locus ceruleus (p. 188) contain melanin pigment. Other inclusions are iron-containing granules found in neurons of the substantia nigra and in the globus pallidus. Very little glycogen is stored in nerve cells.

Mature neurons have processes extending from the cell body for varying distances and branching to varying degrees, depending on the cell type (Fig. 1-4). The axon is one kind of process. Axons in general carry information by means of nerve impulses from the nerve cell body region toward other neurons or effector cells. The axon is therefore the output of the neuron in terms of information flow. A neuron will generally have only a single axon, although the axon may branch. The axon typically arises from a special region of the cell body known as the axon hillock.

The axon hillock is characterized by the absence of Nissl substance. In some neurons, the axon may arise from a dendrite rather than from the cell body. The first portion of the axon may be quite narrow for some distance and then expand to a wider diameter. The narrow region is called the initial segment. If a myelin sheath is present, it begins where the axon widens. The axon may give off branches near the cell body (axon collaterals) that may synapse on neurons nearby. Some axon collaterals turn back toward the cell body; these are called recurrent collaterals. The main part of the axon may extend away from the cell body for a long distance (from centimeters to meters) through a fiber tract of the central nervous system or through a peripheral nerve and end synaptically on other neurons or on effector cells. Neurons with long axons of this kind are termed Golgi type I cells. In Golgi type II cells, the axons are short, terminating on neurons in the immediate vicinity of the cell body. Organelles found in the axon include microtubules and neurofilaments. In general, there are more neurofilaments than microtubules. Some agranular endoplasmic reticulum, vesicles, and mitochrondria are also seen in axons, but granular endoplasmic reticulum and ribosomes appear to be absent.

The dendrite is the other type of process that most neurons possess. Although some neurons lack dendrites, others have several or many (Fig. 1-4). Dendrites generally extend only a short distance (1 mm or less) from the cell body, often branching repetitively to form a characteristic arborization for that particular type of neuron. The cytoplasm of dendrites resembles that of the cell body. There are Nissl bodies, at least in the proximal dendrites. Microtubules and neurofilaments are present, but microtubules generally outnumber neurofilaments. The dendrites of many neurons have fine evaginations called dendritic spines. These serve as points of attachment of certain synapses. However, the main surface of dendrites and of the cell body also receive synaptic terminals. The membrane of the cell body and dendrites thus serves as a receptive region from the standpoint of information flow in the nervous system.

Synaptic endings of axons may take any of a variety of forms (Figs. 1-8 and 1-9). Synapses can generally be subdivided into electrical and chemical types. Electrical synaptic transmission is much more common in the invertebrates and in the lower vertebrates than in mammals, although some electrical synapses do occur in mammals. The morphology of electrical synapses seems to be consistent for various forms. Such synapses involve a gap junction, or narrow cleft, between a presynaptic terminal and the postsynaptic

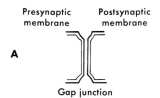

A

Presynaptic membrane   Postsynaptic membrane

Gap junction

Fig. 1-8. Schematic drawings of various types of synapses. **A,** Electrical synapse. This consists of a gap junction (∼ 2 nm) between pre- and postsynaptic membranes. **B,** Chemical synapses. Type I synapses have a widened synaptic cleft (∼ 30 nm), asymmetrical cytoplasmic densities, and spherical vesicles. Type II synapses have a 20 nm synaptic cleft, symmetrical cytoplasmic densities, and sometimes ovoid vesicles. **C,** Synaptic arrangements, including axodendritic, axosomatic, axoaxonal, and dendrodendritic synapses.

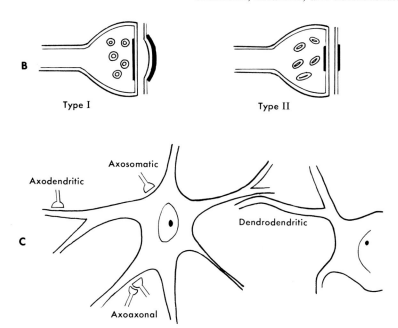

B

Type I   Type II

C

Axodendritic   Axosomatic   Dendrodendritic   Axoaxonal

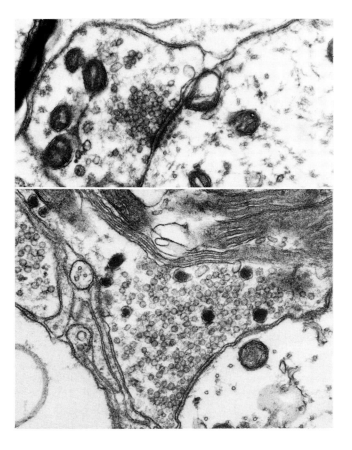

Fig. 1-9. Electron micrographs of synaptic regions. In the upper micrograph, the presynaptic terminal of an axon is shown to the left, and the postsynaptic element is to the right. The presynaptic and postsynaptic elements are separated by a distinct synaptic cleft. The synaptic cleft in this case is actually wider than the adjacent regions of separation between neural and glial elements. This finding of a distinct synaptic cleft was the final proof of the neuron theory. The presynaptic terminal in the upper micrograph contains a number of small, clear synaptic vesicles, as well as several mitochondria. The postsynaptic membrane is thickened, with electron-dense material extending into the cytoplasm. There is also electron-dense material within the synaptic cleft. (×36,600.) The lower micrograph shows another synaptic region. The presynaptic element is at the center, and the postsynaptic element is at the lower right. The synaptic cleft is not distinctly widened, as in the upper micrograph. However, the membranes appear thickened. The presynaptic terminal contains numerous small, clear synaptic vesicles and also several large, granulated vesicles. (×38,200.) (Courtesy Dr. Murray Matthews.)

cell. The cleft spacing is about 2 nm. No special organelles are found in the presynaptic terminal.

Chemical synaptic endings are the most common synaptic structure in the mammalian nervous system. Although chemical synaptic terminals may have any of a variety of forms, all have certain features in common. There is a synaptic cleft between the presynaptic ending and the postsynaptic cell. This synaptic cleft is the final verification of the neuron theory, requiring for its observation the resolution of the electron microscope. The presynaptic ending at the chemical synapse contains numerous synaptic vesicles, which are the storage sites of chemical transmitters (Fig. 1-9). Mitochondria are also abundant in synaptic terminals. The membranes on either side of the synaptic cleft may have associated cytoplasmic thickenings.

At least two kinds of chemical synapses can be recognized (Fig. 1-8). Type I synapses are characterized by a wide synaptic cleft (30 nm), a large junctional surface, and an asymmetrical distribution of cytoplasmic thickenings, with the more prominent thickening being found postsynaptically (Fig. 1-9, *upper*). Type II endings have a synaptic cleft with the same width as the extracellular cleft system of most of the rest of the nervous system (20 nm), a small junctional area, and symmetrically arranged cytoplasmic densities (Fig. 1-9, *lower*). The synaptic vesicles found in type I endings are invariably spherical; those in type II endings are sometimes oval in shape, depending on the preparative techniques used for electron microscopy. In some particular instances, it has been shown that type I synapses are associated with synaptic excitation, whereas type II synapses produce synaptic inhibition. However, it seems likely that the type of synapse and vesicle may relate to the nature of the synaptic transmitter substance rather than to the effect of the transmitter on the postsynaptic membrane. The latter would depend critically on the nature of the receptors located on the postsynaptic membrane (see Chapter 3). Other types of synapses have also been described. In some, the synaptic vesicles are granulated; that is, they contain an electron-dense core. Some synapses of this kind appear to utilize monoamine transmitter.

Another class of axonal terminal is that of neurosecretory cells. These terminals do not end on a postsynaptic cell, but release their secretory products into the circulation. They are therefore a part of the endocrine system. The hormones formed in neurosecretory cells are stored in large vesicles, which often have electron-dense cores. Neurosecretory granules may be so abundant that they can be stained and recognized by light microscopy.

Although synapses are usually formed by axon terminals on cell bodies and dendrites of other neurons or on effector cells, this is by no means the only arrangement of presynaptic and postsynaptic elements. A variety of other possibilities is now recognized. In addition to axosomatic and axodendritic synapses, there are axoaxonal dendrodendritic (Fig. 1-8) and somasomatic synapses. In specific regions of the nervous system, reciprocal synapses (p. 264) have been observed in which the processes of two different neurons make chemical synapses with each other in adjacent patches of dendritic membrane. It is evident that the potential complexities of synaptic interactions are very great.

Types of neurons

One method of classification of neurons depends on the number of their processes. Neurons with only one process, an axon, are called unipolar. These are rare except in the embryonic nervous system. Neurons with two processes (peripheral and central) are bipolar. Examples of this type of cell are found in the retina and in the ganglia of the vestibular and cochlear nerves. Dorsal root ganglion cells have two partially fused processes and are termed pseudounipolar. Cells having a number of processes are multipolar. Neurons of this type include motoneurons of the spinal cord and brainstem, pyramidal cells of the cerebral cortex, and Purkinje cells of the cerebellar cortex.

A special type of neuron lacks an axon, although it has processes that resemble the dendrites of other neurons. Such a cell is called an amacrine (without a long fiber) cell. Examples include the amacrine cells of the retina and the granule cells of the olfactory bulb (see Chapter 7). Synaptic connections with other neurons are made on and by the dendriticlike processes of the amacrine cells.

Neuroglia

Neurons are always found in association with supportive cells. These may be either of ectodermal or mesodermal origin. The ectodermally derived supportive cells of the central nervous system are the neuroglia, which include ependymal cells, astrocytes, and oligodendroglia (Figs. 1-10 and 1-11). Ectodermally derived supportive cells in the peripheral nervous system are the satellite cells of the peripheral ganglia and Schwann cells. Supporting cells from the mesoderm include one glial type, the microglia, as well as connective tissue and vascular tissue cells.

Ependymal cells form a cuboidal epithelium that covers the surfaces of the ventricular system of the brain and the central canal of the spinal cord (Figs. 1-12 and 1-13). Cilia protrude from these cells into the ventricular cavity. Each ependymal cell has a process extending from its base into the central nervous system tissue. Modified ependymal cells cover the choroid plexuses of the cerebral ventricles; these play a major role in the secretion of cerebrospinal fluid. It is possible that other ependymal cells also have a secretory function. Electron micrographs show that ependymal cells contain cytoplasmic fibrils that resemble those of astrocytes.

There are two general kinds of astrocytes, protoplasmic and fibrous (Fig. 1-14). These are likely to be varieties of the same kind of cell, the morphological characteristics depending on whether the cell lies in the gray or in the white matter of the nervous system. The nuclei of astrocytes are ovoid and are larger than the nuclei of oligodendroglia or microglia. There are many processes extending from astrocytes.

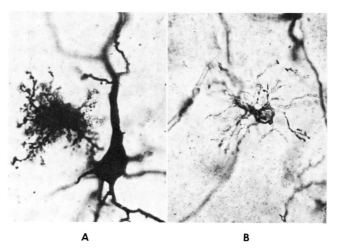

Fig. 1-11. Light micrographs of neuroglial cells. **A,** An astrocyte and a pyramidal cell stained by the Golgi technique. Note the large number of processes of the glial cell. **B,** An oligodendrocyte stained by a heavy-metal technique. The number of processes is smaller than in the case of the astrocyte. Each process may be associated with the formation of a myelin internode.

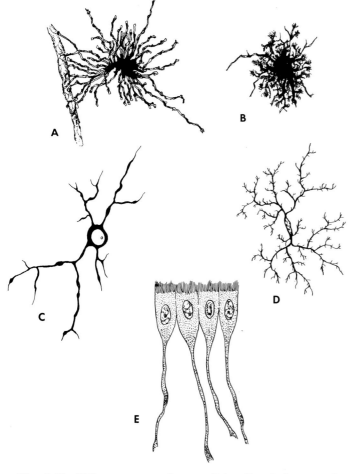

Fig. 1-10. Different types of neuroglial cells of the central nervous system. Fibrous and protoplasmic astrocytes are shown in **A** and **B** respectively. Note the glial footplates in association with a capillary in **A**. An oligodendrocyte is shown in **C.** Each of the processes is responsible for the production of one or more myelin sheath internodes about central axons. A microglial cell is shown in **D**; ependymal cells are shown in **E.**

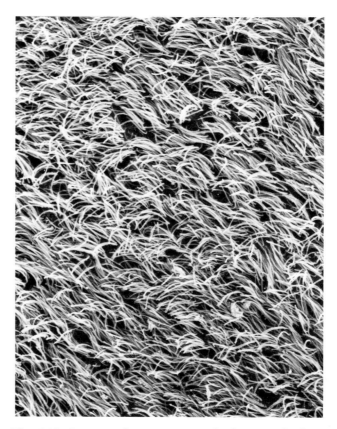

Fig. 1-12. Scanning electron micrograph showing cilia lining the lateral wall of the third ventricle in a normal adult female monkey, *Macaca nemestrina.* (×1,375.) (Courtesy Dr. Penelope W. Coates.)

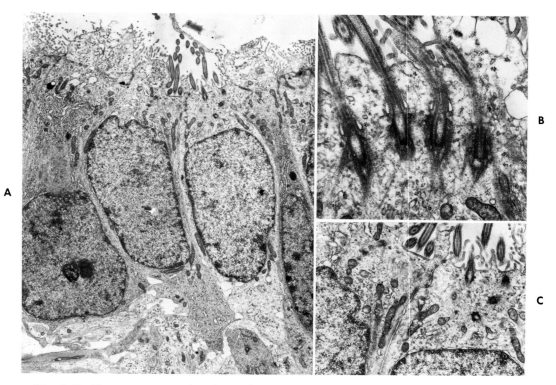

Fig. 1-13. Electron micrographs of ependymal cells. **A,** Row of ependymal cells lining the central canal of the spinal cord. Microvilli and cilia may be seen projecting from the free margins of the cells. (×3,930.) **B,** Basal bodies and attached cilia of an ependymal cell. (×13,350.) **C,** Specialized contact region between the plasma membranes of adjacent ependymal cells (fascia adherens). (×7,630.) (Courtesy Dr. Murray Matthews.)

These are best demonstrated by special staining methods. The processes branch repeatedly and probably represent what light microscopists have called astrocytic fibers, or they may be aggregates of the filaments seen by electron microscopy in the cytoplasm of astrocytes. The distended endings of astrocytic branches encircle capillaries, forming perivascular foot processes. Glia, chiefly astrocytes, cover the nonsynaptic surfaces of neurons. Thus astrocytes are interposed between the blood vessels and nerve cells. The glial cell membranes and the narrow clefts between them probably represent the structural equivalent of a portion of the blood-brain barrier, which restricts the passage of certain substances into the central nervous system. Perhaps more important in this regard are the tight junctions between capillary endothelial cells of nervous tissue. In electron micrographs, the characteristic bundles of filaments coursing through the astrocytic cytoplasm are seen, and glycogen granules are often seen (Fig. 1-14). Following damage to the central nervous system, astrocytes may enlarge and proliferate, forming a glial scar (gliosis).

The oligodendroglia are supporting cells of the central nervous system, having few processes and no cyto-plasmic filaments (Fig. 1-15, A). The appearance of these cells varies with their level of activity. In general, their nuclei are smaller, rounder, and more densely staining (with hematoxylin and eosin) than those of astrocytes. Oligodendroglia are responsible for the myelin sheaths of axons within the central nervous system. A given oligodendroglial cell may provide myelin for a number of axons. They also occur adjacent to neuronal cell bodies, where they are called satellites or perineuronal glia. They do not have perivascular foot processes. One characteristic feature of their ultrastructure is an electron-dense cytoplasm, which is caused in part by an abundance of "rough" endoplasmic reticulum. In damaged areas, oligodendroglia may swell.

Microglia are small cells with elongated or irregular, densely staining nuclei (Fig. 1-15, B). They become phagocytes (gitter cells) when debris is present. During development, these cells migrate into the central nervous tissue along with other mesodermal elements, such as blood vessels. There are relatively few microglial cells present in normal central nervous tissue, but large numbers appear in areas of damage, possibly by way of the circulation as well as by migration

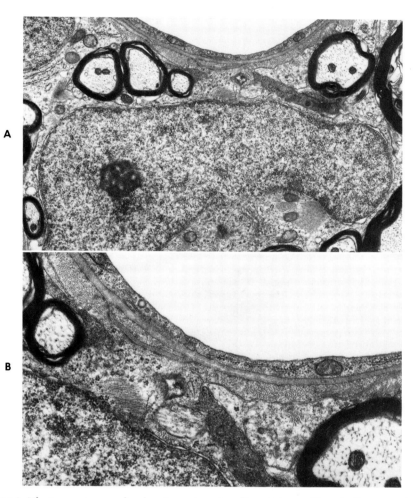

Fig. 1-14. Electron micrographs showing astrocyte adjacent to capillary in the central nervous system. The micrographs represent views of the same electron microscopic field at two different magnifications (**A**, ×8,700; **B**, ×18,350). The nucleus of an astrocyte occupies much of the field in **A.** Just above the astrocyte is a capillary, and several myelinated axons course by it. **B** shows more detail of the cytoplasm of the astrocyte and the relationship of the astrocyte to the capillary endothelium. The cytoplasm of the astrocyte contains numerous filaments cut in longitudinal or cross sections and arranged in sheets; there are also a few glycogen granules. The astrocyte is separated from the capillary endothelial cell by basement membrane. (Courtesy Dr. Murray Matthews.)

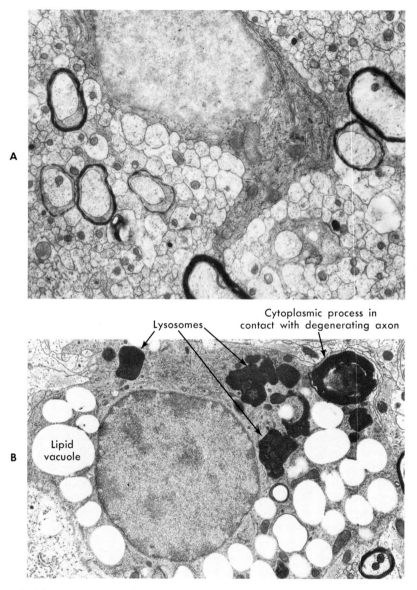

Fig. 1-15. Electron micrographs of glial cells. **A,** Oligodendrocyte. The section was taken through the corticospinal tract of a 15-day-old rat. The field consists primarily of axons cut in cross section. Many of the axons are unmyelinated, and some are in various stages of myelination. The cell extending from the top of the micrograph through the center is an oligodendrocyte. The cytoplasm is characterized by an abundance of rough endoplasmic reticulum and by an electron-dense matrix. The process extending toward the bottom of the micrograph is in continuity with a myelin sheath. (×8,400.) **B,** Microglial cell. The section was made through the lateral geniculate nucleus of a rabbit 4 weeks after removal of the visual cortex. The cell occupying most of the field is apparently engaged in phagocytosis of debris resulting from degeneration. The phagocytic microglial cell is often referred to as a gitter cell (G. *Gitter,* lattice cell), a lipid-laden mononuclear phagocyte. Its cytoplasm contains numerous lipid vacuoles and dense bodies that are presumably lysosomes. A degenerating myelinated axon is being enveloped by the gitter cell. The electron microscopic identification of microglial cells in the normal, noninjured nervous system is controversial. (×8,320.) (Courtesy Dr. Murray Matthews.)

within the nervous system following mitosis. There is evidence that resting microglia may be pericytes, cells located adjacent to capillaries and separated from the nervous tissue proper by a basement membrane.

The peripheral neuroglia are found in ganglia and along nerve trunks. The satellite cells of ganglia form a capsule around the cell bodies of neurons of dorsal root ganglia, cranial nerve ganglia, and autonomic ganglia. Schwann cells form the myelin sheaths of peripheral nerve fibers. However, one Schwann cell is associated with myelin of just one axon. Unmyelinated axons are also found in association with Schwann cells.

Myelin

Many axons are unmyelinated. These are surrounded by the cytoplasm of a supporting cell, the Schwann cell (Fig. 1-16). Several unmyelinated axons may be enclosed or partially enclosed within a single supporting cell; such a group of unmyelinated axons is called a bundle of Remak (Figs. 1-16 and 1-17). In the central nervous system, there may be no glial cell associated with clusters of unmyelinated axons.

Many of the axons of both central and peripheral nervous tissue are surrounded by a myelin sheath (Fig. 1-18). The supporting cells responsible for the production of myelin are the oligodendroglia and the Schwann cells. The main function of the myelin sheath is to increase the velocity of conduction of nerve impulses.

The myelin sheath begins fairly near the cell body of most neurons and extends to a point close to the axon terminals. It is not a continuous sheath, however; it has two kinds of discontinuities. At regular intervals

of about 0.5 to 1.5 mm, the myelin is completely interrupted at the nodes of Ranvier (Fig. 1-19). The internodal segments of myelin are formed by individual supporting cells. The myelin layers of the internodal segments may show the funnel-shaped clefts of Schmidt-Lanterman. Some neurons, such as the bipolar cells of the ganglia of the eighth cranial nerve, have a myelin sheath about the cell body as well as the axon. This arrangement would not be suitable for cells other than primary afferent neurons, because there would be no place on the soma for synaptic endings.

Myelin has long been known to contain lipid compounds. However, these are not simply deposits of lipids situated between an outer membrane and the axon, as was once believed. The modern concept of myelin structure has been developed through the use of several techniques, notably light microscopy with polarized light, x-ray diffraction, and electron microscopy.

Analyses by polarized light and by x-ray diffraction

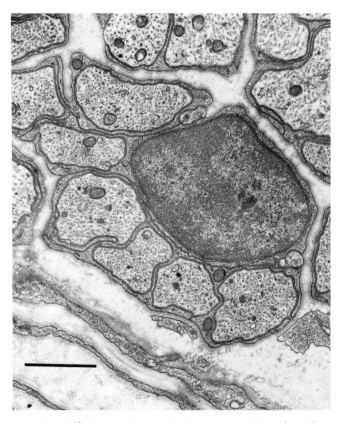

Fig. 1-17. Electron micrograph of a cross section through a gray ramus communicans in the cat. A number of unmyelinated axons are shown. The group at the center is associated with a single Schwann cell (cut through its nucleus). This arrangement is known as a bundle of Remak. Parts of other Remak bundles are also seen. The bar represents 1 μm. (Courtesy Dr. Richard E. Coggeshall.)

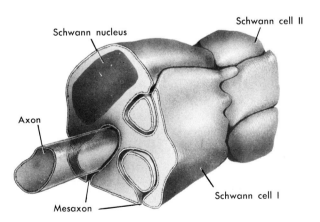

Fig. 1-16. Three-dimensional impression of the appearance of a bundle of Remak. The cut face of the bundle is seen to the left. One of the three unmyelinated axons is represented as protruding from the bundle. Mesaxons are indicated, as is the nucleus of the Schwann cell. To the right, the junction of adjacent Schwann cells is depicted.

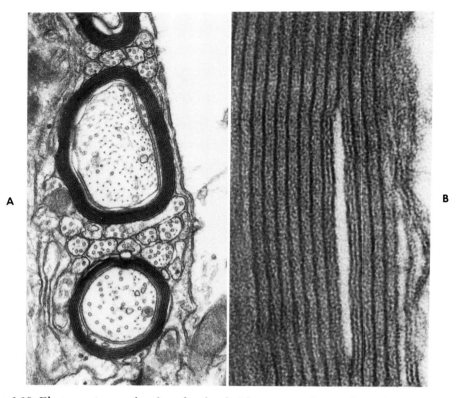

Fig. 1-18. Electron micrographs of myelin sheath. The micrograph at **A** shows three myelinated axons. The outer and inner mesaxons of the largest myelinated axon can be traced. (×21,000.) The periodicity of the myelin sheath is seen to better advantage in the high magnification view in the micrograph at **B**. The major dense lines are formed by fusion of the innermost lamellae of supporting cell plasma membrane, whereas the interperiod (minor dense) lines are formed from the fusion of the outermost lamellae. Note the cytoplasm that has intruded between the two parts of a major dense line near the center of the micrograph. (×168,000.) (Courtesy Dr. Murray Matthews.)

suggested that myelin was composed of concentric layers of radially oriented lipid molecules sandwiched between tangentially oriented protein molecules. The lipids were thought to be in a bimolecular leaflet, with the polar groups directed outward to attach to the protein (the unit membrane). Electron microscopy has confirmed this picture in most details. One difference that has emerged is that the myelin is formed by a continuous spiral of membrane rather than by concentric layers.

The structure of myelin is best appreciated by considering its development (Fig. 1-20). The concept of myelin formation now generally accepted was suggested by Geren in 1954 and was derived from her electron microscopic investigation of myelinization in chick embryos. Before becoming myelinated, axons are found to be partially or completely surrounded by supporting cells—Schwann cells in peripheral nerves or oligodendroglia in the central nervous system. The cytoplasmic membrane of the supporting cell remains distinct from that of the axon, being separated by a

gap. However, when the supporting cell completely encloses the axon, the cytoplasmic membranes of the two encircling arms of the supporting cell may fuse. The outer layers of each membrane become indistinguishable, resulting in a structure known as the mesaxon. Up to this point there has been no difference between the structure of developing myelinated and unmyelinated axons. The further differentiation of myelinated axons occurs as the mesaxon elongates and the supportive cell begins to encircle the axon. This process continues until there are numerous spirals of supporting cell membrane about the axon. The layers are at first separated by cytoplasm of the supporting cell, but this disappears and the membranes fuse. The electron density of the regions of apposition of the outer faces of supporting cell membrane is less than that of the regions where the inner faces join. This results in an alteration of major dense lines and interperiod lines (Figs. 1-18 and 1-21). The explanation for the different electron densities probably lies in differences in the chemical makeup of the protein

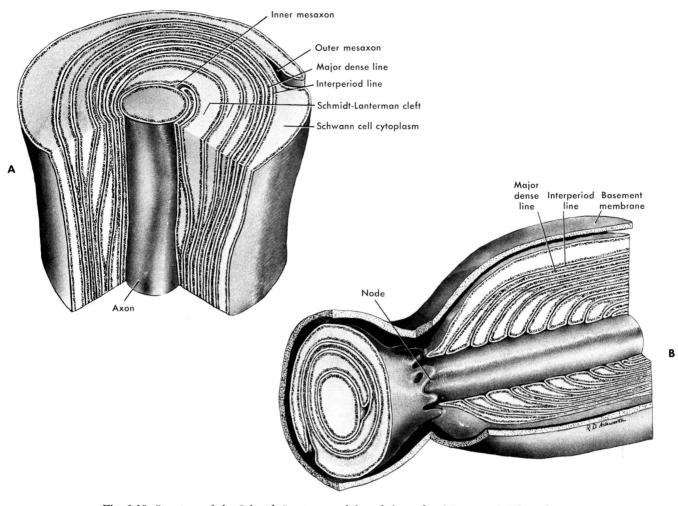

Fig. 1-19. Structure of the Schmidt-Lanterman cleft and the node of Ranvier. A, Three-dimensional representation of a portion of a myelin sheath containing a Schmidt-Lanterman cleft. Note that the cytoplasm of the supporting cell has intruded between the two components of the major dense line and that this intrusion continues in a spiral across the entire width of the myelin sheath, connecting the cytoplasm outside with that inside the myelin. B, Similar representation of a node of Ranvier. The loops of supporting cell membrane in the region to the right of the node are indicated, as are the bare region of the axon and the beginning of the next internode.

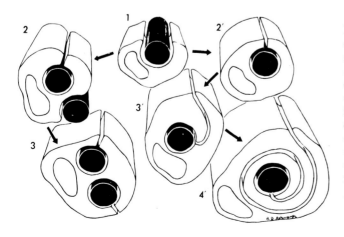

Fig. 1-20. Formation of myelin and bundles of Remak. The drawing shows some of the stages in development of axonal sheaths. The axon becomes partially embedded in a supporting cell, such as a Schwann cell, as indicated in 1. If the axon is destined to remain unmyelinated, it and other axons may become more or less embedded in the same Schwann cell, as in 2 and 3. If the axon will become myelinated, the same initial events occur, 2′, but only a single axon will be myelinated by a given Schwann cell. (In the central nervous system, an oligodendrocyte may myelinate a large number of axons.) The line of fusion of the Schwann cell processes that envelop the axon is the mesaxon. With further development, the mesaxon elongates as the Schwann cell processes grow in a spiral about the axon, as in 3′ and 4′. Eventually, the cytoplasm between adjacent layers of mesaxon is extruded, and the membranes fuse.

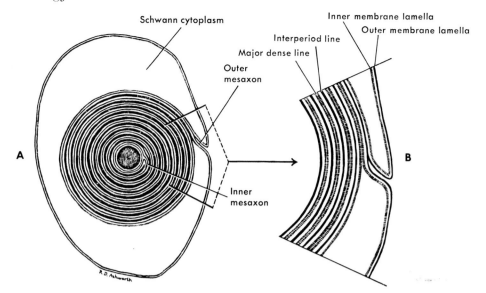

Fig. 1-21. Makeup of the myelin sheath. **B,** Enlargement of the portion of **A** indicated by the broken lines. Note the outer and inner mesaxons.

layers of the outer and inner faces of the unit membrane. The electron light zones between the dense lines presumably represent the lipid component of the membranes.

The mesaxon persists both on the axonal side of the myelin sheath (inner mesaxon) and on the external side (outer mesaxon). Cytoplasm may be seen between the myelin sheath and the supporting cell membrane on either side. The supporting cell nucleus is located outside the myelin. It is thought that in the central nervous system one oligodendroglial cell may provide myelin for several or even many axons.

As the myelin sheath develops, the first layers are formed over a limited area of axon. With growth of the animal, the axon elongates, and successive layers of myelin must cover a greater expanse of axon. There are therefore more myelin lamellae about the center of an internode than near a node of Ranvier (Figs. 1-19 and 1-22). The ends of adjacent lamellae form loops, which are particularly numerous at nodal regions. The nodes of Ranvier are points of junction of neighboring supporting cells. There may be a considerable interdigitation of the lamellar loops of the two supporting cells at a node, but there is nevertheless a fairly free channel from the extracellular space to the nodal membrane. This channel is important for nervous conduction, because it allows ionic exchanges across the axonal membrane.

The clefts of Schmidt-Lanterman are formed by the intrusion of cytoplasm of the supporting cell between myelin lamellae (Fig. 1-19). The cytoplasm may extend in a spiral all the way across the myelin sheath, thus connecting the cytoplasm external to the sheath

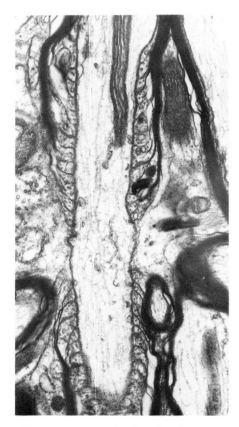

Fig. 1-22. Electron micrograph of node of Ranvier. A longitudinal section through a myelinated axon at a node of Ranvier is seen in the center of the micrograph. Note the bare region of axon at the node and the loops of supporting cell membrane at the ends of each internode. This section is from central nervous system tissue, so the supporting cells are oligodendrocytes. (×15,800.) (Courtesy Dr. Murray Matthews.)

with that internal to the sheath. The spiral of cytoplasm could possibly play a role in the transport of trophic substances or nutrients through the supporting cell.

RESPONSES OF NEURONS TO INJURY

Two of the reactions that neurons undergo in response to injury are of great importance in neurobiology. These are retrograde chromatolysis and wallerian

degeneration (named for its discoverer, A. V. Waller).

When the axon of a neuron is damaged, the cell body may show retrograde chromatolysis, beginning within a day or two. The maximum changes are observed about 1 to 2 weeks after injury. The Nissl substance disperses and is reduced and loses its staining properties, the cell body swells, and the nucleus moves to an eccentric position (Figs. 1-23 and 1-24). The degree of change depends on several factors, such as

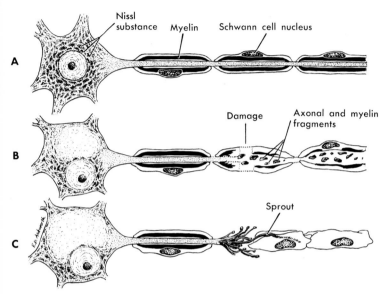

Fig. 1-23. Responses of neurons to injury. **A,** Multipolar neuron, with the cell body and dendrites at the left and a myelinated axon extending to the right. In **B,** an injury has occurred, with damage to the axon at some distance from the cell body of the neuron. The cell body and proximal dendrites display retrograde chromatolysis as a result. The Nissl substance no longer stains, the cell swells, and the nucleus becomes eccentric. The axon and myelin sheath degenerate as well, both distally from the point of injury and proximally at least to the nearest node of Ranvier. The axon and the myelin distal to the injury fragment are in the process of wallerian degeneration. If the damage is not too severe, regeneration may ensue. The Schwann cells whose myelin fragmented may form a pathway along the former peripheral course of the axon. This serves as a guide for the growth of sprouts, **C,** that develop at the terminal of the intact portion of the axon. As a sprout successfully finds its way down the Schwann cell bridge, the remaining sprouts degenerate. The Schwann cells eventually remyelinate the axon.

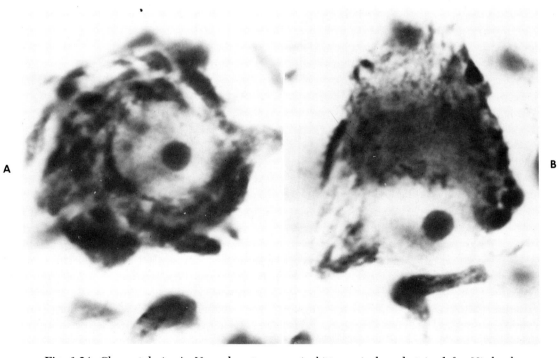

Fig. 1-24. Chromatolysis. **A,** Normal motoneuron in kitten spinal cord stained for Nissl substance. **B,** Chromatolytic motoneuron in the same material. A peripheral nerve had been sectioned.

the time since injury, the distance along the axon from the cell body that the injury occurred, the severity of the injury, and the type of neuron. Some neurons may show no chromatolytic changes after axonal injury, whereas others may degenerate to the point of cell death.

Damage to a neuron may also result in degenerative changes in the axon. If a myelinated axon is injured, its distal segment undergoes wallerian degeneration (Fig. 1-23). The axis cylinder fragments, beginning within a day or two, and is absorbed. The myelin sheath begins to break up into lipoid droplets within the first day following injury. The debris is absorbed, probably largely by phagocytosis. Phagocytes appear in the region of damage by about 1 week; their numbers gradually decrease until they become scarce at about 100 days. The proximal segment of the axon also undergoes wallerian degeneration for a distance that varies with the conditions. If the cell body dies, the entire axon degenerates. Unmyelinated axons also degenerate when sectioned.

In general, the injury of an axon results in no change in the postsynaptic cell. However, there are exceptions to this. For instance, when the motor innervation of a muscle is destroyed, the muscle becomes atrophic and eventually disappears if reinnervation does not occur. A similar phenomenon called transneuronal degeneration has been observed in certain pathways in the central nervous system. The process apparently depends on the removal of some kind of trophic influence by which the axon maintains the condition of the postsynaptic element. The nature of such trophic influences is unknown. The problem of trophic influences is discussed at greater length in Chapter 3.

When damage to a neuron is not overwhelming, it may recover. Chromatolysis reverses over a period of several months. If the axon has been interrupted, recovery entails generation of a new axon. The first evidence of this is the appearance of sprouts from the distal end of the intact portion of the axon (Fig. 1-23). There may be as many as fifty or more sprouts from a single axon. In a crush injury, some of these sprouts may easily find their way along the route followed by the original axon, because the Schwann cells and the endoneural sheaths about them will have remained in their proper relations. The axonal sprouts can then grow along the surfaces of the Schwann cells, and eventually many will reach the appropriate end-organs, whether sensory or motor, which may then be reinnervated. The Schwann cells gradually engulf the axons, forming new myelin sheaths or producing bundles of Remak. There will be only a single axon within each newly developed myelin

sheath, which means that the surplus axonal sprouts from the parent axon must degenerate.

If the continuity of a nerve is lost because of injury, reinnervation becomes more difficult because the axonal sprouts have no direct pathway to follow. Many of the sprouts grow in the wrong direction, some produce spirals, and others develop large bulbous tips. The sprouts, with their Schwann cells and a developing connective tissue scar, may form a neuroma. The neuroma may not only obstruct proper reinnervation of the nerve distal to the point of transection, but it may be painful. An aid to reinnervation across a gap is provided by the activity of Schwann cells in the distal nerve stump. The Schwann cells divide, elongate, and migrate as a bundle toward the proximal nerve stump. If axonal sprouts manage to reach this Schwann cell outgrowth, they may eventually reinnervate the denervated organs. However, the amount of functional recovery would be rather less than in the case of a crush injury. One reason for this is that few axonal sprouts are likely to find their way exactly along the pathway followed originally by their parent fibers. Thus, many axons will reinnervate an inappropriate organ. A motor axon that establishes a connection with a sensory receptor organ will not be able to function. Furthermore, a motor axon that reinnervates a different muscle than the one it originally supplied cannot take part in the same reflex actions that it originally did. Another problem in the case of injuries to long nerves is that the endorgans may atrophy before reinnervation can occur.

The timing of nerve regeneration will vary with the type of injury. Recovery is quicker with crush injuries than with cases of nerve severance. If a nerve is cut and then the ends sutured together, regenerating axons may appear distal to the scar in about a week, whereas they appear distal to a crushed zone within 5 days. After this time, the rate of growth of the tips of the sprouts is about 3 to 4 mm per day in the case of the cut nerve and over 4 mm per day in the crushed nerve. There is further delay once the end-organs are reached by the axons before function is recovered. This delay can be attributed to reversal of any atrophy of the end-organ, reinnervation of the end-organ, and remyelinization and maturation of the axon.

In cases of human nerve injury, the time at which return of motor function can be expected can be determined by measuring the distance from the point of transection to the motor point of the nearest muscle innervated by the nerve distal to the site of injury. A radial nerve injury at the level of the midshaft of the humerus can be taken as an example. This is a common site of injury caused by fracture of the humerus or by improper hypodermic injection of medications deeper than the deltoid muscle. The first muscle to be innervated by the radial nerve distal to the injury is the brachioradial muscle. The motor point is the point at which the nerve enters the muscle and at which transcutaneous electrical stimulation produces muscular contractions with the lowest current strength. A typical distance that the nerve must regrow from the site of injury to enter the motor point is about 11 cm. This distance is divided by the rate of regeneration of the axons. Axons regenerate progressively more slowly as the distance increases from the growing axon tip to the cell body. An average rate of regeneration can be taken as 4 cm per month. For radial nerve injury to the humerus, the expected time of recovery would be about 3 months. Muscle fibers will not survive denervation for more than about 20 to 24 months. Electrical signs of reinnervation of muscle may become apparent on electromyography (the recording of the activity of muscle fibers by needle electrodes inserted into the muscle) before muscle contractions appear that are visible to the eye. The early electromyographic signs of reinnervation are decreasing numbers of spontaneous fibrillation potentials (p. 77) and the appearance of motor unit potentials with voluntary effort (motor unit is defined on p. 77).

Reinnervation in the central nervous system is apparently very limited in higher mammals. Axonal sprouts do occur following injury, but they do not seem to reestablish appropriate functional connections. This may be caused by several factors. The development of a scar at the site of injury may impede the growth of the sprouts. The lack of Schwann cells may prevent the proper direction of the sprouts; it is clear that oligodendroglia do not function like Schwann cells in this regard. However, the major problem may lie in the difficulty of reconnecting the appropriate pathways in a tissue as complex as the central nervous system.

The processes of chromatolysis and wallerian degeneration are often utilized in experimental studies in neuroanatomy for tracing pathways of innervation. For instance, the axons of a functional group of neurons may be sectioned or otherwise damaged. It may then be possible to locate the cell bodies of the neurons from which the axons originate by finding which neurons undergo chromatolysis. Conversely, the neuroanatomist may destroy a group of neuronal cell bodies within, for example, a particular nucleus of the central nervous system. The route taken by the axons may then be traced by staining the degenerating fibers either with a technique designed to demonstrate degenerating myelin or with one for degenerating

axons. In the case of pathways involving unmyelinated axons, the latter approach would be the appropriate one.

ELECTRICAL PROPERTIES OF NEURONS

The activities of neurons are frequently studied by means of electronic instruments (Fig. 1-25). The reason for this is that nervous transmission (as well as synaptic transmission and receptor organ responses) is associated with electrical currents caused by the flow of ions across cell membranes and through extracellular fluid. It is therefore necessary to understand some of the electrical properties of nervous tissue in order to appreciate the way in which neurons transmit information.

There has been some speculation in recent years that neuroglia may contribute to the electrical potentials recorded from the central nervous system. Brief consideration of the electrical properties of neuroglia is given in a later section.

Techniques for studying electrical properties of cells

In the days before electronics, the most sensitive instrument available for measuring small electric currents was the galvanometer. This instrument had sufficient sensitivity to detect the current that is associated with action potentials in nerve fibers, but it was so slow in response that it failed to react to single action potentials. A better frequency response was obtained with the capillary electrometer, but the amplification was not adequate.

One of the most significant advances in biological instrumentation was the application of the cathode ray oscilloscope to the study of nerve impulses by J. Erlanger and H. S. Gasser in the 1920s (Fig. 1-25). The electron beam of this instrument has a negligible inertia, so the frequency response is extremely high. In addition, electronic circuits allow very high amplification. Special techniques have been devised that allow a greatly increased signal-to-noise ratio, and biological signals in the microvolt range can now be recorded without great difficulty.

Another technical achievement has been the development of methods for recording from within single neurons, using microelectrodes so fine that little damage is done to the neuronal membranes through which they are passed (Fig. 1-26). Intracellular recording has allowed a direct measurement of the electrical events occurring in single neurons as they transmit information. The results confirm and extend evidence obtained from recordings made extracellularly either from single neurons or from groups of similar neurons.

Electrical characteristics of the neuron

Because nerve impulses are associated with electrical events, it should not be unexpected that it is possible to construct an electrical circuit model of an axon (Fig. 1-27). For the present, the discussion is restricted to unmyelinated axons, for reasons that will be mentioned later. Initially, the circuit model considered will represent just a short length of axon. The most important electrical circuit elements that must be included in an electrical model of an unmyelinated axon are resistors, capacitors, and batteries.

The extracellular fluid about an axon is usually represented simply as a conductor in circuit diagrams of neurons. The symbol for a conductor is a line,

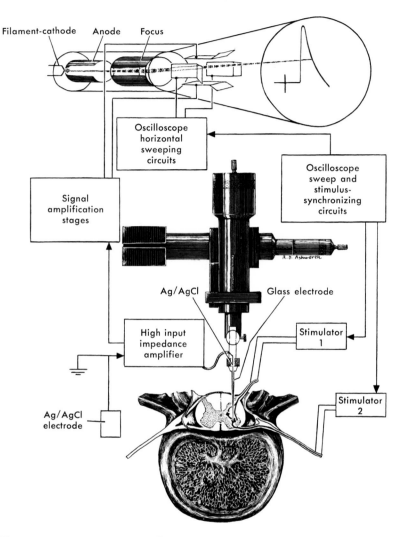

Fig. 1-25. Instrumentation for intracellular recording. In the upper portion of the drawing is the tube of a cathode ray oscilloscope. Voltage ramps are applied to the vertical plates of the tube to cause the oscilloscope sweep to move from left to right across the face of the tube. The rate of rise of these voltage ramps determines the time required for the beam to cross. The electrical activity is amplified, and the amplified signal is applied to the horizontal plates of the oscilloscope. Thus, the x axis signifies time and the y axis voltage in recordings made from nervous tissue. In the center of the drawing is shown a micromanipulator, a mechanical device that allows a microelectrode to be positioned to enter the appropriate part of the nervous system, which is exposed by dissection. The vertical microdrive advances a microelectrode in steps as small as a micron. The recordings made through the microelectrode require a special type of amplifier with a high input impedance. An indifferent electrode is placed on inactive tissue adjacent to the recording site. At the bottom of the figure, the microelectrode is shown penetrating the spinal cord to impale a motoneuron. Nerve fibers are activated by stimulators that consist of electronic devices that generate rectangular voltage pulses that can be applied to nerves through metal electrodes.

representing a wire. A conductor has a low resistance to current flow. The unit of resistance is the ohm. The resistance of a conductor, such as a wire, varies directly with the length and inversely with the cross-sectional area. It also varies with the material used to construct the wire. For instance, copper acts as a better conductor than iron. The relative abilities of materials to conduct current are expressed in terms of a constant, called the resistivity, which has the units of ohm-cm. The resistivity of a material is determined from the resistance of a 1-cm cube of the material. The resistivity of extracellular fluid is about 20 ohm-cm, but because the cross-sectional area of the extracellular fluid is very large, the external resistance along an axon is negligible unless the axon is put into a nonconducting medium. Then the resistance of the small, electrolyte-containing space between the axon and the bathing medium is represented by a resistor (R_e in Fig. 1-27). However, the axoplasm is generally represented by a resistor, because its longitudinal resistance is quite high. The resistivity of axoplasm is about 30 ohm-cm, but the small cross-sectional area of an axon results in a high resistance.

The surface membrane of an axon is composed primarily of lipoprotein. It is semipermeable, permitting a limited exchange of small ions and completely impeding the passage of large molecules, such as protein and most organic anions. Inasmuch as electric currents across the membrane must be carried by ions, such a semipermeable membrane will have a high resistance. A representative value for a neuronal membrane is 1,000 ohm-cm². The resistivity is on the order of 2×10^9 ohm-cm (1,000 ohm-cm²/50 ×

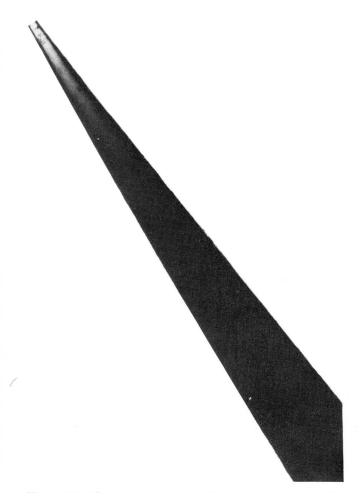

Fig. 1-26. Electron micrograph of microelectrode tip. The microelectrodes that are generally used for intracellular recording are made from glass capillary tubing. The tips are so fine that they cannot be seen at the light microscopic level. The tip shown in this picture was observed with an electron microscope. The outside diameter was found to be less than 0.2 μm. It can be seen that the tip is open. An electrolyte solution is used to fill the microelectrode. Electrical signals can be detected through the electrolyte column, which is exposed only at the end of the glass. Because of the very small dimensions of the electrode, it can be inserted into single nerve cells. (Courtesy R. C. Eggleton.)

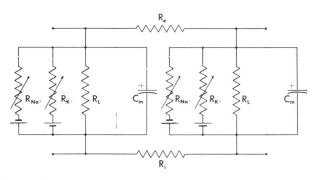

Fig. 1-27. Membrane equivalent circuit. The membranes of nerve cells, together with the adjacent extracellular and intracellular fluids, can be represented by an electrical circuit. In the diagram, the extracellular and intracellular fluids are symbolized by the resistors R_e and R_i respectively. The membrane has an associated transverse resistance as well as a capacitance. The capacitance of the membrane is symbolized by a sequence of capacitors, C_m, arranged in parallel. The transverse membrane resistance is often represented by a sequence of parallel resistors. In this diagram, the contribution of leakage paths for sodium, potassium, and other ions are shown individually as R_{Na^+}, R_{K^+}, and R_L (L, leakage). The batteries associated with the sodium and potassium conductance channels signify the equilibrium potentials for these ions. The sodium equilibrium potential is oriented so that the intracellular fluid would be positive, whereas the potassium equilibrium potential is oriented in the opposite direction. The resting membrane potential is the result of the forces represented by the equilibrium potentials and the constraints to ion flow offered by the resistance of the membrane. Because potassium conductance is more than 10 times greater than sodium conductance, the chief determinant of the resting membrane potential is the potassium equilibrium potential.

10^{-5} cm), because the membrane thickness is about 5 nm.

The membrane of an axon may be regarded as a dielectric separating two conductors, the extracellular fluid and the axoplasm. The surface of an axon, therefore, acts as a capacitor. The specific capacitance for most neuronal membranes is in the range of 1 μF/ cm^2. The dielectric constant is probably about 5.

There is a difference in potential across the resting membrane of an axon. This is called the resting potential. It amounts to about 70 mV, with the interior of the neuron negative to the exterior.

Depolarization and hyperpolarization

A reduction in the relative negativity of a neuron with respect to the exterior is called a depolarization. When the interior becomes more negative, the neuron is said to be hyperpolarized.

A depolarization or hyperpolarization may be produced either by an alteration in the charge held by the membrane capacitor or by the movement of ions through the membrane resistor (Fig. 1-28). For instance, a discharge of the membrane capacitor may be produced in a localized region by bringing a negatively charged electrode near that region. Posi-

tively charged ions adjacent to the outside of the membrane will tend to migrate toward the cathode; positive ions in the axoplasm will tend to move toward the inside of the membrane. The contrary movements will occur with negative ions. This results in a temporary reduction in the gradient of charge across the membrane (a depolarization). The transmembrane potential would be increased (a hyperpolarization) when an anode is brought near the membrane; this would be caused by ion migrations in the reverse direction to those producing depolarization.

A change in the membrane potential can also result from movement of ions across the membrane through its resistive components. Normally, there is a small flux of ions across membrane, but the potential remains constant because the numbers of ions of like charge crossing a unit area of membrane in a given time are equal in the two directions. However, when the permeability is suddenly changed, an asymmetrical ionic flux can occur (that is, there is a larger flux of ions in one direction than in the other). The net transfer of charge across the membrane by ions will change the membrane potential. One mechanism for producing such an asymmetrical ionic flux is that responsible for the action potential. Another is injury to the

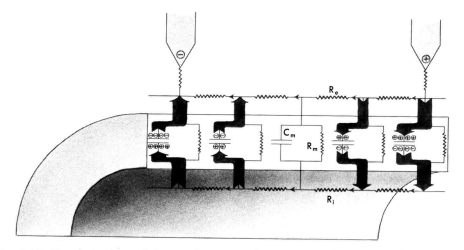

Fig. 1-28. Depolarization and hyperpolarization of a nerve membrane. The drawing shows a cutaway of a nerve fiber membrane. The equivalent circuit elements are shown. R_e and R_i are the resistances of the extracellular and intracellular fluids respectively. C_m and R_m indicate membrane capacitance and membrane resistance. A pair of electrodes is applied to the membrane surface. The one at the left is a cathode; the one at the right is an anode. The paths of current flow are represented by arrows. The amount of current in the various portions of the network depends on the relative resistances in the different parts of the circuit. Some current would flow in the extracellular fluid directly between the anode and the cathode. A small amount of current would flow through the membrane resistance elements (not shown). In addition, a current would flow briefly that would alter the amount of change stored on the membrane capacitive elements. The membrane near the anode would become more polarized, because positive ions would tend to accumulate outside the membrane, inducing an increased storage of anions just beneath the membrane. Conversely, the membrane near the cathode would undergo a reduction in polarization. The anode thus hyperpolarizes and the cathode depolarizes the membrane.

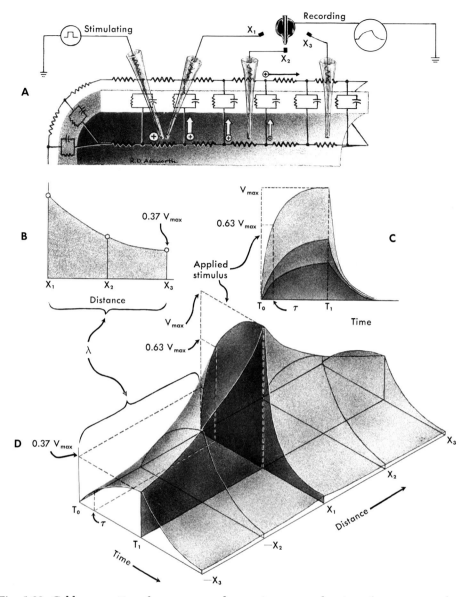

Fig. 1-29. Cable properties of a nerve membrane. A cutaway drawing of a nerve membrane is shown in **A.** To the left is a microelectrode used to alter the membrane potential by passage of a rectangular current pulse. A recording microelectrode is inserted into each of three different positions, indicated by X_1, X_2, and X_3. The location X_1 is at the point of stimulation, whereas X_2 and X_3 are at locations away from this point. The membrane potential is most effectively altered by the applied current pulse just at the point of stimulation, and it is progressively less altered with distance from this point. The change in membrane potential at a given time in response to a current pulse is plotted for X_1, X_2, and X_3 in **B.** The change falls off the 1/e (0.37 times) of its maximum value at a distance known as a length constant. In this case, the length constant is the distance between X_1 and X_3. The membrane potential at a given point along the nerve will increase in response to a rectangular current pulse in an exponential fashion; after the conclusion of the pulse, it will decay exponentially. This behavior is shown for several strengths of current pulses in **C.** The time, T, it takes for the potential to rise to 1−1/e of its maximal value (or 0.63 times the maximum) or to fall to 1/e is called the time constant. The time constant is symbolized by τ. In the case of the nerve fiber in **A,** only the membrane adjacent to the stimulating electrode is subjected to a rectangular current pulse. It is only here that the rise and fall of potential would follow the membrane time constant. The potential changes at points away from this would be slower. An indication of the spread of potential with time and distance in each direction from a stimulating electrode is shown in **D.**

membrane, which results in the flow of an injury current between the outside and inside of the membrane.

Cable properties of axons

When the circuit diagram of a short length of axon is joined to similar diagrams representing adjacent lengths of axon, a complex electrical network is produced that resembles the circuit diagram of a cable, such as might be used to transmit signals beneath an ocean. A property of electrical cables is that signals applied at one point become weaker with distance from that point; that is, the signal decreases. Part of the signal is lost through heating effects, and part is lost by leakage of current through the cable wall. The decrement in the signal may be restored by means of amplifiers stationed along the route of the cable.

When the axon is depolarized (within limits) or hyperpolarized, the change in membrane potential is transmitted along the axon, like a signal applied to a cable (Fig. 1-29). The amount of potential change decreases along the axon with distance from the point at which the signal was applied. Actually, the axon acts like a rather poor cable, in that the potential decreases to $1/e$ of its value within a few millimeters. The decrement is exponentially related to the distance along the axon; that is, for each few millimeters further along the axon the potential falls to $1/e$ of the previous value. The distance for each such decrement is called the space constant of the axon.

If measurements are recorded at a particular point along an axon following a potential change across its membrane, the potential at that point will decay in an exponential fashion with time. The exponential decay curve for this can be characterized in terms of another constant, the time constant of the axon membrane.

It is possible to show that the membranes of neuron cell bodies and dendrites also have cable properties. However, the mathematical description of these is considerably more complex than the description of axon membrane cable properties because of the much greater complexity of the geometry involved.

IONIC BASIS OF THE MEMBRANE POTENTIAL
Squid giant axon

Rapid progress in a field often requires the development of suitable techniques. The study of nervous transmission has been advanced tremendously since World War II because of the introduction to neurophysiology of radioactive tracer techniques and of a variety of electronic devices. Of particular importance was the application of these techniques to the squid

giant axon preparation by a group at Cambridge led by A. L. Hodgkin and A. F. Huxley.

The mantle muscle of the squid is innervated by a giant axon, which is actually a syncytium formed from many neurons. The advantage for electrophysiological studies of the squid giant axon over other types of peripheral nerve fibers is its large size. In some cases an axon may reach a diameter of 1 mm. A number of experimental procedures are possible with squid giant axons that would be difficult or impossible with axons of more common dimensions (less than 10 μm). For instance, the axoplasm may be removed for chemical analysis, and it may be replaced by artificial solutions of varying composition.

Resting potential

As mentioned previously, there is a difference in potential across the cytoplasmic membrane of a neuron that is not engaged in transmitting nerve impulses. This is called the resting potential. It is on the order of 70 mV of interior negativity in the giant axons of intact squids. Other neurons have comparable values of resting potential.

Bernstein, at the turn of the century, suggested that the resting potential originates as a concentration potential caused by the diffusion of potassium ion across the membrane. He believed that potassium is more concentrated inside the cell. If the permeability of the membrane to potassium allowed relatively free diffusion, whereas the permeability to other ions, such as sodium, were negligible, a transmembrane potential would develop. An action potential could be produced in this system by a breakdown of the membrane's selective permeability, discharging the potassium potential (Fig. 1-30). However, Bernstein's hypothesis did not explain the origin of the ionic gradients, nor did it explain the restoration of these gradients after nervous activity.

It has been possible to test Bernstein's ideas on the origin of the resting and action potentials. The squid giant axon has proved to be a particularly valuable preparation for this purpose. Extrusion of the axoplasm has made it possible, for example, to analyze chemically the ionic constitution of the axoplasm so that this may be compared with the extracellular fluid.

Ionic composition of squid axoplasm and extracellular fluid

The ionic constituents of squid giant fiber axoplasm have been determined with considerable accuracy. The major components are listed in Table 1-1. There is also some protein within the axoplasm. Divalent ions (calcium, magnesium) are present in small

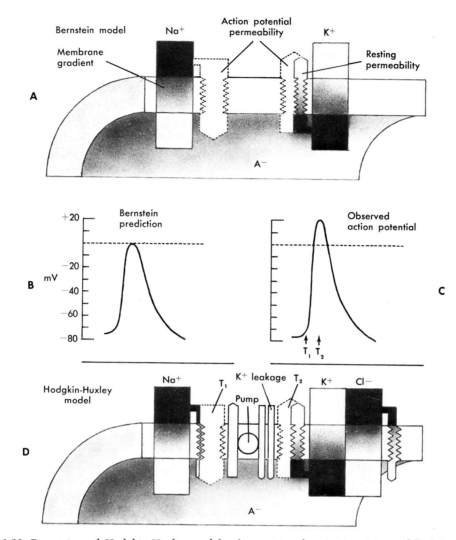

Fig. 1-30. Bernstein and Hodgkin-Huxley models of nerve impulse. **A,** Bernstein model of the nerve impulse. The gradients of the important ions are indicated by shading. Sodium is more concentrated outside the nerve membrane, whereas potassium is more concentrated inside. Bernstein suggested that there is normally no leakage of sodium into the axoplasm, but there is some leakage of potassium to the extracellular fluid, resulting in the resting potential, caused by the large anions, A-, which cannot escape along with the potassium. A nerve impulse would result if the membrane suddenly became permeable to all the important ions *(dotted arrows).* The membrane potential should, in this case, shift toward the zero level, as indicated by the graph at **B.** According to the Hodgkin-Huxley model, there is a resting leakage of both sodium and potassium ions, although the sodium leakage is less. The movements of sodium ions in the resting state include a small inward leak and a component pumped outward; the potassium movements include both outward and inward leaks and the component pumped in. The leakage is compensated for by pumping. These factors are indicated in the drawing at the bottom of the figure. (A chloride leak is also shown.) During the action potential, the permeability to sodium increases initially, at time T_1, causing the membrane potential to approach the sodium equilibrium potential, as shown in **C.** The interior of the axon thus becomes positive for a brief period. The membrane permeability for potassium then becomes increased at time T_2, resulting in a restoration of the potential toward the potassium equilibrium potential, **D.**

Table 1-1. Electrolyte concentrations*

	Na⁺	K⁺	Cl⁻
Squid			
Extracellular	460	20	540
Intracellular	50	400	40-100
Human			
Serum	136-145	3.5-5	100-106
Cerebrospinal fluid	148	2.9	120-130
Intracellular	10†	140†	4†

*Concentrations are given as millimoles (mmole) per liter.
†Estimated.

enough amounts that we can neglect them for this discussion. For comparison, the concentrations of the major ions are also shown for human extracellular fluid and neuroplasm.

Ions responsible for the resting potential

The Nernst equation shows that the distribution of potassium ions across the membrane is nearly that which would be predicted if the system were a passive one, as postulated by Bernstein. The general form of the Nernst equation is

$$E = \frac{RT}{FZ} \log_e \frac{(\text{cation outside})}{(\text{cation inside})}$$

where E is the equilibrium potential for an ion species, R is the gas constant, T is the absolute temperature, F is the Faraday, and Z is the valence. Strictly speaking, the ratio (cation outside)/(cation inside) is in terms of activities rather than concentrations. For the present discussion, a simplified version of the Nernst equation can be used:

$$E = 58 \log_{10} \frac{(\text{cation outside})}{(\text{cation inside})}$$

giving E in millivolts. (This form of the equation assumes that the nerve fiber is studied at room temperature, that the valence of the ion considered is 1, and that the activity coefficients of the ions in axoplasm and in extracellular fluid are the same.) The value of E in this equation defines the expected potential inside the fiber with respect to the extracellular medium, provided that the ions are distributed passively. For example, the equilibrium potential for the observed distribution of potassium ions across the squid axon membrane would be

$$E_{K^+} = 58 \log_{10} (20/400) = -75 \text{ mV}$$

This is close to the resting potential of –70 mV. Nevertheless, the potassium equilibrium potential is consistently somewhat more negative than the resting potential, a fact to which we shall return later.

The concentration gradient of sodium ions is in the opposite direction. The equilibrium potential for sodium, as calculated by the Nernst equation, is about 58 mV, with the interior positive! This indicates that sodium is not distributed passively. Furthermore, work using radioactive tracers has shown that the membrane is somewhat permeable to sodium during the resting state. The permeability to sodium in excised squid axons is less than 0.1 of that to potassium. During activity, the permeability to sodium increases greatly. It is therefore necessary to postulate some type of pumping mechanism to explain the sodium gradient and its maintenance in the face of the small but persistent leakage across the membrane. Potassium is also pumped, although in a direction opposite that of the sodium pumping.

Chloride ions may be at their equilibrium potential when the membrane is at rest. The permeability of the squid axon membrane to chloride is about 0.4 times that to potassium during inactivity. In some neurons, there is a chloride pump, so the chloride equilibrium potential is at a level either more negative or more positive than the resting potential, depending on the direction in which chloride is pumped.

Because the distribution of several ions is involved in the production of the resting potential, a relationship known as the Goldman equation was developed by A. L. Hodgkin and B. Katz from Goldman's constant-field equation to relate membrane potential to ionic concentration gradients. The permeability of the membrane to various ions determines which ion makes the greatest contribution to the resting potential. The Goldman-Hodgkin-Katz equation is

$$E = \frac{RT}{FZ} \log_e \frac{P_{K^+}(K^+)_o + P_{Na^+}(Na^+)_o + P_{Cl^-}(Cl^-)_i}{P_{K^+}(K^+)_i + P_{Na^+}(Na^+)_i + P_{Cl^-}(Cl^-)_o}$$

where E is the resting potential, R, T, F, and Z are as described for the Nernst equation; P is the permeability to the appropriate ion; and (X) is the concentration of the ion. Because the ratio of permeabilities of the squid axon membrane to K⁺, Na⁺, and Cl⁻ is about 1:0.1:0.4, it is evident that the major ion determining the resting potential is K⁺. It is important to note that any large increase in membrane permeability to one of the major ion species (K⁺, Na⁺, or Cl⁻) will increase the degree to which that ion's concentration gradient will determine the membrane potential. For example, a large increase in P_{Na^+} would drive the membrane potential of the squid axon in the direction of +58 mV.

For mammalian nervous tissues, comparable values for the equilibrium potentials for Na⁺, K⁺, and Cl⁻ are obtained, using the appropriate values for the concentrations of these ions in extracellular fluid and in axoplasm (Table 1-1).

Active transport

It is currently believed that cell membranes have the capacity for transporting substances against electrochemical gradients. The process requires energy, which is derived from metabolism, and it is called active transport. There are a number of theories about the mechanism of active transport at the molecular level. One involves the presence within the membrane of special carrier molecules that selectively combine with or release substances such as inorganic ions; the substances are thought to cross the membrane by diffusion or as a result of a configurational change in a membrane moiety while in combination with the carrier. The step in the process that requires energy could be on either side of the membrane. For instance, the structure of the carrier molecule might be altered, causing it to have either an increased or a decreased affinity for a substance. The active transport process that is responsible for the movement of sodium out of the neuron (or other cells) and potassium in is called the sodium-potassium pump.

Sodium-potassium pump

Some excellent work on the sodium-potassium pump has been done using radioactive tracers in giant axons. For example, a squid giant axon may be loaded with radioactive sodium, either by soaking or by injection. The axon can then be placed in seawater, and the rate of efflux of the radioactive ions can be measured. If an inhibitor of oxidative metabolism (for example, cyanide, azide, or dinitrophenol) is placed in the seawater bathing the axon, the rate of sodium efflux falls off dramatically. The efflux may be partially restored by injection into the axon of compounds containing high-energy phosphate bonds, such as adenosine triphosphate. Another agent that is often used to block the sodium-potassium pump is the drug ouabain. The rate of sodium influx by diffusion may also be studied using radioactive tracers. The influx is low during resting conditions, but during nervous activity the influx increases.

The sodium pump is in part dependent on the presence of some extracellular potassium. If the extracellular fluid contains no potassium, the sodium efflux is reduced dramatically, although some efflux does continue. It is believed that the sodium is in part exchanged for potassium. The exchange is not one for one, however; it is thought that about two to three sodium ions are ejected for each potassium ion that is pumped in. The presence of a potassium pump accounts for the discrepancy mentioned previously between the potassium equilibrium potential and the resting potential. The small inward leak of sodium ions causes a slight depolarization of the membrane away from the potassium equilibrium potential. The potassium pump prevents the potassium from leaking out to shift the potassium equilibrium potential to the resting potential, as would happen if potassium were passively distributed.

Origin of the resting potential

The resting potential is essentially the result of the establishment of a charge separation across the nerve cell membrane, caused by the diffusion of potassium ions out of the cell along their concentration gradient. This migration of potassium ions leaves unbalanced negative charges on anions, particularly large organic anions, which are not free to cross the relatively impermeable surface membrane. The presence of a high external concentration of sodium ions that are restrained from crossing the cell membrane serves to prevent osmotic shifts. The resting potential is thus a result of the concentration gradients of the various significant ions in the intracellular and extracellular fluids and the relative permeability of the nerve cell membrane to potassium as compared with other ions. The concentration gradients are presumably established by ion pumps driven by energy derived from metabolism. The ion pumps, especially the sodium-potassium pump, restore any alterations in the gradients that result either from leakage of ions through the resting membrane or from the accelerated leakage that occurs during excitation (see below). In some nerve cells there may be a component of the resting potential that is produced directly by ionic pumping activity. This can happen if more ions are pumped across the membrane in one direction than in the other. For instance, if the sodium-potassium pump causes more sodium ions to leave than potassium ions to enter the cell, the result may be an increased internal negativity. This kind of activity is called an electrogenic pump. The importance of electrogenic pumps is of current research interest.

Function of the resting potential

The resting potential serves as a kind of stored energy. This is most clearly demonstrated with respect to the action potential. Although small depolarizations and any hyperpolarizations are transmitted only a few millimeters along an axon because of its cable properties, action potentials may be transmitted without decrement for distances as great as meters. The only limitation on the distance of transmission of nerve impulses is the length to which an axon can grow. The necessity for the lack of decrement of the action potential has been discussed. For the present, suffice it to say that the energy for the action potential is present in stored form as the resting potential. The actual way in which the energy is stored depends on the differences in ionic concentrations on the two sides of the nerve membranes. Continuing the analogy between an axon and an electrical cable transmission system, the ionic concentration gradients acts like a series of relay amplifiers, allowing long-distance transmission without a decrease in the signal.

ELECTROPHYSIOLOGY OF NEUROGLIA

There have been a number of studies of the electrophysiology of neuroglia. The animal forms investigated have included representatives of invertebrates, lower vertebrates, and mammals. Mammalian neuroglia have been studied in tissue culture, and a number of investigators are now working on the properties of glia in situ in the mammalian central nervous system. The findings in all these systems agree quite well.

Neuroglial cells appear to have high resting potentials. These range up to 90 mV in cells that are presumably minimally damaged. The neuroglia do not develop action potentials when they are depolarized, although very strong shocks (displacing the membrane potential by 200 mV) may result in a prolonged change in membrane potential. There seems to be no direct electrical coupling between neurons and neuroglia. However, there are low resistance pathways between adjacent neuroglia that may be caused by close membrane contacts resembling those at electrical synapses (gap junctions).

The membrane potential of a neuroglial cell appears to be caused almost exclusively by a potassium diffusion potential; that is, the membrane behaves as if it were permeable only to potassium. When the external potassium concentration is altered, the membrane potential changes exactly as predicted from the Nernst equation. It can be calculated that the concentration of potassium within neuroglia is about 100 mEq per liter and of sodium is 25 mEq per liter. This indicates that neuroglia have an ionic composition like neurons and therefore cannot serve as an extracellular space to neurons, as has been suggested in the past.

Activity in adjacent unmyelinated nerve fibers or neuron cell bodies may cause a depolarization of neuroglia. This may be mediated by the release of potassium ions from the neurons during their activity. The effect is a slow one, and it is evidently caused by the release of sufficient potassium into the narrow extracellular cleft system of the central nervous system to produce a significant alteration in potassium concentration.

It is not clear whether the depolarization of neuroglia has a physiological meaning. For example, it is an open question whether the depolarization of a neuroglial cell produces any change in the behavior of the cell, metabolic or otherwise. Furthermore, it is not certain that the currents associated with the depolarization have any effect on neurons. It is possible, however, that the depolarization of neuroglia plays a part in the extracellular records made by neurophysiologists from nervous tissue.

One particularly interesting conclusion may be drawn from these studies. Substances that enter nervous tissue from the circulation probably do so through the narrow clefts between the various cellular elements. The blood-brain barrier appears to consist of the combination of the capillary endothelium, the relatively impermeable neuroglial membranes, and the resistance to diffusion offered by the system of narrow intercellular clefts. Once in the cleft system, small-sized molecules or ions, such as potassium or sodium, probably diffuse fairly freely. It is probable that some substances, including K^+, are transported actively across the neuroglial membranes. Of considerable interest is the finding that glial cells possess an active transport system for synaptic transmitter substances. This implies that glia participate at least indirectly in synaptic function.

There is no good evidence at this time that neuroglia are involved in learning or memory.

NERVE IMPULSE
Changes in electrical properties of an axon during a nerve impulse

The most obvious change in the electrical properties of an axon conducting a nerve impulse is a sequence of alterations in the membrane potential. This series of potential changes is called the action potential (Fig. 1-31). There is an initial abrupt depolarizing

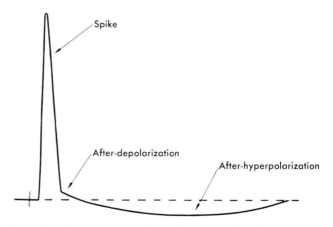

Fig. 1-31. Components of the action potential. The potentials typical of the nerve impulse are seen after the shock artifact. The large initial upward deflection is the spike potential. Following it are the after-depolarization and the after-hyperpolarization. The baseline is indicated by the broken line.

shift in membrane potential, after which it rapidly reverts toward the original state of polarization, then tapers off as a series of two longer lasting potentials— a depolarization followed by a hyperpolarization. The initial peaklike phase of the action potential is the spike potential, and the longer lasting potentials following it are the after-potentials. The first after-potential is the after-depolarization, and the second is the after-hyperpolarization.

Membrane resistance during the action potential

Bernstein suggested that the action potential is produced by a sudden increase in membrane permeability (Fig. 1-30). This hypothesis is supported by work such as that of K. S. Cole and H. J. Curtis, who showed that the membrane impedance* of squid giant axons is reduced during nerve impulses. This could be attributed to a change in membrane resistance, inasmuch as the membrane capacitance did not seem to be altered. However, the permeability change involved appears not to be the unselective one that Bernstein suggested. A sudden increase in permeability to all of the small ions present would reduce the membrane potential toward zero. Hodgkin and Huxley showed by intracellular recording that the action potential results in a transient reversal in the sign of the potential across the membrane. Their modified version of the membrane theory is that there is a transient increase in permeability to sodium ions, followed by an increased potassium permeability. The sodium ions enter the neuron under the influence of a large electrochemical gradient, and they would cause the membrane potential to approach the sodium equilibrium potential. This level is not quite reached, however, because of the delayed increase in potassium permeability. The latter results in a return of the membrane potential toward the resting level (or rather toward the potassium equilibrium potential) as the sodium permeability is inactivated and reverts to its former low level. The evidence for this sodium hypothesis of nervous transmission is discussed later. First, however, some of the basic characteristics of the nerve impulse will be considered.

Threshold. Action potentials are triggered when the membrane potential is depolarized to the critical level known as threshold. The membrane potential may vary over wide limits below threshold without resulting in nervous transmission.

There are many ways by which neurons may be depolarized to threshold. Electrical, mechanical, or chemical stimuli may be used. The easiest type of stimulus to quantitate is electrical.

A convenient type of electrical stimulus is the rectangular pulse. With this wave form, the parameters that may be changed are the strength (measured in volts, amperes, or on some arbitrary scale), the duration, and the frequency at which the stimulus occurs. Often the frequency of stimulation is kept low enough that the effects of successive stimuli are not additive; that is, the nerve is allowed to recover between stimuli. A rectangular pulse produces a depolarization or a hyperpolarization, depending on the sign of the pulse. However, the membrane potential change is not rectangular. This is because the membrane, combined with the conducting media, acts as a capacitor in series with a resistor. The process of charging a capacitor in such a circuit takes time. A very brief pulse may not charge the capacitor completely. Thus, a stimulating pulse of a given strength might not depolarize the membrane as much if the pulse had a brief duration as it would if it had a long duration.

The strength-duration curve shows this effect (Fig. 1-32). This curve may be plotted for various types of excitable tissue. The strength of the stimulus is plotted against the duration of the stimulus for all threshold values. As the duration is shortened, the strength of stimulation must be increased in order to attain threshold; conversely, a long-duration pulse requires only a low strength for evoking an action potential.

There are limits, however, to the range of effective stimulus parameters. For very brief pulses, no stimulus strength is great enough to produce an action potential. With low stimulus strengths, the duration may be increased indefinitely without reaching threshold.

The lowest stimulus strength that will reach threshold when long pulse durations are used is called the rheobase. The minimum duration of a pulse required to evoke an action potential when the stimulus is twice rheobase is called the chronaxie.

Excitability cycle. A nerve impulse leaves in its wake a series of changes in the excitability of the neuron to further stimulation (Fig. 1-33). These changes may in part be related to the permeability changes to cations that are associated with nervous transmission and in part to the after-potential sequence.

A second stimulus, no matter how strong, will not generate a second action potential during the spike potential of an action potential. In the sequence of excitability changes, therefore, the first phase is called

---

*Impedance is a measure of the opposition of a circuit to the flow of alternating current. Circuit elements having impedance include resistors, capacitors, and inductors. The impedance of capacitors and inductors varies with the frequency of the alternating current (inversely for capacitors and directly for inductors).

the absolutely refractory period. It is coextensive in time with the spike potential.

For a time after the absolutely refractory period, the neuron can be discharged a second time, but the stimulus strength must be greater than it originally had to be to reach threshold. This is the relatively refractory period, and it is simultaneous with the early part of the after-depolarization. During the relatively refractory period, the height of the second spike potential is reduced and the conduction velocity is slowed.

The relatively refractory period may be succeeded by a phase of enhanced excitability, the supernormal period. This occurs during the last part of the after-depolarization and is presumably caused by the depolarization.

Following the supernormal period is a long-lasting subnormal period. This coincides with and is caused by the after-hyperpolarization.

Accommodation; cathodal and anodal block. A long-lasting, subthreshold depolarization at first makes a neuron hyperexcitable. In time the enhanced excitability may subside because of a process called accommodation. An excessive depolarization can prevent the discharge of nerve impulses, a phenomenon known as cathodal block. Hyperpolarization can also prevent nerve impulses by keeping the membrane potential away from the threshold; this is called anodal block.

Propagation of the action potential. The action potential is normally triggered at a particular point along a neuron when physiological stimulation is

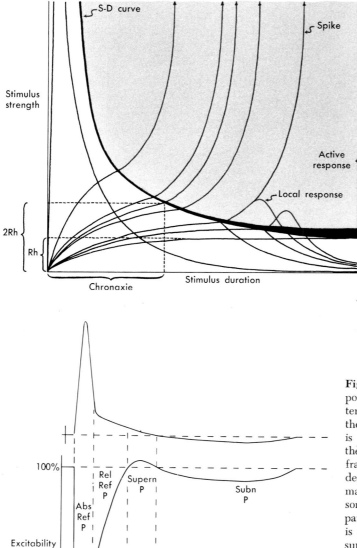

Fig. 1-32. Strength-duration curve. The threshold for evoking a nerve impulse is reached at different times, depending on the strength of stimulation. The basic reason for this is that the membrane potential changes exponentially in response to a rectangular pulse of stimulating current. In the diagram, the stimulus duration is plotted against the stimulus strength. The strength-duration (S-D) curve shows the values of threshold combinations of stimulus parameters. All combinations of values below or to the left of this curve are subthreshold (white area); all combinations above and to the right are suprathreshold (shaded area). Stimuli may have too low a strength or too short a duration to reach threshold. A stimulus that is just strong enough to reach threshold after a long time (several msec) is defined as the rheobase (Rh). The duration of a just-threshold stimulus having a strength of twice the rheobase is called the chronaxie. Note that stimuli near threshold may produce local responses. Furthermore, there is some play in the S-D curve at long durations of stimulus pulses. This is in part caused by alterations in threshold as a result of accommodation.

Fig. 1-33. Excitability cycle. Following the onset of an action potential, the nerve membrane undergoes a sequence of alterations in its excitability. The graph below the drawing of the action potential indicates these changes. Resting excitability is defined as 100%. During the time of the spike potential, the membrane becomes inexcitable. This is the absolutely refractory period (Abs Ref P). During the initial part of the after-depolarization, the membrane is less excitable than it is normally; this is the relatively refractory period (Rel Ref P). In some axons there may be a period coincident with the latter part of the after-depolarization, during which the membrane is actually more excitable than it is at rest. This is called the supernormal period (Supern P). The excitability is less than normal during the time of the after-hyperpolarization. This is called the subnormal period (Subn P).

employed, for example, near a receptor ending in an afferent neuron or near the cell body in a central neuron. It then propagates along the axon to the terminals on the next neuron or the effector organ. Impulses triggered experimentally, as by an electrical stimulus, propagate in both directions along an axon.

The action potential at each point along an axon is produced by changes in ionic permeability of the membrane at that point. The state of each localized area of membrane determines the properties of the action potential at that point. Once threshold is reached, the propagating action potential is quite independent of the stimulus. It is just the same, regardless of the stimulus strength or stimulus type. The nerve impulse, therefore, is said to be all-or-nothing in character.

Ionic basis of the nerve impulse. The sodium hypothesis provides the best available explanation for the mechanism by which the spike potential is produced. Hodgkin and his group have produced evidence for the sodium hypothesis from several lines of investigation. The participation of the membrane and of sodium and potassium ions in nervous conduction has been demonstrated most elegantly in the following kind of experiment. The axoplasm of a squid giant axon may be extruded by a roller and replaced by a perfusion fluid. The axon will still conduct impulses, provided that the right perfusion fluid is used. This indicates that at least the bulk of the axoplasm is unnecessary for conduction. The action potential is reduced in amplitude or blocked when the perfusion fluid contains a high concentration of sodium, whereas it is increased by a low internal sodium concentration. The predicted alterations in the action potential follow changes in extracellular sodium. The spike height, therefore, appears to be controlled by the sodium gradient. Certain cations, notably lithium and some quaternary ammonium ions, can substitute for sodium in the production of spike potentials. However, these cations are not extruded by the sodium pump, and so they are eventually ineffective. It is interesting that the particular anion employed in the perfusion fluid does not seem to matter in most instances.

Radioactive tracers allow an estimate of the quantities of sodium and potassium ions that cross a nerve membrane during an impulse. It should be noted that the increased permeability to an ion will cause an increase in both efflux and influx, but that the net flux will be in the direction of the electrochemical gradient. In cuttlefish giant axons, for example, during a single impulse there is a sodium influx of 10.3×10^{-12} moles/cm^2 of membrane and an efflux of 6.6×10^{-12} moles/cm^2. This is a net influx of 3.7×10^{-12} moles/cm^2. A net efflux of potassium of about the same amount occurs with each impulse. Comparable values have been obtained using squid giant axons.

The entry of about 4 picomoles of sodium per square centimeter of axonal membrane is more than enough to account for the spike potential. If the same area of membrane acts as a capacitor of 1 μF capacitance, the charge needed to alter the membrane potential by 120 mV is

$$Q = VC = 0.12 \times 10^{-6} \text{ coulombs}$$

This is equivalent to 1.2×10^{-12} moles of univalent cation. The excess sodium is probably exchanged with potassium as the permeability to potassium rises; such an exchange would not result in any alteration of potential across the membrane.

In large axons, the ionic shifts caused by a single action potential have relatively little effect on the concentration gradients of the ions. For example, in a squid axon having a diameter of 500 μm, a loss of 4 picomoles/cm^2 of K$^+$ is only one millionth of the total K$^+$. The smaller the fiber, however, the greater is the effect of the ion shifts. For a fiber with a diameter of 0.5 μm, a single action potential results in a loss of one thousandth of the axon's K$^+$. Repetitive stimulation aggravates the losses, but this is somewhat offset by the continued action of the ion pumps or their increased action as a result of changes in ionic concentrations.

Voltage clamp. The timing of the sodium influx and of the potassium efflux was obviously a crucial matter for the substantiation of the sodium hypothesis of nerve conduction by Hodgkin's group. This was made possible by the use of the voltage-clamp technique developed first by Cole. The advantage of this technique is that it simplifies the experimental situation. Normally during an action potential, the membrane potential, resistance, and current are all changing. Furthermore, the current flow includes both a capacitive and a resistive component. The voltage clamp allows the investigator to measure current caused by the nerve impulse just through the membrane resistance, while keeping the voltage constant. This permits a calculation of the change in membrane resistance (or its reciprocal, membrane conductance), and from these values equations can be developed that describe the action potential.

The voltage clamp is an electronic feedback device that enables the experimenter to set the membrane potential at a desired level (Fig. 1-34). The current required to maintain the membrane potential is measured. Because the feedback currents are equal and opposite to the currents crossing the membrane during nervous transmission, it is possible to measure

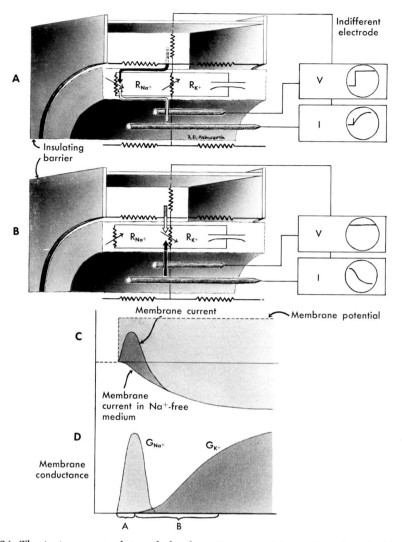

Fig. 1-34. The ionic currents that underlie the action potential were best described by experiments using the voltage clamp. The technique basically consists of the passage of a current through an electrode in the direction opposite that of the currents that would normally cause the action potential. The imposed currents counterbalance the naturally occurring ones, preventing a change in the membrane potential. **A,** A cutaway segment of nerve membrane. Guard partitions extend vertically from the membrane to limit current flow to a radial direction. A large plate electrode is placed along the membrane, and two intracellular electrodes are positioned within the axoplasm. One of the intracellular electrodes is used for passing current; the other records membrane potential. To start the experiment, a current is passed that changes the membrane potential from the resting level to a new level. This voltage step is graphed at the upper right, V. The current required to produce this voltage step is very brief in duration and is indicated by a vertical line in the current record, I. The membrane in this case is depolarized beyond threshold, so current tends to flow into the axoplasm, carried by sodium ions, as shown by the dark arrow at R_{Na^+}. The current from a feedback amplifier, which balances this sodium current, is shown by the open arrow. This is the current in the remainder of the graph, labelled I. As the membrane potential is maintained at the same level, the inward current is succeeded by an outward one carried by potassium ions. This is shown in **B** by the dark arrow at R_{K^+} and by the graph, I. The feedback current is now in the opposite direction (open arrow at R_{K^+}). The time courses of the sodium and potassium currents and the voltage change are better shown in **C.** The darkly shaded region of the current record represents the contribution of the sodium current. The conductance of the membrane for a particular ionic current can be calculated from such current records and from the known voltage steps. **D,** Time courses of the conductance changes of the axon membrane for the sodium and potassium ions. Note that the sodium conductance rises rapidly, then decays back to the original level during a maintained voltage change. The potassium conductance rises slowly, but it remains high during the time the voltage change is maintained. The reversion of the sodium conductance to its original level is caused by a process called inactivation.

these currents. Hodgkin's group demonstrated that a nerve impulse in a voltage-clamped squid axon is associated with an inward current lasting about 1 msec, followed by a long-lasting outward current. The early inward current disappears when the membrane potential is shifted to the sodium equilibrium level, and it reverses to an outward current when the membrane potential exceeds the sodium equilibrium level. The early current also disappears when there is no sodium in the extracellular fluid. It is thus caused by the flow of sodium ions across the membrane. The later current is caused by potassium ions, as shown by comparable experiments.

The ionic currents must be produced by specific changes in the permeability of the membrane to sodium ions and then to potassium ions. The permeability changes may be expressed as changes in the conductance of the membrane with respect to each of these ions.

In addition to its earlier onset, there is an important difference between the sodium conductance change and the potassium change. During a maintained depolarization the sodium conductance reverts to the resting value, whereas the potassium conductance increase remains at a constantly elevated level. The process that causes the reversion of the sodium conductance was termed inactivation by Hodgkin and Huxley. Inactivation persists until the membrane is repolarized. The refractoriness of nerve is caused by the combination of inactivation and a high potassium conductance. Accommodation can also be explained by these processes.

Hodgkin-Huxley equations

Hodgkin and Huxley developed a series of differential equations, based on a theoretical model of nervous transmission, whereby a number of properties of nerve impulses can be predicted (see Appendix II). For example, the shape of a propagated action potential can be mimicked accurately by the Hodgkin-Huxley equations. In modified form they also apply to other excitable tissues, such as cardiac muscle.

Sequence of events in propagated impulses

Based on the experimental evidence of Hodgkin, Huxley, and many others, the sequence of events during a propagated nerve impulse appears to be as follows:

1. The nerve impulse in a given area of membrane or a depolarization produced by a stimulus causes a local circuit current flow along the axon (Fig. 1-35).

2. This discharges the capacity of the neighboring membrane.

3. The depolarization results in an increased sodium conductance (Fig. 1-36). This increase in sodium conductance is dependent only on the depolarization.

4. The increased sodium conductance allows the influx of sodium ions through the membrane along their electrochemical gradient.

5. This further depolarizes the membrane, producing a further increase in sodium conductance.

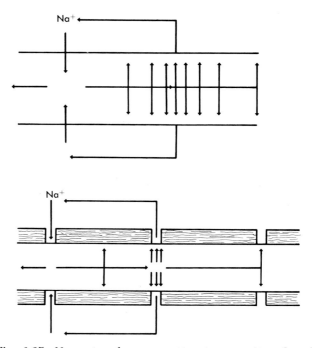

Fig. 1-35. Nerve impulse propagation in unmyelinated and myelinated nerve fibers. Nerve impulse propagation depends on local circuit current flow. As sodium ions enter a region of active nerve membrane, the membrane potential reverses for a brief period of time. Because the interior at the point of activity is positive, a current will flow down the axon toward regions of normal resting potential (interior negative). Some of the current will leak outward across the membrane, with the density of the leakage dependent on the distance along the axon. The return circuit is back through the extracellular fluid. As the outward current depolarizes the membrane beyond threshold, sodium begins to enter the axoplasm, and the active region advances down the membrane. This occurs in a progressive fashion in the case of unmyelinated axons, as indicated in the drawing at the top of the figure. For myelinated axons, the distribution of current outward across the membrane is uneven. More of the current will be concentrated at the nodes of Ranvier than along equal lengths of the internode, because the resistance across the myelin sheath is much higher than across the nodal membrane. Furthermore, the internode is much more readily depolarized than a comparable length of bare membrane would be, because the capacitance is reduced as a result of the thickness of the dielectric. Because of these factors, the threshold membrane potential is reached very quickly at the node of Ranvier, speeding up the conduction velocity greatly in myelinated axons.

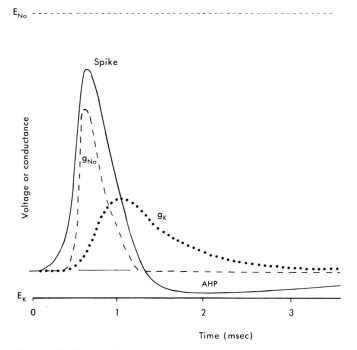

Fig. 1-36. Events during a propagated action potential. Three curves are shown. The solid curve is the spike potential and after-hyperpolarization (AHP) recorded during propagation. The abscissa is time, and the ordinate for this record is voltage. Note that the spike approaches the sodium equilibrium potential (E_{Na}), whereas the AHP approaches the potassium equilibrium potential (E_K). The curve indicated by the dashed line is the time course of the increased sodium conductance (g_{Na}), which is responsible for the spike. The dotted line plots the time course of the increased potassium conductance (g_K). For the conductance curves, the ordinate is in units of conductance (mmho).

6. The process may become regenerative, provided that the potassium conductance has not increased sufficiently to counterbalance the influx of positive charge. When the sodium influx equals the potassium efflux the membrane potential is at threshold. If it exceeds the potassium efflux, the depolarization accelerates and the interior may become positively charged. The sodium influx mechanism is thus a positive feedback (explosive) process (Fig. 1-37, *A*).

7. Inactivation of the sodium conductance mechanism is also produced by depolarization, but at a slower rate than the activation process. However, inactivation becomes progressively more important as the spike approaches its peak.

8. The potassium conductance increases with time, and potassium ions leave the interior of the neuron through the membrane along both their concentration gradient and the now reversed charge gradient.

9. The exodus of potassium ions restores the membrane potential toward the resting level. The potassium efflux mechanism is thus a negative feedback process (Fig. 1-37, *B*). Repolarization causes the inactivation process to begin to revert to the resting condition. The after-potential sequence begins. The Hodgkin-Huxley equations do not attempt to account for the after-potentials in detail. However, the after-depolarization can be attributed to the transient buildup of extracellular potassium after the nerve impulse, and the after-hyperpolarization to a continued increase in permeability to potassium ions following a spike potential.

10. It should be noted that the sodium-potassium pump is not directly involved in the action potential. Any small concentration change in these ions produced

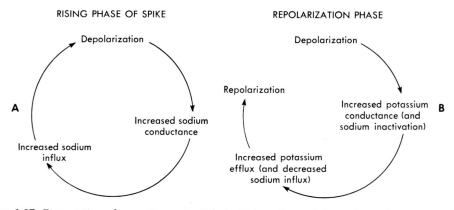

Fig. 1-37. Propagation of an action potential. **A,** Rising phase of the spike is shown to involve a positive feedback mechanism in which depolarization causes an increased sodium conductance, which in turn leads to an increased sodium influx and further depolarization. **B,** Repolarization phase of the spike is shown to result from a negative feedback mechanism. Depolarization causes an increased potassium conductance and sodium inactivation after a delay. The efflux of potassium, coupled with a decreased sodium influx, results in repolarization.

by nerve impulses will eventually be restored by ion pumping, but this occurs over a much greater time span than the action potential.

Molecular basis of conductance changes

Nothing very definite is known about the molecular changes of a nerve membrane that result in the permeability changes that produce the action potential. The dependence of the permeability changes on membrane potential shifts suggests that the movement of charged particles may be involved. One possibility is that calcium ions are present in membrane pores and that these are partially displaced when depolarization occurs. This might then allow the entry of sodium ions through the vacated pores. The known relationship between calcium concentration and membrane excitability would seem to fit this concept. However, Hodgkin's group has evidence against the simplest form of this explanation.

The observation that the poison tetrodotoxin, obtained from the tissues of the pufferfish, blocks selectively the sodium channels involved in nerve impulse propagation and not the potassium channels adds evidence that the molecular rearrangements underlying the sodium and potassium phases of action-potential generation involve different sites in the membrane. Conversely, tetraethylammonium ions block the potassium conductance channels but not the sodium channels.

There is no compelling evidence that acetylcholine is involved in nerve impulse conduction, as suggested by Nachmansohn.

Action potential in myelinated axons

The theory that impulses are conducted in saltatory (jumping) fashion, from node to node, was first proposed by Lillie in 1925. The evidence supporting this theory comes largely from the work of Tasaki and of Huxley and Stämpfli.

Much of the evidence for saltatory conduction is indirect, but it is convincing. For example, the action potential in a single myelinated axon fragments when the fiber is anodally polarized; the portions of the action potential are each all-or-nothing responses, having the properties of typical nerve impulses. Evidently, each fragment originates from a node of Ranvier. Normally, the action potentials from adjacent nodes sum to produce a smooth record, but when the generation of an action potential at one or more nodes is impeded by anodal polarization, the record shows fragmentation into the several spikes contributed by individual nodes.

Stimuli applied along a single myelinated fiber produce a nerve impulse most readily when the point of application is adjacent to a node. Evidently, stimulating currents spread along the axon and excite the fiber just at the node.

If a single fiber is placed so that adjacent nodes are bathed in separate small pools of Ringer's solution and a local anesthetic is applied to one of the nodes, further conduction along the fiber may be prevented. However, if a local anesthetic is applied to the region of an internode, conduction is not affected.

Measurements of the current distribution about myelinated axons during activity show that there is only outward current through internodes, whereas nodal membranes are crossed first by outward and then by inward current (Fig. 1-35). The outward current is produced by local circuit flow preceding the nerve impulses. The inward current is caused by sodium influx, which thus occurs only at the nodes. The outward current is actually very effective in depolarizing the nerve membrane over the short distances involved, so that the action potential in the internodal segment is only slightly smaller in amplitude than that at the nodes.

The conduction velocity in myelinated nerve depends on the time required to charge the capacities of the internodes and the nodes, as well as the time for the sodium conductance change to occur at the nodes. The low capacity of the internodes, the high transverse resistance of the myelin, and the small area involved in a conductance change allow a much more rapid conduction velocity than is possible with even very large unmyelinated fibers.

Most of the experiments that have been done on the properties of nervous transmission in unmyelinated axons have been repeated on node of Ranvier preparations and have been found to yield essentially the same results. For example, the node has a definite threshold, with a strength-duration relationship like that in other nerves, and an excitability cycle.

Pharmacology of nervous transmission

Nerve impulses can be prevented by the action of drugs called local anesthetics, for example, procaine and lidocaine. The mode of action of such drugs appears to be to reduce the membrane permeability to ions and to prevent the ionic conductance changes that are responsible for the action potential. This action is sometimes described as membrane stabilization.

If a local anesthetic agent is injected into the vicinity of a nerve trunk, the concentration of drug at the active sites for the generation of nerve impulses, the nodes of Ranvier for myelinated fibers and the surface membrane for unmyelinated ones, varies with time. As the drug diffuses toward the nerve trunk, the concentration reaches the level necessary to block transmission first about small myelinated nerve fibers, then unmyelinated fibers, and finally large myelinated fibers. With a critical dose of local anesthetic, it is possible primarily to block small fibers. As the anesthetic wears off, conduction reappears in the reverse order according to fiber group; conduction in large fibers is restored first, then in small fibers.

Local anesthetics block the conductance changes for both sodium and potassium in the membrane sites for nerve impulse generation. There are, however, agents that differentially block the sodium conductance mechanism or the potassium conductance mechanism. As mentioned earlier, tetrodotoxin will selectively block the sodium conductance mechanism, and tetraethylammonium ions will selectively block the potassium conductance mechanism. Used singly, tetrodotoxin will prevent spike potentials, whereas tetraethylammonium ions cause a prolongation of spike potentials.

Axoplasmic transport

An intriguing finding that is the subject of a great deal of investigation is the fact that there is a constant movement of material along axons. A major component of this material is protein. Most of the protein required by the axon in maintaining its structural integrity and in renewing the materials involved in synaptic transmission is likely to be produced in the region of the cell body of the neuron. This protein would have to be carried down the axon by axoplasmic flow, because diffusion is too slow a process for elongated cells like neurons. However, some protein may be manufactured in the axon, although not in association with ribosomes. There is probably a relationship between microtubules and axoplasmic flow, inasmuch as chemical agents that produce a disruption or depolymerization of microtubules prevent axoplasmic flow. Such agents include colchicine and the *Vinca* alkaloids (vinblastine and vincristine). The rate of axoplasmic flow has been measured. There are two components: a slow component, which progresses at about 1 to 4.5 mm per day, and a fast component, which travels at a rate of about 400 mm per day (estimates vary over a wide range). The rate of the slow axoplasmic flow corresponds to the maximum rate of regeneration of nerve fibers following injury. It also corresponds to the rate of movement of neurosecretory material, amine storage granules, and other indicators of substances involved in synaptic transmission. Among the chemical compounds associated with the slow axoplasmic flow are some soluble proteins. Substances that are transported rapidly include amino acids, poly-

peptides, and small proteins. It seems clear that axoplasmic flow is among the most important of the properties that allow neurons to perform their special function of communication.

Although much of the axoplasmic flow is in the direction away from the nerve cell body, there is also flow in the reverse direction. For example, horseradish peroxidase placed in the extracellular space around nerve terminals will be picked up and transported in retrograde fashion along the axon to the cell body, where it is accumulated and eventually metabolized (see Appendix I for a description of the use of this agent for tracing neural pathways). It is highly probable that a diversity of substances is transported along axons in this same way, and it is conceivable that this mechanism is of consequence for chemical information transfer and for trophic interactions.

BIBLIOGRAPHY
Neurons and their supportive cells

Bailey, P., and Cushing, H.: A classification of tumours of the glioma group on a histogenetic basis with a correlated study of prognosis, Philadelphia, 1926, J. B. Lippincott Co.

Barr, M. L., Bertram, L. F., and Lindsay, H. A.: The morphology of the nerve cell nucleus according to sex, Anat. Rec. 107:283-297, 1950.

Bodian, D.: Introductory survey of neurons, Cold Spring Harbor Symp. Quant. Biol. 17:1-13, 1952.

Bullock, T. H., and Horridge, G. A.: Structure and function in the nervous systems of invertebrates, 2 vols., San Francisco, 1965, W. H. Freeman and Co. Publishers.

Bunge, R. P.: Glial cells and the central myelin sheath, Physiol. Rev. 48:197-251, 1968.

De Robertis, E.: Histophysiology of synapses and neurosecretion, New York, 1964, Pergamon Press, Inc.

Fernandez-Moran, H., and Finean, J. B.: Electron microscope and low-angle x-ray diffraction studies of the nerve myelin sheath, J. Biophys. Biochem. Cytol. 3:725-748, 1957.

Geren, B. B.: The formation from the Schwann cell surface of myelin in the peripheral nerves of chick embryos, Exp. Cell Res. 7:558-562, 1954.

Gray, E. G., and Guillery, R. W.: Synaptic morphology in the normal and degenerating nervous system, Int. Rev. Cytol. 19:111-182, 1966.

Guth, L.: Regeneration in the mammalian peripheral nervous system, Physiol. Rev. 36:441-478, 1956.

Guth, L., and Windle, W. R., editors: The enigma of central nervous regeneration, Exp. Neurol. (Suppl.) 5:1043, 1970.

Hamilton, W. J., Boyd, J. D., and Mossman, H. W.: Human embryology, Baltimore, 1965, The Williams & Wilkins Co.

Hydén, H.: The neuron. In Brachet, J., and Mirsky, A. E., editors: The cell, vol. 4, New York, 1960, Academic Press, Inc.

Novikoff, A. B.: Lysosomes in nerve cells. In Hydén, H., editor: The Neuron, New York, 1967, Elsevier Publishing Co., pp. 319-377.

Palay, S. L.: Synapses in the central nervous system, J. Biophys. Biochem. Cytol. 2:193-202, 1956.

Peters, A., Palay, S. L., and Webster, H. DeF.: The fine

structure of the nervous system, New York, 1970, Harper & Row, Publishers.

Ramon y Cajal, S.: Neuron theory or reticular theory? Madrid, 1954, Consejo Superior de Investigaciones Cientificas.

Ramon y Cajal, S.: Histologie du système nerveux de l'homme et des vertébrés, Madrid, 1955, Consejo Superior de Investigaciones Cientificas.

Ramon y Cajal, S.: Degeneration and regeneration of the nervous system, New York, 1959, Hafner Publishing Co., Inc.

Ramon y Cajal, S.: Studies on vertebrate neurogenesis, Springfield, Ill., 1960, Charles C Thomas, Publisher.

Shelanski, M. L.: Chemistry of the filaments and tubules of brain, J. Histochem. Cytochem. 21:529-539, 1973.

Shepherd, G. M.: The synaptic organization of the brain; an introduction, New York, 1975, Oxford University Press, Inc.

Young, J. Z.: Fused neurons and synaptic contacts in the giant nerve fibres of cephalopods, Philos. Trans. R. Soc. Lond. [Biol. Sci.] 229:465-503, 1939.

Resting and action potentials

Aidley, D. J.: The physiology of excitable cells, Cambridge, 1971, Cambridge University Press.

Baker, P. F., Hodgkin, A. L., and Shaw, T. I.: The effects of changes in internal ionic concentrations on the electrical properties of perfused giant axons, J. Physiol. (Lond.) 164:353-374, 1962.

Caldwell, P. C., Hodgkin, A. L., Keynes, R. D., and Shaw, T. I.: The effects of injecting "energy-rich" phosphate compounds on the active transport of ions in the giant axons of Loligo, J. Physiol. (Lond.) 152:561-590, 1960.

Cole, K. S., and Curtis, H. J.: Electric impedance of the squid giant axon during activity, J. Gen. Physiol. 22:649-670, 1939.

Eccles, J. C.: The physiology of nerve cells, Baltimore, 1957, The Johns Hopkins University Press.

Erlanger, J., and Gasser, H. S.: Electrical signs of nervous activity, Philadelphia, 1937, University Press.

Gasser, H. S., and Grundfest, H.: Action and excitability in mammalian A fibers, Am. J. Physiol. 117:113-133, 1936.

Gotch, F.: The submaximal electrical response of nerve to a single stimulus, J. Physiol. (Lond.) 28:395-416, 1902.

Graham, H. T.: The subnormal period of nerve response, Am. J. Physiol. 111:452-465, 1935.

Graham, H. T., and Lorente de Nó., R.: Recovery of blood-perfused mammalian nerves, Am. J. Physiol. 123:326-340, 1938.

Graham, J., and Gerard, R.: Membrane potentials and excitation of impaled single muscle fibers, J. Cell Physiol. 28:99-117, 1946.

Hodgkin, A. L.: The conduction of the nervous impulse, Springfield, Ill., 1964, Charles C Thomas, Publisher.

Hodgkin, A. L., and Huxley, A. F.: Currents carried by sodium and potassium ions through the membrane of the giant axon of Loligo, J. Physiol. (Lond.) 116:449-472, 1952.

Hodgkin, A. L., and Huxley, A. F.: The components of membrane conductance of the giant axon of Loligo, J. Physiol. (Lond.) 116:473-496, 1952.

Hodgkin, A. L., and Huxley, A. F.: The dual effect of membrane potential of sodium conductance in the giant axon of Loligo, J. Physiol. (Lond.) 116:497-506, 1952.

Hodgkin, A. L., and Huxley, A. F.: A quantitative description of membrane current and its application to conduction and excitation in nerve, J. Physiol. (Lond.) 117:500-544, 1952.

Hodgkin, A. L., Huxley, A. F., and Katz, B.: Measurements of current-voltage relations in the membrane of the giant axon of Loligo, J. Physiol. (Lond.) 116:424-448, 1952.

Hodgkin, A. L., and Katz, B.: The effect of sodium ions on the electrical activity of the giant axon of the squid, J. Physiol. (Lond.) 108:37-77, 1949.

Hodgkin, A. L., and Keynes, R. D.: Active transport of cations in giant axons, from Sepia and Loligo, J. Physiol. (Lond.) 128:28-60, 1955.

Hodgkin, A. L., and Rushton, W. A. H.: The electrical constants of a crustacean nerve fibre, Proc. R. Soc. Lond. [Biol.] 133:444-479, 1946.

Hutchison, H. T., Werrbach, K., Vance, C., and Haber, B.: Uptake of neurotransmitters by clonal lines of astrocytoma and neuroblastoma in culture. I. Transport of γ-aminobutyric acid, Brain Res. 66:265-274, 1974.

Huxley, A. F., and Stämpfli, R.: Evidence for saltatory conduction in peripheral myelinated nerve fibres, J. Physiol. (Lond.) 108:315-339, 1949.

Huxley, A. F., and Stämpfli, R.: Direct determination of membrane resting potential and action potential in single myelinated nerve fibres, J. Physiol. (Lond.) 112:476-495, 1951.

Huxley, A. F., and Stämpfli, R.: Effects of potassium and sodium on resting and action potentials of single myelinated nerve fibres, J. Physiol. (Lond.) 112:496-508, 1951.

Katz, B.: Nerve, muscle, and synapse, New York, 1966, McGraw-Hill Book Co.

Keynes, R. D.: The ionic movements during nervous activity, J. Physiol. (Lond.) 114:119-150, 1951.

Kuffler, S. W., and Nicholls, J. G.: The physiology of neuroglial cells, Ergeb. Physiol. 57:1-90, 1966.

LaVail, J. H., and LaVail, M. M.: The retrograde intraaxonal transport of horseradish peroxidase in the chick visual system; a light and electron microscopic study, J. Comp. Neurol. 157:303-358, 1974.

Ling, G., and Gerard, R. W.: The normal membrane potential of frog sartorius fibers, J. Cell Physiol. 34:383-396, 1949.

Moore, J. W., Narahashi, T., and Shaw, T. I.: An upper limit to the number of sodium channels in nerve membrane, J. Physiol. (Lond.) 188:99-106, 1967.

Nachmansohn, D.: Chemical and molecular basis of nerve activity, New York, 1959, Academic Press, Inc.

Narahashi, T., Anderson, N. C., and Moore, J. W.: Comparison of tetrodotoxin and procaine in internally perfused squid giant axons, J. Gen. Physiol. 50:1413-1428, 1967.

Ochs, S., and Ranish, N.: Characteristics of the fast transport system in mammalian nerve fibers, J. Neurobiol. 1:247-261, 1969.

Ochs, S., Sabri, M. I., and Ranish, N.: Somal site of synthesis of fast transported materials in mammalian nerve fibers, J. Neurobiol. 1:329-344, 1970.

Tasaki, I.: Nervous transmission, Springfield, Ill., 1953, Charles C Thomas, Publisher.

CHAPTER **2**

Receptors and receptor mechanisms

The information utilized by the central nervous system for decision making is derived from the environment, either external or internal. The detection of this information is the function of the receptor organs. There is a variety of receptor types that are capable of sensing different forms of stimuli—mechanical, thermal, chemical, photic; and in certain fish there are electroreceptors.

Receptor organs transmit the information they detect to the central nervous system by means of nerve impulses. Thus, receptor organs act like the transducers commonly employed in physiological and other experiments. Transducers are devices that convert one form of energy to another. They are often used to detect mechanical, photic, or other events and to signify by means of an output device the presence and extent of such events. Receptor organs behave in a similar fashion, but the recording device employed is the central nervous system rather than a penwriter or meter.

CLASSIFICATION OF RECEPTORS

There are a number of ways in which the receptor organs may be classified. C. S. Sherrington divided them into exteroceptors, interoceptors, and proprioceptors, according to whether they provide information related to the external environment, the activity of the viscera, or the position of the body in space. Another classification is the following:

Special	Vision, audition, taste, olfaction, balance
Superficial	Touch, pressure, warmth, cold, pain
Deep	Position, vibration, deep pressure, deep pain
Visceral	Hunger, nausea, visceral pain

No doubt other systems of classification would serve as well.

The emphasis in this chapter is placed on the superficial receptors found in the skin and on the deep receptors of muscle and joints. Consideration is given to the special sensory and visceral receptors in later chapters.

RECEPTOR SPECIFICITY

A given receptor type is generally specialized so that it is particularly sensitive to one kind of stimulus. A number of factors may contribute to this specialization, including the position of the receptor in the body, the cellular organization of the receptor, and the chemical composition of the surface membrane of the receptor or of its organelles.

Johannes Müller, in his doctrine of specific nerve energies, suggested that sensory discrimination depends on the differential sensitivity of receptors for particular forms of stimuli. This concept has been challenged by a group of investigators led by G. Weddell. Although there is no question about the specificity of receptors such as the eye and the ear, there is some room for doubt concerning the specificity of cutaneous receptors. Investigators in the past tried to assign particular functions to a variety of cutaneous receptor organs by applying different kinds of stimuli to intact human skin, localizing small areas that seemed to respond only to a single sensory modality, and then examining the sensory spots histologically to find out what kind of receptor was present that could account for the sensation. Weddell and others have shown that a number of mistakes were made using this approach. They feel that it is more likely that cutaneous sensations involve the stimulation of several kinds of receptors concurrently and that the central nervous system interprets and differentiates the various patterns of input in terms of specific sensations.

Although the central nervous system no doubt plays an important role in deciphering patterns of nervous input from receptors contributing information about a stimulus, it is still likely that receptor specificity is a major factor in sensory discrimination. Studies utilizing records from single afferent fibers from cutaneous receptor organs have shown that a given receptor may respond in a highly selective way.

GENERALIZATIONS ABOUT RECEPTOR MECHANISMS

The discussion in this section is concerned with some general properties of receptor mechanisms. A more detailed consideration is given in the next sections to the mechanisms utilized by some specific examples of receptor organs that have been well studied.

Discharges in afferent fibers

The characteristics of the different types of sensory receptors may be investigated in a number of ways. One of the most fruitful involves the recording of activity in single afferent fibers from particular kinds of sensory receptors (Fig. 2-1). This method was pioneered in the laboratory of E. D. Adrian and has been used successfully by many workers. In addition to afferent impulses, it is sometimes possible under favorable conditions to record receptor potentials from the region of the sensory receptor.

Receptor potentials

The application of an appropriate stimulus to a sensory receptor produces a depolarization, called a

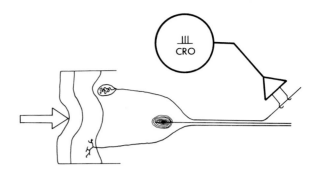

Fig. 2-1. Recording discharges from single afferent fiber. A group of nerve fibers is shown innervating several types of receptor organs in the skin. A single afferent fiber has been dissected from the nerve bundle so that afferent nerve impulses from just one type of sensory receptor can be recorded on a cathode ray oscilloscope *(CRO)*. The stimulus is symbolized by the arrow.

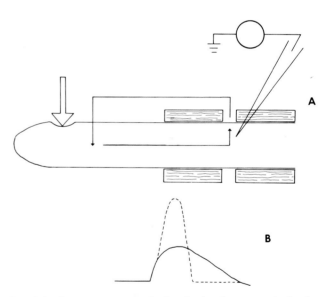

Fig. 2-2. Receptor potential. In **A** the bare terminal of a myelinated afferent fiber is represented as a mechanoreceptor. A stimulus is applied, as symbolized by the open arrow. The distortion of the membrane causes an increased permeability to ions, including sodium. Current flows into the terminal, along the axoplasm, and out of the fiber. Some of the current would depolarize the membrane at a trigger point, such as the first node of Ranvier, where a nerve impulse will be evoked if the depolarization exceeds threshold. This depolarization is called a receptor potential. The microelectrode impaling the terminal is recording the receptor potential. In practice, it is seldom possible to record receptor potentials intracellularly. However, extracellular recordings can often be made. In **B** the receptor potential is indicated by the solid line, and an action potential is shown by the broken line. The receptor potential in this case is at threshold.

receptor potential (Fig. 2-2). The receptor potential may or may not be large enough to reach threshold for evoking an action potential in the afferent axon, depending on the intensity of the stimulus.

The mechanism by which receptor potentials are produced varies with the particular receptor organ under consideration. A photochemical reaction is involved in the case of the retinal cones and rods, whereas the immediate cause of the receptor potential of a pacinian corpuscle is the mechanical deformation of the axon terminal within the corpuscle. In general, the rising phase of a receptor potential is caused by an increased permeability to certain ions, including sodium; the decay is probably the passive recharging of the axonal membrane capacity.

A distinction should be made between receptors in which the receptor potential and the afferent nerve impulses are established within the same cell and those in which a receptor potential is produced in one cell, which in turn elicits impulses in an adjacent nerve terminal (Fig. 2-3). An example of the former is the pacinian corpuscle, and an instance of the latter is the hair cells of the cochlea. The receptor potential in the first case produces a local circuit flow of current, which triggers the nerve impulse in an area of membrane adjacent to the receptor membrane. Transmission between cells in the second case probably

involves a large enough current flow to effectively bridge the gap between the cells. Although not established at the present time, it is possible that in some receptors a chemical transmitter substance is released, as in chemical synaptic transmission (see Chapter 3).

Receptor adaptation

If a stimulus is maintained, a train of afferent impulses may result. Generally, the frequency of discharge is highest initially and gradually falls off as time passes; the receptor is said to adapt to the stimulus (Fig. 2-4). When the frequency drops to zero soon after the onset of stimulation, despite the continuation of the stimulus, the receptor is rapidly adapting; if it continues to discharge throughout the period of stimulation, the receptor is slowly adapting. The mechanism of adaptation may vary with the type of receptor. For mechanical stimuli, adaptation may reflect changes in the mechanical properties of the tissues about the sensory ending. However, an

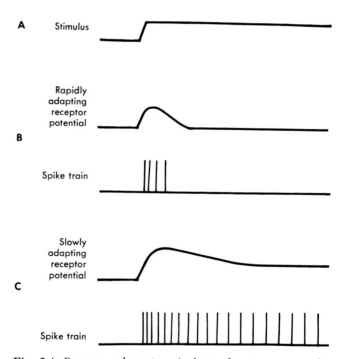

Fig. 2-4. Receptor adaptation. **A** shows the time course of a stimulus applied to a sensory receptor. The stimulus is rapid in onset and is maintained for a long period of time. **B** shows the time course of a receptor potential at the terminal and of a burst of nerve impulses in the afferent fiber of a rapidly adapting receptor. **C** shows the time course of a receptor potential at the terminal and a train of nerve impulses from the afferent fiber supplying a slowly adapting receptor. Note the overshoot in the size of the receptor potential and in the frequency of the spike train of the slowly adapting receptor. This is referred to as a dynamic response, whereas the plateau in receptor potential height and in spike frequency that follows this period is called the static response.

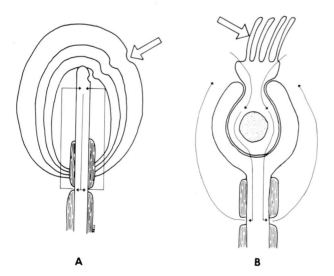

Fig. 2-3. Receptor potentials from one-element and two-element receptors. In **A** the receptor potential is produced by a stimulus indicated by the arrow. The currents depolarize a trigger point in the same element, in this case the nearest node of Ranvier, where a nerve impulse will be evoked if the receptor potential exceeds threshold. In **B** the stimulus produces current flow through the membrane of a hair cell. The current crosses to another element, a sensory nerve terminal in contact with the hair cell, where the nerve impulse may be evoked.

additional mechanism involves neural accommodation. This may be the most important mechanism for adaptation in receptors, other than mechanoreceptors.

Stimulus intensity

The intensity of a stimulus may be signaled in one of two ways. The stronger the stimulus, the greater is the frequency of discharge of the receptor organ (Fig. 2-5). With slowly adapting receptors, the duration of stimulation is also signaled by the duration of discharge. A strong stimulus lasting a long time will evoke a long train of impulses at a high frequency. Another way in which a strong stimulus makes its effects known is by eliciting discharges in many receptor organs. For instance, a light pressure stimulus applied to an area of skin will set up receptor potentials in many receptors, but these will reach threshold in only

the most sensitive receptors located in the immediate vicinity of the stimulus. A stronger stimulus will cause more receptor potentials to reach threshold, and so more afferent fibers will be discharged. The central effects of stimuli of greater intensity will be increased because of the combined actions of these afferents.

The relationship between the response of a sensory receptor and the intensity of a stimulus can be determined experimentally. Curves have been fitted to such stimulus-response relationships. Sometimes a straight line will provide the best fit, but often the curve is nonlinear. A common curve found for many receptors is a power function. The general equation for a power function is

$$\text{Response} = (\text{Constant})(\text{Stimulus})^n$$

where the exponent, n, varies from case to case. Typically, n is less than 1, and the curve that results shows the response to rise rapidly at first and then to plateau as the stimulus becomes more intense. One result of such a stimulus-response relationship is that with weak stimuli a small change in stimulus strength produces a considerable change in the response. However, for large stimuli the response is small for relatively great stimulus differences. The range of responsiveness of a receptor is in effect widened to cover very small and very large stimulus intensities.

Stimulus direction

A receptor may respond to a stimulus that displaces the receptor in one direction but not in another. Such a receptor will signal the spatial directionality of a stimulus. For example, some joint receptors might be activated by flexion of a joint but not by extension. Other receptors do not distinguish directionality. Pacinian corpuscles, for instance, are activated by

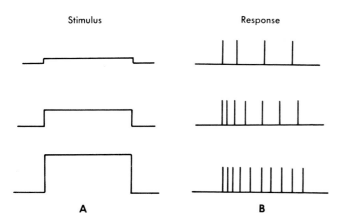

Fig. 2-5. Coding of stimulus intensity. **A,** Three stimuli of progressively greater intensity. **B,** Responses of a single receptor are shown by the spike trains recorded from its afferent fiber. As stimulus intensity increases, the number and frequency of spikes in the afferent increase.

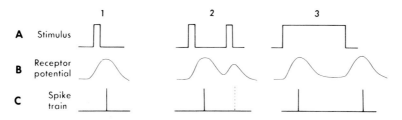

Fig. 2-6. Receptor fatigue. **A,** Time courses of stimuli applied to a rapidly adapting sensory receptor; **B,** receptor potentials; and **C,** afferent nerve impulses. **1,** The stimulus evokes a receptor potential that is above threshold for evoking a nerve impulse. In **2,** two successive stimuli are applied. The first produces a suprathreshold receptor potential; the second stimulus causes the generation of a smaller receptor potential than did the first stimulus. This is caused by a type of refractoriness of the receptor membrane. The second receptor potential may or may not be above threshold for evoking a nerve impulse *(broken vertical line)*. This depends on the strength of the second stimulus and on the interval between the stimuli. **3** shows that a prolonged stimulus may evoke receptor potentials and nerve impulses both at the onset and offset of the stimulus. This kind of receptor will not sense stimulus direction. The pacinian corpuscle is an example of such a receptor (see pp. 49-52).

pressure waves, but the pressure wave can strike the corpuscle in any direction (Fig. 2-6).

Receptor fatigue

Repetitive stimulation of a sensory receptor may produce successively smaller receptor potentials. This is termed receptor fatigue (Fig. 2-6). The mechanism for this may involve different processes according to the type of receptor. One process that may occur is a kind of refractory state of the sensory nerve terminal. Another is the bleaching of photosensitive pigment in the retina. The result of receptor fatigue would be a decrease in the probability of discharge in the afferent fiber, because the receptor potential in response to a given strength of stimulus might drop below threshold.

Spontaneous activity

Many afferent fibers are found to discharge even when no obvious stimulation of their receptor organs has occurred. This type of discharge is called spontaneous.

The physiological importance of spontaneous discharge has been emphasized by Ragnar Granit. For one thing, a continuous afferent input into the central nervous system keeps the excitability of the various pathways high. This activity is probably of great importance for the maintenance of the waking state, inasmuch as the deprivation of sensory input may result in somnolence. Another role of spontaneous afferent activity may be to allow a greater range of change in the discharge pattern with various kinds of stimuli; if an ongoing spontaneous background discharge were occurring, a decrease as well as an increase in stimulation could be signaled.

Central control of sensation

Many afferent systems are under the control of pathways originating in the brain. This centrifugal control is undoubtedly of great importance to the organism, for it provides a means of sorting out essential from trivial information. For instance, the ticking of a clock may not disturb the sleep of a person at all, whereas noises of a lower intensity produced by a potential burglar may cause the person to awaken. Specific examples of centrifugal control systems are mentioned in the discussion of the muscle spindle and of various afferent pathways.

Receptive fields

A single afferent fiber may supply one or more receptor organs. The area that when stimulated causes a discharge in the afferent fiber is said to be its receptive field (Fig. 2-7). In general, single afferent fibers have relatively discrete receptive fields. The receptive

fields of several afferents may overlap because receptor organs supplied by the fibers may be topographically intermingled.

The size of the receptive field of a particular type of receptor may be different, depending on the location of the receptor. For instance, many cutaneous receptors have small receptive fields if they are

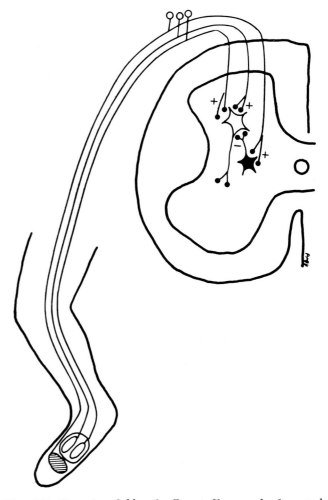

Fig. 2-7. Receptive fields of afferent fibers and of central neurons. Several receptive fields for afferent fibers are shown by the ovals connected with peripheral processes of dorsal root ganglion cells. The central processes of the afferent fibers end synaptically on interneurons of the spinal cord. All of the afferent fibers are excitatory. However, one of the interneurons inhibits the other. The afferents from the receptive fields, shown by the open ovals on the foot, are excitatory to the more dorsally located interneuron, and so these account for part of the excitatory receptive field of the interneuron. The remainder of the excitatory receptive field of the interneuron is indicated by the larger outlined area; other afferent fibers ending on the interneuron account for the difference. The shaded oval area would be an inhibitory receptive field, because the pathway involves an interneuron that inhibits the neuron whose activity is being described. However, this same area is an excitatory receptive field for the inhibitory interneuron.

located on the distal part of an extremity, but the receptive fields of comparable receptors located on the proximal extremity or on the trunk may be much larger. Because sensory discrimination is much better developed on the distal parts of the extremities, there is reason to attribute this in part to the finer sizes of the receptive fields of the sense organs in this part of the body. Another factor, however, is that the density of innervation is also greatest on the distal extremities, and so there are many more receptors for a given area of skin on the fingers, for instance, than on the back.

Central neurons, which receive information from afferent fibers, are also described in terms of receptive fields. The sizes of the receptive fields of central neurons vary considerably. This is to be expected because each central neuron may receive connections from more than one afferent fiber. Some receive excitatory connections from afferents connected with receptors covering a wide area, whereas others receive connections from receptors localized to very small areas. Another difference between the receptive fields of central neurons and of afferents is the occurrence of central inhibition. Afferents may be excited or not excited by their receptor organs. Central neurons appear to receive only excitatory synaptic connections directly from afferents; however, afferent information may be relayed through one or more interneurons, which may produce excitation or inhibition. A discussion of central inhibition is found in Chapter 4.

Surround inhibition

Occasionally, an excitatory receptive field of a central neuron is surrounded by an inhibitory receptive field. This arrangement may be of significance for sensory discrimination. For instance, a moving stimulus may cross an inhibitory receptive field before entering the excitatory one. The detection of the arrival of the stimulus within the excitatory field would presumably be enhanced by the contrast provided by the prior activation of receptors within the surrounding inhibitory field.

STRETCH RECEPTOR

Many of the principles of operation of receptor organs are well illustrated by the crayfish stretch receptor (Fig. 2-8). Similar organs are found in lobsters and other crustacea, but the crayfish stretch receptor has been the subject of the most intense investigation.

Morphology of the crayfish stretch receptor

The crayfish stretch receptor serves well as a model receptor organ because of its structural arrangement.

The cell body of the receptor neuron lies peripherally, adjacent to a bundle of muscle fibers. The dendrites of the neuron penetrate the muscle bundle, so the stretch of the muscle will distort the dendrites. The axon runs from the receptor neuron cell body through a peripheral nerve to the central nervous system. The peripheral nerve also contains efferent axons, which terminate synaptically both on the muscle fibers and on the receptor neuron.

Excitation of the stretch receptor

Because of the large size of the cell body of the receptor neuron and its proximity to the point of generation of the receptor potential, it is easy to obtain intracellular records of the receptor potential and to relate these to mechanical stimuli applied to the dendrites by stretch of the muscle.

When the muscle bundle is stretched slightly, the receptor neuron becomes depolarized. The depolarization, or receptor potential, is graded according to the degree of stretch, and it lasts for the duration of the stretch. However, the peak depolarization is not maintained. Instead, the depolarization undergoes a gradual decline. If the depolarization reaches some 10 to 20 mV from the resting potential, action potentials may be triggered. The number and frequency of these depends on the amount of depolarization and its duration. There are also differences between stretch receptor organs, some of which are more slowly adapting than others. Following each spike is an afterhyperpolarization. As this subsides, the membrane depolarizes again until it reaches threshold for ex-

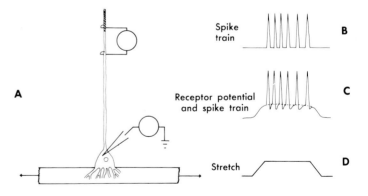

Fig. 2-8. Crayfish stretch receptor. **A,** Stretch receptor neuron, with its dendrites embedded in a bundle of muscle fibers and its axon dissected for recording afferent discharges. A microelectrode impaling the cell body can be used to record the receptor potential produced by stretch of the muscle bundle. The inhibitory nerve and its endings are not shown. **B,** Time course of a stretch stimulus; **C,** receptor potential and superimposed spike train; and **D,** the afferent discharges. The receptor potential and spike train are characteristic of a slowly adapting receptor.

citing another nerve impulse. Presumably, the continued distortion of the dendrites provides a maintained tendency toward depolarization, which is only transiently interrupted by the after-potential sequence. After stretch is terminated, the membrane potential may become hyperpolarized beyond the resting level before resuming that level.

The observations that the receptor potential declines in size following an early peak size and that the membrane becomes hyperpolarized following the cessation of stretch may be related to the characteristic of many slowly adapting receptors to show dynamic as well as static responses. It has frequently been observed that a receptor will show a disproportionate increase in its firing rate during the onset of a stimulus and a disproportionate decrease in firing rate when the stimulus is terminated. These are known as dynamic responses. The firing rate during the steady state is known as the static response. (An example of dynamic and static responses is illustrated in Fig. 2-4.) In stretch receptors, the cause of the dynamic response, as well as of any progressive adaptation of the static response, may well be mechanical and brought about by slow changes in the properties of the muscle and associated connective tissue.

Centrifugal control

The stretch receptor organ is under the control of the central nervous system. There are two means by which this control is exerted. The muscle is provided with an excitatory innervation. When the muscle is excited to contract, this produces a distortion of the stretch receptor neuron's dendrites and consequently a receptor potential. Thus, the stretch receptor neuron can be fired by either stretch or contraction of its attached muscle bundle. In addition, the stretch receptor neuron is contacted by an inhibitory fiber. The central nervous system is able to prevent the firing of the receptor cell through the action of this inhibitory linkage. The crayfish stretch receptor has provided experimentalists with a convenient preparation for the study of inhibitory processes, and in addition it serves to demonstrate the principle of the centrifugal control of receptor organs, which applies to the mammalian as well as to the invertebrate nervous system. Although many mammalian receptor organs do not receive direct innervation from the central nervous system, some do (for example, the muscle spindle and the hair cells of the cochlea). In any case, sensory input is often controlled centrally at the level of the first synapse.

Table 2-1. Cutaneous receptor organs

Class	Functional category	Morphological category	Frequency range	Size of axon	Probable sensory role	Type of skin
Mechanoreceptor						
Position (and velocity) detectors	Type I	Merkel's cell ending; touch corpuscle	DC	Aβ	Touch-pressure	Hairy; glabrous
	Type II	Ruffini's corpuscle	DC	Aβ	Touch-pressure	Hairy; glabrous
Velocity detector	Hair follicle	Tylotrich and guard hairs	Intermediate	Aβ	Movement, flutter	Hairy
		Down	Low	Aδ	Slow movement	Hairy
	Field	?	Intermediate	Aβ	Movement, flutter	Hairy
	C	? Free	Low	C	Slow movement	Hairy
	RA (rapidly adapting)	Meissner's corpuscle	5 to 40 Hz	Aβ	Movement, flutter	Glabrous
Transient detector	Hair follicle	Tylotrich and guard hairs	High	Aβ	Rapid movement	Hairy
	Pacinian (phasic, tap)	Pacinian corpuscle	60 to 300 Hz	Aβ	Vibration, tap	Subcutaneous
Thermoreceptor	Warm	? Free endings	Dynamic and static warming	C	Warmth	Hairy; presumably glabrous
	Cold	Free endings	Dynamic and static cooling	Aδ or C	Cooling	Hairy; glabrous
Nociceptor	High-threshold mechanoreceptor	? Free	DC	Aδ or C	Pressure-pain	Hairy; glabrous
	Thermal	? Free	DC	Aδ or C	Pain	Hairy; glabrous
	Polymodal	? Free	DC	C	Pain	Hairy; glabrous

STRUCTURE AND FUNCTION
OF CUTANEOUS RECEPTOR ORGANS

The cutaneous exteroceptors of mammals, including man, may be classed according to the type of stimulus to which they respond (Table 2-1). There are mechanoreceptors, thermoreceptors (temperature receptors), and nociceptors (receptors that respond only to severe stimuli that produce or threaten damage to the skin).

Mechanoreceptors can be subdivided into slowly adapting and rapidly adapting varieties. A more useful approach, however, is that suggested by P. R. Burgess and E. R. Perl. This is a classification of mechanoreceptors according to their probable roles as position, velocity, or transient detectors. Position detectors signal static displacement (p), for example, of the skin. Velocity detectors respond to the velocity of displacement (dp/dt), but not to displacement as such. When a displacement is completed, the velocity of displacement decreases to zero, and the receptor is no longer activated. Transient detectors discharge in association with stimulus acceleration (d^2p/dt^2) or jerk (d^3p/dt^3). In the older terminology, the position detectors would be the slowly adapting receptors, whereas the velocity and the transient detectors would together be the rapidly adapting receptors.

Thermoreceptors can also be subdivided. The two classes of specific thermoreceptors are cold and warm receptors. In addition, certain kinds of mechanoreceptors are also affected by thermal changes; however, the role of these in thermal sensation and in thermoregulation is unknown. Specific thermoreceptors characteristically show both a dynamic and a static sensitivity to thermal changes.

Nociceptors include afferents that are specifically excited by either noxious mechanical stimuli or noxious thermal stimuli. In addition, polymodal nociceptors are activated by both noxious mechanical and noxious thermal changes as well as by chemical damage.

Mechanoreceptors

Position detectors. Cutaneous receptors with type I and type II endings appear to serve as position detectors. It should be recognized, however, that the responses of these receptors show both a dynamic and a static phase and that the dynamic phase signals stimulus velocity. Therefore these endings serve both as position and velocity detectors. They respond to very small displacements of the skin, having thresholds in the range of 5 to 15 μm. These are sometimes referred to as touch or pressure receptors, but the senses of touch and pressure are difficult to define. Type I endings are associated with touch cor-

puscles in many species (Fig. 2-9, *A*). Touch corpuscles are recognized grossly on the hairy skin as a domelike mound having a diameter of several hundred micrometers. The epidermis over the corpuscle is thicker than that of the surrounding skin, and the dermal core of the corpuscle contains a dense meshwork of collagen. A rich vascular supply causes the touch corpuscle to have a reddish coloration. The touch corpuscles are often associated with hair follicles; thus they have sometimes been called hair disks. However, the term touch corpuscle is preferable because it is believed that there is no functional interaction between the hair and the type I ending. Type I endings are also found in the glabrous skin, but here the domelike appearance is lacking. The common structural feature of the type I endings of hairy and glabrous skin is the layer of specialized cells on which the nerve terminates. These cells are called Merkel's cells. They are located within the epidermis just above the basement membrane (Fig. 2-9, *B*). By electron microscopy, it has been shown that Merkel's cells contain granulated vesicles. Processes extend from these cells in a superficial direction to indent the cytoplasm of overlying epidermal cells. Each type I ending is innervated by a single large myelinated fiber (although one fiber may innervate several touch corpuscles). The fiber branches just below the basement membrane. Unmyelinated terminal branches penetrate the basement membrane to end in relation to Merkel's cells. There are areas of membrane specialization suggestive of synaptic junctions between the cell and its adjacent nerve terminal. It is possible that the granulated vesicles contain a chemical transmitter that is released by the Merkel's cells onto the nerve ending.

The receptive field of a type I ending is immediately over the touch corpuscle(s). Movement of the skin adjacent to the corpuscle has no effect unless the stimulus spreads to the corpuscle, and stretch of the skin does not activate the receptor. Thus, type I endings should provide a very discrete stimulus localization (although some ambiguity will result from the multiple endings of many type I receptors). A characteristic feature of the slowly adapting discharges of type I endings during a maintained stimulus is the irregular nature of the discharge. This may result from a synaptic coupling between Merkel's cells and the nerve terminals. Another property of type I endings is their tendency to discharge during cooling of the skin.

Type II endings are also found both in hairy and glabrous skin. The probable morphological form of the receptor is the Ruffini ending (Fig. 2-10). A Ruffini ending consists of multiple branched unmyelinated

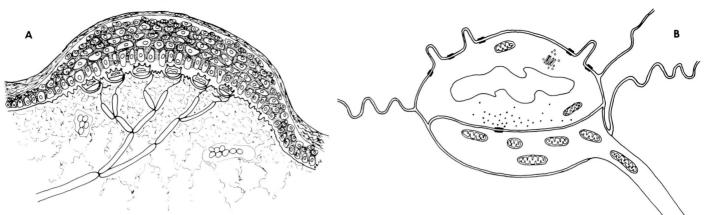

Fig. 2-9. **A,** Touch corpuscle. The skin over a touch corpuscle is thickened, as is the dermal core beneath it. A large, myelinated fiber innervates the corpuscle. Branches of the fiber lose their myelin, penetrate the basement membrane, and end on a series of special cells called Merkel's cells. The touch corpuscle signals highly localized mechanical stimuli. It has a low threshold and is slowly adapting. **B,** Merkel's cell. The nerve fiber terminal is shown approaching a Merkel's cell from below. The Merkel's cell contains the usual organelles but in addition has numerous granulated vesicles. There are specialized areas of contact between the Merkel's cell and the nerve ending. These may serve as low-resistance paths for current. Alternatively, the granules may represent a chemical transmitter that might be responsible for communication between Merkel's cell and nerve fiber. The processes extending from the upper surface of the Merkel's cell and indenting epidermal cells just superficial to it may be distorted by mechanical stimuli. (After Iggo and Muir, 1969.)

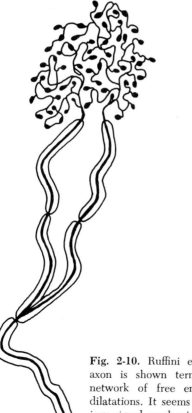

Fig. 2-10. Ruffini ending. The myelinated axon is shown terminating in a complex network of free endings, with numerous dilatations. It seems likely that Ruffini endings signal mechanical events. In joint capsules they are slowly adapting.

terminals of a large myelinated fiber. They are found in the skin within the dermis. The type II receptor responds both to displacement of the skin directly over the receptor and also to stretch of the adjacent skin. Thus, a type II receptor can be activated by a stimulus applied at some distance, provided that it is strong enough to distort the skin in the region of the terminal. However, there is only one receptor associated with a given nerve fiber. Thus, type II endings should also provide useful information about stimulus location as well as about stimulus intensity. A characteristic that helps differentiate type II from type I endings is the regular discharge of the type II ending.

The function of the velocity component of the discharges of type I and type II endings is not clear. One possibility is that this may give clues as to the timing and localization of the stimulus, because these properties are recognized soon after stimulus onset. On the other hand, the static response during a maintained stimulus would signal stimulus intensity and duration.

Velocity detectors. A variety of types of cutaneous receptors are chiefly responsive to stimulus velocity. These are best discussed separately for hairy and glabrous skin.

In hairy skin, many of the velocity-sensitive mechanoreceptors are associated with hair follicles (Fig.

2-11). Several different kinds of hair follicles can be recognized in common laboratory animals. These include the very long and coarse tylotrich hairs, the intermediately long and thick guard hairs, and the short, fine down hairs. Guard and down hairs are abundant in human hairy skin. Some of the afferents connected with tylotrich, guard, and down hairs are velocity sensitive. In addition, there is a category of velocity detector that responds either to movement of a number of hairs or of the skin. The morphology of these receptors is unknown, but they are called field receptors. Another velocity-sensitive receptor in hairy skin is connected to an unmyelinated afferent fiber. These receptors are called C mechanoreceptors. It is interesting that a large fraction of unmyelinated afferents supply sensitive mechanoreceptors of this kind, especially in the skin of the proximal parts of the extremities. The receptor terminal configuration is unknown, but it may well be a free ending (Fig. 2-12).

The important velocity-sensitive endings in glabrous skin are Meissner's corpuscles (Fig. 2-13, *A* and *B*). These are found in the palmar and plantar surfaces in dermal papillae, and in humans they are most numerous in the skin over the fingertips. A given Meissner's corpuscle may receive terminals from several different large myelinated fibers.

In general, the velocity-sensitive receptors with large myelinated afferents are likely to be involved in the sensation of flutter, or low-frequency vibration. These receptors can be activated best by repeated stimuli at rates of about 5 to 40 Hz. Such receptors are probably very useful in detecting movement of a stimulus across the skin or of the skin across a surface. They presumably would have the capability of detecting stimulus location and rate of movement. The down hair receptors have a very low threshold, but their receptive fields are relatively large; thus they would have less capability for defining stimulus location than would some other types of receptors. The C mechanoreceptors respond best to very slow stimulus movements. They are also quite sensitive but have large receptive fields. The various velocity detectors can be considered to be tuned to different frequency ranges of stimuli.

Transient detectors. These receptors signal stimulus acceleration or a higher derivative of position (jerk). Some of the tylotrich and guard hair receptors fall into this category, as does the best studied receptor in the skin. This is the pacinian corpuscle (Fig.

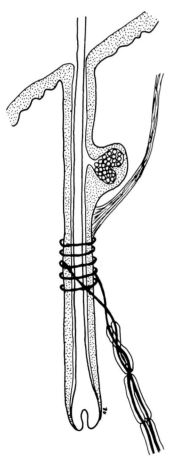

Fig. 2-11. Hair follicle receptor. Finely myelinated nerve fibers are shown terminating on a hair follicle. These would discharge in response to movements of the hair, thus signaling a form of touch.

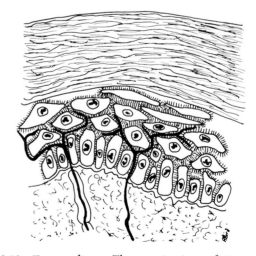

Fig. 2-12. Free endings. The terminations of two afferent fibers as free endings in the skin are shown. The fiber on the left is a finely myelinated axon, while that on the right is unmyelinated. The endings penetrate the basement membrane and ramify among the cells of the lower layers of the epidermis. Endings of this type may signal touch, pain, or temperature, depending on the nature of the membrane of the particular terminals.

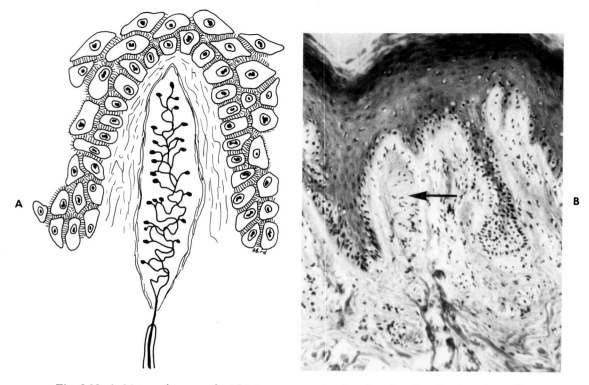

Fig. 2-13. **A,** Meissner's corpuscle. This is an encapsulated ending found in the dermal papillae of the skin. It is likely that Meissner's corpuscles are involved in detecting fine, discriminative touch. **B,** Section through skin. Several dermal pegs are shown, one of which contains a Meissner's corpuscle *(arrow).*

2-14). These encapsulated receptor organs, first described by Vater and by Pacini, are found widely distributed in subcutaneous tissue, fascial planes around joints and tendons, and in the mesentery. They vary in shape, but are commonly ovoid. They may have lengths of up to several millimeters. Typically, each is innervated by a single large myelinated nerve fiber. The myelin sheath is lost soon after the axon penetrates the corpuscle.

The corpuscle is composed of numerous concentric layers of connective tissue cells. Around the outer portion of the corpuscle the connective tissue is loosely organized, with an abundance of extracellular fluid in spaces between cellular layers. Near the center of the corpuscle the spacing of the connective tissue cells is much closer, and the cell processes no longer encircle the entire corpuscle. Instead, processes of the connective tissue cells form plates stacked on one side or the other of the centrally placed axon. This arrangement provides an extracellular fluid channel, or cleft, on either side of the axon. Presumably, this allows the nerve fiber access to ions or to nutrients. The structure of the terminal portion of the axon is characterized by the absence of myelin and the presence of an abundance of mitochondria.

A maintained deformation results in activation of a

pacinian corpuscle both at its onset and at its termination. The corpuscle detects pressure waves but does not distinguish their direction. Thus, the activity of a pacinian corpuscle can be an on-off response to a mechanical stimulus. However, this behavior should be distinguished from the on-off activity of retinal cells, because the behavior of the latter is caused by the pattern of synaptic activity within the retina, whereas the activity of pacinian corpuscles depends entirely on the structure of the receptor organ.

There have been many studies of the activity of pacinian corpuscles. The receptor potential can be recorded from the intact corpuscle or from one denuded of most of its capsule. Action potentials in the afferent fiber can be blocked with a local anesthetic, leaving an apparently unaltered receptor potential. The receptor potential is characterized by a rapid depolarization, which then decays back more slowly to the original level of membrane potential. The depolarization is presumed to result from an increased permeability to small ions, especially Na^+, of the membrane region of the axon, which acts as the receptive element. The decay phase of the receptor potential is presumed to be passive recharging of the membrane capacity. However, a process similar to refractoriness also occurs, because a second mechanical stimulus

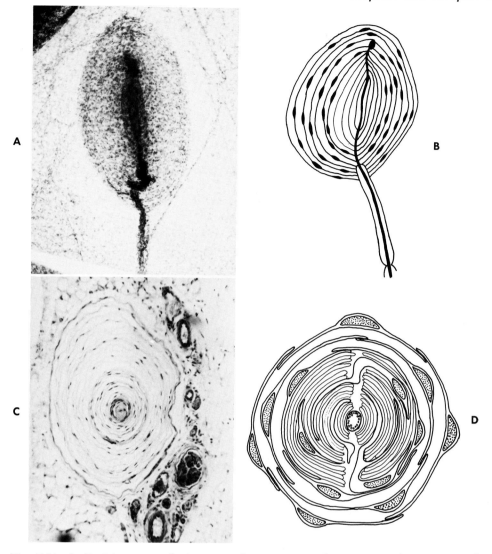

Fig. 2-14. **A,** Pacinian corpuscle in a squash preparation of mesentery. The nerve can be seen entering the corpuscle at the bottom, first following a spiral course and then running along the axis of the corpuscle. **B,** Schematic drawing of pacinian corpuscle in longitudinal section. **C,** Cross section through pacinian corpuscle. **D,** Cross section through the central core region of a pacinian corpuscle. The concentric layers of the capsule are seen, but the nerve and central zone of the capsule are difficult to distinguish at this magnification. The axon is seen at the center. The connective tissue cells within the core region do not form a complete covering of the axon. Instead, the layers are hemicylindrical, with a distinct gap on each side of the axon. The gap appears to be in continuity with the extracellular space outside the corpuscle.

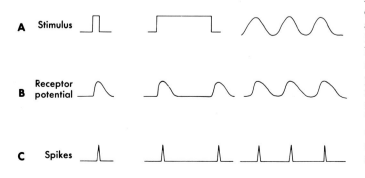

Fig. 2-15. Responses of a pacinian corpuscle. The time course of several mechanical stimuli applied to a pacinian corpuscle are shown in **A.** The receptor potentials and consequent afferent nerve impulses are shown in **B** and **C.** At the left, a brief mechanical stimulus is shown to evoke a short-lasting receptor potential, which in turn triggers a single nerve impulse in the afferent fiber. At the middle, a longer lasting mechanical stimulus produces receptor potentials and resultant spikes at the onset and at the offset of the stimulus. The receptor is rapidly adapting and responds just to transients. At the right, a sinusoidal mechanical stimulus (vibratory stimulus) evokes a series of receptor potentials and spikes at the frequency of the stimulus.

within a short interval of the first will not produce as large a receptor potential. This refractory state of the receptor membrane is at least partially responsible for the fact that pacinian corpuscles are rapidly adapting. Another contributing factor is the poor mechanical coupling between the connective tissue of the corpuscle and the nerve ending. Only transients of pressure pass effectively to the level of the nerve fiber, whereas slowly changing pressures are absorbed by the connective tissue.

Pacinian corpuscles probably play an important role in sensory perception. In animal experiments, it has been found that the effects of stimulation of single corpuscles can readily be detected in recordings from the cerebral cortex.

Thermoreceptors

Specific thermoreceptors respond to small changes in cutaneous temperature in either the cooling or the warming direction. They show both a dynamic and a static response to thermal changes. The thresholds may be changes as small as 0.1° C. Cold receptors discharge maximally at skin temperatures below the normal surface temperature of around 35° C. Warming will slow their discharge, although noxious heating may produce a "paradoxical discharge." Cold receptors appear to be free endings within the basal epidermis. Their afferents are small myelinated fibers in primates. Warm receptors show an increased discharge when the skin temperature is elevated to levels up to about 43° C. Temperatures in the noxious heat range (over 45° C) tend to inactivate the discharge of warm receptors. Cooling also slows the discharge. The terminal configuration of warm receptors is unknown, but may be free endings. The afferent fibers of warm receptors are unmyelinated.

Nociceptors

There are several kinds of nociceptors. One class is the high-threshold mechanoreceptor. These endings respond to intense mechanical stimulation ranging from near noxious pressure to frankly damaging intensities. Particularly effective stimuli include pinprick and crushing of the skin with toothed forceps. The receptor terminals are presumably free endings, and the axons are small myelinated or unmyelinated fibers. Other nociceptors are activated by intense thermal stimuli, such as noxious heat (above 45° C) or intense cold. These are also activated by noxious mechanical stimuli. The terminals may be free endings, and the afferent axons are small myelinated or unmyelinated fibers. The polymodal nociceptors are apparently a special category of ending that responds to noxious mechanical, thermal, and chemical stimuli. Again, these may be free endings. The afferents are unmyelinated.

STRUCTURE AND FUNCTION OF MUSCLE RECEPTORS

There are several kinds of receptor organs to be found in or about skeletal muscle. The main ones are muscle spindles, Golgi tendon organs, pressure-pain endings, and occasional pacinian corpuscles (Table 2-2).

Pacinian corpuscles

The behavior of pacinian corpuscles in the fascial planes of muscle is similar to that of the ones in skin. They respond to pressure transients and vibration.

Pressure-pain endings

These appear to be bare nerve endings located in fascia. The afferent fibers from their endings are small myelinated group III and unmyelinated group IV fibers. The pressure-pain endings appear to respond both to mechanical and to noxious stimuli and thus to signal deep pressure and pain in muscle.

Golgi tendon organs

Special bare nerve endings are found ramifying about bundles of collagen fibers of tendons at the ends of muscles or within the muscle bellies. These

Table 2-2. Muscle and joint receptors

Receptor type	Location	Adaptation rate	Probable function
Muscle			
Pacinian corpuscles	Fascial planes	Rapid	High frequency vibration
Pressure-pain endings		Slow	Pressure or pain in muscle
Golgi tendon organs	Tendons	Slow	Reflex (clasp knife; see Chapter 4)
Primary endings	Muscle spindles	Slow	Reflex (stretch reflex, tendon jerk; see Chapter 4)
Secondary endings		Slow	Reflex (flexion reflex; see Chapter 4)
Joints			
Paciniform endings	Joint capsule	Rapid	Changes in joint position
Ruffini endings	Joint capsule and ligaments	Slow	Joint pressure
Free endings		Slow	Joint pain

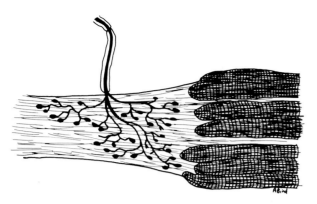

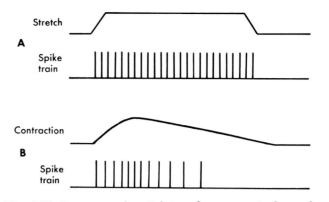

Fig. 2-16. Golgi tendon organ. A large, myelinated nerve fiber approaches a tendon, loses its myelin sheath, and ends with a profuse branching pattern. Each fine branch terminates in apposition to a bundle of collagen fibers. Any stimulus that causes an increase in tension in the tendon will tend to distort the endings and excite the afferent fiber. The tension is effectively increased by stretch of the muscle, contraction of the muscle, or both simultaneously. The Golgi tendon organ is slowly adapting.

Fig. 2-17. Responses of a Golgi tendon organ. **A** shows the effect of stretch of a muscle on the discharge of a Golgi tendon organ. The first trace shows muscle length; the second is a record from the afferent fiber of a Golgi tendon organ. During stretch, the afferent fires repetitively. **B** shows the effect of a contraction of the muscle. The tension of the tendon is recorded in one trace; the other shows the discharge of the afferent fiber during the contraction.

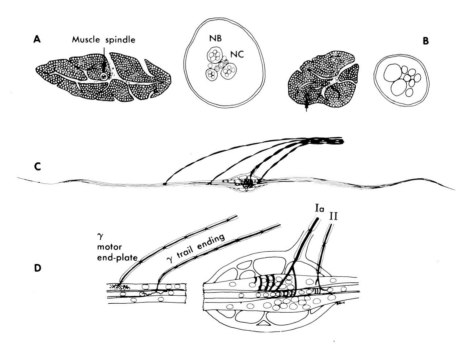

Fig. 2-18. Structure of the muscle spindle. The upper row of drawings shows the appearance of a muscle spindle cut in cross section. In **A** the section passes through the lymph space near the central, or equatorial, region of the spindle. The nuclei of the nuclear bag *(NB)* and nuclear chain *(NC)* intrafusal muscle fibers are shown in the high-power view. The nuclear bag fibers contain a cluster of nuclei. The nuclear chain fibers have a row; only one nucleus appears in a cross section. In **B** the section is away from the equatorial region of the spindle. **C** shows the innervation of the spindle. The sensory endings are in the equatorial region within the lymph space, which presumably offers some protection against inadvertent stimulation. The motor endings are on the polar regions of the spindle. **D** is an expanded view showing the innervated areas. At the left are two forms of motor endings made by gamma motor axons. On the right are the primary and secondary endings made by group Ia and group II fibers respectively. Note that the primary ending includes terminals on both nuclear bag and nuclear chain fibers, whereas the secondary ending is chiefly associated with nuclear chain fibers. All of the intrafusal muscle fibers receive innervation, although this is not shown in the drawing.

are called Golgi tendon organs (Fig. 2-16). The afferent fibers are among the largest fibers in peripheral nerve tissue. They have been designated group Ib afferents.

The group Ib afferents from Golgi tendon organs are silent when there is little tension on their tendon. However, when tension is increased, either by stretch of the muscle or by contraction of the muscle against resistance, the Golgi tendon organ terminals are distorted and an afferent discharge is produced (Fig. 2-17). A combination of stretch and contraction is a particularly effective stimulus. The receptor is slowly adapting, so the discharge continues throughout the duration of the increase in tension. The rate of the discharge reflects the amount of tension.

The central effects of the discharge of Ib afferents are discussed later. However, it should be noted that there is no evidence that the discharge reaches the level of consciousness.

Muscle spindle

The third most complex sense organ (after the eye and the ear) is the muscle spindle. Some of the early work on muscle spindles was done by Sherrington and by Ruffini. A great deal of research has been devoted in recent years both to the anatomy and to the physiology of these organs.

Structure of muscle spindles. A typical muscle spindle in mammalian muscle is composed of two types of modified muscle fibers, a capsule, and both afferent and motor innervation (Fig. 2-18).

The muscle fibers are termed intrafusal fibers to distinguish them from the ordinary skeletal muscle (extrafusal) fibers. One type of intrafusal fiber is called the nuclear bag type because it contains a clump of nuclei near its midpoint; the other kind of intrafusal fiber is called the nuclear chain type because it has a single row of nuclei. The nuclear bag fibers are often longer than the nuclear chain fibers; when this is true, the capsule extends only the length of the nuclear chain fibers. The nuclear bag fibers are connected loosely to the connective tissue about the extrafusal fibers at one end of the muscle spindle; at the other end they attach either to connective tissue or to the muscle tendon. The capsule is expanded near the middle of the spindle, and there is a space within it called the lymph space about the intrafusal fibers.

It is very important that the ends of the spindle are attached to the extrafusal muscle; the middle part of the spindle is not. Muscle spindles are arranged in parallel with extrafusal muscle fibers. This means that a stretch of the whole muscle will increase the tension on the muscle spindle, whereas a contraction of the whole muscle will decrease the tension of the spindle, unless the spindle itself contracts.

The muscle spindle is innervated both by afferent and by motor fibers. Two kinds of afferent fibers end on intrafusal fibers: group Ia and group II. Group Ia fibers are the largest of the peripheral myelinated fibers; group II fibers are middle-sized myelinated fibers. A single group Ia fiber reaches each spindle and divides into one branch per intrafusal fiber; each of these branches ends by a coil about the middle of the respective intrafusal fiber. The endings of group Ia fibers are called primary endings; they used to be called annulospiral endings, from the form of their terminals. Group II innervation is variable. There may be none, one, or several group II endings in a spindle. The terminals are located on either or both sides of the primary ending. They are concentrated on nuclear chain intrafusal fibers, although a few small endings may occur on nuclear bag fibers. The form of the ending is often annulospiral, but it may be a multiply branched structure. The old terminology of flower-spray ending has now been dropped and replaced by the term secondary ending.

The motor innervation of the intrafusal fibers is by gamma motor fibers. These end on both nuclear bag and nuclear chain fibers. The terminals on polar regions of intrafusal fibers tend to resemble closely the endplates made on extrafusal muscle fibers by alpha motor axons. The terminals of gamma motor axons on the juxtaequatorial regions are multiple, small dilatations spread over a large area of the muscle fiber membrane; these are called trail endings. Each intrafusal fiber may receive terminals from several gamma axons, and each gamma axon may distribute to several intrafusal fibers. There are at least two functional categories of gamma motor fibers, dynamic and static. The former increase the sensitivity of the primary endings to the velocity of stretch; the latter increase the static discharge of both primary and secondary endings at any given muscle length, while actually reducing the dynamic response of the primary ending.

Receptor potential of muscle spindle. The receptor potential of frog muscle spindles was studied in 1950 by Bernard Katz. Although frog muscle spindles are less complex than those in mammals, some valuable inferences can be made from Katz's work.

Katz found that a graded stretch of the spindle produced a graded depolarization of the afferent terminals. When tension was low, there was an irregular discharge of impulses in branches of the afferent fiber within the spindle. Sometimes a discharge was set up in the afferent fiber proper; this would then be carried into the central nervous system. Other discharges were blocked and hence would have no central action.

When an increasing depolarization was produced by progressive stretch, more impulses were propagated into the afferent fiber and fewer were blocked.

A rapid stretch, which was then maintained at a constant level, produced a biphasic response—an initial burst of impulses followed by a steady discharge at a lower rate. The first phase is the dynamic response, and the second the static response.

The depolarization triggering the discharges is the receptor potential. This can be studied in isolation from the nervous impulses by the application of local anesthetic. A step stretch was found by Katz to produce a biphasic depolarization, the initial greater depolarization reverting to a lower amplitude, maintained depolarization. Thus, the receptor potential showed a dynamic and static phase, accounting for the pattern of the nervous discharges. The ionic mechanism responsible for the depolarization is presumably an increased permeability to small ions, especially to Na$^+$, of the membrane of the afferent terminal.

Operation of muscle spindles. When a muscle is stretched, the afferent fibers from muscle spindles show an increased discharge rate. Thus the muscle spindle, like the Golgi tendon organ, is a stretch receptor. However, the behavior of muscle spindle afferents is much more complex than is that of Golgi tendon organ afferents.

Only a slight stretch is required to cause the receptor potentials of muscle spindles to exceed threshold (Fig. 2-19). Even in apparently slack muscle, there may be a spontaneous discharge of muscle spindle afferents, in contrast to Golgi tendon organ afferents, which generally require some initial tension of the muscle before discharging. As the muscle is stretched, the discharge rates in both group Ia and group II afferent fibers from muscle spindles accelerate. The firing rates after a new muscle length is reached reflect the degree of stretch. This increase

in the rate of discharge of muscle spindle afferents as a function of stretch of the muscle is called the static response of the muscle spindles. With a sufficient stretch, the group Ib afferents from Golgi tendon organs also fire at a rate that is a function of the tension developed within the muscle because of stretch; that is, Golgi tendon organs also have a static response to stretch. The group Ia fibers from muscle spindles also display a dynamic response to stretch. During the onset of stretch the rate of discharge of these afferents greatly exceeds that rate characteristic of the afferent in the steady state after the new length of the muscle is achieved. The discharge adapts following the completion of stretch. When the muscle length is restored to the original value, the group Ia fiber may stop discharging transiently before resuming the spontaneous discharge rate. Group II afferent fibers from muscle spindles have only a small dynamic response. It is possible that the difference in the behavior of the two types of afferent fibers from muscle spindles is related to their different points of attachment to the intrafusal fibers within the spindles, because the mechanical properties of nuclear bag and nuclear chain fibers during stretch may be different. Golgi tendon organ afferents show little dynamic response.

The dynamic responsiveness of group Ia fibers suggests that muscle spindles detect muscle length as well as the rate of change of muscle length. This property of these afferents is utilized clinically in the testing of reflexes originating from their activation by the pro-

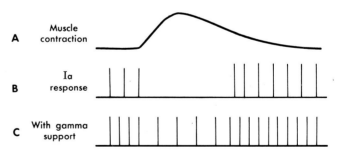

Fig. 2-20. Response of a muscle spindle afferent to muscle contraction with and without activation of gamma motor fibers. **A** shows muscle tension during a twitch produced by stimulation of alpha motor axons supplying the muscle. **B** shows the response of the group Ia afferent fiber from the primary ending of a muscle spindle contained within the muscle. Note that the afferent discharge ceases during the contraction, because of the unloading effect on the spindle as the extrafusal muscle fibers shorten. In **C**, gamma motor axons are excited in addition to the alpha motor axons. The spindle is not unloaded as much by contraction of the extrafusal muscle fibers, because the intrafusal muscle fibers also shortened. This allows the continuation of the discharge of the Ia fiber despite contraction of the muscle.

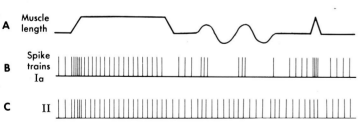

Fig. 2-19. Responses of afferent fibers from a muscle spindle. **A** shows changes in the length of the muscle containing the muscle spindle. The muscle length is changed with various wave forms of stretch and release of stretch. **B** shows the response of a group Ia afferent fiber from the primary ending of the spindle. Note the high dynamic sensitivity of this type of ending. **C** shows the response of a group II afferent fiber from a secondary ending of the spindle. Note the low dynamic sensitivity.

duction of quick stretches of muscle. A common test of this kind is the demonstration of the knee jerk reflex by tapping the patellar tendon with a rubber hammer. The reflex pathway involved is discussed in Chapter 4.

Another difference in the behavior of muscle spindle and Golgi tendon organ afferents is shown by their contrasting responses during muscular contraction. Whereas Golgi tendon organ afferents have an accelerated discharge rate during contraction, muscle spindle afferents undergo a reduced discharge rate or stop firing altogether (Fig. 2-20). The reason for this is the disposition of muscle spindles, which lie parallel to extrafusal muscle fibers. During contraction the extrafusal muscle fibers shorten, causing a reduction in the degree of stretch of the muscle spindles. This is equivalent, as far as the muscle spindles is concerned, to reduction in the degree of stretch of the whole muscle. When the contraction is over, the renewed tension on the muscle spindle will cause a renewed discharge of its afferent fibers. The discharge rate in group Ia fibers will initially exceed the original one because of the dynamic responsiveness of these endings.

The unloading effect of muscular contraction on the discharge rates of muscle spindle afferents can have important reflex consequences. The input from these afferents during a period of maintained posture would result in a steady level of reflex activity. If a muscular action is initiated, one result may be the sudden withdrawal of the input from the muscle spindles. There is a mechanism that can be used by the central nervous system to prevent this. Muscle spindles receive a motor innervation in addition to the sensory ones. The gamma motor axons can cause the contraction of the intrafusal muscle fibers in a fashion similar to that by which alpha motor axons cause the contraction of extrafusal muscle fibers. If the polar regions of the muscle spindle contract through the action of gamma motor axons, the middle region of the spindle, where the sensory endings are found, undergoes an increase in tension. This effect is enhanced by the paucity of contractile protein in this region of the intrafusal muscle fibers. The increased tension in the sensory region of the muscle spindle results in an accelerated discharge rate of the afferent fibers. With suitable timing, it is possible for the discharges of gamma motoneurons to speed up the discharge rate just enough to compensate for the unloading effect of a contraction of the extrafusal fibers. If the gamma motor drive is still greater, the input from muscle spindles may even be increased despite the unloading effect. This ability of the central nervous system to regulate the discharge rate of a receptor organ is a good example of the process of centrifugal

control of input to the central nervous system. It also represents another difference in the behavior of muscle spindles and the Golgi tendon organ.

The central effects of afferent discharges in group Ia and II fibers are discussed later.

STRUCTURE AND FUNCTION OF JOINT RECEPTORS

The fibrous capsules of joints are innervated by three types of sensory endings. Two are specialized endings supplied by myelinated nerve fibers. These include the spraylike terminals called Ruffini endings and the lamellated, encapsulated structures known as paciniform corpuscles, or Golgi-Mazzoni endings (Table 2-2). Paciniform endings resemble pacinian corpuscles, except that they are smaller. The third type of sensory ending is formed by unmyelinated fibers. Its structure is that of a feltlike plexus with some free terminations. Many of these unspecialized endings are associated with blood vessels, but some are distributed within the connective tissue. The ligaments associated with joints are supplied by Golgi tendon organs, some Ruffini endings, and free endings. There are no paciniform endings in ligaments, but the tissue around joints may contain pacinian corpuscles. Besides the sensory endings, there are motor fibers of the sympathetic nervous system to smooth muscle of the blood vessels in and about joints.

Sensory discharges in afferents from joints

Both rapidly and slowly adapting responses have been recorded from joint afferents (Fig. 2-21). The

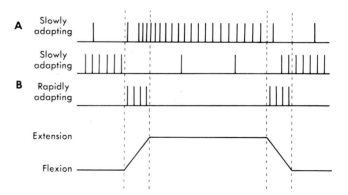

Fig. 2-21. Responses of joint afferents. At the bottom of the figure, the ramp indicates the stimulus, which is a change in joint position from flexion to extension. The two slowly adapting receptors, whose responses are illustrated in **A**, differ only in that one fires during extension and the other pauses. The reverse firing pattern is seen when the joint is flexed. Each receptor shows a small dynamic response, as well as a static response. The rapidly adapting receptor, whose activity is shown in **B**, fires just during the movement.

rapidly adapting responses are from the paciniform endings. These signal transients, as do the pacinian corpuscles elsewhere. Slowly adapting discharges are produced by Ruffini endings. The Ruffini endings do not discharge until the joint is bent to near its limit. Some will discharge during extension and others during flexion. However, few, if any, true joint receptors appear to discharge while joint position is maintained in an intermediate position. Thus, Ruffini endings are presumably incapable of signaling joint position. Instead, they may contribute to a form of deep pressure sensation.

Little is known about the responses of the free endings in joint capsules. Presumably these mediate pain, although other functions have not been ruled out. The Golgi tendon organs in ligaments act similarly to those in tendons, as described in the section on muscle receptors (pp. 52-54).

RECEPTOR TYPES AND SENSORY PERCEPTION

A variety of sensory modalities have been associated with stimuli applied to the skin, to muscle, or to joints. Those having the greatest clinical relevance include awareness of mechanical stimuli (touch, pressure, vibratory sensibility), temperature gradients (cold, warmth), pain, and position.

Mechanoreception

Touch and pressure presumably differ chiefly in the intensity of the mechanical stimulus that elicits them. If this is true, then deep structures signal only pressure stimuli, because the force required to activate receptors below the skin is generally relatively strong. Velocity and transients of mechanical stimulation are detected by rapidly adapting receptors. These include hair follicle receptors, pacinian corpuscles, and Meissner's corpuscles. A special care of this kind of stimulus is the action of a vibrator, such as a tuning fork. It seems likely that pacinian corpuscles are the main receptors that respond to high-frequency vibratory stimuli. Meissner's corpuscles are likely to be responsible for the sensation of flutter associated with lower frequencies of vibration. Steady signals interpreted as touch or pressure are sensed by such slowly adapting receptors as touch corpuscles and possibly Ruffini endings. It should be emphasized that the types of mechanoreceptors found in different regions of the skin, such as hairy or glabrous skin, may be quite different structurally, yet the sensations elicited from these regions are quite similar. Deep pressure sensation produced by squeezing muscle is probably mediated by pressure-pain endings, which are supplied by finely myelinated nerve fibers.

Temperature reception

Both cold and warmth receptors have been studied in animal experiments. Cold receptors seem to be more common than warmth receptors. Temperature receptors are innervated by both myelinated and unmyelinated fibers. It is likely that free endings form one kind of temperature receptor.

Pain

Pain endings in skin are supplied by both myelinated and unmyelinated fibers. The receptors are likely to be free endings, extending into the epidermis, within the connective tissue of the dermis, and about blood vessels. Muscle pain is mediated by pressure-pain endings, which have small myelinated or unmyelinated axons, and by afferents about blood vessels. Joint pain is presumed to be mediated by free endings in the connective tissue about the joint and associated with blood vessels.

Position sense

The position of a body part in space is detected by a variety of means. However, the term position sense generally refers to detection of parts of the extremities in the absence of visual or gravitational cues. Although cutaneous information may play a role, it is likely that the major input is from muscle receptors of the slowly adapting type. There is increasing evidence that muscle receptors such as muscle spindles play a part in position sense.

ACTION OF LOCAL ANESTHETICS

In Chapter 1 the differential blocking action of local anesthetics on nerve fibers of various sizes was mentioned. The injection of local anesthetic in the vicinity of a nerve trunk will block transmission first in small myelinated fibers, then in unmyelinated fibers, and finally in large myelinated fibers. Recovery is in the reverse order. Because the sensations of pain and temperature are conveyed by small-caliber fibers, these are lost first as local anesthetic action develops. The function of gamma motor axons is lost simultaneously. As the concentration of local anesthetic builds up, large fibers are blocked, with the resultant loss of touch, pressure, and conduction in alpha motor axons. A carefully titrated dose of local anesthetic and other drugs can result in blockade of small fibers without significant interference with the functioning of large fibers. Drugs such as phenol and ammonium sulphate will preferentially destroy small fibers and are used in conjunction with local anesthetics to perform nerve blocks for more lasting pain relief than can be afforded by local anesthetics alone.

In contrast to the effect of the local anesthetics,

ischemia blocks conduction in the large fibers first. Therefore, when a tourniquet, such as a blood pressure cuff inflated to above arterial systolic pressure, is applied to a limb, pain sensation persists longer than touch sensation.

BIBLIOGRAPHY

Adrian, E. D.: The basis of sensation, New York, 1964, Hafner Publishing Co., Inc.

Alexandrowicz, J. S.: Muscle receptor organs in the abdomen of *Homarus vulgaris* and *Palinurus vulgaris*, Q. J. Micr. Sci. 92:163-202, 1951.

Andres, K. H., and Duering, M. von: Morphology of cutaneous receptors. In Iggo, A., editor: Handbook of sensory physiology, vol. 2, Somatosensory system, New York, 1973, Springer Publishing Co., Inc., pp. 3-28.

Barker, D.: The innervation of the muscle-spindle, Q. J. Micr. Sci. 89:143-186, 1948.

Barker, D., editor: Symposium on muscle receptors, Hong Kong, 1962, Hong Kong University Press.

Bekesy, G., von: Sensory inhibition, Princeton, N. J., 1967, Princeton University Press.

Bessou, P., and Perl, E. R.: Response of cutaneous sensory units with unmyelinated fibers to noxious stimuli, J. Neurophysiol. 32:1025-1043, 1969.

Boyd, I. A.: The structure and innervation of the nuclear bag muscle fibre system and the nuclear chain muscle fibre system in mammalian muscle spindles, Philos. Trans. R. Soc. Lond. [Biol. Sci.] 245:81-136, 1962.

Boyd, I. A., and Roberts, T. D. M.: The histological structure of the receptors in knee-joint of the cat correlated with their physiological response, J. Physiol. (Lond.) 124:476-488, 1954.

Brown, A. G., and Iggo, A.: A quantitative study of cutaneous receptors and afferent fibres in the cat and rabbit. J. Physiol. 193:707-733, 1967.

Burgess, P. R., and Perl, E. R.: Myelinated afferent fibres responding specifically to noxious stimulation of the skin, J. Physiol. (Lond.) 190:541-562, 1967.

Burgess, P. R., and Perl, E. R.: Cutaneous mechanoreceptors and nociceptors. In Iggo, A., editor: Handbook of sensory physiology, vol. 2, Somatosensory system, New York, 1973, Springer Publishing Co., Inc., pp. 29-78.

Burgess, P. R., Petit, D., and Warren, R. M.: Receptor types in cat hairy skin supplied by myelinated fibers, J. Neurophysiol. 31:833-848, 1968.

Catton, W. T.: Mechanoreceptor function, Physiol. Rev. 50:297-318, 1970.

Chambers, M. R., Andres, K. H., Duering, M. von, and Iggo, A.: The structure and function of the slowly adapting type II mechanoreceptor in hairy skin, Q. J. Exp. Physiol. 57:417-445, 1972.

Clark, F. J., and Burgess, P. R.: Slowly adapting receptors in the cat knee joint; can they signal joint angle? J. Neurophysiol. 38:1448-1463, 1975.

Diamond, J., Gray, J. A. B., and Inman, D. R.: The relation between receptor potentials and the concentration of sodium ions, J. Physiol. (Lond.) 142:382-394, 1958.

Douglas, W. W., and Ritchie, J. M.: Non-medullated fibres in the saphenous nerve which signal touch, J. Physiol. (Lond.) 139:385-499, 1957.

Eklund, G., and Skoglund, S.: On the specificity of the Ruffini-like joint receptors, Acta Physiol. Scand. 49:184-191, 1960.

Eldred, E., Yellin, H., Gadbois, L., and Sweeney, S.: Bibliography on muscle receptors; their morphology, pathology and physiology, Exp. Neurol. (Suppl.) 3:1-154, 1967.

Eyzaguirre, C.: The motor regulation of mammalian spindle discharges, J. Physiol. (Lond.) 150:185-200, 1960.

Fulton, J. F., and Pi-Suñer, J.: A note concerning the probable function of various afferent end-organs in skeletal muscle, Am. J. Physiol. 83:554-562, 1928.

Gardner, E.: Conduction rates and dorsal root inflow of sensory fibres from the knee joint of the cat, Am. J. Physiol. 152:436-445, 1948.

Goodwin, G. M., McCloskey, D. I., and Matthews, P. B. C.: The contribution of muscle afferents to kinesthesia shown by vibration induced illusions of movement and by the effects of paralysing joint afferents, Brain 95:705-748, 1972.

Granit, R.: Receptors and sensory perception, New Haven, Conn., 1955, Yale University Press.

Granit, R., editor: Muscular afferents and motor control, Nobel Symposium I, New York, 1966, John Wiley & Sons, Inc.

Gray, J. A. B., and Sato, M.: Properties of the receptor potential in pacinian corpuscles, J. Physiol. (Lond.) 122:610-636, 1953.

Hagbarth, K. E., and Vallbo, A. B.: Single unit recordings from muscle nerves in human subjects, Acta Physiol. Scand. 76:321-334, 1969.

Harrington, T., and Merzenich, M. M.: Neural coding in the sense of touch; human sensations of skin indentation compared with the responses of slowly adapting mechanoreceptive afferents innervating the hairy skin of monkeys, Exp. Brain Res. 10:251-264, 1970.

Hensel, H.: Cutaneous thermoreceptors. In Iggo, A., editor: Handbook of sensory physiology, vol. 2, Somatosensory system, New York, 1973, Springer Publishing Co., Inc., pp. 79-110.

Hensel, H., Iggo, A., and Witt, I.: A quantitative study of sensitive cutaneous thermoreceptors with C afferent fibers, J. Physiol. (Lond.) 153:113-126, 1960.

Horch, K. W., Clark, F. J., and Burgess, P. R.: Awareness of knee joint angle under static conditions, J. Neurophysiol. 38:1436-1447, 1975.

Hubbard, S. J.: A study of rapid mechanical events in a mechanoreceptor, J. Physiol. (Lond.) 141:198-218, 1958.

Hunt, C. C.: Relation of function to diameter in afferent fibers of muscle nerves, J. Gen. Physiol. 38:117-131, 1954.

Hunt, C. C., and Kuffler, S. W.: Further study of efferent small nerve fibres to mammalian muscle spindles; multiple spindle innervation and activity during contraction, J. Physiol. (Lond.) 113:283-297, 1951.

Hunt, C. C., and Kuffler, S. W.: Stretch receptor discharges during muscle contraction, J. Physiol. (Lond.) 113:298-315, 1951.

Hunt, C. C., and McIntyre, A. K.: An analysis of fibre diameter and receptor characteristics of myelinated cutaneous afferent fibres in the cat, J. Physiol. (Lond.) 153:99-112, 1960.

Iggo, A.: Cutaneous thermoreceptors in primates and subprimates, J. Physiol. (Lond.) 200:403-430, 1969.

Iggo, A., and Muir, A. R.: The structure and function of a slowly adapting touch corpuscle in hairy skin, J. Physiol. (Lond.) 200:763-796, 1969.

Jänig, W.: The afferent innervation of the central pad of the cat's hindfoot, Brain Res. 28:203-216, 1971.

Katz, B.: Action potentials from a sensory nerve ending, J. Physiol. (Lond.) 111:248-260, 1950.

Katz, B.: Depolarization of sensory terminals and the initiation of impulses in the muscle spindle, J. Physiol. (Lond.) **111:** 261-282, 1950.

Kuffler, S. W.: Synaptic inhibitory mechanisms; properties of dendrites and problems of excitation in isolated sensory nerve cells, Exp. Cell Res. (Suppl.) **5:**493-519, 1958.

Kuffler, S. W., Hunt, C. C., and Quilliam, J. P.: Function of medullated small nerve fibers in mammalian ventral roots; efferent muscle spindle innervation, J. Neurophysiol. **14:**29-54, 1951.

Leksell, L.: The action potential and the excitatory effects of the small ventral root fibres to skeletal muscle, Acta Physiol. Scand. (Suppl. 31) **10:**1-84, 1945.

Livingston, R. B.: Central control of receptors and sensory transmission systems. In Field, J., editor: Handbook of physiology, sec. 1, Neurophysiology, vol. I, Washington, D.C., 1959, American Physiological Society, pp. 741-760.

Loewenstein, W. R.: On the specificity of a sensory receptor, J. Neurophysiol. **24:**150-158, 1961.

Loewenstein, W. R., and Skalak, R.: Mechanical transmission in a pacinian corpuscle; an analysis and a theory, J. Physiol. (Lond.) **182:**346-379, 1966.

Matthews, P. B. C.: Muscle spindles and their motor control, Physiol. Rev. **44:**219-288, 1964.

Matthews, P. B. C.: Mammalian muscle receptors and their central actions, Baltimore, 1972, The Williams & Wilkins Co.

Pease, D. C., and Quilliam, T. Q.: Electron microscopy of the pacinian corpuscle, J. Biophys. Biochem. Cytol. **3:**331-342, 1957.

Perl, E. R.: Myelinated afferent fibres innervating the primate skin and their response to noxious stimuli, J. Physiol. (Lond.) **197:**593-615, 1968.

Rose, J. E., and Mountcastle, V. B.: Touch and kinesthesis. In Field, J., editor: Handbook of physiology, sec. 1, neurophysiology, vol. 1, Washington, D.C., 1959, American Physiological Society, pp. 387-492.

Ruffini, A.: On the minute anatomy of the neuro-muscular spindles of the cat, and their physiological significance, J. Physiol. (Lond.) **23:**190-208, 1898.

Sherrington, C. S.: On the anatomical constitution of nerves to skeletal muscles; with remarks on recurrent fibres in the ventral spinal nerve-root, J. Physiol. (Lond.) **17:**211-258, 1894.

Sinclair, D. C.: Cutaneous sensation, London, 1967, Oxford University Press.

Sweet, W. H.: Pain. In Field, J., editor: Handbook of physiology, sec. 1, Neurophysiology, vol. I, Washington, D.C., 1959, American Physiological Society, pp. 459-506.

Talbot, W. H., Darian-Smith, I., Kornhuber, H. H., and Mountcastle, V.: The sense of flutter-vibration; comparison of the human capacity with response patterns of mechanoreceptive afferents from the monkey hand, J. Neurophysiol. **31:**301-334, 1968.

Vallbo, A. B., and Hagbarth, K. E.: Activity from skin mechanoreceptors recorded percutaneously in awake human subjects, Exp. Neurol. **21:**270-289, 1968.

Weddell, G., Pallie, W., and Palmer, E.: The morphology of peripheral nerve terminations in the skin, Q. J. Micr. Sci. **95:**483-501, 1954.

Winkleman, R. K.: Nerve endings in normal and pathologic skin, Springfield, Ill., 1960, Charles C Thomas, Publisher.

Zotterman, Y.: Thermal sensations: In Field, J., editor: Handbook of physiology, sec. 1, Neurophysiology, vol. I, Washington, D.C., 1959, American Physiological Society, pp. 431-458.

CHAPTER 3

Peripheral nervous system

ORGANIZATION OF THE PERIPHERAL NERVOUS SYSTEM

The peripheral nervous system includes various types of sensory receptors, the nerve fibers that convey information from these receptors to the central nervous system, and the motor fibers that direct the activity of effector organs. The behavior of receptor organs has been considered in Chapter 2. The present discussion is concerned primarily with the organization of spinal cord roots and peripheral nerve trunks. The component of the peripheral nervous system known as the autonomic nervous system is considered later in this chapter.

Spinal roots

From each segment of the spinal cord there arise a pair of dorsal roots and a pair of ventral roots. The dorsal roots contain solely afferent fibers; that is, all the fibers normally carry information from receptor organs into the spinal cord. The ventral roots contain efferent or motor fibers; these fibers are concerned with the control of effector organs. A division in function of the two types of spinal roots was first clearly demonstrated by the work of Bell and Magendie in the early nineteenth century.

An exception to the concept that the ventral root is exclusively motor is the presence of occasional myelinated afferent fibers in ventral roots of the cat. These are too few to be regarded as important. However, recently it has been found that there are large numbers of unmyelinated afferent fibers in the ventral root and that many of these supply nociceptors. Thus, the ventral root appears to contain a major sensory component, although the central effects of the ventral root afferents are not yet known.

Dorsal root ganglia

Associated with each dorsal root is a dorsal root ganglion (Fig. 3-1). Within a dorsal root ganglion are the pseudounipolar nerve cell bodies that give rise to afferent fibers. A single process is connected with the soma of each dorsal root ganglion cell. After reaching a distance of up to several millimeters from the ganglion cell, this process bifurcates. The larger of the two branches courses toward the periphery through the spinal nerve of that segment to contact a sensory receptor organ. The smaller of the two branches enters the spinal cord through the dorsal root. A fiber originating from a large dorsal root ganglion cell becomes myelinated near the cell body; there are often several nodes of Ranvier on the unbranched part of the process. Small ganglion cells give rise to unmyelinated fibers. Surrounding each ganglion cell

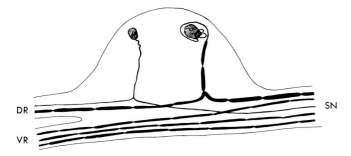

Fig. 3-1. Organization of a dorsal root ganglion. The dorsal *(DR)* and ventral *(VR)* roots of a spinal segment are shown approaching a dorsal root ganglion from the left of the figure. The dorsal root contains only afferent fibers. These are the central processes of the pseudounipolar dorsal root ganglion cells, two of which are shown within the ganglion. The smaller dorsal root ganglion cell has a relatively straight process and gives rise to an unmyelinated nerve fiber. The larger dorsal root ganglion cell has a convoluted process that forms a glomerulus, and it gives rise to a myelinated nerve fiber. The peripheral processes of the dorsal root ganglion cells enter the spinal nerve *(SN)* at the right. Here the afferent fibers become mixed with motor fibers that had been in the ventral root.

body is a sheath composed of interlocking satellite cells. The axon penetrates this sheath. In the case of large ganglion cells, the axon may follow a tortuous course near the soma, forming a glomerulus. The axons of small ganglion cells follow a straighter course. The dorsal root ganglion is invested with and contains fibrous connective tissue, which is continuous with the connective tissue of peripheral nerve.

Peripheral nerves

In general, peripheral nerves carry both afferent and motor fibers. Branches supplying the skin contain not only afferent fibers from cutaneous sensory receptors but also motor fibers of the autonomic nervous system to sweat glands, blood vessels, and piloerector muscles. Likewise, branches of nerves entering muscles contain, besides motor fibers to muscle fibers and blood vessels, afferent fibers from muscle spindles, Golgi tendon organs, and pressure-pain endings.

COMPOUND ACTION POTENTIAL
Action potentials in bundles of nerve fibers

In Chapter 1, the action potential of the single nerve fiber was described. The action potential consists of a spike followed by a series of after-potentials. A stimulus may be below threshold, at threshold, or above threshold for triggering an action potential. The wave form of the action potential is not changed as the stimulus strength is increased beyond threshold; that is, the action potential is either present or absent, all-or-nothing.

Often in experimental work and sometimes in clinical situations, it is possible to record action potentials from single nerve fibers (Fig. 3-2, *A*). However, the techniques required, such as a tedious dissection of a

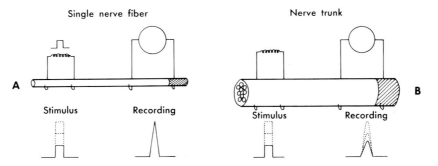

Fig. 3-2. Recording an action potential. **A** shows a procedure used for recording activity from a single nerve fiber. Stimulating and recording electrodes are applied extracellularly to the fiber, which has been dissected from a nerve trunk. The stimulus, if above threshold, can be varied over a wide range without affecting the form of the nerve impulse recorded at a distance along the fiber. In **B** a similar set of electrodes is applied to a nerve trunk. As the stimulus is graded, however, the compound action potential recorded from the end of the nerve is also graded.

nerve bundle and the introduction of a microelectrode, are frequently not applicable experimentally or may be damaging in the case of human subjects. Instead of recording from single nerve fibers, it is often necessary to observe the activity of groups of nerve fibers. An action potential recorded simultaneously from a number of axons is called a compound action potential.

Workers such as J. Erlanger and H. S. Gasser demonstrated that there are differences in the wave forms of compound action potentials that depend on the experimental circumstances (Fig. 3-2, *B*). For instance, the size of the spike potential grows, within limits, as the stimulus strength is raised from threshold to higher values. Furthermore, the spike potential may display several peaks when it is recorded at a distance from the stimulating electrodes, whereas only a single peak may be present at a position near the stimulus. Clearly, the compound action potential is not all-or-nothing.

The explanation for many of the differences between the action potentials of single axons and those of bundles of axons is straightforward. Nerve fibers are not uniform in size. They range from small unmyelinated fibers with diameters of about 1 μm to myelinated fibers over 20 μm in diameter. The threshold to electrical stimulation varies inversely with diameter. The largest fibers are the most readily activated by electrical stimuli, because more of the stimulating current can enter them. The conduction velocities of action potentials in large fibers are larger than the conduction velocities of impulses recorded from small fibers. The conduction velocity is a function of fiber diameter, being directly proportional in the case of myelinated fibers.

When a bundle of nerve fibers is stimulated with weak electrical shocks, the largest fibers will be activated by the smallest stimulating currents. The threshold for the whole nerve bundle is that of its largest fiber. The action potentials of one or a few large fibers in a small bundle can be shown to display all-or-nothing behavior. However, as the stimulus strength is raised, the action potentials of an increasingly larger number of axons are summed, masking the behavior of the individual action potentials. The size of the compound action potential is now proportionate to the number of summed action potentials. The summation is not linear, however, because the extracellularly recorded action potentials of single nerve fibers vary in size with the fiber diameter. Large fibers produce more current flow in the extracellular fluid during an action potential than do small fibers. Thus, as the stimulus strength applied to a nerve bundle is increased, the increment in the size of the

action potential caused by the recruitment of action potentials in progressively smaller fibers decreases.

The contribution of different-sized axons to the compound action potential also depends on the placement of the recording electrodes relative to the stimulating electrodes (Fig. 3-3). If both sets of electrodes are at the same point on the nerve trunk, the compound action potential size will consist of a summation of the spikes in all the fibers stimulated, regardless of the fiber diameter. However, if the recording electrodes are placed at a distance from the stimulating electrodes, the effect of the range of conduction velocities of different-sized fibers comes into play. The action potential in the largest axons will arrive at the recording electrodes first; the action potentials in progressively smaller fibers will arrive later. If the spectrum of fiber size were uniform, the compound action potential recorded at a distance from the point of stimulation might be expected to resemble a prolonged spike potential. However, the spectrum of nerve fiber sizes is not uniform. There are groups of large, middle-sized, and small myelinated fibers and a group of tiny unmyelinated fibers. In certain nerves, there is a special group of autonomic preganglionic axons having a conduction velocity between that of the usual myelinated fiber component and the unmyelinated component.

The original terminology used to describe the several groups of nerve fibers was alphabetical. The mye-

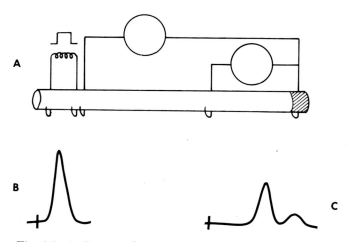

Fig. 3-3. **A,** Compound action potentials recorded at different distances from the point of stimulation. Stimulating electrodes are placed at one end of a nerve trunk. There are two different recording sites, one near the stimulating electrodes and one toward the opposite end of the nerve. The synchronous compound action potential (**B**) was recorded after conduction over a short distance, whereas the compound action potential having dual peaks (**C**) was recorded after propagation over a relatively long distance. The two peaks correspond to the activity of two groups of nerve fibers having different diameters and hence different conduction velocities.

linated fibers commonly found in peripheral nerves and contributing the earliest arriving component of the compound action potential at a recording site were called A fibers. These A fibers were further subdivided into large, middle-sized, and small groups of fibers and were given labels from the Greek alphabet. However, we will follow a more recently devised system, which is described later. The small myelinated preganglionic fibers of the autonomic nervous system that contributed to a second large hump in the compound action potential were called B fibers. The unmyelinated fibers that produced the latest portion of the compound action potential were called C fibers.

Properties of different nerve fiber types

It was found experimentally that there are a number of functionally meaningful differences between fibers belonging to different fiber groups as defined by the criteria of size and conduction velocity. The A fibers were shown to include the myelinated somatic afferent and motor fibers. As already stated, B fibers are autonomic preganglionic axons. The C fibers include both autonomic postganglionic axons and unmyelinated afferent fibers.

Special properties of B and C fibers. It has been possible to record the compound action potentials of B and C fibers by selecting nerves that lack fibers of larger diameter or by blocking the action potential of the larger fibers, using one of several available techniques (electrical, pressure, and cold-block methods have been employed). An unusual property of the action potentials of B fibers is the absence of an after-depolarization. This is correlated with the lack of a supernormal period in the excitability cycle of these fibers. The after-hyperpolarization of B fibers is large. C fibers may have an after-depolarization, and they generally have a large after-hyperpolarization. The difference in after-potentials between A fibers and these smaller axons may in part reflect changes in the intracellular ionic composition during activity in the smaller fibers.

Subdivisions of group A fibers. Much of our knowledge of the basic mechanisms of reflex action in the spinal cord is derived from the study of the effects of volleys in A fibers. Some current work is directed toward the study of the action of C fibers, and no doubt our knowledge of the reflex actions of these fibers will soon become more complete. However, technically it is easier to stimulate and to record from A fibers; thus the greatest progress has been made using these fibers.

Afferent fibers of type A have been divided into three groups on the basis of fiber diameter and conduction velocity (Table 3-1). The group I fibers are found only in muscle nerves and include the large axons from primary endings of muscle spindles (group Ia) and those from Golgi tendon organs (group Ib). Muscle nerves also contain group II fibers, chiefly from secondary endings of muscle spindles, and group III fibers, chiefly from pressure-pain endings. Cutaneous nerves contain A-beta and A-delta fibers from various kinds of receptors. The A-beta and A-delta

Table 3-1. Fiber types and their functions

Type	Group	Sub-group	Diameter (μm)	Conduction velocity (m/sec)	Tissue supplied	Function
Afferent						
A	I	Ia	12-20	72-120	Muscle	Afferents from muscle spindle primary endings
		Ib			Muscle	Afferents from Golgi tendon organs
	II		6-12	36-72	Muscle	Afferents from muscle spindle secondary endings
	Beta				Skin	Afferents from pacinian corpuscles, touch receptors
	III		1-6	6-36	Muscle	Afferents from pressure-pain endings
	Delta				Skin	Afferents from touch, temperature, and pain receptors
C	IV		$\simeq 1$	0.5-2	Muscle	Afferents from pain receptors
	Dorsal root				Skin	Afferents from touch, pain, and temperature receptors
Motor						
A	Alpha		12-20	72-120	Muscle	Motor supply of extrafusal skeletal muscle fibers
	Gamma		2-8	12-48	Muscle	Motor supply of intrafusal muscle fibers
B			$\simeq 3$	3-15	Ganglia	Preganglionic autonomic fibers
C	Sympathetic		$\simeq 1$	0.5-2	Cardiac and smooth muscle; glands	Postganglionic autonomic fibers

fibers are equivalent in size to group II and III fibers in muscle nerve.

Motor fibers of type A are divided into two groups, alpha and gamma. The alpha motor fibers innervate skeletal muscle fibers; the gamma motor fibers supply the intrafusal muscle fibers of muscle spindles (Table 3-1).

For large A fibers the numerical value of the conduction velocity is approximately six times the diameter of the fiber. For instance, a fiber with a diameter of 10 μm will have a conduction velocity of about 60 m/sec. The multiplier for small A fibers is closer to 4. Thus the conduction velocity of an A fiber with a diameter of 2 μm is about 8 m/sec.

Electrical excitability

The electrical stimulus strength required to excite a peripheral nerve fiber depends on the diameter of the fiber. The most excitable A axons, therefore, are the group I afferent fibers and the alpha motor fibers. It should be emphasized, however, that a fiber may have a low threshold to electrical stimulation and yet have a high threshold to natural stimulation, whether this be by activation of a sensory receptor organ or by a response of its cell body to synaptic excitation. The converse may also be true.

Recording compound action potentials

The activity of groups of nerve fibers may be recorded in any of several ways. The easiest to interpret are known as diphasic and monophasic recordings (Fig. 3-4). The nerve is placed in an insulating medium, such as mineral oil or air, so that the currents traveling extracellularly are concentrated in a thin layer of fluid around each axon. Two recording electrodes are placed in contact with the surface of the nerve, and a compound action potential is set up in the nerve either by means of a pair of stimulating electrodes or by some other type of stimulation. If the recording desired is diphasic, both of the recording electrodes are placed on the surface of the intact nerve. There is no potential difference between the two electrodes when the nerve is at rest. When the action potential approaches one of the recording electrodes, the potential of that electrode becomes negative with respect to the other electrode. With continued propagation of the nerve impulse, it reaches a point along the nerve at which the potential detected by each electrode is the same. Then, as the action potential approaches the second electrode, the potential at the first electrode becomes relatively positive. Finally, the nerve impulse is conducted to a region of the nerve that does not influence the potential adjacent to either electrode, and the potential difference becomes zero again.

For monophasic recording, one of the electrodes is placed in contact with a cut or damaged part of the nerve. There will be a difference in potential between the two electrodes when the nerve is at rest, because one electrode "sees" the negative interiors of the axons (as well as the extracellular environment between axons), whereas the other electrode detects only the

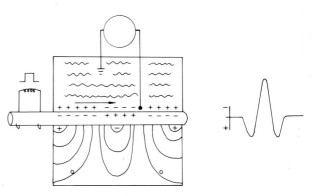

Fig. 3-5. Recording a compound action potential in a volume conductor. A nerve trunk is placed in a conductive medium. One recording electrode is placed adjacent to the nerve, and an indifferent electrode is in contact with the electrolyte at some distance from the nerve. A nerve impulse is evoked by the stimulating electrodes. As the action potential approaches, passes by, and then recedes from the active electrode, a triphasic (positive-negative-positive) deflection is recorded, as shown at the right. The distribution of the electrical field potential about the active region of the nerve is plotted in the region of volume conductor drawn below the nerve trunk. The extracellular fluid is negative adjacent to the region of activity, whereas it is positive ahead of and behind this region. The triphasic action potential can be regarded as the movement of this field potential past the recording electrode.

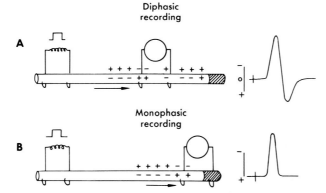

Fig. 3-4. **A**, Arrangement of stimulating and recording electrodes for diphasic recording of a compound action potential. The action potential is seen at the right. Only the low-threshold fibers were stimulated, so the spike is synchronous. **B**, Arrangement of the recording electrodes for monophasic recording. Note that one electrode is placed on the killed end of the nerve. The monophasic spike is seen at the right.

potential of the extracellular fluid. An action potential in the nerve can reach only the electrode in contact with normal nerve; when this occurs, the potential difference between the two electrodes is reduced and a monophasic action potential is recorded.

Another method of recording may be used when nerve activity must be studied from large organs, such as the brain or spinal cord. This is known as recording from a volume conductor (Fig. 3-5). The interpretation of potentials recorded in volume is very difficult except in particularly favorable circumstances. In general, if an electrode is placed near a long bundle of nerve fibers in a volume conductor, and an action potential propagates past the electrodes, the following sequence of potential changes may be recorded. As the action potential approaches the electrode, a positive potential develops; this is caused by the flow of current from the vicinity of the electrode toward the region of active membrane. When the action potential is near the electrode, a negativity is recorded; the currents are now directed toward the region of the electrode. Finally, as the action potential is propagated away from the electrode, a positive potential is recorded; the currents have shifted in direction again. The wave form is triphasic.

The particular sequence of potentials recorded depends, however, on many geometric factors, such as how far away the electrode is from the active nerve fibers, the direction of propagation of the nerve impulses, and so on. Another problem is that many potentials recorded from the central nervous system are caused by synaptic activity and not by action potentials. Inasmuch as synaptic potentials may be either hyperpolarizing or depolarizing, many complicated recording problems may develop. However, potentials recorded in volume from peripheral nerves are relatively easy to interpret.

Clinical studies of compound action potentials

Diseases of peripheral nerve fibers may be associated with a reduction in the conduction velocity of nerve trunks. This can be assessed for motor fibers by timing the interval between a stimulus and the onset of electromyographic evidence of muscle activity. For examining the activity of sensory fibers, it is possible to record in volume the compound action potential of nerves situated near the body surface in response to percutaneous stimulation at a distant point on the same nerve. In practice the motor conduction velocity is used more often than the sensory conduction velocity, because the potentials recorded through the skin from nerve trunks are small and must be averaged by computerlike devices to extract the signal from the noise. The motor conduction velocity is most useful in determining if the dysfunction of a nerve is caused by compression of the nerve at a particular point along its course, usually where the nerve runs under a ligament over a joint. A case of weakness of the intrinsic muscles of the hand supplied by the median nerve can be taken as an example. These muscles lie in the thenar eminence and are used in opposing the thumb to the other fingers and in flexing the thumb. The conduction velocity of the median nerve passing across the wrist is measured and compared both with the contralateral nerve and with tables of normal velocities. Decreased conduction velocity across the segment of the nerve, with normal velocities across the segments more proximal, strongly suggests compression of the nerve under the carpal ligament at the wrist (carpal tunnel syndrome). The compression can be relieved by cutting the pathologically thickened transverse carpal ligament. If the conduction velocities of all segments of the nerve are low, a degenerative process of the nerve is suggested. Another diagnostic test that can be carried out in some cases of suspected degenerative disease is nerve biopsy. A biopsy can be taken of fascicles of nerves, generally cutaneous branches supplying skin with a large overlap from other nerves; these nerves can then be studied with light and electron microscopy.

PROPERTIES OF SYNAPTIC TRANSMISSION
Synapse

The area of functional contact between a nerve ending and another cell was termed the synapse by C. S. Sherrington. Working primarily with the spinal cord and using indirect techniques, Sherrington and his collaborators and students collected a large amount of information about the properties of synapses. Further information on synaptic organization and behavior resulted from studies on peripheral junctions, such as the neuromuscular junction and the sympathetic ganglion, again with indirect techniques. However, rapid progress has been made in recent years through the use of intracellular recording techniques. Outstanding work has been done on the spinal cord by J. C. Eccles and his co-workers and on the neuromuscular junction by B. Katz and his associates. Another useful preparation for the study of synaptic transmission is the squid giant synapse.

Characteristics of synaptic transmission

There are a number of features by which transmission across a synapse differs from the conduction of nerve impulses along nerve fibers. Among these are the following:

1. There is a synaptic delay in transmission from presynaptic terminals to the postsynaptic cell. This delay amounts to some tenths of a millisecond in mammalian tissue, and it cannot be accounted for by conduction along fine terminal branches. In lower forms, the synaptic delay may be 1 or more milliseconds.
2. Transmission across a synapse occurs in only one direction.
3. Synaptic transmission is very susceptible to the effects of hypoxia, drugs, and fatigue.
4. The postsynaptic cell may discharge repetitively to a single volley in the presynaptic pathway. With complicated pathways, the postsynaptic cell may show a prolonged discharge, known as after-discharge, following the cessation of stimulation of the presynaptic path.
5. A single presynaptic volley may not cause any discharge of the postsynaptic cell, whereas repetitive stimulation of a single presynaptic pathway or concurrent stimulation of more than one pathway may. The effects of presynaptic stimulation may, therefore, show temporal or spatial summation.
6. Inhibition of synaptic transmission may occur without prior excitation. Inhibitory synaptic actions are discussed in Chapter 4.

Chemical transmission

The properties of synaptic transmission become easier to understand when one realizes that there is a fundamental distinction between the conduction of nerve impulses and synaptic transmission.

Nerve impulses are produced by an electrochemical reaction within the nerve membrane. The propagation of the reaction along a nerve fiber is caused by the local spread of ionic current that depolarizes neighboring areas of membrane and so triggers the nerve impulse at each point along the membrane.

The spread of local ionic currents along a nerve fiber is aided by the cablelike structure of the fiber. The current flows along the axoplasm and then across the nerve membrane. However, current flow from the one nerve cell across a synapse to another cell cannot take place without a special geometry of the synaptic region. For this reason, the electrical activity of one neuron usually has only a slight effect on the electrical activity of a nearby cell. There are a number of known cases of electrically transmitting synapses, but most of these are in the invertebrates and lower vertebrates.

Synaptic transmission is thus brought about in most mammalian synapses by a chemical mechanism (Fig. 3-6). The terminals of nerve fibers contain stores of a chemical known as a transmitter substance. A fraction of this transmitter substance is released when a nerve impulse reaches the region of the presynaptic terminals. The transmitter then diffuses across the synaptic cleft to the postsynaptic membrane, where a reaction takes place with special receptor sites.

Synaptic delay is the sum of the time required for transmitter release, diffusion of the transmitter substance across the synaptic cleft, and the reaction of the transmitter with special receptor molecules. The receptor reaction is terminated by enzymatic destruction of the transmitter, by diffusion of the transmitter out of the synaptic cleft, or by reuptake of the transmitter by the presynaptic ending. Conduction across a chemically transmitting synapse is unidirectional, because the transmitter substance and the mechanism of its release are located only presynaptically, whereas

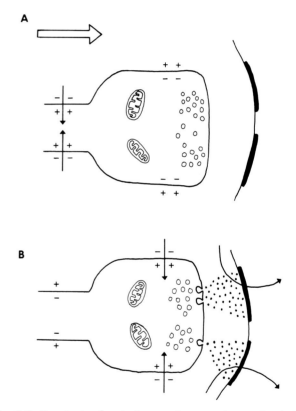

Fig. 3-6. Events in chemical synaptic transmission. In **A** the action potential is shown approaching a synaptic terminal containing transmitter stored in synaptic vesicles. In **B** the arrival of the nerve impulse triggers the release of transmitter into the synaptic cleft. The transmitter diffuses across the cleft and reacts with receptor molecules associated with the postsynaptic membrane. The resultant change in membrane permeability to ions, such as sodium and potassium, causes the flow of a synaptic current. In this case, the current is inward across the subsynaptic membrane, then outward across the adjacent inactive membrane, resulting in a depolarization called the excitatory postsynaptic potential. Following these events, the transmitter action is terminated, either by enzymatic destruction, diffusion, or reuptake into the presynaptic terminal.

the receptor molecules are located chiefly on the postsynaptic membrane. The chemical nature of the synaptic transmission makes the process susceptible to changes that affect biochemical reactions, such as blocking agents.

Transmitter substances

The identity of the chemical agent responsible for synaptic transmission is known only for certain synapses (Fig. 3-7). It is acetylcholine, for instance, at the neuromuscular junction and at the synapses of motor axon collaterals on Renshaw cells in the spinal cord. However, the transmitter substances at most synapses are unknown. It is likely that in the near future many different biologically active compounds will be identified as chemical transmitters at particular synapses. Candidate transmitters include norepinephrine, serotonin, gamma-aminobutyric acid, histamine, glycine, glutamic acid, and substance P, in addition to acetylcholine.

To demonstrate that a substance is a chemical transmitter, the substance must be shown to (1) be produced in presynaptic neurons and stored in synaptic terminals, (2) be released from the presynaptic terminals when they are activated, (3) mimic the effect of synaptic activity when applied to the postsynaptic membrane artificially, and (4) be removed from the postsynaptic receptor site.

Properties of postsynaptic potentials

The action of a chemical transmitter substance on the membrane of a postsynaptic cell appears in general to be the alteration of membrane permeability to small ions. Other conceivable actions that may be shown to be important include changes in cellular metabolism and interference with the actions of transmitters released from other synapses. However, the synapses that have been investigated in depth so far seem to operate by increases in membrane permeability.

If the membrane permeability to sodium alone were increased, the membrane potential would shift in the direction of the equilibrium potential for sodium, as it does in the case of the spike potential. An increased permeability to chloride ions might result in no alteration in membrane potential, whereas potassium currents would tend to hyperpolarize the membrane (Fig. 3-8). However, there is no evidence that permeability changes need be restricted to just one ion species. When the membrane permeability is changed for more than one type of ion, the membrane potential shifts toward a level that can be predicted from the Goldman equation. For instance, if the permeability to both sodium and potassium were to increase, the membrane potential would change toward a level between the sodium and potassium equilibrium potentials; that is, somewhere between +60 and –80 mV. The exact level would depend on the new values for P_{Na}^+ and P_K^+.

The alteration in permeability of the postsynaptic membrane in response to excitatory chemical transmitters seems to involve at least the sodium and potassium ions. The membrane potential undergoes a depolarization called an excitatory postsynaptic potential (Fig. 3-9). The level toward which the membrane potential shifts is close to zero membrane potential. This particular level may result simply from a fortuitous balance of the changes in P_{Na}^+ and P_K^+.

Activity of an excitatory synapse thus results in a tendency for the membrane potential of the post-

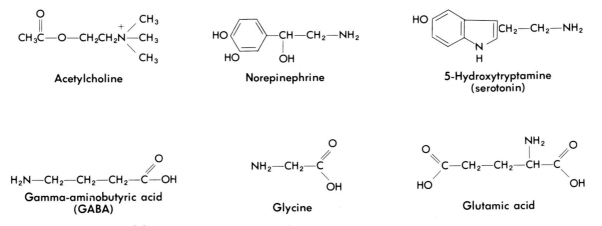

Fig. 3-7. Candidate chemical transmitter substances. Some of the compounds whose chemical formulas are shown, such as acetylcholine and norepinephrine (also called noradrenaline), have been proved to be transmitter substances at particular synapses. The same substances are also thought to be transmitters at other synapses, although the evidence is as yet inconclusive. The other agents are also likely to be transmitters elsewhere in the nervous system.

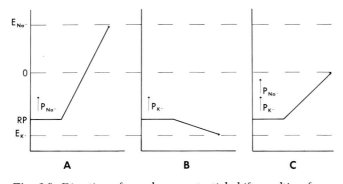

Fig. 3-8. Direction of membrane potential shift resulting from changes in permeability to particular ions. The graphs show the membrane potential (ordinate) plotted against time (abscissa). The levels of the sodium and potassium equilibrium potentials (E_{Na^+} and E_{K^+}) and of the resting potential *(RP)* are given. **A** shows that the membrane potential will shift toward the sodium equilibrium potential if the permeability to sodium is increased. **B** shows the shift toward the potassium equilibrium potential when the permeability to potassium is selectively increased. **C** indicates that the membrane potential will move toward some intermediate level, such as zero potential, if the permeabilities for both sodium and potassium are increased simultaneously.

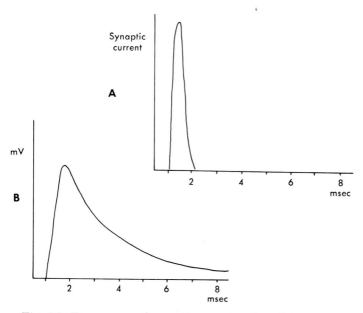

Fig. 3-9. Time course of synaptic current and excitatory post-synaptic potential. The graph in **A** shows the amount of synaptic current plotted against time. The excitatory transmitter was released just after the start of the abscissa. The action of the transmitter is terminated within 2 msec, as shown by the cessation of the synaptic current at this time. In **B** the membrane potential change resulting from the synaptic current is plotted against time. The excitatory postsynaptic potential reaches a peak soon after the peak of flow of the synaptic current. After the synaptic current has ceased, the membrane potential decays passively to the resting level. The time course of decay depends on the membrane electrical characteristics and the location of the synapses involved in relation to the position of the recording electrode.

synaptic cell to approach zero. However, the chemical transmitter substance will generally not act long enough for the membrane potential to shift more than a fraction of the way between the resting level and zero. For many synapses, the action of a chemical transmitter substance has been shown to last no more than a few milliseconds. However, the transmitter need not cause such a dramatic change in membrane potential to evoke an action potential, because threshold may be at a level only some 10 or 15 mV less than resting potential.

An important consideration is the spread of synaptic currents over the membrane of the postsynaptic cell (Fig. 3-10). The chemical transmitter acts only in the immediate vicinity of the release sites from a presynaptic terminal. Ionic currents flow through the membrane just at the region where the membrane permeability has increased. The currents then distribute throughout the cytoplasm of the postsynaptic cell, with a capacitative component crossing the membrane in an outward direction to enter the external return circuit in the extracellular environment of the neuron. This outward capacitative current is responsible for depolarizing the membrane of the postsynaptic cell at all points beyond the subsynaptic region. Because the neuronal membrane acts as a leaky capacitor, the synaptic currents become progressively less effective with distance from the synapse. For example, very

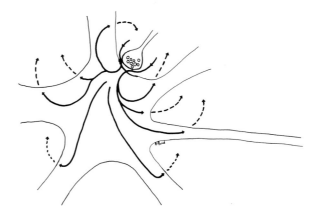

Fig. 3-10. Distribution of synaptic current. Some of the lines of current flow during excitatory synaptic activity are shown. A single synapse is active. Current enters the subsynaptic membrane at this point because of the membrane permeability change caused by transmitter released from the synaptic ending. The current then flows through the cytoplasm of the neuron into the dendrites and the axon. The outward flow of current is largely capacitative. This outward current flow depolarizes the membrane of the neuron. The return path of the current is through the extracellular fluid. The exact distribution of the current will depend on the geometry of the neuron and the membrane properties at a given time for each region of the neuron.

little change occurs in the membrane potential of much of the axon during excitatory synaptic transmission. However, synaptic currents are transmitted well along the lengths of dendrites, and the membrane potential of the axon hillock may be changed effectively by synapses located on the cell body and even well out on dendrites.

SQUID GIANT SYNAPSE
Structure

A useful experimental model for the study of excitatory synaptic transmission is the squid giant synapse (Fig. 3-11). Giant synapses are formed by the connections between the branches of a giant fiber entering the stellate ganglion and each of several giant fibers leaving the ganglion. The largest of these efferents is the giant axon used in studies of the nerve impulse. The giant fiber system forms a mechanism for activating the mantle and related muscles to provide the squid with jet propulsion for escaping from predators.

The advantage of the giant synapse preparation is that both the presynaptic and the postsynaptic elements are large enough to allow their penetration by one or more electrodes. This allows the recording of

transmembrane potentials of each element at the synapse and also permits the passage of currents to alter the potential across either the presynaptic or postsynaptic membrane. A disadvantage of the squid giant synapse preparation is that the chemical transmitter at this synapse is as yet unknown. A candidate transmitter is glutamic acid.

Synaptic delay

Several features of chemical synaptic transmission are very well illustrated in experiments utilizing the squid giant synapse (Fig. 3-12).

With recording microelectrodes in both the presynaptic and postsynaptic elements of the squid giant synapse, it has been possible to show that a true synaptic delay occurs between the arrival of the presynaptic action potential and the onset of the excitatory postsynaptic potential. The amount of delay is on the order of 1 or 2 msec, depending on the temperature. The action potential in either element is recorded in the other element as a small deflection having essentially the same amplitude as the potential recordable from the extracellular space adjacent to the synapse. The currents associated with the action potential in the presynaptic element, therefore, travel almost exclusively in the extracellular fluid and do not cross the membrane of the postsynaptic element.

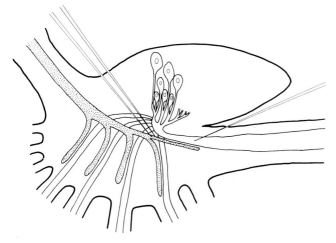

Fig. 3-11. Structure of the squid giant synapse. The stellate ganglion of the squid is shown. Cell bodies of some of the neurons that form the syncytial giant fibers are shown at the top of the ganglion. The axon that these cells form is the giant axon used also for studies of the nerve impulse. It forms the postsynaptic element of the squid giant synapse. A single microelectrode is shown impaling it, although several electrodes can be inserted into this large fiber. Other giant fibers are indicated leaving through the various connectives of the ganglion. The presynaptic element of the giant synapse is shown by the stippling. This is a giant fiber originating from another ganglion. Two microelectrodes are shown inserted into the presynaptic axon near the synapse.

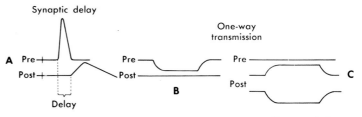

Fig. 3-12. Properties of synaptic transmission illustrated by squid giant synapse. The upper trace in each set of records is from the presynaptic element of the squid giant synapse; the lower traces are from the postsynaptic element. In **A** the presynaptic element is invaded by a nerve impulse evoked by stimulation of the fiber at a distance from the synapse. The spike is shown beginning a short time after the stimulus artifact. An excitatory postsynaptic potential is recorded from the postsynaptic element, as shown in the lower trace. The time between arrival of the nerve impulse at the presynaptic terminal and the start of the postsynaptic potential is the synaptic delay. In **B** a hyperpolarizing pulse has been applied to the membrane of the presynaptic element through one microelectrode, and the potential change as shown is recorded by the other microelectrode in the presynaptic element. The lower trace shows that this large potential change in the presynaptic element does not affect the postsynaptic element. In **C** both depolarizing and hyperpolarizing pulses are applied to the postsynaptic element. Neither affects the presynaptic element. **B** and **C** show the lack of electrical coupling across the synapse.

One-way transmission

When hyperpolarizing current pulses are applied across the presynaptic membrane, there is little or no change in the membrane potential of the postsynaptic element. Similarly, alterations of the postsynaptic membrane potential in either the depolarizing or the hyperpolarizing direction cannot be detected by recording from the presynaptic element. There is clearly no significant electrical coupling across the squid giant synapse. Information crosses the synapse strictly by chemical means and only when the presynaptic element is depolarized sufficiently.

Susceptibility to hypoxia, drugs, and fatigue

Synaptic transmission fails when insufficient oxygen is available. This is well demonstrated by the squid giant synapse, which must be perfused with oxygenated seawater when it is isolated from the animal.

A number of drugs known to affect synaptic transmission involving particular transmitters have been tried on the giant synapse preparation without success. It can be anticipated that additional pharmacological manipulations of the synapse will be employed when the transmitter is identified. The major agents that do have an action include divalent cations, such as calcium and magnesium, nerve poisons, like tetrodotoxin, and tetraethylammonium ions.

An increase in the concentration of calcium ions in the extracellular fluid enhances synaptic transmission, whereas an increase in the concentration of magnesium ions depresses it. Tetrodotoxin, while having no direct effect on synaptic potentials, does block nerve action potentials by preventing activation of the mechanism permitting an influx of sodium ions in response to depolarization. Tetraethylammonium ions specifically block the potassium efflux mechanism. These agents have been used to study excitation-secretion coupling.

If the presynaptic fiber of the squid giant synapse is activated repetitively, the amount of transmitter released by each impulse decreases, so that in time the excitatory postsynaptic potential may be reduced below threshold for evoking a postsynaptic action potential. This process is a type of fatigue and may be caused by the depletion of stored transmitter.

Excitation-secretion coupling

If the presynaptic terminal is depolarized by a current pulse and then an action potential is allowed to propagate into the depolarized ending, the size of the action potential is smaller than normal (Fig. 3-13). This presumably is caused by the reduced electrochemical gradient to sodium, the development of an increased membrane permeability to potassium,

and some inactivation of the sodium influx mechanism. The excitatory postsynaptic potential is smaller than normal or absent, depending on the amount of depolarization. If the presynaptic action potential invades a hyperpolarized terminal, the size of the spike is larger than normal, and the resultant excitatory postsynaptic potential is also enhanced. It appears that the release of transmitter is a function of the size of the presynaptic action potential.

As a means of providing better control of the degree and duration of depolarization of the presynaptic terminals at the squid giant synapse, it is possible to block the action potential with tetrodotoxin and to alter the potential artificially. A problem encountered in experiments in which this is done is that the potassium permeability increases with depolarization. The increased membrane conductance prevents the maintenance of depolarization beyond about 1 msec. To prevent this short-circuiting effect, tetraethylammonium ions can be injected into the presynaptic element (Fig. 3-14). This allows an applied current to produce a long-lasting depolarization. In experiments of this kind, it has been shown that an excitatory postsynaptic potential results only if the amount of depolarization reaches a threshold level (around 40 mV from the resting potential) and if it does not exceed a very much more depolarized level. If the depolarization is, for example, to 200 mV, the excitatory postsynaptic potential is delayed until after the depolarization is terminated.

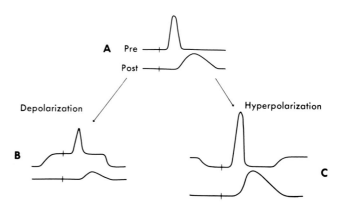

Fig. 3-13. Effect of changes in the amplitude of the presynaptic spike potential on transmitter release. The size of the presynaptic spike potential can be altered by the application of current pulses to the presynaptic terminal membrane. In **A** the control sizes of presynaptic spike and of the resulting excitatory postsynaptic potential are shown. In **B** the presynaptic membrane is depolarized by current passed from a microelectrode impaling the fiber. The spike potential invading the terminal is reduced in size, as is the excitatory postsynaptic potential. The opposite effect is shown in **C**, when a hyperpolarizing pulse is applied to the presynaptic membrane.

The best interpretation of these findings appears to be as follows. The depolarization of the presynaptic ending, if large enough, results in the influx of calcium ions into the ending. In some manner, the calcium ions trigger the release of transmitter from storage granules through the presynaptic membrane and into the synaptic cleft. The mechanism persists in the absence of a sodium current (in tetrodotoxin-poisoned preparations) or of a potassium current (in preparations injected with tetraethylammonium ions). How-

ever, the calcium current can be prevented if the membrane is depolarized to the calcium equilibrium potential. The permeability to calcium is enhanced by depolarization, so as soon as the potential is returned below the calcium equilibrium potential, a large influx of calcium occurs. Magnesium ions apparently compete with calcium ions for the active sites in the transmitter secretion mechanism. However, they are ineffective in causing transmitter release and, in fact, interfere with the secretion process.

NEUROMUSCULAR TRANSMISSION
Twitch versus tonic fibers

The vertebrate neuromuscular junction may also be considered as a model for excitatory synaptic transmission. A great deal of experimental work has been done on frog and mammalian neuromuscular junctions, and some work has been done on similar junctions in a variety of other animals. In vertebrates, the function of efferent terminals on skeletal muscle is to evoke a contraction of the muscle. This is accomplished indirectly through the production of an excitatory synaptic potential, often called an end-plate potential. In the skeletal muscle fibers that contract in all-or-nothing fashion with a twitch, the end-plate potential generally reaches threshold for the production of an action potential, which then propagates along the muscle fiber. The action potential in turn triggers a contraction. The triggering agent appears to be the depolarization associated with the action potential, because localized contractions can be produced by the application to the membrane of a microelectrode acting as a cathode. Animals such as the frog have another variety of muscle fiber, the tonic fiber, which contracts in a graded fashion. In these fibers, the end-plate potential is itself the triggering agent for the contraction. There is no propagated action potential. The polarization is spread along the fiber by virtue of the distribution of many neuromuscular junctions all along the muscle membrane. Inasmuch as there is evidence that most mammalian muscles lack tonic fibers, the discussion that follows is concerned primarily with the structure and function of neuromuscular junctions on twitch fibers. In the mammal, the only known tonic muscle fibers are in the extraocular muscles and in the muscles of the middle ear.

Structure of the neuromuscular junction

Although the light microscopic appearance of neuromuscular junctions varies somewhat with the species, there are a number of common features (Fig. 3-15). As the nerve approaches the muscle fiber, it loses its

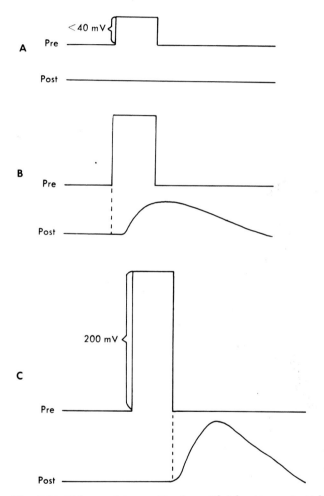

Fig. 3-14. Release of transmitter by artificial action potentials. The spike mechanism in this squid giant synapse preparation is blocked by a combination of tetrodotoxin (which prevents the sodium influx from occurring) and tetraethylammonium ions (which block the delayed efflux of potassium). The presynaptic membrane can then be depolarized to any level desired and the depolarization maintained. It is found (**A**) that depolarizations less than 40 mV from the resting level do not result in the liberation of transmitter, as judged by the absence of any excitatory postsynaptic potential in records from the postsynaptic element *(lower trace)*. Depolarizations greater than 40 mV cause the release of transmitter (**B**). However, if the membrane is depolarized to 200 mV (**C**), the transmitter is not released until the termination of the depolarization.

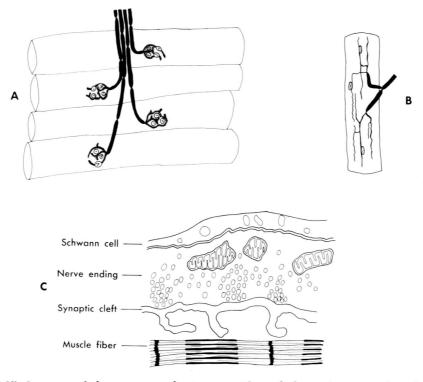

Fig. 3-15. Structure of the neuromuscular junction. The end-plates of a mammalian skeletal muscle are shown in **A**, and the end-brushes of a frog skeletal muscle in **B**. These views are at the light microscopic level. The ultrastructure of a neuromuscular junction is shown in **C**. The nerve terminal is covered by a Schwann cell. The nerve ending contains many synaptic vesicles, which tend to cluster at intervals along the presynaptic membrane. The synaptic cleft separates the nerve terminal and the muscle membrane. The latter is folded at regular intervals. These folds tend to occur opposite regions of the nerve ending in which the vesicles aggregate.

myelin sheath. The terminal appears to be partially embedded in the muscle fiber. Between the nerve ending and the muscle is a structure called the subneural apparatus. This resembles a palisade. The subneural apparatus is best demonstrated using histochemical techniques for the staining of acetylcholinesterase, the enzyme responsible for the destruction of the transmitter at the neuromuscular junction, acetylcholine.

The electron microscope has greatly assisted the interpretation of many of the structural features of the neuromuscular junction. The nerve terminal is seen to be quite separate from the muscle fiber, the synaptic cleft being around 50 nm. The nerve ending is covered externally to the junction by a Schwann cell. The sarcolemma beneath the nerve ending is folded at regular intervals. The membrane of the folds and adjacent to the folds has been shown to have acetylcholinesterase associated with it. Thus, the sarcolemma, with its folds, forms the subneural apparatus. The cytoplasm of the nerve terminal re-

sembles that of other presynaptic endings in containing a concentration of mitochondria and large numbers of synaptic vesicles. Often the synaptic vesicles seem to be clustered near a region of density of the presynaptic membrane. These specialized areas tend to be located opposite the folds of the subneural apparatus.

End-plate potential

Excitation of a motor axon results in the generation of an end-plate potential in each of the muscle fibers on which the motor axon terminates. The term end-plate potential is used for the excitatory synaptic potentials recorded at most neuromuscular junctions on skeletal muscle, whether the morphological arrangement resembles a "plate" (Fig. 3-15, *A*) or a "brush" (Fig. 3-15, *B*). The end-plate potential is a transient depolarization of the muscle fiber membrane, and it is due to the release of acetylcholine from the motor nerve terminal. The depolarization may exceed 50 mV from the resting potential level, which is typically about –90 mV in skeletal muscle. This large a depolarization is well beyond threshold, so the end-plate potential normally triggers an action potential in the muscle fiber. Even repetitive stimulation of the motor nerve will result in a muscle action potential following each nerve impulse, despite a reduction in the amplitude of the end-plate potential because of a depletion of the acetylcholine stores. Each muscle action potential in turn causes a contraction of the muscle fiber through the process known as excitation-contraction coupling. The depolarization of the muscle membrane associated with the muscle action potential releases calcium within the muscle fiber, and this initiates a series of events leading to the activation of the contractile proteins. The maximum rate at which muscle action potentials can occur and still contribute measurable increments in muscle tension is limited, however, and varies with the particular muscle type.

For the study of end-plate potentials using an intracellular recording technique, it is necessary to prevent the muscle fiber from contracting, because a twitch may either dislodge the microelectrode or result in damage to the muscle fiber membrane. One way to do this is to reduce the sensitivity of the muscle membrane at the neuromuscular junction to acetylcholine. This can be done by application of curare, a drug that combines with the acetylcholine receptors without activating them (see p. 75). Curare reduces the amplitude of the end-plate potential because it competes for the active sites on the acetylcholine receptors. With the proper dose, the end-plate potential can be investigated in the absence of a muscle action potential, because the end-plate potential can be reduced to a level below threshold for the muscle membrane. However, a larger dose of curare may completely eliminate the end-plate potential.

The end-plate potential recorded from curarized muscle can be shown to originate in a very restricted region of the muscle membrane. The region is just that part occupied by the neuromuscular junction. If the recording microelectrode impales the muscle fiber at the neuromuscular junction, the end-plate potential observed has its maximum amplitude and fastest time course here. When the microelectrode is moved slightly away from the junctional region, the end-plate potential recorded is smaller in amplitude and slower in time course. This finding is just what is predicted if the end-plate potential is produced at a discrete location and the depolarization spreads passively along the muscle fiber membrane. The passive spread of potential along a leaky cable results in a decay in the recorded amplitude of the potential and a slowed time course (see p. 26).

Ionic mechanism producing the end-plate potential

The end-plate potential results from the reaction of acetylcholine with receptors on the surface of the muscle membrane at the neuromuscular junction. The receptors appear to be located on the external surface of the muscle membrane, because injection of acetylcholine into the cytoplasm of the muscle fiber has no effect, whereas release of acetylcholine from a micropipette just outside the muscle membrane mimics the action of the motor nerve. The reaction between acetylcholine and the receptors causes a change in the permeability of the muscle membrane to a number of small ions, but most importantly to sodium and potassium ions. The simultaneous influx of sodium ions and efflux of potassium ions produces a shift of the membrane potential toward the zero level (Fig. 3-8). If the membrane potential is artificially displaced to a positive value, the end-plate potential reverses in sign, indicating that a membrane potential of near zero is the equilibrium potential for the combination of ions that are involved in the generation of the end-plate potential.

Quantal release of acetylcholine

The release of acetylcholine by a nerve impulse in the motor axon is dependent on the presence of calcium ions in the extracellular fluid. This calcium dependence appears to be a universal requirement for secretory processes and has already been discussed in relation to transmission at the squid giant synapse (pp. 70-71). The amount of transmitter release can be changed by altering the concentration of calcium in the extracellular fluid. Alternatively, inasmuch as the effect of calcium is antagonized by magnesium ions, the amount of transmitter released can be manipulated by changes in the magnesium concentration. For example, the end-plate potential may be increased in size if the calcium concentration is elevated or if the magnesium concentration is reduced; conversely, the end-plate potential can be diminished in size by either a reduction in calcium or an elevation in magnesium concentration.

When the amount of acetylcholine is sufficiently reduced by the appropriate adjustments in calcium or magnesium concentration or both, the end-plate potentials evoked by successive nerve impulses vary in size. One nerve impulse may result in no end-plate potential at all; another may produce a small one. The sizes of the end-plate potentials do not, however, appear to vary over a continuum. Instead, they have any of several discrete sizes. Furthermore, the sizes are multiples of the smallest amplitude end-plate potential. For this reason, Katz suggested that acetylcholine released at the neuromuscular junction is quantal in nature. If any acetylcholine is released, it is released in a sufficient amount to produce an end-plate potential of a small size, approximately 1 mV, or a larger end-plate potential of 2, 3, or 4 mV. These potentials are not due to the release of single molecules of acetylcholine. This small a quantity of acetylcholine does not produce any detectable change in the muscle membrane potential; it would take several thousand molecules of acetylcholine to cause an end-plate potential of 1 mV. Katz and his co-workers have further suggested that each packet of acetylcholine is stored in a synaptic vesicle. Thus, the nerve impulse releases the contents of a number of synaptic vesicles into the synaptic cleft. With depression of neuromuscular transmission by an altered calcium or magnesium concentration, the number of vesicles that release acetylcholine in response to a nerve impulse may vary from none to one or a few. However, the nerve impulse at a normal neuromuscular junction causes the release of the contents of about 200 synaptic vesicles. A further discussion of quantal release may be found in Appendix II.

Miniature end-plate potentials

It is possible to record activity from skeletal muscle fibers even in the absence of nerve impulses in the motor fibers. This activity takes the form of small potentials that have all the electrical and pharmacological properties of end-plate potentials, except that they are small and occur in a random fashion without the need of nerve activity. These have been called miniature end-plate potentials

There is ample evidence that the miniature end-plate potentials represent a leakage of packets of acetylcholine from the motor nerve terminal. The amplitude of a miniature end-plate potential is the same as the amplitude of a quantum sized end-plate potential recorded at a junction treated with a solution containing a reduced calcium or elevated magnesium concentration. Evidently, synaptic vesicles release acetylcholine not only in response to the invasion of the synaptic terminal by a nerve impulse but also occasionally by some kind of spontaneous process. Katz has suggested that synaptic vesicles must attach to the presynaptic membrane at specific release sites in order for release to occur. Perhaps there must be a molecular matching between points on the outer surface of the membranes of the synaptic vesicles and on the inner surface of the presynaptic membrane for release to occur. In the absence of nerve activity, random collisions between the synaptic vesicles and the presynaptic membrane occur that occasionally result in an appropriate match of these sites and in

acetylcholine release. The nerve impulse, perhaps through the influx of calcium ions, may cause a greatly increased number of presynaptic membrane sites and hence an increased number of successful collisions by synaptic vesicles. Evidence for this concept comes from the observation that the rate at which miniature end-plate potentials occur can be influenced by changes in the membrane potential of the presynaptic terminal.

Relationship between miniature end-plate potentials and presynaptic polarization

When the membrane potential of the motor axon terminal at a neuromuscular junction is reduced, the frequency of miniature end-plate potentials as recorded from the muscle fiber is increased (Fig. 3-16). The relationship is not a linear one, however. Liley found that there was a tenfold increase in frequency for every 15 mV of depolarization. He then showed that the depolarization associated with an action potential in the motor axon terminal would speed up the frequency of the miniature end-plate potentials sufficiently to result in the release of a burst of several hundred acetylcholine quanta, thus accounting for the end-plate potential.

Neuromuscular pharmacology

As mentioned, the chemical synaptic transmitter substance at the neuromuscular junction is acetylcholine (Fig. 3-17). The acetylcholine is synthesized by the enzyme choline acetyltransferase. It is stored in synaptic vesicles in the motor axon terminal, and it is released from the storage sites, either in response to the invasion of a nerve action potential into the presynaptic ending or spontaneously. The acetylcholine diffuses across the synaptic cleft and reacts

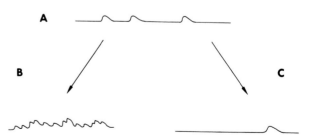

Fig. 3-16. Effect of presynaptic membrane potential on the frequency of miniature end-plate potentials. In **A** the resting rate of miniature end-plate potentials is shown, as recorded from a muscle cell by a microelectrode. In **B** the rate of the miniature end-plate potentials is seen to be greatly elevated by a depolarization of the presynaptic terminal membrane (either by an applied current or by an elevated potassium concentration). In **C** the miniature end-plate potential rate is slowed by hyperpolarization of the terminal.

with acetylcholine receptors associated with the post-synaptic membrane. The reaction between acetylcholine and the acetylcholine receptors appears to result in conformational changes in the muscle membrane structure, which in turn cause an enhanced permeability of the membrane to sodium and potassium ions. The action of the acetylcholine is stopped by several processes. Some of the acetylcholine is probably taken up by the nerve ending by an active transport mechanism. Some may diffuse out of the synaptic cleft into the extracellular space. However, the most significant process at the neuromuscular junction is the hydrolysis of the acetylcholine by the enzyme acetylcholinesterase present at the surface of the muscle membrane. The reaction products of the hy-

drolysis are acetate and choline, neither of which has any significant effect on acetylcholine receptors.

Several drugs can mimic the action of acetylcholine at the neuromuscular junction (Table 3-2). One of these is nicotine, which in low doses has an excitatory action on skeletal muscle (in high doses, it blocks neuromuscular transmission). There are a variety of other substances, including several choline esters, that also have an excitatory or cholinomimetic action on the neuromuscular junction.

A number of important drugs have an influence on neuromuscular transmission (Table 3-2). The sites of possible drug action include the synthesis and storage mechanism, the release mechanism, the acetylcholine receptors, and the acetylcholinesterase. For instance, hemicholinium-3 blocks the synthesis of acetylcholine, presumably by competing for sites of choline uptake. Botulinus toxin, the agent that causes botulism from food contaminated by *Clostridium botulinum*, prevents the release of acetylcholine from motor axon terminals. Curare, the poison used by South American Indians on the tips of blowgun

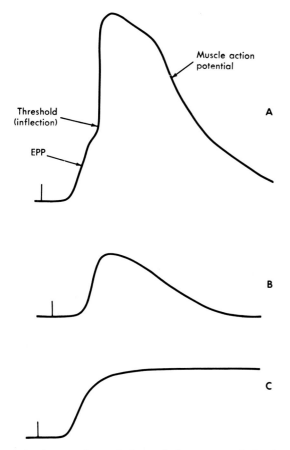

Fig. 3-17. Pharmacology of the end-plate potential. In **A** an end-plate potential *(EPP)* is shown as recorded in a preparation placed in a physiological bathing solution. The end-plate potential is well above threshold for triggering a muscle action potential. The threshold level is indicated by the inflection on the rising phase of the potential sequence. In **B** the end-plate potential is seen alone, because a portion of the acetylcholine receptors has been rendered insensitive to acetylcholine by the addition of curare to the bathing solution. In **C** the end-plate potential has been greatly prolonged by the further addition of an anticholinesterase to the bathing solution.

Table 3-2. Agents that enhance and depress neuromuscular transmission

Substance	Mechanism
Enhancers	
Acetylcholine	Activates acetylcholine receptors
Nicotine (small doses)	Activates acetylcholine receptors
Cholinomimetic drugs	Activate acetylcholine receptors
Anticholinesterases	Prolong the action of acetylcholine
Increased Ca^{++} or decreased Mg^{++}	Increases the amount of acetylcholine released by nerve impulse
Depressors	
Acetylcholine (in presence of anticholinesterase), nicotine (large dose), cholinomimetics (large doses)	Either excessively depolarize muscle membrane (inactivating spiking mechanism) or desensitize acetylcholine receptors or both
Hemicholinium	Interferes with acetylcholine synthesis by blocking uptake of choline by nerve terminal
Local anesthetics	Prevent nerve impulses and thus prevent transmitter release
Botulinus toxin, decreased Ca^{++} or increased Mg^{++}	Decrease the amount of acetylcholine released from nerve terminal
Curare (*d*-tubocurarine)	Competitively blocks acetylcholine receptors

arrows, prevents the reaction of acetylcholine with the acetylcholine receptors by competition for the active sites. Finally, there are several compounds, including eserine and neostigmine, that combine with acetylcholinesterase to prevent it from hydrolyzing acetylcholine. Such agents are called anticholinesterases.

The effect of these various drugs on neuromuscular transmission is generally predictable. Hemicholinium-3, botulinus toxin, and curare all block neuromuscular transmission, although by quite separate mechanisms. Anticholinesterases generally enhance neuromuscular transmission, although this may not be readily demonstrable because there is generally a one-to-one relationship between motor axon discharge and activation of a motor unit contraction. The effect of anticholinesterases in enhancing transmission is best seen in junctions that are fatigued or partially blocked, for example, by curare.

Anticholinesterases have also been employed in investigations of the phenomenon of desensitization in neuromuscular transmission. In the presence of anticholinesterase, acetylcholine may accumulate in excess of normal at the postsynaptic membrane, and the reaction between acetylcholine and the receptor molecules is prolonged. It is believed that the conformational change induced by this reaction (and the subsequent permeability increase) is transient, but that an inactive coupling between acetylcholine and receptor occurs that actually interferes with the further synaptic action of the acetylcholine. This process is called desensitization. Removal of the excess acetylcholine usually leads to a return of the normal functional state.

Recycling of synaptic vesicle membrane

Evidence has recently been reported for a recycling of synaptic vesicle membrane at the neuromuscular junction. Stimulation of the nerve causes a reduction in the population of synaptic vesicles but an increase in the surface area of the terminal. It is presumed that the synaptic vesicles fuse with the surface membrane during the exocytotic process of transmitter release. After a period of stimulation, coated vesicles and membranous cisternae appear in the cytoplasm of the ending. Following a rest period, the cisternae are replaced by new synaptic vesicles. In the meanwhile the surface area of the terminal returns to normal. Horseradish peroxidase molecules, which serve as an electron-dense marker, when introduced into the extracellular space around the synaptic ending appear in the coated vesicles and cisternae shortly after nerve stimulation. Later, they appear in the synaptic vesicles, which suggests that these form from the other organelles. Further stimulation causes the syn-

aptic vesicles to release the peroxidase. Coated vesicles appear to be the initial intermediary in the recycling process. They probably form from membrane adjacent to the release site and then several coalesce to form a cistern. Synaptic vesicles pinch off from the cisternae. In this fashion membrane is conserved, reducing the need for resynthesis and also for disposal. On a longer time scale, however, new synaptic vesicles presumably arrive at the synaptic ending after axoplasmic transport from the neuronal soma, and old membrane is probably removed from the ending by retrograde axoplasmic transport, to be broken down in the soma by lysosomal action.

TROPHIC EFFECTS

Information that contributes in some essential way to the normal maintenance of the innervated cells must be transferred from axon terminals to the innervated cells. This is shown experimentally by the fact that denervation can result in atrophy of an organ, such as muscle, after a certain delay. However, the information transfer occurs between nerve fibers and receptor organs as well as across synapses in the direction of synaptic transmission. Thus, it is not likely that the mechanism involved is related to the release of transmitter substance at synaptic endings. It is possible that the mechanism is related to the general problem of embryonic organizing substances.

The best-studied instance of a trophic influence operating between a nerve and another structure is the neuromuscular junction. Perhaps this is because of the simplicity of the synaptic arrangement as well as the clinical importance of denervation atrophy of muscle. In many muscles, there is a single neuromuscular junction on each muscle fiber. When one axon is interrupted, the entire motor innervation of as many as several hundred muscle fibers may be lost (Fig. 3-18). The entire motor unit is paralyzed. However, the muscle is still contractile unless atrophy becomes advanced. This can be shown by direct stimulation of the muscle.

In some disease states, denervation results from the death of the parent motoneuron. As a motoneuron degenerates, it may discharge spontaneously in an apparently random fashion. With each discharge, the motor unit it supplies will contract, producing a twitch that can be detected visually if the muscle is a surface one or by electromyography if not. This type of sporadic contraction is called a fasciculation (Fig. 3-18).

Whatever the cause of denervation of muscle, after denervation a number of characteristic changes occur in the functional properties of the muscle. The individual muscle fibers develop a hypersensitivity to

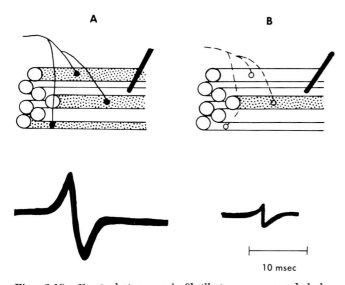

Fig. 3-18. Fasciculations and fibrillations as recorded by electromyography. **A** shows a bundle of muscle fibers, including a motor unit (fibers innervated by a single motor axon). The activity of the motor unit produced by spontaneous discharges of a dying motoneuron is recorded by a wire electrode inserted into the muscle. The motor unit potential shown below is large and complex because of the contribution of a number of individual muscle fiber action potentials. **B** shows a denervated bundle of muscle fibers. The fibrillation potential below is recorded from an individual muscle fiber discharging spontaneously as a result of the changes occurring following denervation. The action potential of the single muscle fiber is small and brief, in contrast to a motor unit potential.

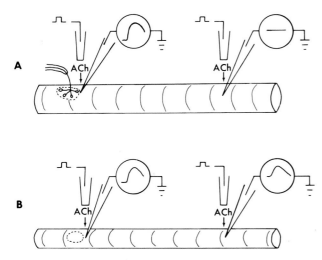

Fig. 3-19. Spread of acetylcholine sensitivity along a muscle membrane following denervation. In **A** the motor innervation of a muscle fiber is intact. Application of a pulse of acetylcholine by microelectrophoresis produces depolarization of the muscle membrane (acetylcholine potential) only when the acetylcholine is released near the end-plate. After denervation, **B**, acetylcholine potentials may be produced all along the muscle membrane.

acetylcholine and substances resembling it (Fig. 3-19). The hypersensitivity appears to be caused by an increased area of the muscle fiber membrane that contains receptor sites activated by acetylcholine. Normally, most of the acetylcholine receptor molecules are confined to the area immediately adjacent to the endplate. After denervation, the sensitivity of the membrane to applied acetylcholine does not change in the region of the end-plate, but spreads along the surface membrane until eventually the entire fiber responds to the drug. This appears to be one mechanism of denervation hypersensitivity.

In addition to an increased sensitivity to acetylcholine, the individual muscle fibers begin to contract spontaneously. The contractions within a motor unit are asynchronous, and so they cannot be detected simply by inspection of the skin over superficial muscles. The best method for detecting these fibrillations is by electromyography (Fig. 3-18).

Because the nerve fibers to a denervated muscle rapidly lose their ability to conduct action potentials as they begin to undergo wallerian degeneration, the electrical responsiveness of the muscle will change. In normal muscle, electrical stimulation frequently produces a contraction indirectly through the nerve, because the intramuscular nerve fibers tend to have a lower threshold to electrical stimulation than do the muscle fibers. This effect is particularly likely if an effort is made to stimulate the muscle in a region known to be traversed by the nerve fibers. The region of greatest sensitivity to percutaneous stimulation of a nerve with faradic currents is known as the motor point, and tests and measurements involving the motor point are made to determine the extent of denervation and the progress of reinnervation in patients who have sustained nerve injuries. Charts of the locations of the motor points were made by the German neurologist Erb. With the use of such charts the reactions of the muscle are observed during faradic stimulation and galvanic stimulation. Faradic stimuli, named after the English physicist Faraday, strictly speaking are the interrupted currents produced by an induction coil, but in terms of practice they are pulses of direct current. Galvanic currents, named after the Italian physiologist Galvani, are direct currents, such as those produced by batteries, with either the anode or cathode applied near the muscle. Using galvanic currents, the normal muscle contracts with a brisk twitch when the circuit is closed. The threshold is normally lowest if the cathode or negative pole is applied to the motor point. The denervated muscle contracts more slowly, with a writhing movement. In addition, anodal currents become relatively more effective in eliciting contraction. These changes and the changes in chronaxie after denervation are spoken of as the reaction of degeneration. They appear about 2 weeks after the injury producing denervation. After complete denervation, the only way to evoke a contraction is by raising the stimulus strength to a point sufficient to activate muscle fibers directly. If a strength-duration curve is plotted and the chronaxie is determined, it will be found that the apparent chronaxie of normal muscle is much shorter than that of denervated muscle. This is understandable because nerve fibers have a shorter chronaxie than do muscle fibers, and it is the nerve chronaxie that is largely being tested in normal muscle. In clinical practice, electromyographic recording of muscle fiber fibrillation potentials with fine needle electrodes inserted into the muscle has largely replaced galvanic testing as a more sensitive and convenient test for denervation and reinnervation.

Another approach to the question of the trophic effect of nerve on muscle has been a series of experiments in which slow and fast muscles were cross reinnervated. Following regeneration of the nerves, slow muscle receiving innervation that had formerly supplied a fast muscle now becomes faster. Conversely, fast muscle reinnervated by a nerve that had supplied slow muscle now becomes slower. Besides the physiological change in contraction time, there are numerous biochemical changes in the cross-reinnervated muscle. For instance, the levels of activity of glycolytic and oxidative enzymes change from those appropriate to the original muscle type to those characteristic of the opposite muscle type.

Evidently the trophic action of nerve on muscle, whatever its mechanism, is continuously active in determining the properties of the muscle. A question for the future is the extent to which muscle and other effector tissue may help determine the connectivity and properties of central nervous tissue.

AUTONOMIC NERVOUS SYSTEM

The autonomic nervous system is concerned with the regulation of visceral functions. It may be divided into the peripheral autonomic nervous system and the central autonomic control centers. The latter are considered in later chapters.

The peripheral autonomic nervous system is classically described as a motor system that controls the activity of smooth muscle, cardiac muscle, and glands. Afferent fibers from visceral structures are associated with reflex mechanisms utilizing discharges in nerve fibers of the autonomic nervous system. To prevent confusion in terminology, however, these afferent fibers are called visceral afferents.

The autonomic nervous system may be subdivided into sympathetic (thoracolumbar) and parasympathetic (craniosacral) portions (Fig. 3-20). These systems differ in a number of ways: in their sites of origin, in the relationship of the location of their peripheral ganglia with respect to the target organs that their fibers innervate, in the transmitter substances secreted at their target organs, and in their actions on their target organs, which are often opposed. In general, the sympathetic nervous system mediates visceral activities that resemble the responses observed in an animal behaving in a "fight or flight" manner. For instance, when there is a general sympathetic discharge, an animal will respond by acceleration of the heart, elevation of the blood pressure, dilation of the pupils, and piloerec-

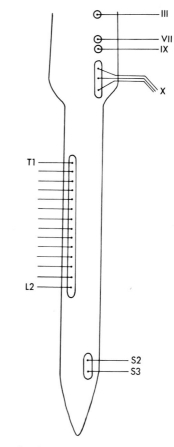

Fig. 3-20. Levels of origin of the preganglionic fibers of the autonomic nervous system. On the left, the origin of the sympathetic nervous system preganglionic fibers is shown to be the intermediolateral cell column of the spinal cord segments from T1 to L2. On the right, the parasympathetic preganglionic fibers are shown to include a cranial portion and a sacral portion. The cranial parasympathetic preganglionic fibers travel with cranial nerves III, VII, IX, and X. The sacral parasympathetic preganglionic fibers arise from the S2 and 3 spinal cord segments (or S3 and 4 in some cases).

tion. On the other hand, the parasympathetic system mediates many of the more placid functions of the viscera. For example, parasympathetic activity is involved in the processes of slowing of the heart and pupillary constriction. Parasympathetic activity is also associated with digestion of food, such as secretion of various digestive glands and intestinal contractions that move food along the digestive tract.

Sympathetic nervous system

Information carried by the sympathetic nervous system to peripheral effector organs, such as smooth muscle of the gut or cardiac muscle, travels along a two-neuron path. The synapse between the two neurons occurs within sympathetic ganglia. The term used for the proximal neuron is preganglionic; the axon of the second neuron is called postganglionic.

The cell bodies of sympathetic preganglionic neurons are located within the spinal cord (Fig. 3-21). They are found at levels between the upper thoracic segments (sometimes eighth cervical) and the upper lumbar segments. The location within the gray matter of sympathetic preganglionic neuron somata includes the intermediolateral cell column. The axons of these preganglionic neurons are finely myelinated fibers of the B type. They leave the cord through the nearest ventral root and enter a neighboring paravertebral sympathetic ganglion through the appropriate white communicating ramus. A given axon may synapse on a ganglion cell of the same ganglion; it may instead turn rostrally or caudally into the sympathetic trunk that joins adjacent paravertebral ganglia and synapse on a ganglion cell at some distance; or it may enter a splanchnic nerve connecting the paravertebral ganglion with a prevertebral ganglion and end on a ganglion cell within it. Generally, a given preganglionic fiber will branch and end on each of several ganglion cells, often in several different ganglia.

The paravertebral ganglia are arranged in an approximately segmental fashion. However, the ganglia derived from some of the embryonic segments become fused during development. For this reason, there are often just three cervical ganglia: the superior, incorporating the first four embryonic segmental ganglia, and the middle and inferior, representing two segments each. The superior cervical ganglion mediates pupillary dilatation and to some extent opening of the upper eyelid (by the superior tarsal muscle). The fused inferior cervical and first thoracic ganglion, called the stellate ganglion, sends postganglionic axons to the arm. The degree of fusion is less at lower levels. There are generally ten or eleven thoracic, four lumbar, four sacral, and one

coccygeal ganglia. The latter is called the ganglion impar (unpaired ganglion) because it serves both sides of the body; the other ganglia are paired.

The ganglia on each side of the body are connected by the sympathetic trunk. This is a fiber bundle that contains preganglionic and postganglionic axons traveling either rostrally or caudally. The sympathetic trunk thus serves as a distribution system. Besides the connections with the sympathetic trunk, each paravertebral ganglion may have other connections. These include white communicating rami in the case of the thoracic and the first two or three lumbar ganglia. As mentioned, the white rami carry preganglionic axons from the ventral roots of the thoracic and upper lumbar spinal cord. These axons originate from the preganglionic cell bodies

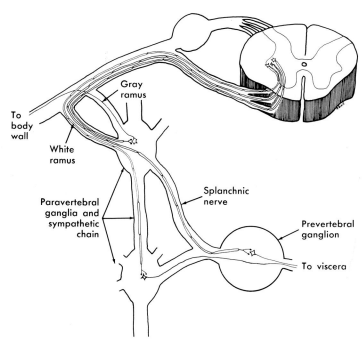

Fig. 3-21. Distribution of the sympathetic nervous system. Sympathetic preganglionic neurons are shown in the intermediolateral cell column of the thoracic spinal cord. The axons of these cells leave the cord through a ventral root and enter a sympathetic paravertebral ganglion through a white communicating ramus. Some of the preganglionic fibers synapse within the ganglion of the same segmental level, and some travel up or down the sympathetic chain to an adjacent ganglion. Postganglionic fibers arising from ganglion cells may join a spinal nerve by passing through a gray communicating ramus; these supply smooth muscle and glands of the body wall (including extremities). Other postganglionic fibers travel through a splanchnic nerve to innervate viscera of the body cavities. Some preganglionic fibers travel through splanchnic nerves to prevertebral ganglia, where they synapse. Postganglionic fibers originating from prevertebral ganglia supply smooth muscle and glands of the viscera.

in the intermediolateral cell column of the same segments. In addition, each ganglion may have a gray communicating ramus, which is the pathway followed by postganglionic fibers entering spinal nerves to be distributed to structures of the body surface. There may also be one or more splanchnic nerves, which carry preganglionic and postganglionic axons to the various autonomic plexuses of the viscera. Some of the splanchnic nerves are large enough to be named, for example, the superior, middle, and inferior cardiac nerves from the respective cervical sympathetic ganglia. The greater splanchnic, lesser splanchnic, and least splanchnic nerves arise from the fifth through the ninth, and tenth to eleventh, and the last thoracic ganglia respectively. The greater and lesser splanchnic nerves join the coeliac plexus, while the least splanchnic nerve ends in the renal plexus.

Parasympathetic nervous system

There are two widely separated portions of the parasympathetic nervous system. The cranial part is associated with several of the cranial nerves. The other part originates from the sacral spinal cord (S2 and 3 or S3 and 4). In general, the cranial parasympathetic nervous system supplies structures of the head, neck, thorax, and part of the abdomen, whereas the sacral parasympathetic nervous system innervates the remainder of the abdomen and the pelvis. The dividing line between the territories of the cranial and sacral supplies within the abdomen is about the level of the transverse colon. The descending colon and rectum are supplied by sacral parasympathetics. The extremities do not appear to receive a parasympathetic innervation.

In contrast to the sympathetic nervous system, in which postganglionic fibers may be of considerable length, the parasympathetic nervous system is organized in such a way that its ganglia are adjacent to the organs innervated, and the postganglionic fibers are relatively short (Fig. 3-22).

The cranial nerves that contain parasympathetic preganglionic fibers are the oculomotor, facial, glossopharyngeal, and vagus nerves. The central nervous system nuclei of origin of these fibers are considered in Chapter 6. Many of the preganglionic fibers synapse in one of the parasympathetic ganglia of the head. The preganglionic axons in the oculomotor nerve, for example, pass through the motor root of the ciliary ganglion to synapse within the ganglion. The postganglionic axons emerge from the ganglion in the short ciliary nerves and enter the eye. They supply some of the intrinsic muscles of the eye and the blood vessels. The other parasympathetic ganglia of

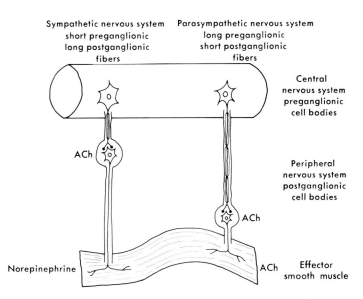

Fig. 3-22. Relative lengths of preganglionic and postganglionic fibers of sympathetic and parasympathetic nervous system and neural transmitters. The preganglionic neurons of the sympathetic nervous system have axons of relatively short length, whereas the postganglionic axons are relatively long. The situation is reversed in the parasympathetic nervous system, where the preganglionic axons are long and the postganglionic axons short. The synaptic transmitter used by both systems at the junction between preganglionic and postganglionic neurons is acetylcholine. The postganglionic neuron of the sympathetic nervous system uses norepinephrine as its transmitter (usually), and that of the parasympathetic postganglionic neuron is acetylcholine.

the head include the sphenopalatine ganglion (receiving preganglionic fibers of the facial nerve and supplying the glands of the nasal and pharyngeal mucous membranes), the submaxillary ganglion (facial preganglionics, supplying the submaxillary and sublingual glands), and the otic ganglion (receiving preganglionic fibers from the glossopharyngeal nerve and supplying the parotid gland). The vagus nerve is not associated with a parasympathetic ganglion in the head but with ganglia and plexuses in the walls of the many organs that it innervates. For instance, its preganglionic fibers end synaptically on ganglion cells of the myenteric and submucosal plexuses of the wall of the intestinal tract. The preganglionic fibers of the sacral division have a similar relationship to the lower abdominal and pelvic viscera.

Structure of autonomic ganglia

There is little if any difference in the structure of sympathetic and parasympathetic ganglia at the gross or light microscopic level, although the parasympathetic plexuses in the walls of viscera include only scattered nerve cell bodies in contrast to the more compact ganglia.

The autonomic ganglion typically consists of a collection of multipolar neurons, their associated satellite glial cells, and a connective tissue capsule. Attached to the ganglion are nerve bundles consisting of preganglionic nerve fibers entering the ganglion, postganglionic fibers arising from nerve cells within the ganglion, and afferent and efferent fibers of passage. As a rule, the preganglionic autonomic fibers are small myelinated fibers (B fibers), and the postganglionic ones are unmyelinated (C fibers). However, there are exceptions to this generalization. The ganglion serves as a point of synaptic connection between preganglionic and postganglionic neurons in the pathways of autonomic outflow. Numerous synapses on the long dendrites of the main population of neurons within the ganglion have been observed with the electron microscope. There are also some synapses on the cell bodies. The majority of these synapses are undoubtedly between preganglionic and postganglionic neurons, but there may also be functional contact between the processes of postganglionic neurons. Furthermore, there is evidence for the presence of interneurons within the ganglion. It is probable that ganglia serve an integrative function in addition to their role in the relaying of autonomic information to effector cells.

Synaptic transmission in autonomic ganglia

Much of the work that has been done on synaptic transmission in autonomic ganglia has focused on the mammalian or the amphibian sympathetic ganglion as a model system. The basic features that have recently been described from studies using intracellular recordings from postganglionic neurons are similar for both the mammal and the amphibian.

A volley in preganglionic fibers produces the following sequence of postsynaptic potentials in some ganglion cells: an excitatory postsynaptic potential of brief latency, followed by an inhibitory or excitatory postsynaptic potential of long latency (Fig. 3-23).

In the rabbit superior cervical sympathetic ganglion, graded stimulation of the sympathetic trunk produces a graded early excitatory postsynaptic potential, indicating convergence of several preganglionic fibers on a single postganglionic neuron. Maximal stimulation of the preganglionic fiber bundle can fire a given cell once or twice. Many cells generate late inhibitory and excitatory postsynaptic potentials, especially with repetitive stimulation of the preganglionic fibers. It is sometimes possible to elicit a slow inhibitory postsynaptic potential without the

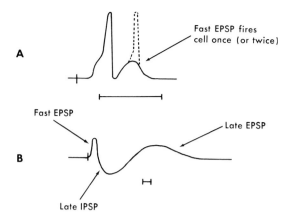

Fig. 3-23. Responses of a postganglionic neuron to a preganglionic volley. **A** shows the response of a postganglionic neuron to a volley in preganglionic axons. The preparation is bathed with a physiological electrolyte solution. The chief response seen is an excitatory postsynaptic potential (EPSP) that elicits one or two action potentials. The latency of the EPSP is brief, as indicated by the time mark. **B** shows the response of the same neuron on a slower sweep. The time mark represents the same interval as in **A**. In this case, synaptic transmission is depressed by curare. The short latency EPSP follows the shock artifact. After this, there is an inhibitory postsynaptic potential (IPSP) and a late excitatory postsynaptic potential.

initial brief latency excitatory postsynaptic potential. This suggests the possibility of specific inhibitory pathways to particular autonomic ganglion cells.

Another line of investigation has been the analysis of synaptic transmission in the avian ciliary ganglion. Although this is an example of a parasympathetic ganglion, it is not clear how representative it is. The preganglionic fibers in the ciliary ganglion of the chick form large, calyxlike synapses on the postganglionic cells. The membrane of the presynaptic element encloses nearly half the spherical cell body of the postganglionic cell. Intracellular recordings have shown that transmission across this synapse occurs by two mechanisms; in addition to chemical transmission, there is electrical transmission across this synapse.

Pharmacology of ganglionic transmission

The synaptic transmitter responsible for the excitation of postganglionic neurons by preglanglionic fibers is acetylcholine. This is true for both sympathetic and parasympathetic ganglia.

There are two types of receptors sites for acetylcholine (Fig. 3-24). These can be distinguished by studying the types of compounds, in addition to acetylcholine, that will activate them and by determining which drugs block their activation. The names classically given to the two kinds of cholinergic receptors

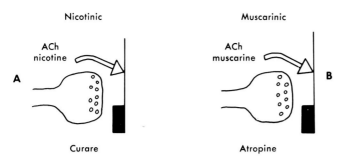

Fig. 3-24. Two kinds of acetylcholine receptors. The synaptic endings shown both release acetylcholine (ACh). The postsynaptic membrane in **A** responds both to ACh and to nicotine, but not to muscarine. The response of the receptors can be blocked by curare. The receptors are described as nicotinic. The postsynaptic membrane in **B** responds to ACh and to muscarine, but not to nicotine. The response can be blocked by atropine. The receptors are called muscarinic.

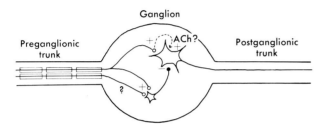

Fig. 3-25. Possible synaptic actions within a sympathetic ganglion. Preganglionic fibers are shown terminating synaptically on a postganglionic neuron and on an interneuron. The transmitter released by the preganglionic endings is acetylcholine. This excites the neurons by a nicotinic action. It is possible that acetylcholine from the same preganglionic terminal produces the late excitatory postsynaptic potential by an action on muscarinic receptors. The inhibitory transmitter may be dopamine that is released from the endings of the interneuron.

(activated by acetylcholine) are nicotinic and muscarinic, the former being activated by nicotine and the latter by muscarine, two alkaloids extracted from plants. Nicotinic receptors can be blocked by curare; muscarinic receptors are rendered inactive by atropine. A variety of other drugs have actions at one or both of these kinds of receptors.

Some of the sites in the body that are known to have nicotinic synapses include the neuromuscular junctions on skeletal muscle and the synapses between preganglionic and postganglionic neurons within autonomic ganglia. An important muscarinic synapse is that between postganglionic neurons of the vagus nerve and cardiac muscle fibers. Although the nicotinic synapses mentioned are excitatory and the muscarinic one is inhibitory, there is no necessary connection between the type of cholinergic

synapse and the sign of the synaptic action. For instance, there are excitatory muscarinic synapses on smooth muscle and on gland cells.

The nicotinic synapse between preganglionic and postganglionic neurons in autonomic ganglia is the one responsible for the production of brief latency excitatory postsynaptic potentials (Fig. 3-25). This is the most significant of the two kinds of excitatory events in the ganglion cells. The late excitatory postsynaptic potentials seem also to be produced by acetylcholine, but the receptors are muscarinic, being blocked by atropine and not by curare. The mechanism by which the late excitation is produced is not clear, although diffusion of acetylcholine within the ganglion to sensitive areas on the membranes of the postganglionic cells away from the synapse made by preganglionic axons is a possibility. The action of acetylcholine in autonomic ganglia is terminated primarily by the hydrolysis of the transmitter by acetylcholinesterase.

The inhibitory postsynaptic potentials in postganglionic neurons appear to be produced by another synaptic transmitter, perhaps dopamine. Inhibition within autonomic ganglia may thus be adrenergic (produced by a compound resembling epinephrine). It seems likely that the inhibition in ganglia is mediated by the interneurons that have been observed among the postganglionic neurons. These interneurons resemble chromaffin cells and hence may secrete a catecholamine, such as dopamine.

Structure of postganglionic synapses on effector cells

Postganglionic axons may be seen to enter layers of smooth muscle, the parenchyma of glands, or heart muscle. However, there are no discrete synaptic regions in these structures. It appears that the postganglionic fibers release transmitter at regions of the axons that are bare of their Schwann cell sheath. Otherwise, there is no fine structural correlate of regions of synapse. The transmitter presumably diffuses in the extracellular space and acts at receptor sites within the effector organs, often at a considerable distance from the nerve. Evidently, a given nerve fiber may have an action on a large number of effector organ cells.

Synaptic transmission at postganglionic junctions

Both excitatory and inhibitory postsynaptic potentials have been recorded from effector cells following activation of postganglionic nerve fibers. For instance, stimulation of the sympathetic postganglionic fibers to the vas deferens has been shown to cause the generation of excitatory postsynaptic potentials in the smooth muscle cells of that organ. The excitatory potentials resemble those of the skeletal neuromuscular junction, except that they are slower and the time courses of excitatory potentials in a given smooth muscle cell vary greatly because the sites of generation are distributed at varying distances from the point of recording.

The effect of the parasympathetic postganglionic fibers in the pathway from the vagus nerve to the heart is inhibitory. The inhibitory postsynaptic potential produced by these postganglionic cells can be recorded from cardiac muscle fibers of the atrium. The characteristics of the inhibitory postsynaptic potential have been well studied. It is caused by an increased permeability of the membrane for potassium ions. Its action is to slow the development of the pacemaker potential, which triggers the cardiac action potential to initiate contraction.

Pharmacology of postganglionic transmission

In general, the synaptic transmitter substance utilized by postganglionic neurons of the parasympathetic nervous system is acetylcholine. There may be exceptions to this, however. The receptors on the effector cells for parasympathetic action are muscarinic (see the section on the pharmacology of ganglionic transmission, p. 81). Thus, the action of acetycholine released by postganglionic fibers of the vagus can be blocked by atropine.

The transmitter used by most postganglionic neurons of the sympathetic nervous system is norepinephrine. The synapses employing norepinephrine are called adrenergic synapses. As with acetylcholine, there are two different kinds of receptors, named alpha and beta receptors, for adrenergic agents such as norepinephrine (Fig. 3-26). They are distinguished by the potency of certain drugs in activating them and by the ability of certain agents to block their activation. Norepinephrine has a greater action at alpha receptors than at beta receptors in comparison with other adrenergic compounds, such as isoproterenol. Beta receptors are more powerfully activated by isoproterenol than by norepinephrine. An example of a drug that can block alpha adrenergic receptors is phenoxybenzamine. One that blocks beta receptors is propranolol.

There are several mechanisms by which the action of norepinephrine is normally terminated. An important one is the reuptake of norepinephrine into the synaptic ending by a process of active transport. Norepinephrine may also be broken down by monamine oxidase, which is located within the presynaptic terminals, or by inactivation by the enzyme catechol-

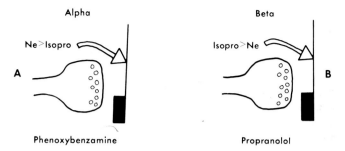

Fig. 3-26. Two kinds of adrenergic receptor. There are at least two types of receptors that respond to agents resembling epinephrine (adrenaline). These are called alpha and beta adrenergic receptors. In the drawing, both the synapses release an agent that acts on adrenergic receptors. However, for a test of the type of receptor, drugs that act on the receptors are administered. An important drug for differentiating between alpha and beta adrenergic receptors is isoproterenol. In general, norepinephrine (Ne) exerts a much greater action on alpha receptors than does isoproterenol (Isopro), whereas the reverse is true for beta receptors. Epinephrine has an action intermediate between that of norepinephrine and isoproterenol. Another way to distinguish between actions on alpha and beta receptors is by use of blocking agents that are specific for one or the other kind of receptor. Phenoxybenzamine blocks alpha receptors and so is called an alpha blocker; propranolol is a beta blocker.

o-methyltransferase, located in the extracelluar spaces of various organs and in glial cells.

Although most sympathetic postganglionic neurons release norepinephrine at their junctions with effector organs, it is said that the terminals on sweat glands release acetylcholine. However, there is now evidence for both a cholinergic and an adrenergic mechanism at sweat glands.

Denervation supersensitivity

When ganglia or autonomic effector organs are denervated, the receptors on the postsynaptic membranes become supersensitive to the agent that was formerly the transmitter substance and to related compounds. There may be several underlying mechanisms. The apparent increase in number of acetylcholine receptors on denervated muscle has been mentioned in the section on trophic effects (p. 77). A similar increase in the numbers of receptors has recently been demonstrated at autonomic synapses following denervation. Another factor, at least at synapses utilizing norepinephrine, is the removal of the active transport mechanism for the reuptake of norepinephrine into the presynaptic ending. Without the presynaptic ending, an applied dose would presumably be more effective. Other mechanisms may also play a role.

Clinical applications

The neuropharmacology of the autonomic nervous system is of great importance in medical practice (see also Chapter 9 and 10). The subject of the clinical use of drugs that act at peripheral, ganglionic, and central autonomic synapses for the control of hypertension and other autonomic disorders is beyond the scope of this book; however, there are several points about procedures carried out on the peripheral autonomic nerves and ganglia that should be stressed here.

Portions of the autonomic outflow can be selectively blocked by the percutaneous injection of local anesthetics around the sympathetic ganglia. This procedure is usually carried out to produce vasodilatation and improve blood flow in an arm or leg for therapeutic or diagnostic purposes. The stellate ganglion is blocked by percutaneous injection at the root of the neck just below the carotid tubercle of the C6 vertebra (see Chapter 5). This produces partial block of sympathetic activity to the ipsilateral face and arm. The lumbar sympathetic ganglia are blocked at L1, 2, 3, and 4 by paravertebral injections carried out lateral to the vertebral column. This produces a partial block of sympathetic activity to the leg. These blocks produce a warm, dry limb. Stellate block also produces Horner's syndrome of miosis, ptosis, and enophthalmos (constricted pupil, drooping lid, and slightly sunken eyeball, which is usually less noticeable).

Permanent sympathetic denervation can be produced by surgical sympathectomy. An important point is that, whenever possible, only the preganglionic fibers are cut. This procedure interrupts centrally mediated vasoconstrictor and sweating responses during central sympathetic discharge but leaves the target organ innervated by postganglionic fibers. This prevents the target organs from developing denervation supersensitivity and from hyperreacting to catecholamines circulating in the bloodstream, which may be one reason for the failure of sympathetic denervation to control the symptoms for which it was performed.

The sympathetic nerves may also be blocked or cut to interrupt the afferent sensory fibers that travel with them and carry pain impulses from the viscera. Such denervations are not much used at present but have been carried out for relief of pain of visceral malignancies and for relief of angina (cardiac pain produced by ischemia caused by coronary blood flow insufficiency).

"Referred" pain is probably mediated by sensory fibers traveling with the peripheral autonomic nerves. Referred pain designates pain produced by ischemia or pressure on the viscera and is felt as somatic pain in an adjacent part of the body. For example, myocardial ischemia or infarction may be felt as severe aching pain radiating from the chest into the left arm or as pain radiating upward into the lower jaw. The site of interaction of visceral and somatic sensory activity that gives rise to referred pain is not definitely known. Visceral afferents in the sympathetic nerves and cutaneous afferents can interact within the dorsal horn of the spinal cord by excitation of cells giving rise to the ascending tract mediating pain, the spinothalamic tract (see Chapter 7). Inasmuch as such tract cells are rarely likely to be excited by visceral input except when visceral pathology occurs, the individual probably associates the activation of such cells with cutaneous pain. When visceral pain does occur, it is interpreted as pain originating from the body surface rather than from the viscera.

Causalgia is a clinically important and neurophysiologically interesting condition, possibly with an interaction of the sympathetic motor and somatic sensory afferent fibers in peripheral nerves. Causalgia is the burning and frequently excruciating pain that can develop in the cutaneous distribution of a peripheral nerve following crushing or partial section of the nerve. The condition was vividly described by the neurologist Weir Mitchell, with G. R. Morehouse and W. W. Keen, in a book recording their observations of nerve injuries sustained by Union soldiers in the Civil War, *Gunshot Wounds and Other Injuries of Nerves*, published in Philadelphia in 1864. The book is also interesting for their deductions about spinal cord functions at a time when the reflex activity of the spinal cord was very poorly understood.

Causalgia is more prone to develop after injuries of the median nerve in the arm and the tibial nerve in the leg than after injuries of the other nerves in the limbs. The pain of causalgia can very frequently be relieved by sympathetic nerve block. The reason for this is not known with certainty. The best explanation at present is based on results of experiments in which it was found that action potentials of efferent fibers could set up activity in afferent fibers by depolarizing the afferent fibers at the site of a crush injury.

Excitation of neurons by the depolarization of adjacent neurons is called ephaptic transmission. Although ephaptic effects can be produced experimentally, it is not known if they actually do occur in normal or disease states. However, a hypothesis concerning causalgia is that the tonic barrage of descending impulses in sympathetic fibers evokes ascending impulses in pain fibers at the site of the injury and that sympathetic nerve block stops the ephaptic transmission.

The pain of causalgia can also be suppressed by selective stimulation of the A fibers in the injured nerve, which produces a buzzing sensation and abolishes the pain for minutes or hours. The mechanism of this effect is not understood but may involve the inhibition of cells of the pain pathway (see Chapter 7).

BIBLIOGRAPHY

Axelrod, J.: The metabolism of catecholamines in vivo and in vitro, Pharmacol. Rev. **11:**402-408, 1959.

Birks, R. I., Huxley, H. E., and Katz, B.: The fine structure of the neuromuscular junction of the frog, J. Physiol. (Lond.) **150:**134-144, 1960.

Birks, R., and MacIntosh, F. C.: Acetylcholine metabolism of a sympathetic ganglion, Can. J. Biochem. **39:**787-827, 1961.

Blair, E. A., and Erlanger, J.: A comparison of the characteristics of axons through their individual electrical responses, Am. J. Physiol. **106:**524-564, 1933.

Bryant, S. H.: Transmission in squid giant synapses; the importance of oxygen supply and the effects of drugs, J. Gen. Physiol. **41:**473-484, 1958.

Burn, J. H., and Rand, M. J.: The cause of the supersensitivity of smooth muscle to noradrenaline after sympathetic degeneration, J. Physiol. (Lond.) **147:**135-143, 1959.

Burnstock, G., and Holman, M. E.: Spontaneous potentials at sympathetic nerve endings in smooth muscle, J. Physiol. (Lond.) **160:**446-460, 1962.

Clifton, G. L., Vance, W. H., Applebaum, M. L., Coggeshall, R. E., and Willis, W. D.: Responses of unmyelinated afferents in the mammalian ventral root, Brain Res. **82:**163-167, 1974.

Coggeshall, R. E., Coulter, J. D., and Willis, W. D.: Unmyelinated axons in the ventral roots of the cat lumbosacral enlargement, J. Comp. Neurol. **153:**39-58, 1974.

Couteaux, R.: Localization of cholinesterases at neuromuscular junction, Int. Rev. Cytol. **4:**335-375, 1955.

del Castillo, J., and Katz, B.: Quantal components of the end-plate potential, J. Physiol. (Lond.) **124:**560-573, 1954.

del Castillo, J., and Katz, B.: Statistical factors involved in neuromuscular facilitation and depression, J. Physiol. (Lond.) **124:**574-585, 1954.

Eccles, J. C.: The physiology of synapses, Berlin, 1964, Springer-Verlag

Eccles, R. M., and Libet, B.: Origin and blockade of the synaptic responses of curarized sympathetic ganglion, J. Physiol. (Lond.) **157:**484-503, 1961.

Fatt, P., and Katz, B.: Spontaneous subthreshold activity at motor nerve endings, J. Physiol. (Lond.) **117:**109-128, 1952.

Gasser, H. S., and Grundfest, H.: Axon diameters in relation to the spike dimensions and the conduction velocity in mammalian A fibers, Am. Physiol. **127:**393-414, 1939.

Goodman, L. S., and Gilman, A.: The pharmacological basis of therapeutics, New York, 1965, The Macmillan Co.

Grundfest, H.: The properties of mammalian B fibers, Am. J. Physiol. **127:**252-262, 1939.

Guth, L.: "Trophic" influences of nerve on muscle, Physiol. Rev. **48:**645-687, 1968.

Hagiwara, S., and Tasaki, I.: A study of the mechanism of impulse transmission across the giant synapse of the squid, J. Physiol. (Lond.) **143:**114-137, 1958.

Hancock, M. B., Foreman, R. D., and Willis, W. D.: Convergence of visceral and cutaneous input onto spinothalamic tract cells in the thoracic spinal cord of the cat, Exp. Neurol. **47:**240-248, 1975.

Heuser, J. E., and Reese, T. S.: Evidence for recycling of synaptic vesicle membrane during transmitter release at the frog neuromuscular junction, J. Cell Biol. **57:**315-344, 1973.

Hillarp, N. A.: Peripheral autonomic mechanisms. In Field, J., editor: Handbook of physiology, sec. 1, neurophysiology, vol. II, Washington, D.C., 1960, American Physiological Society, pp. 979-1006.

Hursh, J. B.: Conduction velocity and diameter of nerve fibers, Am. J. Physiol. **127:**131-139, 1939.

Katz, B.: Nerve, muscle and synapse, New York, 1966, McGraw-Hill Book Co.

Katz, B.: The release of neural transmitter substances, Springfield, Ill., 1969, Charles C Thomas, Publisher.

Katz, B., and Miledi, R.: The measurement of synaptic delay, and the time course of acetylcholine release at the neuromuscular junction, Proc. R. Soc. Lond. (Biol.) **161:**483-495, 1965.

Katz, B., and Miledi, R.: A study of synaptic transmission in the absence of nerve impulses, J. Physiol. (Lond.) **192:**407-436, 1967.

Katz, B., and Miledi, R.: Tetrodotoxin-resistant electric activity in presynaptic terminals, J. Physiol. (Lond.) **203:**459-487, 1969.

Katz, B., and Miledi, R.: Further study of the role of calcium in synaptic transmission, J. Physiol. (Lond.) **207:**789-801, 1970.

Katz, B., and Thesleff, S.: A study of the "desensitization" produced by acetylcholine at the motor end-plate, J. Physiol. (Lond.) **138:**63-80, 1957.

Katz, B., and Thesleff, S.: The interaction between edrophronium (Tensilon) and acetylcholine at the motor end-plate, Br. J. Pharmacol. **12:**260-264, 1957.

Kuntz, A.: Autonomic nervous system, Philadelphia, 1953, Lea & Febiger.

Liley, A. W.: The effects of presynaptic polarization on the spontaneous activity at the mammalian neuromuscular junction, J. Physiol. (Lond.) **134:**427-443, 1956.

Lloyd, D. P. C., and Chang, H. T.: Afferent fibers in muscle nerves, J. Neurophysiol. **11:**199-208, 1948.

Martin, A. R.: Quantal nature of synaptic transmission, Physiol. Rev. **46:**51-67, 1966.

McLennan, H.: Synaptic transmission, Philadelphia, 1963, W. B. Saunders Co.

Miledi, R., and Slater, C. R.: The action of calcium on neuronal synapses in the squid, J. Physiol. (Lond.) **184:**473-498, 1966.

Norberg, K. A., and Sjoquist, F.: New possibilities for adrenergic modulation of ganglionic transmission, Pharmacol. Rev. **18:**743-751, 1966.

Ranson, S. W.: The structure of the spinal ganglia, and of the spinal nerves, J. Comp. Neurol. **22:**159-175, 1912.

Rexed, B., and Therman, P. O.: Calibre spectra of motor and sensory nerve fibers to flexor and extensor muscles, J. Neurophysiol. **11:**133-139, 1948.

Sherrington, C. S.: Notes on the arrangement of some motor fibers in the lumbosacral plexus, J. Physiol. (Lond.) **13:**621-772, 1892.

Sherrington, C. S.: Experiments in examination of the peripheral distribution of the fibers of the posterior roots of some spinal nerves, Philos. Trans. R. Soc. Lond. **190:**45-186, 1898.

Takeuchi, A., and Takeuchi, N.: Further analysis of relationship between end-plate potential and end-plate current, J. Neurophysiol. **23:**397-402, 1960.

Takeuchi, A., and Takeuchi, N.: Electrical changes in pre-

and postsynaptic axons of the giant synapse of Loligo, J. Gen. Physiol. **45**:1181-1193, 1962.

Thesleff, S.: The effects of acetylcholine, decamethonium and succinylcholine on neuromuscular transmission in the rat, Acta Physiol. Scand. **34**:386-392, 1955.

von Euler, U. S.: Autonomic neuroeffector transmission. In Field, J., editor: Handbook of physiology, sec. 1, neurophysiology, vol. I, Washington, D.C., 1959, American Physiological Society, pp. 215-237.

Werman, R.: A review-criteria for identification of a central nervous system transmitter, Comp. Biochem. Physiol. **18**:745-767, 1966.

White, J. D., Smithwick, R. H., and Simeone, F. A.: The autonomic nervous system; anatomy, physiology and surgical applications, New York, 1952, The Macmillan Co.

CHAPTER 4

The spinal cord

STRUCTURE

The central nervous system is composed of the brain and the spinal cord. The brain lies within the skull; the spinal cord lies in the vertebral canal. The two structures join at the level of the foramen magnum. Peripheral nerves are connected with the spinal cord through the spinal roots. The dorsal roots contain primary afferent fibers, which innervate sensory re-ceptor organs. The cell bodies of the primary afferent fibers are in dorsal root ganglia. The ventral roots contain motor (efferent) fibers. These pass either directly to skeletal muscle, in the case of somatic motor fibers, or synapse within autonomic ganglia, in the case of autonomic preganglionic fibers.

The spinal cord is typical of central nervous system tissue in that it consists of both white and gray matter. White matter is characterized by the presence of axons and oligodendroglia and by the absence of neuron cell bodies. Many of the axons are myelinated by the oligodendroglia, and the color of white matter comes from the abundance of myelin. Fibrous astrocytes may also be found in white matter. Gray matter contains axons, both myelinated and unmyelinated, but it is characterized by the presence of neuronal cell bodies and the bulk of dendrites. There are in addition oligodendroglia and protoplasmic astrocytes in gray matter. The color of gray matter is determined in part by the neuronal and neuroglial components and the relative paucity of myelin; it is also in part determined by the higher vascularity of gray as opposed to white matter.

The neuronal cell bodies of gray matter are usually not uniformly distributed. In some areas, the cell bodies form layers. This is true in the spinal cord, especially in the dorsal regions of the spinal cord gray matter, but layering is even more striking in several regions of the brain. In other areas, cell bodies of neurons having a similar function may form a cluster or a column. Either grouping of central nervous system neurons is called a nucleus (to be distinguished from the organelle). In the peripheral nervous system, a similar grouping of neurons is called a ganglion.

Between nerve cell bodies within nuclei there is a tangle of nerve cell processes and associated neuroglial processes. This tangle is called the neuropil. The nerve cell processes include dendritic branches from the neurons of the nucleus and axon terminals from other regions of the central nervous system. The terminals synapse on the cell bodies and dendrites of the neurons of the nucleus. Thus, the neuropil is rich in synapses. The neuroglial processes in the neuropil include oligodendroglial sheaths forming myelin about some myelinated fibers, but perhaps the main constituent is astrocytic processes. There is some evidence that these form organized compartments within the neuropil, selectively grouping sets of axon terminals and their synapses from other elements of the neuropil.

Embryology

The adult spinal cord is derived with little change in basic plan from the neural tube of the embryo. As outlined in Chapter 1, the neural tube is formed by an infolding of the surface ectoderm of the neural plate. The neural groove deepens, then the neural folds pinch off to form the neural tube. Cells adjacent to the neural groove separate to become the neural crest. Cells of the neural crest form the dorsal root ganglia, and those of the neural tube form the spinal cord proper (Fig. 4-1).

The layering of the neural tube begins with the ependymal layer, the cells immediately around the lumen of the neural tube. This is the germinal layer of the neural tube. Primitive cells of the ependymal layer undergo mitosis and give rise to precursor cells of neurons and neuroglia. Many of the precursor cells migrate outward from the ependymal layer to form the mantle layer. As neurons differentiate, their axons grow out away from the cell bodies. Neurons forming propriospinal connections or tracts that will ascend to the brain project their axons into the outer, or marginal, layer. Motoneurons send their axons into the developing ventral roots.

The lumen of the neural tube soon becomes the diamond-shaped central canal. The groove on each side is called the sulcus limitans. The developing gray matter dorsolateral to the sulcus limitans is called the alar plate. The alar plate becomes associated with sensory functions. Its mantle layer develops into the dorsal horn, and afferent fibers from the neurons of the dorsal root ganglion grow in through the developing dorsal roots to terminate within the alar plate region. The gray matter ventrolateral to the sulcus limitans is called the basal plate. Its mantle layer is primarily motor in function, because it contains the developing motoneurons. The regions just dorsal and ventral to the central canal are the roof and floor plates respectively.

As development progresses, the mantle layer of the neural tube becomes the gray matter of the spinal cord; the marginal layer becomes the white matter. The subdivisions of gray and white matter are discussed later. After the neural tube closes completely, the lengthwise growth of the spinal cord is limited. The elongation of the vertebral canal is greater than that of the spinal cord during fetal life and infancy. This process results in the termination of the spinal cord at about the level of the interspace between the first and second lumbar vertebrae in the adult. In the infant the cord terminates about a vertebral segment lower.

Meninges and cerebrospinal fluid

Like the rest of the central nervous system, the spinal cord is covered by three protective connective tissue coats, the meninges (Fig. 4-2). These are the dura mater, the arachnoid, and the pia mater. There is often a quantity of fat, called the epidural fat,

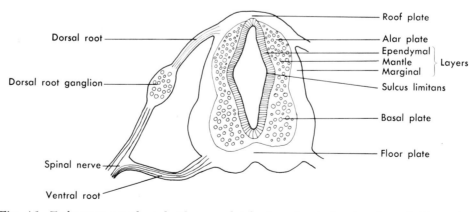

Fig. 4-1. Embryonic spinal cord. The neural tube has closed, forming the primitive spinal cord. The drawing shows the dorsal root, dorsal root ganglion, ventral root, and spinal nerve connecting the spinal cord with the peripheral nerves. The central canal shows a sulcus limitans, which separates the alar and basal plates. The roof and floor plates are above and below the central canal. The layers of the neural tube include the ependymal, mantle, and marginal layers.

outside the dura. There is also a plexus of veins within the vertebral canal outside the dura. Beneath the dura is a narrow cleft, the subdural space. Between the arachnoid and the pia is the subarachnoid space. This contains cerebrospinal fluid because it is continuous with the subarachnoid space about the brain (see Chapter 5).

The dura mater is composed of a dense layer of fibrous connective tissue. It is relatively avascular. The arachnoid is made up of a delicate sheath of fibrous connective tissue, as is the pia mater. The pia is closely adherent to the nervous tissue, dipping into each crevice and following its surface exactly, whereas the arachnoid is loosely adherent, bridging over any folds or crevices. Strands of connective tissue bridge the subarachnoid space, linking the arachnoid and pia. Numerous blood vessels enter and leave the spinal cord through the pia-arachnoid. Along the lateral edges of the spinal cord the pia thickens to form a pair of denticulate, or dentate, ligaments. The denticulate ligament is attached to the dura at each segmental level a half segment lower than the pair of exiting dorsal and ventral roots, thus providing support for the spinal cord. Also at the caudal end of the cord the pia thickens to form another supportive structure, the filum terminale. This passes caudally, merges with dura, and inserts on the coccyx. Support for the cord is also provided by the spinal roots, which pick up sleeves of dura as they leave the vertebral cord. The dura fuses with the epineurium of the spinal nerves.

The subarachnoid space is narrow along the length of the spinal cord. However, it becomes distended at levels below the caudal end of the cord. The lumbar cistern is formed by the distended region of subarachnoid space about the roots in the lower lumbar portion of the vertebral canal. The lumbar cistern is the most available site for obtaining samples of cerebrospinal fluid. The procedure used for this is

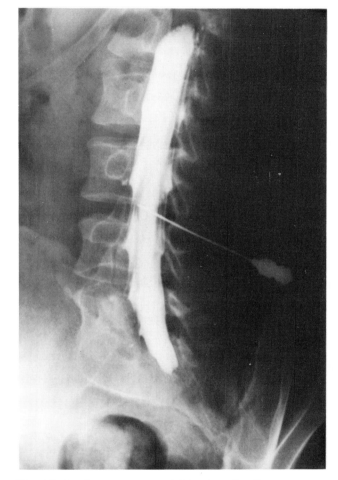

Fig. 4-3. Lumbar puncture and injection of radiopaque water-insoluble contrast medium into the spinal subarachnoid space (myelography). Note that the tip of the needle is touching and laterally displacing two nerve roots of the cauda equina descending parallel to each other. The nerve roots appear within the contrast medium as filling defects, dark streaks that are outlined by the contrast medium. The pedicles of the right side of the vertebral column are seen end-on as oval shadows in this oblique view of the spine. Note the course of the roots as they descend ventrally and laterally to loop around the pedicles of the vertebrae before exiting through intervertebral foramina. The scalloped lateral expansions of the column of contrast medium are the axillary pouches of the nerve roots (lateral extensions of the subarachnoid space).

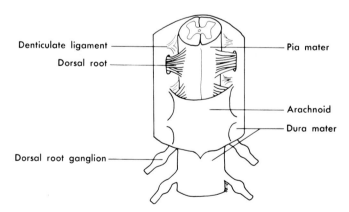

Fig. 4-2. Spinal cord meninges. The meningeal coverings of the spinal cord are shown. The outermost and thickest is the dura mater. There is a potential subdural space beneath this. The second covering of the cord is the arachnoid. Beneath this is the subarachnoid space, which contains cerebrospinal fluid. The innermost covering of the spinal cord is the pia mater. This is tightly adherent to the surface of the cord. Along the lateral margins of the cord, the pia thickens to form the denticulate ligaments. These attach the pia to the dura at most segmental levels, the connection being made between the exit points of the successive roots through the dura.

called a lumbar puncture, or spinal tap (Fig. 4-3). It consists of inserting an 18- to 20-gauge needle, using sterile technique, into an appropriate interspace between lumbar vertebrae, through the dura, and into the subarachnoid cistern. The German physician Quincke originally described the use of lumbar puncture in children. Quincke suggested that the puncture be made between the third and fourth lumbar (L3-4) vertebrae. L3-4 as the site for lumbar puncture has been reprinted in textbooks since then, but most neurosurgeons and neuroradiologists electively puncture the spinal subarachnoid space between L5 and S1, which is where the gap between the laminae is widest. The subarachnoid space at this level is filled with the roots of the cauda equina. The roots are generally pushed aside by the tip of the needle. If they are punctured, a brief lightninglike pain is felt, which is relieved by withdrawing the needle slightly. The subarachnoid space can also be tapped by a needle introduced into the large intervertebral foramen between the first and second cervical vertebrae, and the cisterna magna can be punctured by a needle inserted at the margin of the foramen magnum.

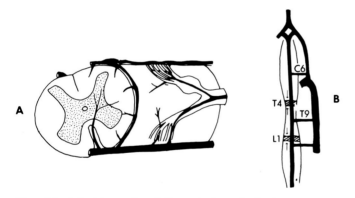

Fig. 4-4. Arterial supply of the spinal cord. **A,** Arrangement of the ventral and dorsal radicular arteries and their connections with the ventral and dorsal spinal arteries. The anastomosis between ventral and dorsal spinal arteries is also shown. The distribution of the terminal branches of the ventral spinal artery to the ventral and lateral white matter and to most of the gray matter is indicated, as is the supply of the dorsal columns by the two dorsal spinal arteries. **B,** Schematic of the main arterial branches feeding into the ventral spinal artery. The connections with the vertebral arteries and the large radicular arteries are shown, and the direction of blood flow is indicated by arrows. The hatched regions are watershed areas, the spinal cord segments most easily deprived of their arterial blood supply. The large radicular artery, which enters the spinal cord in the lower thoracic or upper lumbar region, is the artery of Adamkiewicz. It enters on the left side in 60% of individuals, generally between T8 and L1 (T9 shown). The dorsal spinal arteries and their tributaries are not shown. (After Schechter and Zingesser, 1966.)

Vascular supply

The majority of the blood supply to the spinal cord enters through several large radicular arteries, which are branches of the aorta (Fig. 4-4). Although the vascular pattern is extremely variable, in general there is one large branch that enters the cervical area, another in the midthoracic area, and another in the lumbar area (the artery of Adamkiewicz, which usually enters the cord on the left side). The spinal cord is also supplied by branches of the vertebral arteries, which fuse and form the ventral and dorsal spinal arteries, and by a series of smaller radicular arteries. The radicular arteries are branches of the intercostal and lumbar arteries, accompanying respectively the ventral and dorsal roots of certain segments. There are about six to eight each of ventral and dorsal radicular arteries. The ventral radicular arteries feed into the ventral spinal artery, which courses along the ventral median sulcus. This vessel also receives branches of the vertebral arteries at its rostral end. The caliber of the ventral spinal artery varies with the segmental level of the cord, being largest in the lumbosacral region and smallest in the thoracic region. Branches of the ventral spinal artery penetrate the cord from the ventral median sulcus to supply the ventral funiculi, the ventral horns, and the base of the dorsal horns. The ventral spinal artery also contributes to the vascular supply of the lateral columns and, by way of anastomoses with the dorsal spinal arteries, the dorsal part of the cord.

The dorsal radicular arteries join the dorsal spinal arteries, one of which is located along the dorsolateral surface of each side of the cord. The dorsal spinal arteries derive a part of their vascular supply also from branches of either the posterior inferior cerebellar arteries or the vertebral arteries. The dorsal spinal arteries supply blood to the dorsal funiculi and dorsal horns, and they provide anastomotic connections with branches from the ventral spinal artery.

Veins of the spinal cord run longitudinally in the pia. Radicular veins, which run with the nerve roots, drain the pial veins into the internal vertebral venous plexus, which lies in the epidural fat in the epidural space (Fig. 4-5). This is a dense plexus of veins. The anterior longitudinal vertebral sinuses are two large venous channels that lie in the anterolateral gutters of the spinal canal on the posterior surfaces of the vertebral bodies and on the intervertebral disks. Bleeding from these channels may be troublesome during surgical excision of herniated lumbar disks if their location is not appreciated and they are torn. The internal vertebral venous plexus drains into the dorsospinal branches of the paired intercostal veins. Blood also drains into these veins from the external venous plexus, which consists of a posterior plexus around the spines and lamina, and an anterior plexus around the body. In addition, there is a plexus of veins, called the basivertebral veins, within the vertebrae. The venous system of the vertebrae can be visualized by the technique of intraosseous venography, the injection of water-soluble contrast material opaque to x-rays into the marrow of a vertebral spine, and by then taking serial radiographs.

Within the abdominal cavity the intercostal veins are replaced by the lumbar veins, which drain into the right and left ascending lumbar veins. The right ascending lumbar vein enters the thorax and becomes the azygos vein; the left ascending lumbar vein becomes the hemiazygos vein. The hemiazygos crosses the vertebral column at about T8-9 to join the azygos vein. The azygos and the accessory hemiazygos of the left side of the thorax drain into the right and left brachiocephalic trunk, or superior vena cava system.

The functional significance of the vertebral venous system is twofold. Changes in intra-abdominal and intrathoracic pressure are communicated to the spinal subarachnoid space by way of these veins and affect the cerebrospinal fluid (CSF) pressure. A marked rise of CSF pressure can be seen if the abdomen is compressed when a lumbar puncture has been performed

and a manometer is connected to the lumbar needle. A further discussion of vascular effects on CSF dynamics is given in Chapter 5. The effects of changes in pressure in the veins draining the brain on CSF pressure are generally greater than the effects of the spinal veins.

The second important aspect of the vertebral veins was emphasized by Bateson, and the interconnections of these veins with the azygos system are sometimes called Bateson's plexus. This system is a parallel drainage channel and a bypass for the superior vena cava and inferior vena cava venous system. Pelvic carcinomas, particularly of the prostate gland, are thought to spread throughout the vertebral column by entry into this plexus of veins.

Vertebral and spinal cord segmental levels

There are generally 31 pairs of spinal nerves in humans (Fig. 4-6). These are made up of dorsal and ventral roots from each segment of the cord, except the first cervical, which often lacks a dorsal root. The roots are distributed along the cord as follows: eight cervical, twelve thoracic, five lumbar, five sacral, and one coccygeal. The spinal nerves exit from the vertebral canal through the intervertebral foramina. The first cervical nerves leave between the skull and the

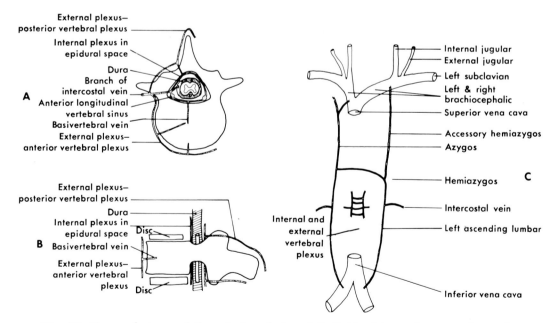

Fig. 4-5. Venous drainage of the spinal cord. **A** and **B,** Epidural internal venous plexus, the perivertebral external venous plexus, and the basivertebral veins of the vertebral bodies. All of these venous channels drain into the dorsospinal branches of the intercostal veins. **C,** Diagram of the drainage of the internal vertebral venous plexuses into the ascending lumbar and azygos venous systems. For simplicity, only one pair of intercostal veins is shown, and the anastomoses of the vertebral plexus with the ascending lumbar-azygos veins and of the ascending lumbar veins with the inferior vena cava are shown schematically.

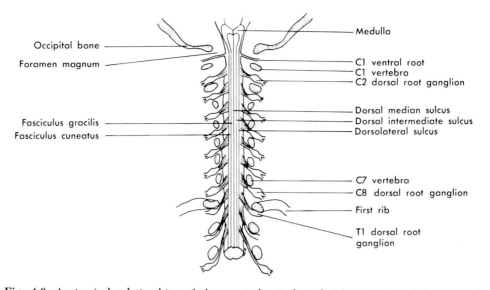

Occipital bone

Foramen magnum

Fasciculus gracilis

Fasciculus cuneatus

Medulla

C1 ventral root
C1 vertebra
C2 dorsal root ganglion

Dorsal median sulcus
Dorsal intermediate sulcus
Dorsolateral sulcus

C7 vertebra
C8 dorsal root ganglion

First rib

T1 dorsal root ganglion

Fig. 4-6. Anatomical relationships of the cervical spinal cord. The junction of the cervical spinal cord with the medulla at the foramen magnum is shown at the top of the figure. The first cervical roots exit from the vertebral canal between the occipital bone and the first cervical vertebra. The remaining cervical roots leave above the vertebra of the same number, except C8, which leaves between the C7 and the T1 vertebrae. All lower roots leave the central canal below the vertebrae of the same number. Note the progressive discrepancy between the position of the spinal segment and the level of the vertebra of the same number at successively more caudal levels. The pedicles of the vertebrae are indicated by the shaded oval profiles. The dorsal column of the spinal cord is subdivided into the fasciculus gracilis and fasciculus cuneatus at levels above the midthoracic segments.

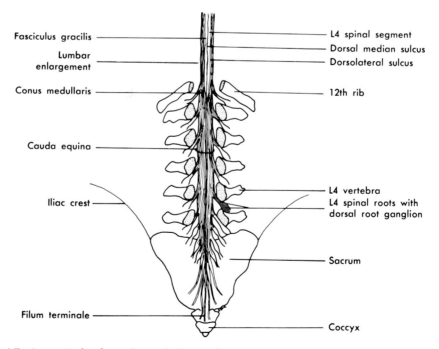

Fasciculus gracilis

Lumbar enlargement

Conus medullaris

Cauda equina

Iliac crest

Filum terminale

L4 spinal segment
Dorsal median sulcus
Dorsolateral sulcus

12th rib

L4 vertebra
L4 spinal roots with dorsal root ganglion

Sacrum

Coccyx

Fig. 4-7. Anatomical relationships of the caudal end of the spinal cord and cauda equina. The lumbosacral enlargement and conus medullaris of the spinal cord are shown adjacent to the twelfth rib. The vertebral canal below the L1 vertebra contains the cauda equina and the filum terminale, in addition to meninges. At this level of the spinal cord, the dorsal column consists only of the fasciculus gracilis.

first cervical vertebra; the eighth cervical nerve exits between the C7 and T1 vertebrae. All the other spinal nerves leave through the foramen below the vertebra having the same number.

The relationships of the spinal cord to the overlying vertebrae are of considerable clinical importance (Fig. 4-7). In common laboratory animals such as the cat and dog, the spinal cord extends the length of the spinal canal. However, in humans the vertebral column grows during childhood at a faster rate than the spinal cord. At birth the tip of the spinal cord lies at the level of the L2-3 vertebral body. In the adult the vertebral column has elongated so that the tip of the spinal cord lies at L1-L2. The remainder of the space in the lumbar canal is filled by the cauda equina (horse's tail), the nerve roots descending from the spinal cord and exiting at the intervertebral foramina.

An important clinical feature of the topographic anatomy of the motoneurons of the spinal cord is the relationship of the cord segments to the vertebral body overlying them. The muscles supplied by motoneurons of the second cervical segment of the spinal cord lie approximately under the lamina and on the body of the second cervical vertebra. However, because the length of the vertebral column is greater than that of the spinal cord, the spinal segments fall progressively behind the vertebral column as it descends, and the nerve roots exiting between the intervertebral foramina pass from the cord at progressively downward angles. Generally, in the middle or lower cervical cord the spinal cord segment related to a spinal nerve root exiting between two vertebrae lies opposite the body of the vertebra that is one or two segments higher. For example, the C8 segment (hand muscles) lies opposite the C6 body. In the upper and midthoracic areas there is a disparity of two vertebrae between the cord segment and the intervertebral foramen of exit. In the case of the roots of the cauda equina the lower lumbar cord segments and all of the sacral cord segments are crowded together opposite the T12-L1 vertebral bodies. Therefore, a small injury to the spinal cord area opposite this vertebral body level can have an extremely devastating effect neurologically by damaging a large number of lower motoneurons related to leg movement and sacral autonomic bowel, bladder, and sexual functions. Some useful segmental-vertebral relationships are given in Table 4-1.

The spinal cord is suspended in the dural canal by two denticulate ligaments that pass from the dura and attach to the pia-arachnoid of the cord. These tether the spinal cord to some degree within the dural canal. The spinal cord, particularly the cervical cord, moves when the neck is flexed or extended. When the

Table 4-1. Segmental-vertebral relationship

Cord segment	Vertebral body	Spinous process
C8	C6-7	C6
T6	T4-5	T3
L1	T11	T10
Sacral	T12-L1	T12-L1

neck is flexed, the cord is stretched and pulled over the ventral surface of the spinal canal, which may have osteoarthritic ridges on it. When the neck is extended, the cord is compressed and may buckle slightly. Infolding of the ligamentum flavum overlying the dura may compress the cord when the neck is in this position. The medulla and cervical-medullary junction also participate in these movements. It is of great interest that intrinsic regulatory mechanisms lying in the medulla, such as those controlling respiration, blood pressure, and heart rate, can continue to function with great regularity despite deformation in their shape produced by head and neck movements.

External anatomy

The spinal cord has a generally cylindrical form, but it is flattened somewhat ventrodorsally. There are two regions of enlargement, the cervical and lumbar; it is from these that the nerve fibers innervating the forelimbs and hindlimbs originate. The caudalmost part of the cord tapers rapidly, ending as the conus medullaris.

The spinal cord is composed of white and gray matter. The white matter surrounds the gray, so that only the former is visible from the outside of the cord. The white matter may be divided into several columns, or funiculi. A funiculus is a large bundle of nerve fibers of diverse function. The funiculi of the spinal cord are the dorsal, lateral, and ventral. The landmarks by which the funiculi are divided are the dorsolateral and ventrolateral sulci. A sulcus is a shallow groove on the surface of central nervous system tissue. The dorsolateral and ventrolateral sulci follow the dorsal and ventral root entry and exit zones respectively. The left and right sides of the cord are demarcated by the dorsal median sulcus and the ventral median fissure. A fissure is a deep groove on the surface of the central nervous system. In the cervical and upper thoracic spinal cord, the dorsal funiculi are subdivided by still another groove, the dorsal intermediate sulcus. The two parts of the dorsal funiculus at levels above the midthoracic spinal cord are called the fasciculus gracilis and the fasciculus cuneatus. A fasciculus is a fiber bundle within the central nervous system having a smaller size than a funiculus. A fasciculus generally has a relatively discrete function. The fasciculus gracilis is medial to the fasciculus cuneatus. Below the midthoracic level the fasciculus cuneatus is not present, so the dorsal funiculus is composed of the fasciculus gracilis only.

Cross section

In cross section, the white and gray matter of the spinal cord are clearly demarcated, even in unstained tissue (Fig. 4-8). The gray matter forms an H-shaped structure, which is surrounded by the various funiculi of the white matter. Near the midpoint of the cord is the central canal. The crossbar of the H-shaped gray matter passes both dorsally and ventrally to the central canal as the gray commissures. Fibers may cross between the two sides of the spinal cord within the gray commissures or in the ventral white commissure. On each side of the cord the gray matter extends vertically, forming the dorsal and ventral horns. The gray matter at the intersection of dorsal and ventral horns at the level of the central canal is often called the intermediate region.

The relative proportions of gray and white matter

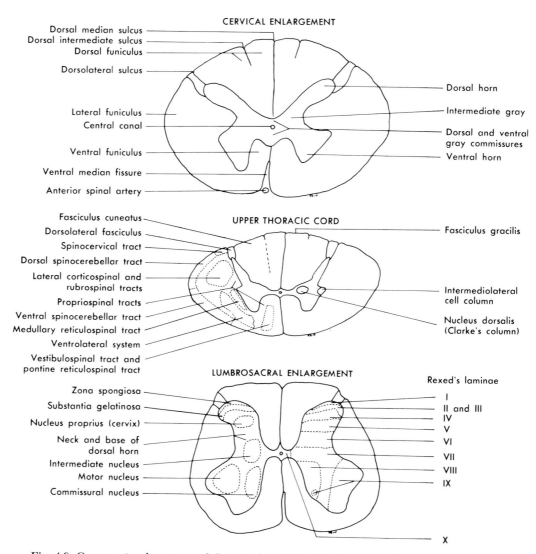

Fig. 4-8. Cross-sectional anatomy of the spinal cord. The labels associated with the cross section of the cervical enlargement indicate the important general landmarks of the cord surface, white matter, and gray matter. The regions indicated at the left of the thoracic cross section are the approximate locations of the principal ascending and descending tracts in the white matter. The special nuclei of the thoracic and upper lumbar cord, the intermediolateral cell column, and the nucleus dorsalis are shown at the right. The gray matter in the cross section of the lumbosacral enlargement is subdivided into the important nuclei on the left and Rexed's laminae on the right.

vary with the segmental level. The gray matter is largest in the cervical and lumbar enlargements. This is related to the large increase in numbers of neurons that are used in the control of the upper and lower extremities. The white matter in general increases in amount from caudal to rostral levels. This is reasonable, inasmuch as all of the pathways connecting the spinal cord with the brain must be present at the highest cervical level, whereas only those required for a given level and below are present at successively lower segments. However, the number of intrinsic fibers of the cord, the propriospinal fibers, varies with the level, and there is an increase in the bulk of the white matter in the enlargements because of these.

Composition of white matter

The white matter of the spinal cord contains bundles of axons having particular functions. A bundle of fibers connecting one part of the central nervous system with another and having a uniform function is called a tract. Some of the spinal cord tracts are myelinated, some unmyelinated, and some mixed. The general categories of tracts in the spinal cord are the propriospinal tracts, the long ascending tracts, and the long descending tracts. Propriospinal tracts serve to interconnect different levels of the spinal cord. The long ascending tracts connect the spinal cord with the brain, and the long descending tracts connect the brain with the spinal cord. The location of the cells of origin and the destination of the long tracts is often indicated by the names given these tracts. For instance, fibers originating from cells in the spinal cord, ascending to the brain, and terminating synaptically in the cerebellum are called spinocerebellar tracts. Fibers arising from neurons of the cerebral cortex and descending through the spinal cord to end synaptically on spinal neurons are called corticospinal tracts. Sometimes there are two or more tracts interconnecting the same structures. These are often distinguished on the basis of their relative positions within the spinal cord. The dorsal spinocerebellar tract is found in the dorsal part of the lateral funiculus, whereas the ventral spinocerebellar tract is located in the ventral part of the lateral funiculus.

The major long ascending and descending pathways are mentioned briefly here (Fig. 4-8); they are discussed in more detail in later chapters.

The dorsal funiculi contain few propriospinal fibers. Most of the axons in the dorsal funiculi are branches of primary afferents. Some of these terminate within a few segments of the level of their entry into the spinal cord through a dorsal root. Others end in the spinal cord gray matter at some distance from their entry point. A special category of such fibers comprises those that form the fasciculi gracilis and cuneatus. These fasciculi are long ascending pathways to the brain. They are formed from ascending branches of primary afferent fibers from certain types of sensory receptors. Afferents in the fasciculus gracilis originate from the lower part of the body, including the lower extremities. Afferents in the fasciculus cuneatus originate from the upper part of the body, including the upper extremities. It is because of its place of origin that the fasciculus cuneatus exists only at the midthoracic level of the spinal cord and more rostrally.

At the intersection between the dorsal and lateral funiculi, just dorsal to the most dorsolateral extent of the dorsal horn, is a bundle of small myelinated and unmyelinated fibers known as the dorsolateral fasciculus (of Lissauer). This is largely a propriospinal bundle, although it contains branches of unmyelinated afferent fibers as well. The propriospinal component interconnects the substantia gelatinosa of the dorsal horn at different levels of the spinal cord. The substantia gelatinosa (discussed below) is a region of gray matter located near the most dorsal part of the dorsal horn. The unmyelinated afferent fibers in the dorsolateral fasciculus are also thought to terminate within the substantia gelatinosa.

The lateral and ventral funiculi contain large numbers of propriospinal fibers, many of which are myelinated. In addition, they contain several long tracts. Some of the ascending tracts are the dorsal and ventral spinocerebellar tracts in the lateral funiculus and the ventrolateral system in both the lateral and ventral funiculi. The ventrolateral system makes synaptic terminations at many levels of the brainstem, including the reticular formation, the inferior olivary nucleus, the tectum, and the thalamus. These structures are discussed in later chapters. Some of the descending tracts include the lateral corticospinal tract, the rubrospinal tract and the medullary reticulospinal tract in the lateral funiculus and the ventral corticospinal tract, the vestibulospinal tracts, the pontine reticulospinal tract, and the tectospinal tract in the ventral funiculus.

Composition of gray matter

Certain features are common to the gray matter at all levels of the spinal cord (Figs. 4-8 and 4-9). The gray matter may be divided into the dorsal and ventral horns, which correspond to the vertical bars of the H-shaped gray matter. The area between the dorsal and ventral horns is called the intermediate region. The dorsal horn may be further divided into horizontal strata, known in older terminology as the zona spongiosa, the substantia gelatinosa of Rolando,

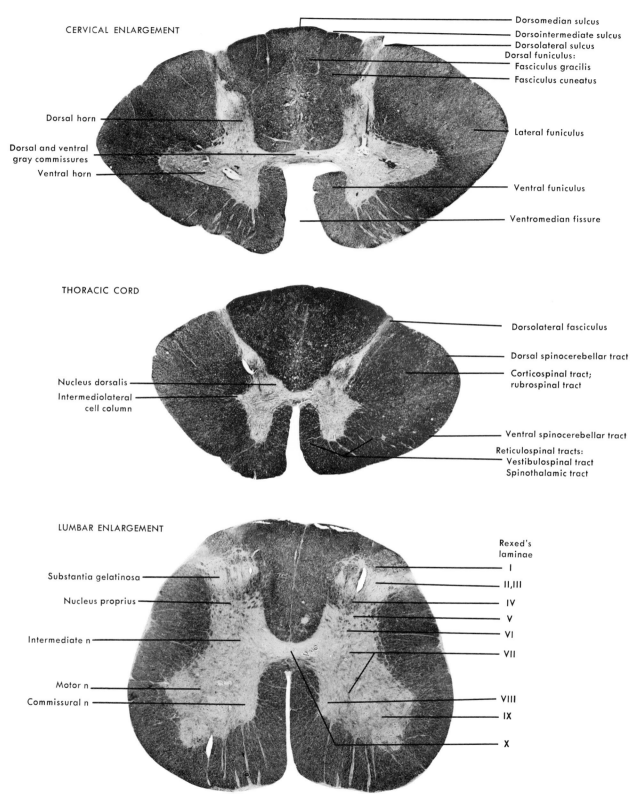

CERVICAL ENLARGEMENT

Dorsomedian sulcus
Dorsointermediate sulcus
Dorsolateral sulcus
Dorsal funiculus:
Fasciculus gracilis
Fasciculus cuneatus

Dorsal horn

Lateral funiculus

Dorsal and ventral
gray commissures
Ventral horn

Ventral funiculus

Ventromedian fissure

THORACIC CORD

Dorsolateral fasciculus

Dorsal spinocerebellar tract

Corticospinal tract;
rubrospinal tract

Nucleus dorsalis
Intermediolateral
cell column

Ventral spinocerebellar tract

Reticulospinal tracts:
Vestibulospinal tract
Spinothalamic tract

LUMBAR ENLARGEMENT

Rexed's
laminae

Substantia gelatinosa

I

II,III

Nucleus proprius

IV

V

Intermediate n

VI

VII

Motor n
Commissural n

VIII

IX

X

Fig. 4-9. Transverse sections of human spinal cord.

the nucleus proprius, the cervix, and the base. The intermediate region contains the cell group known as the intermediate nucleus. The ventral horn includes a number of motoneuronal nuclei, as well as many interneurons, some of which probably serve as relay cells for the descending pathways in the ventral part of the white matter. It also contains in its medial portion a commissural nucleus.

A new terminology for the various layers of the gray matter of the cord was introduced by Rexed. He divides the gray matter into laminae I to X. The laminae I to VI occupy the dorsal horn. Part of VII roughly corresponds to the intermediate region. Lamina VII also forms much of the ventral horn. The medial aspect of the ventral horn in the enlargements includes lamina VIII. The motoneurons are in groups corresponding to functional relations, and they are classed as lamina IX. The zone around the central canal is considered lamina X.

Certain changes in composition of the gray matter according to segmental level should be mentioned. There is a special group of cells in the upper cervical cord (C1 to 3) located just lateral to the dorsal horn within the lateral funiculus. This is a relay nucleus, called the lateral cervical nucleus, for the spino-cervical tract (see Chapter 7).

There is another special group of cells located in a column in lamina VII and extending from the first thoracic to the third lumbar level. It is called the nucleus dorsalis (column of Clarke).

Sympathetic preganglionic neurons have their cell bodies located in the intermediolateral cell column (a dorsolateral extension of lamina VII) in the thoracic and upper lumbar cord. Parasympathetic preganglionic neurons are located in a similar position within the spinal cord gray matter, but at the S2 and 3 (or S3 and 4) segmental levels. The parasympathetic motor nucleus does not form a prominent intermediolateral cell column like that of the sympathetic motor nucleus.

Motoneurons supplying skeletal muscle are found in cell columns at all levels of the cord, but they are most numerous in the cervical and lumbar enlargements (Figs. 4-8 to 4-10). A number of workers have described the composition of the motoneuronal cell columns. In general, the motoneurons innervating skeletal muscle controlling the distal joints of an extremity are located in the dorsal part of the ventral horn, whereas motoneurons to the proximal musculature are placed more ventrally. There is also a segregation of motoneuronal nuclei according to function, those motoneurons responsible for flexion of joints being separated from those producing extension.

SPINAL MOTONEURON AS A MODEL CENTRAL NEURON

Many of the basic features of central nervous system activity have been first or best described in studies of the behavior of spinal cord alpha motoneurons. Although the activity of other types of neurons may vary sharply from that of the motoneuron, it can nevertheless be stated that the motoneuron serves as a kind of baseline and that the activity of other kinds of cells is often discussed in reference to that of motoneurons.

Structure of the alpha motoneuron

Alpha motoneurons are the largest of the cell types in the spinal cord (Fig. 4-10). Some cells giving rise to ascending tracts, such as the ventral spinocerebellar tract, may be of the same size, but no spinal neurons are larger. In the cat, the cell bodies of motoneurons range up to about 70 μm in diameter (long axis). A motoneuron has a number of dendrites, perhaps six to twelve. The dendrites tend to run longitudinally in the spinal cord, although there is some transverse spread as well. A given dendrite may exceed 1 mm in length. The axon of an alpha moto-

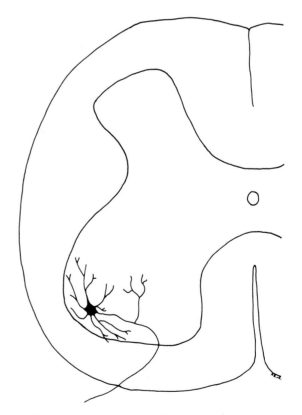

Fig. 4-10. Alpha motoneuron. The drawing shows the cell body, dendrites, axon, and recurrent collateral of an alpha motoneuron as it would appear in a Golgi stain.

neuron generally runs medially to join a bundle of exiting ventral root fibers. The level of the rootlet containing a motor axon is usually close to the level of the motoneuron cell body, although it may be displaced somewhat caudally. Although some motor axons lack branches, it is not uncommon for a motor axon to have one or more collaterals. These collaterals are often recurrent; that is, they travel dorsolaterally back toward the motoneuron cell body.

The surface membrane of the motoneuron is covered with numerous synapses. Perhaps a third to half of the surface membrane lies beneath synaptic terminals. The remaining surface membrane is covered by glial processes. The synapses on the surface of a motoneuron are not homogeneous in structure. Many small synaptic boutons are found in contact with the membrane of both the cell body and the dendrites. Some of these boutons have spherical and others flattened vesicles. There are also occasional synaptic endings containing granulated or dense-cored vesicles, and rarely there are large synaptic terminals, some of which receive axoaxonal synapses.

The ultrastructure of the motoneuron is typical of that of many kinds of neurons. The granular endoplasmic reticulum and the Golgi apparatus are prominent.

Passive electrical properties of the motoneuron membrane

The membrane of the alpha motoneuron has been studied biophysically on numerous occasions. The passive electrical properties of motoneurons have been examined by passing current pulses through a microelectrode and recording the voltage change through the same microelectrode or through the second barrel of a double-barreled microelectrode. Recently, sinusoidally varying currents have been used as well as pulses.

When plots are made of the voltage changes produced by various currents passed across the motoneuron membrane, it is possible to assign a value of resistance to the motoneuron. This value is a kind of average resistance, because the currents are distributed in a complicated manner through the cell body and dendrites. The value for membrane resistance in motoneurons is a little greater than 1 megohm. In some motoneurons, the membrane resistance changes during a prolonged current pulse. This might be expected for depolarizing pulses, which can cause a delayed increase in potassium conductance, just as in axonal membranes (see Chapter 1). This type of conductance change is known as delayed rectification. However, some motoneurons undergo a reduction in their membrane resistance during prolonged hyper-

polarization. This is termed anomalous rectification. There is as yet no satisfactory explanation of anomalous rectification.

Through an analysis of transient changes in membrane potential by applied current pulses, using an elaborate theory taking into account the complex geometry of the motoneuron, one can assign the motoneuron a value of about 5 msec for its membrane time constant. Again, this is a kind of average value. If a potential change occurred uniformly over the soma and dendrites of the motoneuron and if this potential were allowed to decay passively back to the resting potential, the potential would reach 1/e of its initial value in about 5 msec. However, it should be emphasized that potential changes that are produced just at the level of the cell body of a motoneuron decay passively much more rapidly, whereas potentials developed exclusively in the distal dendrites and recorded at the level of the cell body decay much more slowly.

The analysis of passive electrical properties of motoneurons has also been applied to a determination of the expected effect of the dendrites on the spatial decrement of signals. It is now thought that the distalmost dendrites are within 1.5 length constants of the cell body. This means that signals applied even at the extreme ends of the dendrites can be expected to produce significant changes in the membrane potential of the cell body and axon hillock region.

Excitation of motoneurons

Motoneurons can be excited to fire action potentials in a number of ways. Direct electrical stimulation will excite a motoneuron, just as it will excite an axon. Stimulation of the axon of a motoneuron will result in the invasion of the motoneuron by an action potential that propagates backward into the motoneuron cell body and dendrites. Such a backward-conducted nerve impulse is called an antidromic action potential (Fig. 4-11). Normally, however, motoneurons discharge in response to excitatory postsynaptic potentials produced by the activity of synapses from other neurons. Action potentials produced in this way are called orthodromic (Fig. 4-12).

No matter which method is employed for exciting a motoneuron, the action potential in the motoneuron is triggered in a specially sensitive region, which is probably the axon hillock. When this trigger zone discharges, the action potential not only propagates down the axon, but also spreads across the cell body and into the dendrites of the motoneuron. Apparently, the somadendritic membrane (soma, cell body) has a higher threshold than does the axon hillock. Because

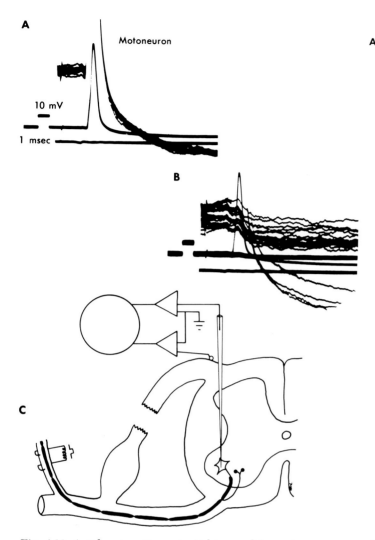

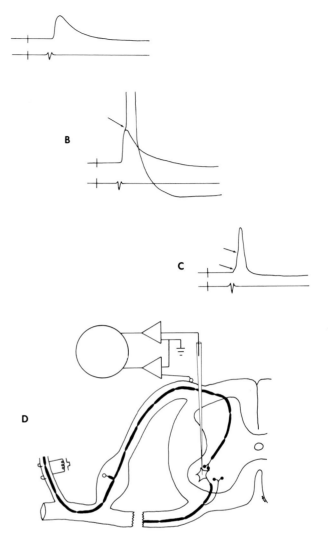

Fig. 4-11. Antidromic action potential in an alpha motoneuron. The dorsal roots are cut so that stimulation of a nerve supplying muscle results in activity reaching the spinal cord only through the ventral roots. This is called an antidromic volley, because the normal impulse traffic in ventral roots is in the direction away from the spinal cord. A microelectrode is inserted into a motoneuron that sends its axon to the muscle whose nerve is stimulated. The volley invading the motoneurons of that muscle nerve is recorded by a gross electrode placed on the dorsal surface of the spinal cord. The potentials recorded by the microelectrode are shown in the upper two traces in A and B; the volley recorded by the gross electrode is in the lower trace. The amplifier gain is high for the upper trace and low for the middle trace. A shows the antidromic action potential. Note the inflection on the rising phase of the spike potential in the low-gain record. The after-hyperpolarization is well seen in the high-gain record. In B the stimulus strength is reduced to threshold for the motor axon to this particular motoneuron, although it is still well above threshold for other motor axons. The action potential occurs intermittently. When no action potential occurs, an IPSP is observed. This results in recurrent inhibition, which is caused by the activity of Renshaw cells excited by action potentials invading the recurrent collaterals of motor axons. The stimulating and recording arrangement is shown in C.

Fig. 4-12. Orthodromic excitation of an alpha motoneuron. The ventral roots are cut, so activation of the axons of a muscle nerve results in an afferent volley reaching the spinal cord through the normal, or orthodromic, pathway. Antidromic invasion is prevented. Activation of group Ia afferent fibers results in monosynaptic excitation of the alpha motoneurons belonging to the same muscle as that supplied by the nerve stimulated or to synergistic muscles. The monosynaptic EPSP in the upper trace of A was evoked in this fashion. The afferent volley recorded from the dorsal surface of the spinal cord is shown in the lower trace. The stimulus strength was submaximal, activating only a fraction of the group Ia fibers of the nerve. When the stimulus strength was increased to fire all of the group Ia fibers, the EPSP became larger because of spatial summation. It now exceeded threshold for firing the motoneuron in part of the trials, as seen in B. The firing level is indicated by the arrow. The records in A and B were made with a high-amplifier gain, so the peak of the spike in B is not seen. However, the full spike is shown in C, which was recorded when the amplifier gain was reduced. The lower of the two arrows shows the EPSP. The upper arrow indicates the inflection on the rising phase of the spike, caused by the slowing of conduction as the action potential invaded the nerve cell body from the initial segment. The stimulating and recording arrangement is shown in D.

of the higher threshold of the soma-dendritic membrane, invasion of the nerve impulse from the axon hillock may be delayed slightly, resulting in an inflection on the rising phase of the action potential as recorded by a microelectrode placed in the cell body. The delay can be prolonged or a block in invasion can be produced if the motoneuron membrane is made less excitable, as when it is hyperpolarized. The delay is minimal when action potentials are evoked orthodromically, because the depolarization produced by synaptic currents makes the soma-dendritic membrane more excitable.

The after-potentials following the spike potential in the axon hillock membrane are small, resembling those typical of myelinated axons of the peripheral nervous system. This can be shown by blocking the soma-dendritic spike and recording from the soma or, rarely, by recording from the axon hillock region. The spike in the soma-dendritic membrane, however, is followed by a very large and prolonged after-hyperpolarization. This large after-potential is thought to be a major factor in limiting the firing frequency of motoneurons, because it is associated with a substantial subnormal period.

Excitatory postsynaptic potentials of motoneurons

A number of nervous system pathways have been found to excite motoneurons synaptically. The excitatory postsynaptic potentials (EPSPs) recorded from motoneurons seem to resemble in most respects the end-plate potentials that can be recorded from skeletal muscle in response to activation of motor axons (see Chapter 3). For instance, the equilibrium potential for the EPSPs of motoneurons is probably about 0 mV, just as is that of the end-plate potential. This means that the membrane is probably made more permeable to ions such as sodium and potassium during the generation of the EPSP. The synaptic currents that flow in through the motoneuron membrane beneath the excitatory synapses spread through the cell body and dendrites and out across the inactive part of the motoneuron membrane, depolarizing it (see Fig. 3-10). Inasmuch as the axon hillock region is the trigger zone of the motoneuron, having the lowest threshold for discharge of any part of the membrane, the most important fraction of the synaptic current is that which depolarizes the axon hillock. In some motoneurons the threshold for firing is not absolutely constant. Rapidly rising EPSPs may reach threshold at a lower level of depolarization than do slowly rising EPSPs. This is apparently because of accommodation of the membrane of the axon hillock.

Although EPSPs produced by many different pathways have been studied in recordings from motoneurons, the most useful EPSPs for analysis have been those generated following activation of the largest afferent fibers (group Ia) from muscle spindles. These afferents terminate directly on motoneurons, forming a pathway with a single synapse, or monosynaptic pathway. A monosynaptic pathway is much more readily investigated than a polysynaptic one. Polysynaptic pathways involve a series of two or more sets of synaptic connections. In the case of polysynaptic pathways to motoneurons from primary afferent fibers, the afferents terminate on interneurons, which then synapse with the motoneurons.

The monosynaptic EPSPs produced in motoneurons by electrical stimulation of the large muscle spindle afferents have a characteristic time course. The rising phase is quick, lasting about 1 msec. The falling phase is more prolonged, occupying some 10 to 15 msec. The rising phase is accounted for by a transient increase in membrane permeability to ions, such as sodium and potassium, in response to the release of a chemical transmitter from the terminals of the group Ia fibers. The nature of the chemical transmitter is as yet unknown. The falling phase of the monosynaptic EPSP can be accounted for by the passive recharging of the membrane, because the time constant of decay of the EPSP is similar to the motoneuron membrane time constant. This suggests that the monosynaptic EPSP may be generated by synapses placed relatively uniformly over the soma-dendritic membrane of the motoneuron, because the passive decay of the EPSP would be faster than the overall membrane time constant if the synapses were located primarily on the soma and slower if they were primarily on the distal dendrites.

Unitary monosynaptic excitatory postsynaptic potentials

It is now technically feasible to investigate the action of a single group Ia afferent fiber in generating a monosynaptic EPSP in a motoneuron. Studies of this kind have shown that such EPSPs, called unitary EPSPs, differ in several respects from the monosynaptic EPSP produced by stimulating the whole muscle nerve (Fig. 4-13). They are, of course, smaller. The monosynaptic EPSP produced by stimulation of the whole nerve is a summation of all the unitary EPSPs produced by the individual Ia afferent fibers of the nerve. Furthermore, the unitary EPSPs have a spectrum of time courses. Some resemble in time course the summed EPSP. However, not infrequently a unitary EPSP will be much more rapid or much slower. The implication is that the fast unitary monosynaptic EPSPs are generated by one or more synapses made by the afferent fiber on the region of the motoneuron soma, whereas the slow unitary EPSPs are produced by an afferent whose synapses are located on the distal dendrites.

Repeated stimulation of a single group Ia afferent produces a unitary monosynaptic EPSP of variable size. It appears that the size varies stepwise, like the variation in size of the end-plate potential during repetitive stimulation of a motor nerve (see Chapter 3). This variation has been analyzed for the unitary EPSPs in motoneurons, and it seems clear that synaptic transmission in the central nervous system is quantal, just as it is at peripheral synapses. Inasmuch as central synapses are characterized by synaptic vesicles in the presynaptic terminals, as is the neuromuscular junction, it seems reasonable to conclude that the synaptic transmitter in the monosynaptic pathway to motoneurons is associated with synaptic vesicles in the terminals of group Ia fibers.

The motoneuron membrane shows a series of spontaneous fluctuations having the time course of synaptic potentials and the size of unitary monosynaptic EPSPs in the absence of any overt stimulation. These fluctuations have been called synaptic noise. Some of these are caused by transmitter release from group Ia afferent fibers, but many are no doubt caused by transmitter release from the terminals of interneurons

ending on the motoneuron. There are at least two mechanisms to explain this spontaneous release of transmitter. Some of the EPSPs are caused by nerve impulses invading the synaptic terminals. Many afferent fibers and interneurons are spontaneously active, and this transmitter release would be a direct consequence of such activity. In addition, there is likely to be a spontaneous quantal release of transmitter at central synapses, just as there is at the neuromuscular junction. An attempt has been made to distinguish between these two mechanisms by blocking nerve impulse activity within the spinal cord. This has been done by the application of tetrodotoxin (see pp. 37 and 70). This procedure blocks much of the synaptic noise, but not all. The residuum of synaptic noise is presumably the result of spontaneous transmitter release in the absence of nerve impulse traffic.

Spatial and temporal summation

As is discussed again later, monosynaptic EPSPs are generated in motoneurons only when certain muscle nerves are stimulated. The muscle nerves involved are those that supply the muscle innervated by the motoneurons and also the synergistic muscles. Thus, if two different muscle nerves are stimulated and they each supply a synergistic muscle, each afferent volley

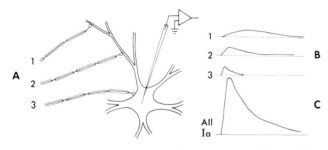

Fig. 4-13. Unitary EPSPs. **A,** Three group Ia afferent fibers are shown terminating synaptically on an alpha motoneuron. Fiber *1* ends distally on a dendrite, fiber *2* more proximally on a dendrite, and fiber *3* on the cell body. The unitary EPSPs evoked by each of these fibers and recorded by a microelectrode placed in the cell body of the motoneuron are shown in **B.** The time courses of the EPSPs are markedly different. The farther the synaptic region is from the point of recording, the slower the wave form of the EPSP. If a comparable amount of synaptic transmitter is released at each point, the potentials would also become progressively smaller for more distant synapses. However, the unitary EPSPs are drawn as equal in height, because there is evidence that more transmitter may be liberated at synapses located distal to the cell body than at synapses on the cell body. The effect of spatial summation of the unitary EPSPs of the various group Ia fibers in producing the EPSP seen when the whole muscle nerve is stimulated is shown in **C.** The size of the summed EPSP is essentially the sum of the sizes of the unitary EPSPs, and the time course is a kind of average of that of the unitary EPSPs.

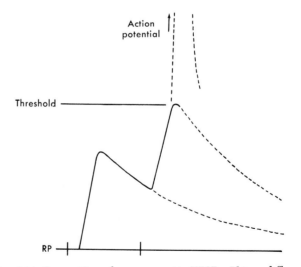

Fig. 4-14. Summation of monosynaptic EPSPs. If two different nerves to synergistic muscles are stimulated, the monosynaptic EPSPs recorded from a motoneuron to one of the muscles will sum, provided that the interval between the stimuli is less than the duration of the first EPSP. This is shown in the drawing. The second EPSP reaches a greater peak depolarization than the first. If the first EPSP is subthreshold, the motoneuron may still be fired by the second EPSP, as indicated. This phenomenon is called spatial summation. A similar effect may be seen with repetitive stimulation of a single nerve. This is called temporal summation.

will evoke an EPSP in a motoneuron belonging to either muscle. When two such volleys arrive at the spinal cord simultaneously, the monosynaptic EPSP recorded in the motoneuron will be the sum of the EPSPs produced by either volley alone (Fig. 4-14). If the two volleys arrive at different times, their effects will still sum if the second EPSP begins during the first one. The addition of two EPSPs from activation of different pathways is called spatial summation. The significance of spatial summation is that the effects of two or more pathways to a motoneuron can often fire the motoneuron when a single pathway might be ineffective.

A similar buildup of the degree of depolarization of a motoneuron by EPSPs occurs when a given pathway is activated two or more times in succession, again provided that the successive EPSPs occur within the duration of preceding ones. This effect is called temporal summation. Frequently, repetitive stimulation of a pathway is effective when a single stimulus is not. Besides temporal summation, repetitive stimulation of a pathway causes changes in the amount of synaptic transmitter released, as is discussed in the next section.

Alterations in the monosynaptic EPSP by repetitive stimulation

The monosynaptic EPSP evoked in a motoneuron by stimulating a whole muscle nerve changes in size somewhat according to the frequency of stimulation. In general, the EPSP is largest when low rates of stimulation are used and becomes progressively smaller as the frequency increases. However, the relationship is nonlinear.

If the muscle nerve is activated repetitively at a high rate and then the monosynaptic EPSP is evoked intermittently at a slow rate, its size is transiently increased as compared with the control size. This increase in size of the EPSP following repetitive (or tetanic) stimulation is called posttetanic potentiation. The potentiation lasts for minutes. The mechanism of the potentiation is not clear; several possible ones are discussed on p. 119. However, the process is of great interest because it represents a means by which activation of a synapse enhances transmitter release by that synapse in response to later activation. The synapse has, in effect, a short-lasting memory of prior activity.

Relationship between properties of motoneurons and muscle

The term motor unit means the motoneuron and all of the skeletal muscle fibers it supplies. The term muscle unit refers to the muscular component of a motor unit. When a motoneuron discharges, normally all of the muscle fibers it innervates, which may number several hundred, twitch. When muscle is stimulated repetitively, the twitches may sum, depending on the frequency. With high rates of stimulation, the muscle contraction is said to be tetanic. The individual twitches are no longer observed; instead, the contraction is maintained at a plateau level throughout the period of stimulation. The frequency at which this occurs depends on the speed of the twitch. A smooth tetanic contraction is first observed at a lower frequency for muscles with a slow twitch than for muscles with a rapid twitch.

It appears that the electrophysiological properties of motoneurons match the properties of the muscle fibers they innervate. Motoneurons that innervate muscle fibers that twitch slowly tend to discharge at lower rates than do those that supply muscle fibers that twitch rapidly. The limits of the discharge rates of different motoneurons approach the rates that are required by the muscle fibers they innervate to reach a smooth tetanic contraction. One of the factors that helps determine the discharge rates of motoneurons is the amplitude and duration of the after-hyperpolarization following their spikes. Motoneurons to slow muscle tend to have large, prolonged after-hyperpolarizations; those to fast muscle have smaller, shorter lasting after-hyperpolarizations.

There is now available rather detailed information about the organization of the motor units of certain muscles in experimental animals and about the relationship between the functional properties of the motoneurons and of the muscle units they supply. The best-studied neuromuscular apparatus is the medial gastrocnemius muscle of the cat. The organization of the motor supply of this muscle will be discussed, but it should be recognized that many of the conclusions reached are widely applicable to other muscles and other species.

The muscle units in the medial gastrocnemius muscle can be subdivided into three classes: FF (fast, easily fatigued), FR (fast, fatigue-resistant), and S (slow, fatigue-resistant). The FF and FR types are characterized by a rapid contraction time. However, the FF units develop more tension than do the FR units. Both types have an abundance of myofibrillar ATPase activity when they are stained histochemically. However, they can be distinguished on the basis of other histochemical staining properties (Table 4-2). These two classes of fiber are distinguishable on the basis of how rapidly they fatigue with repetitive stimulation, but there are fibers with intermediate properties, and the proportions of these fiber types in a given muscle may vary with the use

Table 4-2. Properties of motor units in cat medial gastrocnemius muscle

Properties of motoneurons	Type of muscle unit		
	Type FF	Type FR	Type S
Axon conduction velocity	Rapid	Rapid	Slow
Input resistance	Small	Small	Large
After-hyperpolarization	Short	Short	Long
Muscle fibers contraction speed	Fast	Fast to intermediate	Slow
Tetanic fusion frequency	High	High	Low
Fatiguability	High	Low	Fatigue resistant
Histochemical profile			
Myofibrillar ATPase	High	High	Low
Acid stable-ATPase	Intermediate	Intermediate	High
Reduced diphosphopyridine nucleotide dehydrogenase	Low	Intermediate to high	High
Succinic dehydrogenase	Low	Intermediate to high	High
Glycogen	High	High	Low
Number of motor axons	124	78	78
Innervation ratio	800	450	550
Average tetanic tension per unit	69 g	22 g	5 g
Total tetanic tension	8,600 g	1,700 g	380 g

of the muscle by the animal and other factors. The motoneurons that supply FF and FR muscle units have rapidly conducting axons, a small input resistance (implying large size), and a brief after-hyperpolarization. The type S muscle units are distinctly different; they have a slow contraction time, and they develop less tension than do the other muscle unit types. However, S units are less dependent on anerobic glycolysis, and the fibers are more abundantly supplied with capillaries than are the fast units. As a consequence, type S units are extremely resistant to fatigue. Their motoneurons have slowly conducting axons, a high input resistance (indicating a small size), and a long-lasting hyperpolarization. The relationship between motoneuron size and the participation of motoneurons in reflex actions is discussed below.

The organization of the muscle units within the gastrocnemius muscle of the cat has been studied by repetitively activating single motor units by intracellular stimulation of motoneurons. The repetitive contractions result in glycogen depletion, which can be recognized in histochemically stained sections of the muscle. All of the fibers of a stimulated muscle unit will show glycogen depletion, whereas no other

muscle units will. A given muscle unit is found to occupy a territory within a fraction of the muscle belly, but that territory is shared with about 50 other muscle units. There are about 280 alpha motor axons in the cat medial gastrocnemius nerve. Of these, about 124 supply type FF units, 78 supply type FR units, and 78 supply type S units. The average number of muscle fibers supplied by a given axon is about 800 for FF units, 450 for FR units, and 550 for S units. The sum of the average contractile tension produced by each of the muscle units accounts for the total tension that can be developed by the cat medial gastrocnemius muscle (about 10 kg).

The innervation ratios for motor units within other muscles may be quite different. For instance, the muscles that provide for the fine movements of the fingers and the extrinsic muscles of the eyes have small muscle units consisting of only a few muscle fibers. There is generally an inverse relationship between the number of muscle fibers per motoneuron and the degree of fineness of muscular control required. Another variable from muscle to muscle is the proportion of the fibers that belong to the different classes of motor units. Some muscles, like the medial gastrocnemius, have a mixture of types of motor unit, but other muscles, like the soleus, may contain a rather homogeneous population of one type. Slow postural muscles, like the soleus, consist essentially entirely of type S muscle units. Such muscles are often called red muscles because of the color given to them by the S muscle fibers, which contain a large amount of myoglobin, and by a rich vascular supply. Other muscles are pale or white, by contrast.

Size principle. An important generalization that has emerged from the studies of Henneman and his colleagues is called the size principle. The motoneurons that are most easily activated during a variety of reflex activities are those with the smallest axonal diameter. Because the axon diameter presumably reflects neuron size, the motoneurons that participate most readily in reflexes are small motoneurons. These supply type S muscle units. During activity, the greatest use is thus made of motor units characterized by fatigue resistance. Another property is that the contractile tension exerted by each type S muscle unit is small, and so the contraction of the entire muscle as it is activated by small motoneurons is finely graded. By the time the larger motoneurons are recruited during intense reflex activity, the amount of contractile tension added by each motor unit is a small fraction of the total muscle tension, so the graded nature of the contraction remains fine. Inhibition is also organized on the size principle: large motoneurons are more readily inhibited than are small motoneurons. Thus, small motoneurons are responsible for the bulk of the muscular activity of the body, and large motoneurons are called on only rarely when very strenuous activity is required.

Inhibition

The term inhibition as applied to synaptic transmission refers to an active process by which excitatory transmission is prevented. Eccles defined inhibition as follows:

> Nerve impulses exert an inhibitory action when they cause a depression of the generation of impulses by nerve or muscle cell, which is attributable to a specific physiological process and which does not arise as a consequence of its previous activation.

Thus, the decrease in excitability of a neuron caused by a large after-hyperpolarization is not attributable to inhibition; it is caused by previous activity of the cell.

There are at least two types of central nervous system inhibition, including postsynaptic and presynaptic. In a sense, the terms are inadequate because both mechanisms involve synaptic transmission and presumably chemical transmitter substances. However, the nomenclature was developed because of the locations of the inhibitory synapses on the membrane of the postsynaptic cell. Postsynaptic inhibition is mediated by synapses placed directly on the membrane of the postsynaptic cell. With pre-

synaptic inhibition, the inhibitory synapses are located on the presynaptic endings of excitatory nerve fibers going to the postsynaptic cell. In other words, the inhibitory endings are presynaptic to excitatory endings, which in turn are presynaptic to another cell.

Postsynaptic inhibition. The inhibitory transmitter substance responsible for postsynaptic inhibition produces a hyperpolarization of the postsynaptic membrane. The hyperpolarization seems to be caused by an increase in membrane permeability to potassium and chloride. The equilibrium potential for chloride ions is probably at or near the resting potential, but that for potassium ions is some 20 mV more negative than the resting potential. An increase in permeability to both of these ions should result in a shift in membrane potential toward, but not to, the potassium equilibrium potential. The level will be a balance between the chloride and potassium equilibrium potentials. This shift is considered to be the cause of the inhibitory postsynaptic potential (IPSP), which may be recorded intracellularly during the time of activity of inhibitory nerve impulses (Fig. 4-15).

If a current is passed across the membrane in such a way as to hyperpolarize the cell, the inhibitory potential is reduced in size and even reversed at successive stages of polarization. On the other hand, a depolarization of the cell will increase the size of the inhibitory potential. In short, the inhibitory potential tends to approach a particular level, which is intermediate between the potassium and chloride equilibrium potentials. The amplitude and direction of the IPSP will vary predictably as the membrane potential is shifted in relationship to the equilibrium potential of the IPSP.

The equilibrium potential for chloride ions may be altered experimentally by injecting chloride ions into the interior of a neuron, by using a current, or simply by diffusion. An increase in the internal chloride ion concentration will lower the chloride equilibrium potential. The inhibitory potential still approaches a level between the chloride and potassium equilibrium potential. If enough chloride is injected, the inhibitory potential is smaller or even reversed at resting potential. The original state returns as the chloride concentration reverts to normal.

Mechanism of postsynaptic inhibition. The ionic shifts that drive the inhibitory potential toward a particular level, depending on the chloride and potassium equilibrium potentials, occur only during the initial part of the inhibitory potential. These currents alter the charge on the membrane capacitance, just as do the currents responsible for the EPSP, and the resting potential is restored only after a period of time (Fig. 4-16).

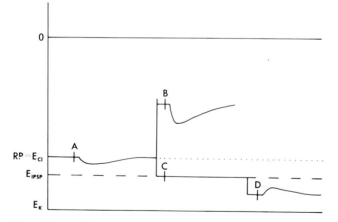

Fig. 4-15. Inhibitory postsynaptic potential (IPSP). **A,** Hyperpolarization of a motoneuron membrane during the action of an inhibitory volley. The equilibrium potentials for chloride (E_{Cl}) and for potassium (E_K) are shown, as well as the resting potential (RP) and the equilibrium potential for the IPSP (E_{IPSP}). If the membrane is depolarized, **B,** the ionic driving force during the inhibitory action is greater, so the IPSP becomes larger. If the membrane is hyperpolarized to the E_{IPSP}, **C,** the ions flowing during the inhibitory action do not change the membrane potential. If the membrane is hyperpolarized beyond the E_{IPSP}, **D,** the IPSP is reversed.

The hyperpolarization, which lasts throughout the IPSP, would carry the membrane potential away from threshold for the production of an action potential. Thus, an EPSP would have to be large enough not only to depolarize the neuron from resting potential to threshold potential, but also to depolarize the membrane from the level of the inhibitory potential to the resting potential.

However, during the period of time that the ionic currents generating the inhibitory potential are flowing, there is another factor that limits the potency of an excitatory volley. The membrane becomes hyperpolarized by a reduction in membrane resistance. Synaptic currents that would normally produce a large excitatory potential are much less effective during this time. In effect, the excitatory potential is shunted and is thus less capable of depolarizing the neuron to threshold.

Types of postsynaptic inhibition. There appear to be at least two kinds of postsynaptic inhibition. Both have the same ionic mechanism, but they can be distinguished by their location in the nervous system, their duration, and their susceptibility to strychnine poisoning. The IPSPs of the spinal cord have a relatively brief duration of 10 to 50 msec, and they are reduced or eliminated in strychnine intoxication. The effect may, in fact, account for strychnine convulsions. On the other hand, many of the IPSPs of the brain (cerebral cortex, hippocampus, and cerebellar cortex) have a duration of over 100 msec. The effect of strychnine on these brain IPSPs is variable. Some appear to be blocked; others seem to be strychnine resistant.

Reciprocal inhibition. The fact that group Ia afferent fibers from muscle spindles produce monosynaptic EPSPs in motoneurons supplying the same muscle that contains the muscle spindles or its synergists

has already been discussed. When group Ia fibers from the antagonistic muscle are stimulated, an IPSP can be recorded from the motoneuron. The time course of the IPSP is similar to that of the monosynaptic EPSP. It has a brief rising phase of about 1 msec and a slower decay of about 10 msec. The rising phase occurs during the synaptic currents produced by the action of the transmitter substance released by the inhibitory terminals. The decay phase is presumably caused by a passive discharge of the potential. However, the IPSP differs from the monosynaptic EPSP in that its latency is nearly a millisecond longer. This and other evidence indicate that the inhibitory pathway is not monosynaptic. Instead, it is disynaptic, there being an interneuron interposed in the pathway. The group Ia afferent fibers excite a population of interneurons, which in turn re-

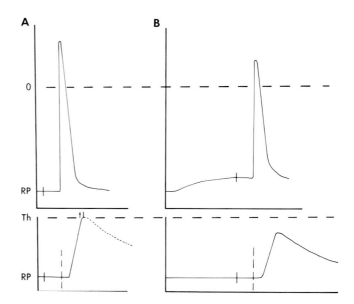

Fig. 4-17. Presynaptic inhibition resulting in EPSP depression. The upper traces in **A** and **B** represent events in the presynaptic terminals of group Ia afferent fibers; the lower traces show a monosynaptic EPSP recorded from an alpha motoneuron. The EPSP in **A** is at threshold *(Th)*, sometimes firing an impulse (indicated by the vertical line by the arrow). In **B** a depolarization of the presynaptic terminal is shown in the upper trace. This results from the action of a presynaptic inhibitory volley (shock artifacts not shown) set up before the excitatory volley. The depolarization causes a reduction in amplitude of the presynaptic action potential. This in turn causes a reduction in the amount of excitatory transmitter substance released by the nerve endings and hence a reduction in the size of the EPSP (lower trace). Note that the depolarization in the presynaptic terminal has no direct effect on the postsynaptic membrane (the rate of miniature synaptic potentials should be increased, but not enough to sum and change the membrane potential). The reduced EPSP is now below threshold, so the excitatory transmission is inhibited. *RP*, resting potential levels.

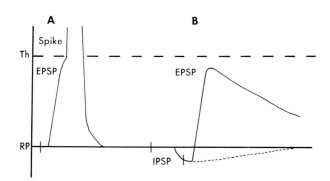

Fig. 4-16. Mechanism of postsynaptic inhibition. A monosynaptic EPSP is shown in **A** to exceed threshold and thus to fire an alpha motoneuron. In **B** the EPSP is lowered below threshold by the action of an IPSP.

lease an inhibitory transmitter at their terminals on motoneurons.

A variety of studies have produced two candidate substances, one of which may be the inhibitory transmitter substance released on motoneurons by group Ia activated inhibitory interneurons. One of these substances is glycine; the other is gamma-aminobutyric acid. Both of these substances tend to depress motoneurons when released near them from micropipettes by microelectrophoresis; however, the action of glycine is more readily blocked by strychnine.

Presynaptic inhibition. Another type of central nervous system inhibition is called presynaptic inhibition. As mentioned, the term used depends on the location of the synapses involved.

The mechanism of presynaptic inhibition is quite different from that of postsynaptic inhibition. The postsynaptic membrane is not affected in any detectable way during presynaptic inhibition. The inhibition is produced by a reduction in the amount of transmitter substance released by the excitatory nerve terminals (Fig. 4-17). This is brought about by a depolarization of the presynaptic terminals of the excitatory fibers.

Depolarization and transmitter release. The way in which a depolarization of presynaptic terminals can reduce transmitter release has been studied in several isolated tissue preparations. The best evidence, perhaps, is from work on the isolated squid giant synapse preparation. In this synapse, the presynaptic terminal is so large that several microelectrodes can be inserted into it. One or more can also be placed within the postsynaptic cell. The membrane potential of the presynaptic element can be altered by passing current through one electrode, and the new level is recorded through another electrode. The amplitude of the spike potential in the presynaptic fiber can be recorded at several levels of membrane potential, and this amplitude may be correlated with the size of the excitatory potential recorded from the postsynaptic cell. It has been found that a depolarization reduces the size of the presynaptic spike potential and of the excitatory postsynaptic potential. The reverse occurs with a hyperpolarization.

The effect of polarizing currents on the release of transmitter substance can be understood if the amount of transmitter released depends on the size of the presynaptic spike potential. There is considerable evidence that this is the case (see Chapter 3).

Potentials associated with presynaptic inhibition. The depolarization of afferent terminals that is associated with presynaptic inhibition can be recorded in several ways. Because presynaptic inhibitory synapses occur on primary afferent fibers, it is possible

to show that these fibers become depolarized simply by recording from them in filaments of dorsal roots. The potentials thus recorded are called dorsal root potentials (Fig. 4-18). The same process causes a potential change that can be recorded from the spinal cord as the positive intermediary cord potential. Several other techniques, including intracellular recording from primary afferent fibers, have been used to detect the depolarization. This type of inhibition is likely to be of considerable physiological interest, because it lasts longer than the spinal cord type of postsynaptic inhibition (duration of hundreds, rather than tens, of milliseconds). Presynaptic inhibition is strychnine resistant; it is reduced by picrotoxin, another convulsant. The transmitter responsible for producing presynaptic inhibition is unknown. The pathway seems to be polysynaptic.

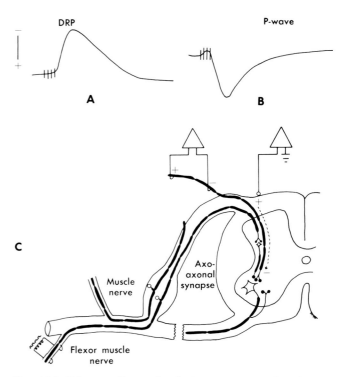

Fig. 4-18. Primary afferent depolarization associated with presynaptic inhibition. Presynaptic inhibitory volleys cause a depolarization of the terminals of primary afferent fibers. This depolarization spreads electrotonically back out the afferent fibers at least as far as the dorsal root, where it can be recorded as a dorsal root potential *(DRP)*, **A.** An electrode placed on the dorsal surface of the cord will record a positive potential known as a positive intermediary cord potential *(P-wave)*, **B.** The recording arrangement is drawn in **C.** The current flow associated with the primary afferent depolarization travels in the extracellular fluids from the dorsal part of the cord toward the region of afferent termination. Thus, the dorsal region of the cord becomes positive and the ventral part negative during the primary afferent depolarization, as indicated by the dotted line in **C.**

SPINAL CORD INTERNEURONS
Structure

Interneurons are central neurons other than moto-neurons. A special category of spinal interneuron is the tract cell that sends an axon to the brain. Interneurons within the spinal cord vary in size from the very small cells of the substantia gelatinosa to the cells of origin of the ventral spinocerebellar tract, which are as large as alpha motoneurons (Fig. 4-19). The dendrites are oriented in different ways, depending on the location and presumably the function of the interneurons. The dendrites of interneurons of the substantia gelatinosa are found primarily in a sagittal plane, whereas more deeply situated interneurons have their dendrites spread transversely across the cord gray matter.

The distribution of the axons of spinal interneurons determines their sphere of influence. The small interneurons of the substantia gelatinosa send axons only to other regions of the substantia gelatinosa, either of the same or the contralateral side. Some of the large interneurons in Rexed's laminae IV and V give

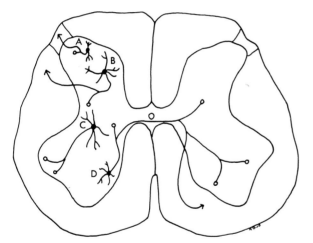

Fig. 4-19. The cell bodies, dendrites, and the axons of several kinds of spinal interneurons in the spinal cord gray matter, as seen in Golgi-stained preparations. The terminations of axons within the gray matter are indicated by the open circles; ascending axon collaterals are shown by the arrowheads. Interneuron *A* belongs to the substantia gelatinosa (laminae II to III). Its axon either terminates within the substantia gelatinosa near the cell or projects through the dorsolateral fasciculus (of Lissauer) to the substantia gelatinosa at a different segmental level. The interneuron *B* lies in the nucleus proprius (laminae IV to V). In addition to local terminals, many of the cells in this region send an axon collateral up the dorsal part of the lateral funiculus as part of the spinocervical tract. Interneuron *C* is in the intermediate nucleus (lamina VII) and projects to the motor nucleus. The cell labeled *D* is in the commissural nucleus (lamina VIII); its axon has terminals both in the ipsilateral and in the contralateral gray matter, and a branch ascends as part of the ventrolateral system to the brainstem.

rise to fibers of a tract that ascends the ipsilateral side of the cord in the lateral funiculus. In addition, interneurons in the same laminae project axons ventrally within the gray matter of the cord. Interneurons at the base of the dorsal horn, in the intermediate region, and in the medial part of the ventral horn send axons contralaterally. Many of these form ascending tracts. In addition, collaterals of these axons synapse both ipsilaterally and contralaterally in the cord gray matter. Interneurons in the lateral part of the ventral horn appear to distribute axons ipsilaterally within a few segments of their cell bodies.

Distribution of primary afferents

Primary afferent fibers are distributed throughout much of the ipsilateral spinal cord gray matter. However, the distribution of afferents is by no means uniform. Afferents from sensory receptors of the skin appear to terminate chiefly or entirely in the dorsal horn. These afferents synapse just with interneurons. Muscle afferents end deep within the dorsal horn, in the intermediate region, and in the ventral horn. As already discussed, group Ia afferent fibers end both on motoneurons and on certain types of interneurons. Other classes of muscle afferents, such as group Ib afferents from Golgi tendon organs, synapse just with interneurons. Some types of interneurons do not seem to receive any synaptic connections from primary afferent fibers.

Electrical activity of interneurons

Intracellular records from interneurons have revealed that these cells generate excitatory and inhibitory postsynaptic potentials in the same fashion as motoneurons when pathways synapsing on them are activated. They also show spontaneous synaptic noise in the absence of intentional stimulation. When monosynaptic excitatory pathways to interneurons are studied, it is possible to show that the characteristics of the monosynaptic EPSPs resemble those of the monosynaptic EPSPs recorded in motoneurons in response to stimulation of group Ia afferent fibers. Thus, in many respects interneurons behave like motoneurons. However, there are points of difference for particular types of interneurons.

Some interneurons generate a prolonged EPSP in response to activation even of a monosynaptic pathway (Fig. 4-20). It is not clear why such EPSP's last longer than those recorded from motoneurons; but whatever the mechanism, long-lasting EPSPs are of great significance, both in the spinal cord and in the brain. Such EPSPs may exceed threshold for exciting an interneuron for a time longer than the refractory period and thus cause a repetitive dis-

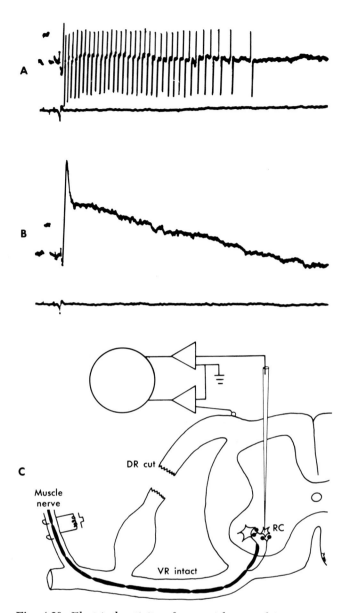

charge. Many interneurons fire repetitively in response to a single afferent volley. The importance of this is that such behavior allows interneurons to act as a kind of amplifier, because each action potential generated by an interneuron would exert its own effect at the synaptic terminals of the interneuron. A burst discharge would guarantee temporal summation of the effects of the interneuron, whether these are excitatory or inhibitory.

In addition to the long-lasting EPSP, a subsidiary reason for the ability of many interneurons to fire repetitively is that their action potentials do not terminate with a large after-hyperpolarization, as do those of motoneurons. There is, therefore, no substantial subnormal period to interfere with repetitive discharge.

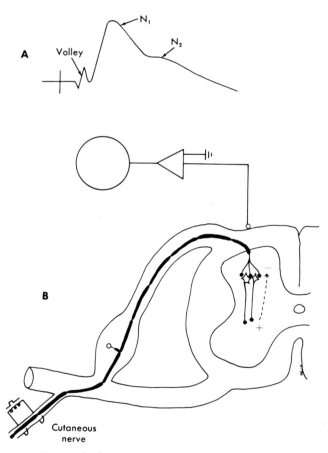

Fig. 4-20. Electrical activity of a special type of interneuron, the Renshaw cell. Renshaw cells *(RC)* are located in the ventral part of lamina VII, between the motor nucleus and lamina VIII. Stimulation of motor axons in a peripheral nerve or in a ventral root causes synaptic activation of Renshaw cells because the antidromic volley in the motor axons invades recurrent collaterals that terminate on these special interneurons. An extracellular recording from a Renshaw cell is shown in **A.** The response to a single stimulus to a peripheral nerve (dorsal roots cut) is a repetitive discharge of the Renshaw cell. A few moments later, the microelectrode impaled the same Renshaw cell, and the EPSP shown in **B** was recorded in response to the same motor axon volley. The Renshaw cell was apparently damaged enough by the impalement that the ability of the cell to fire spikes was lost. Note that the EPSP has an initial rapid phase followed by a slow phase. The initial high rate of discharge of the Renshaw cell in **A** is no doubt caused by the initial part of the EPSP, whereas the discharge train lasts as long as the slow phase of the EPSP exceeds threshold. The recording arrangement is shown in **C.**

Fig. 4-21. Cord dorsum negative potentials during activity of dorsal horn interneurons. Stimulation of a cutaneous nerve causes the excitation of a large population of interneurons in the dorsal horn of the spinal cord. In **A** the volley is entering the spinal cord, followed by two successive negative waves (N_1 and N_2), which are associated with EPSPs and spikes generated by the volley in dorsal horn interneurons. The recording arrangement is shown in **B.** Note that the current flow during the excitation of dorsal horn interneurons is from ventral to dorsal, so that a gross electrode placed on the dorsal surface of the cord will record a negative potential.

The synaptic activity and discharges of a population of interneurons in the dorsal horn can be recorded from the dorsal surface of the spinal cord in response to stimulation of either a dorsal root or a cutaneous nerve (Fig. 4-21). The potential recorded takes the form of a series of negative waves called N waves. N waves can also be recorded as negative potentials by a microelectrode inserted into the dorsal horn. Inasmuch as muscle afferents end on interneurons situated more deeply in the gray matter, as well as on motoneurons, the synaptic activity of these is not readily recorded from the dorsal surface of the spinal cord. However, a negative potential can be recorded from the depths of the cord by a microelectrode.

Actions of interneurons and the final common pathway

Spinal cord interneurons exert a variety of actions. Their discharge may cause excitation or inhibition. The inhibition may be of the presynaptic or postsynaptic type. The interneurons act on other neurons, either other spinal interneurons, motoneurons, or cells of the brain. In the case of presynaptic inhibition, the action of interneurons is on the terminals of primary afferent fibers.

As a general rule, pathways for the conduction of information through the central nervous system involve synaptic relays on one or more interneurons. Very complex pathways may involve a series of many interneurons. Some of these may be located in the spinal cord and others in the brain. The outcome of such information transfer on the behavior of the organism must eventually be determined by the effect of such a pathway on a set of motoneurons. If alpha motoneurons are excited to discharge, muscle contracts. If the motoneurons are prevented from firing because of inhibition, muscle either does not contract or it relaxes, depending on the initial state of the muscle. Because the final decision about the outcome of information transfer through the central nervous system rests with the alpha motoneuron, Sherrington called the motoneuron the final common pathway.

THE REFLEX

The central nervous system is responsible for the coordination of much of our activity. It ensures the smooth performance of movements by causing the proper muscles to contract or to relax in the best sequence. When the needs of the body change, the nervous system produces the appropriate alterations in function of the various systems of the body—cardiovascular, respiratory, digestive, and so on. Sherrington

called this executive role played by the nervous system its integrative action.

Some of the activities of the nervous system are built in by virtue of the synaptic connections made by particular neurons with other neurons. Excitation of a pathway of this type results in the performance of some relatively stereotyped action. Such an action is often called a reflex. The term reflex originated from the writings of Descartes, who suggested that some actions were caused by the reflection of light from the retina to the nervous system, which then caused a muscular response. Sherrington studied a number of reflexes that can be supported by the spinal cord without any connection with the brain. Thus, reflexes are possible in relatively simple neural structures. Reflexes may also be elicited by way of pathways to the brain. However, as the nervous system becomes more complex, the behavior that results from activation of nervous pathways becomes less stereotyped. The conditioned reflex is an example of a higher order of neural activity, and the highest order is that which underlies thought processes.

In the following sections a number of reflex mechanisms are considered. These are representative of the types of activity that can be studied at various levels of the nervous system, although for the most part they have been studied best in the spinal cord. In addition to the basic reflex pathways, some consideration is also given to processes such as posttetanic potentiation, which can alter synaptic transmission and hence reflex activity.

Reflex connections of group Ia afferent fibers

Monosynaptic reflex pathway. The group Ia fibers from primary endings of muscle spindles make up the afferent limb of the monosynaptic reflex pathway (Fig. 4-22). These fibers enter the spinal cord through the dorsal roots and send branches rostrally and caudally in the spinal cord. Collaterals from these branches penetrate the gray matter of the cord and end in the intermediate region and in the motor nucleus. The fibers that terminate in the motor nucleus form direct connections between peripheral receptor organs and alpha motoneurons. The axons of the alpha motoneurons traverse the ventral roots to innervate extrafusal muscle fibers. This pathway involves, therefore, only a single synapse within the central nervous system; thus it is called the monosynaptic reflex pathway.

A great deal of spinal cord neurophysiology has been concerned with the properties of this pathway because it is simple and easily accessible to experiment. Particularly significant contributions were made

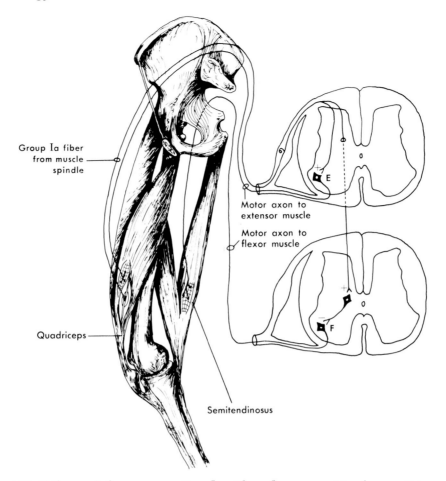

Group Ia fiber
from muscle
spindle

Motor axon to
extensor muscle

Motor axon to
flexor muscle

Quadriceps

Semitendinosus

Fig. 4-22. Pathway of the monosynaptic reflex. The reflex arc consists of an excitatory and an inhibitory component. The excitatory portion is monosynaptic. Group Ia afferent fibers from the primary endings of muscle spindles enter the cord through dorsal roots, traverse the gray matter, and end synaptically on alpha motoneurons to the same muscle as that containing the muscle spindles and to the synergistic muscles (the knee extensor, *E*, quadriceps, is illustrated here). The inhibitory component is disynaptic. Group Ia fibers end on interneurons of the intermediate region of the spinal cord gray matter (in lamina VII) to excite them. The interneurons synapse on motoneurons of the antagonistic muscles to inhibit them (the knee flexor, *F*, semitendinosus, is illustrated here). This reflex arc is thus characterized by reciprocal innervation of muscles opposing each other at a joint.

by D. P. C. Lloyd. It is also of great clinical importance because this pathway is often used in the ordinary tests of reflex activity, such as the knee jerk.

Several methods are available for measuring activity in the monosynaptic reflex pathway. The discharge of large numbers of alpha motoneurons fired synchronously may be recorded monophasically from a cut ventral root (Fig. 4-23). This technique has the advantage that it may be used as a test of the excitability of a population of motoneurons. A single volley of afferent impulses results in the discharge of a certain proportion of motoneurons. This discharge is caused by the monosynaptic EPSP, whose properties have already been discussed. If another

volley of afferent impulses in the nerve to a synergistic muscle, called a conditioning volley, precedes the test volley, the number of motoneurons that discharge may change. This means that the conditioning volley has altered the reflex excitability of the motoneuronal pool. Some of the motoneurons that did not discharge when the test volley was used alone may now discharge because of the action of the conditioning volley. These motoneurons were in the subliminal fringe, but they have been brought to the firing level by the excitatory action of the conditioning impulses. The cause of the change in excitability of the motoneurons was the production of an EPSP by the conditioning volley, which sums with that produced

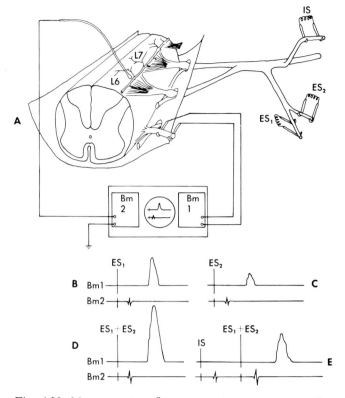

Fig. 4-23. Monosynaptic reflex testing. A monosynaptic reflex spike can be recorded from a ventral root when group Ia afferent fibers are stimulated in a muscle nerve. The reflex discharge is a compound action potential *(Bm1)* in a bundle of alpha motor axons. The lower beam *(Bm2)* is a recording from the dorsal surface of the cord, showing the afferent volley. The size of the reflex spike is proportional to the number of motoneurons participating in the reflex discharge. An afferent volley in a muscle nerve will typically excite monosynaptically all of the alpha motoneurons belonging to the same muscle and most of those supplying synergistic muscles. However, only a fraction of the motoneurons to the same muscle will be excited to threshold, and none of the motoneurons to antagonistic muscles will be discharged. The motoneurons that are excited, but to a level below threshold, are said to belong to the subliminal fringe. Those that fire are in the discharge zone. The monosynaptic reflex spike is often used as a test of the excitability of the population of motoneurons to a muscle. If a conditioning volley in group Ia afferent fibers to a synergistic muscle is combined with a test volley and each volley fires only a small number of motoneurons, the spatial summation of EPSPs evoked by the two volleys may enhance the size of the reflex spike. This is called facilitation, illustrated in **B** to **D**. The stimulating and recording arrangement is shown in **A**. The monosynaptic reflex spikes evoked by the conditioning *(ES₁)* and testing *(ES₂)* volleys are shown in **B** and **C** respectively. When the two volleys are combined, as in **D**, the resultant reflex discharge is larger than the sum of the discharges produced by the two volleys stimulated independently. If an inhibitory volley, such as a volley in group Ia afferent fibers of the antagonistic muscle nerve *(IS)*, precedes the test monosynaptic reflex spike, the number of motoneurons that discharge will be decreased. The reflex spike will thus be smaller, as illustrated in **E**. The timing of the facilitatory and inhibitory conditioning volleys can be varied with respect to the test volley. This allows a determination of the time course of excitation or inhibition.

by the test volley. This is a case of spatial summation. Conversely, an IPSP or a presynaptic inhibitory volley will reduce the reflex excitability, as tested by the monosynaptic reflex.

When the effects of conditioning volleys on individual motoneurons are studied, one of several techniques may be used. Single alpha motoneuronal axons may be dissected in ventral roots; the probability of discharge is then employed as an indication of motoneuronal excitability. A more direct method is intracellular recording from motoneurons. This allows the recording of excitatory or inhibitory postsynaptic potentials, although there is the possible disadvantage of some damage to the neuron because of the penetration by the microelectrode. Another approach that can be used clinically is to record discharges from single motor units by electromyography.

Myotatic unit. Muscles may be classified according to their function. When several muscles cooperate in a function, such as extension of a joint, they are said to be synergists. When they are opposed in a function, they are called antagonists.

The group Ia afferent fibers from a muscle have been found to excite by a monosynaptic reflex pathway the alpha motoneurons to the same muscle and to its synergists. Thus, all the muscles that cooperate in a particular action are linked together reflexly by this pathway, which is very powerful and rapid in action. On the other hand, the same group Ia fibers inhibit motoneurons supplying antagonistic muscles. The inhibitory pathway is disynaptic, the interneuron having its cell body in the intermediate gray matter of the spinal cord.

The group of synergistic and antagonistic muscles about a joint is called the myotatic unit, and the pattern of excitatory innervation of synergists and inhibitory innervation of antagonists is referred to as reciprocal innervation. The function of reciprocal innervation is clearly to enable a group of synergists to reinforce the action of one another and to eliminate the opposition of antagonistic muscles to a particular movement.

Initiation of monosynaptic reflex and clinical applications. The monosynaptic reflex pathway may be activated by one of several methods. The usual laboratory technique is to stimulate electrically the lowest threshold fibers of a muscle nerve. This approach is also of value in certain types of clinical tests.

However, a more physiological stimulus is a stretch of a muscle and its contained muscle spindles. This distorts the primary endings about intrafusal fibers and produces an increase in the rate of firing of the group Ia afferent fibers (see Chapter 2). If the stretch is a rapid one, a nearly synchronous burst of impulses reaches the motoneurons of that muscle and its synergists. The excitatory potentials set up by these impulses are generally large enough to discharge the motoneurons belonging to the muscle whose afferents were stimulated, but not those to the synergistic muscles. The motoneuronal discharge is then detected by noting the phasic contraction of the extrafusal muscle fibers. This is the basis for the clinical tests of the so-called deep-tendon reflexes, such as the knee jerk and the ankle jerk. In the neurologic examination, a reflex hammer is used to strike a tendon (such as the patellar or Achilles tendon). This results in a rapid stretch of the muscle and a reflex contraction. It also causes a temporary relaxation of the antagonistic muscles because of the inhibition produced by the afferent volley in their motoneurons. In disease states, a reflex contraction may not be elicitable, or it may be excessively strong. In the latter case, a spread of reflex contractions to synergistic muscles may occur.

The monosynaptic reflex pathway is employed by the nervous system not only for the production of phasic movements but also for maintenance of posture. This can be demonstrated by the stretch reflex. If the tension of a muscle is recorded by a myograph, it can be shown that the muscle develops both active and passive tension as it is stretched.

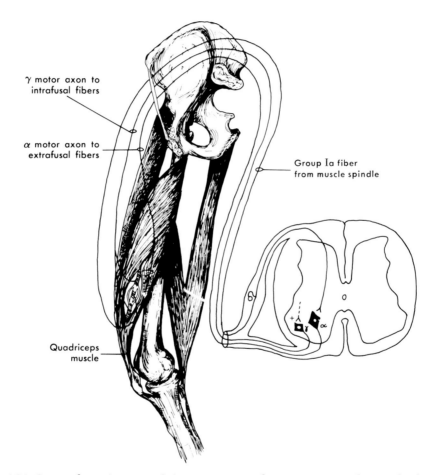

Fig. 4-24. Gamma loop. A gamma (γ) motoneuron is shown innervating the intrafusal muscle fibers of a muscle spindle. Excitation of gamma motoneurons by pathways, such as segmental reflex paths or tracts descending from the brain (indicated by the broken line approaching the gamma motoneuron cell body), will cause the contraction of the polar regions of muscle spindles. This results in stretch of the equatorial regions of the spindles, with distortion of the afferent terminals belonging to group Ia and II fibers. The group Ia fibers that discharge will excite alpha (α) motoneurons to the same and to synergistic muscles through the monosynaptic reflex pathway and inhibit alpha motoneurons to the antagonistic muscles. The gamma loop mechanism may help in the initiation of movements, acting as a servomechanism. In addition, it prevents the unloading effect that would ensue if the extrafusal muscle contracted without simultaneous shortening of the muscle spindles.

The amount of passive tension can be estimated by repeating the stretch after the nerve is servered. The reflex mechanism involved in the active component of the tension is the monosynaptic reflex pathway. The stretch reflex would assist in maintaining posture, because any movement of a joint would produce a stretch of the muscles that act to oppose the movement. In some disease states, the stretch reflex is hyperactive. This results in strong opposition of muscles to stretch when joints are passively moved.

Gamma loop. Movements, whether voluntary or involuntary, may be initiated in one of two ways. Alpha motoneurons may be excited directly by excitatory synaptic bombardment, or they may be excited indirectly by the gamma loop mechanism (Fig. 4-24). If gamma motoneurons are excited to discharge, a contraction of intrafusal muscle fibers will result in shortening of the muscle spindles of the appropriate muscles. This will cause an increased discharge rate of group Ia afferent fibers and hence excitation of the motoneurons to the same muscles (plus inhibition of motoneurons to antagonistic muscles).

The gamma loop mechanism is probably involved in most smoothly coordinated movements. If the contraction of intrafusal fibers precedes or keeps pace with the contraction of extrafusal muscle fibers, a high discharge rate may be maintained in group Ia afferents, resulting in a continuous excitation of alpha motoneurons. Movements produced by activation just of alpha motoneurons would be expected to have a less coordinated character, because extrafusal fiber contractions would unload muscle spindles and thus produce a decrease in Ia activity (see Chapter 2).

Presynaptic inhibition of group Ia pathways. A long-lasting depolarization of group Ia terminals may

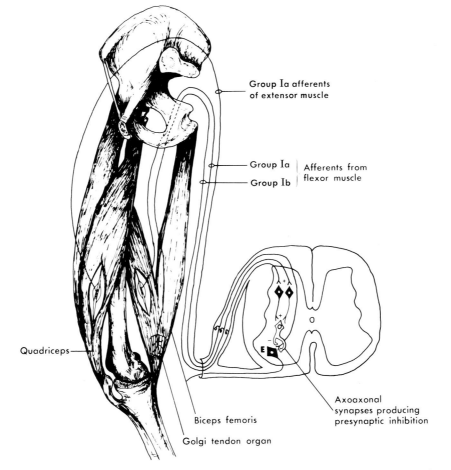

Group Ia afferents
of extensor muscle

Group Ia | Afferents from
Group Ib | flexor muscle

Quadriceps

Axoaxonal
synapses producing
presynaptic inhibition

Biceps femoris

Golgi tendon organ

Fig. 4-25. Pathway for presynaptic inhibition of group Ia afferent fibers. A group Ia afferent fiber from an extensor muscle is shown receiving axoaxonal synapses from an interneuron. Group Ia afferent fibers of flexor muscles receive similar axoaxonal synapses. The depolarization of the afferent terminals by the interneuron reduces the amount of transmitter released by the terminal, resulting in presynaptic inhibition. The afferent fibers producing the presynaptic inhibition are group Ia and Ib fibers belonging to muscle nerves. The location of the interneurons in the pathway for presynaptic inhibition is unknown.

be produced by stimulation of certain pathways. The depolarization causes a reduction in the amount of transmitter that will be released when afferent volleys reach the depolarized terminals. This results in presynaptic inhibition, because there will be a diminished amount of postsynaptic activity.

The pathways that cause presynaptic inhibition of group Ia activity include group Ia and Ib afferent fibers from muscle and a bulbospinal pathway (Fig. 4-25). No doubt others will be found.

The action of presynaptic inhibitory volleys can be studied in a number of ways. For instance, the depolarization of the group Ia afferent fibers can be detected by intracellular recording from such fibers. The inhibitory action can be determined either by monosynaptic reflex testing or by demonstrating a reduction in the size of the intracellularly recorded monosynaptic EPSP.

Significance of presynaptic inhibition of group Ia afferents. The importance of presynaptic inhibition in reflex actions is not yet evident. However, the central neurons can derive at least one important benefit from presynaptic as opposed to postsynaptic inhibition. Presynaptic inhibition prevents an excitatory pathway from activating a neuron, in this case a motoneuron. Yet the excitability of the motoneuron is unaltered by the inhibitory volley. This leaves the motoneuron free to respond to other pathways. Presynaptic inhibition may thus serve as a switching mechanism. In the case of the group Ia monosynaptic reflex pathway, presynaptic inhibition would tend to eliminate the stretch reflex, allowing the motoneurons to participate in other activities.

Group Ia information reaching the brain. There are pathways by which information from group Ia fibers from muscle spindles reaches the brain (see Chapters 7 and 8). Recent evidence indicates that input from muscle spindles may play a role in position sense and kinesthesis. In addition, such information may play a major role in the subconscious modulation of spinal cord reflexes by way of descending pathways from the brain to the spinal cord.

One of the brain areas affected by volleys in group Ia afferents is the sensorimotor cortex. A substantial amount of activity can be recorded from a zone adjacent to the motor cortex in response to stimulation of group Ia fibers. Evidently this activity is involved in modifying the discharges of neurons of the motor cortex.

Another brain area known to receive muscle spindle information from group Ia fibers is the cerebellum. This information is relayed by cells of the spinocerebellar tracts. These cells, which lie within the spinal cord gray matter, are excited mono-

synaptically by group Ia fibers. Details about the spinocerebellar tracts may be found in Chapter 8. Inasmuch as one of the major functions of the cerebellum lies in the smoothing and controlling of spinal cord reflex actions, it seems reasonable that the cerebellum is provided with information originating from the muscle spindles.

Flexion reflex

Function of flexion reflex. Limb movements that occur because of the contraction of flexor muscles are of benefit in a number of behavioral patterns. For instance, flexion of a limb is important when damage might otherwise result, as when the foot encounters a sharp object. Flexion of limbs is also a part of the activity involved in progression. Sherrington and his students were among the early investigators of the flexion reflex.

This reflex may be elicited easily in "spinal" animals; that is, in those with limbs innervated by the part of the spinal cord below a complete transection. The reason for this will be apparent later. Many kinds of stimuli, particularly to the skin, will evoke the flexion reflex. However, it is perhaps most easily produced by harmful stimuli. The muscles that contract during withdrawal of a limb from a nociceptive stimulus are defined as physiological flexor muscles. Several muscles considered extensors from an anatomical point of view, such as the extensor digitorum longus muscle of the leg, are flexors from the physiological point of view. The motion of dorsiflexion of the foot is part of the flexion reflex; the opposite motion, plantar flexion, may be considered an extension in physiological terms.

Pathway of flexion reflex. The receptors that give rise to activity in the flexion reflex pathway include not only nociceptors, but also touch, pressure, and other types of receptors (Fig. 4-26). This suggests that the flexion reflex may be initiated during other activities than withdrawal from harmful stimuli; presumably, the reflex is used for walking, running, and other activities. Besides the cutaneous receptors, afferent input to the flexion reflex comes from secondary endings of muscle spindles, pressure-pain endings in fasciae, and some joint receptors.

The afferent fiber diameters of myelinated axons carrying information to the flexion reflex pathway range from 1 to 12 μm, including groups II and III. It is reasonable to expect that unmyelinated fibers (group IV) also contribute to the flexion reflex.

Within the spinal cord the flexion reflex afferents (FRA) divide into ascending and descending branches, collaterals of which enter the gray matter. These collaterals terminate in the dorsal horn on interneurons.

The interneurons project to other interneurons or to motoneurons. Thus, information reaches motoneurons through a polysynaptic pathway.

The pattern of innervation of motoneurons determines the character of the reflex. The interneuronal pathways are arranged so that the last interneurons projecting to extensor motoneurons are inhibitory ones; therefore, the FRA inhibit postsynaptically extensor motoneurons. The pathway to flexor motoneurons is made up of excitatory interneurons; thus, flexor motoneurons are excited by the FRA. The resultant activity in the limb from which the stimulated FRA arise is a flexion movement, caused by the

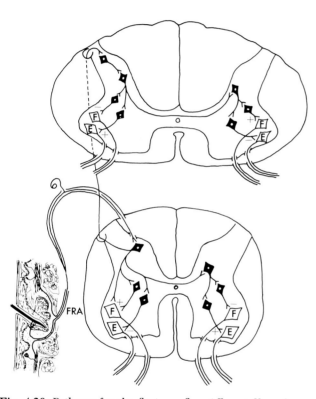

Fig. 4-26. Pathway for the flexion reflex. Afferent fibers from a variety of sensory receptor organs can initiate flexion reflexes. These receptors may be in the skin, muscle, or joints. The afferents enter the spinal cord and excite interneurons of the dorsal horn. The interneurons act on motoneurons, either directly or through relay paths involving other interneurons. The eventual effects are an excitation of alpha motoneurons to the flexor muscles *(F)* and an inhibition of alpha motoneurons to the extensor muscles *(E)* of the limb stimulated. If the reflex excitability of the spinal cord is high and the stimulus strong, there may be a spread of the reflex to the contralateral limb. In this event, however, the excitation is of extensor motoneurons, and the inhibition is of flexor motoneurons. In highly excitable spinal cords, the action may spread to the other pair of limbs. The reflex actions in this set of limbs would be just opposite of those in the first set: extension of the limb ipsilateral to the stimulus and flexion of the limb on the contralateral side. *FRA*, flexion reflex afferents.

relaxation of extensor muscles and the contraction of flexor muscles.

The limb opposite to that in which the FRA are stimulated behaves in the reverse fashion. The extensor muscles contract and the flexor muscles relax, resulting in the crossed extension reflex. This behavior would be appropriate, for example, in an animal that had just stepped on a thorn. The injured foot would be withdrawn, while the other limb of the pair would extend to keep the body from toppling. A very strong stimulus to the FRA results in activity in all four limbs. The pattern of the flexion reflex also varies with the particular FRA that are excited. For example, the reflex is different when receptors in the foot are stimulated from the reflex that occurs when receptors in the skin over the thigh are excited. The variation in the pattern of a reflex according to the source of afferent input was termed local sign by Sherrington.

Other connections made by FRA. The flexion reflex afferents produce a variety of actions within the spinal cord in addition to those on motoneurons. For instance, stimulation of one set of FRA will result in presynaptic inhibition of other FRA. The purpose of this is not yet clear. One suggestion is that a large volley produced by a strong stimulus, for example, to the skin, will excite a set of interneurons within the spinal cord. One of the consequences of this will be the presynaptic inhibition of other pathways from the skin that are only weakly stimulated at the moment. The strongly excited pathway will convey the information required for an action, whereas the nervous system will no longer receive extraneous information not relevant to that action. An interesting case that may be explained on this basis is the interference that a given cutaneous stimulus may exert on the perception of another cutaneous stimulus. For instance, the perception of pain from a focal region of the skin may be reduced by tactile stimulation of an adjacent area of skin. This interference could as well take place at other levels of the central nervous system than the first synapse. However, it is likely that intercepting information at the earliest point in a pathway may be the most economical way of stopping its action.

As stated above, information from the FRA reaches the level of consciousness. The pathways for this include one for information related to mechanical stimulation of the skin and joints and another for pain and temperature. The main pathway for relaying information concerned with mechanical stimulation is the dorsal column pathway (fasciculi gracilis and cuneatus); pain and temperature data are transmitted through the ventrolateral system. Some information concerning mechanical stimulation is also conveyed by a pathway, called the spinocervical tract, in the dorsal part of the lateral funiculus. In addition, mechanical stimuli activate some fibers of the ventrolateral system. (These pathways are discussed in Chapter 7.) However, it is likely that not all mechanically activated afferents should be classed as FRA.

The FRA also send information to the cerebellum through the spinocerebellar and spino-olivary tracts. Presumably, the cerebellum requires information about the ongoing activity in the flexion reflex system in order to coordinate movements properly.

Control of the flexion reflex. When the FRA are stimulated in an animal in which a transection has been made through the midbrain, little or no flexion occurs (Fig. 4-27).The flexion reflex is thus difficult to elicit in the decerebrate preparation. If the spinal cord is cut to make a spinal preparation, or if the spinal cord is cooled, making a functional transection, the flexion reflex appears. Apparently there is a pathway descending from the brainstem that in the decerebrate animal tonically inhibits the flexion reflex pathway. This tonic descending pathway has been under study in Sweden by Lundberg and his associates.

The tonic descending inhibitory pathway is less active in the intact animal than in the decerebrate preparation. It appears that the inhibitory pathway itself is under the control of the part of the brain that is above the midbrain level.

In summary, the flexion reflex involves a segmental mechanism, which includes an afferent pathway from a variety of receptors and a set of interneurons. The activity of this mechanism results in an excitation of flexor motoneurons and an inhibition of extensor motoneurons of the limb that is stimulated. The motoneurons of other limbs are affected in an appropriate manner. The flexion reflex pathway is under the control of an inhibitory system originating in the brainstem. This inhibitory system is, in turn, under the influence of still higher centers.

Spinal cord control mechanisms

Negative feedback. A number of physiological mechanisms can be described in terms used for servomechanisms. One commonly used term is negative feedback. The principle involved in a negative feedback device is that a part of the output of the system is rechanneled or fed back into the system in such a way as to reduce the activity of the system. For instance, an elevation of blood glucose will ordinarily produce the secretion of insulin, which will in turn set in operation processes that will lower blood glucose levels.

Stretch reflex as negative feedback. The operation of the stretch reflex in maintaining the position of a joint may be regarded as a negative feedback device.

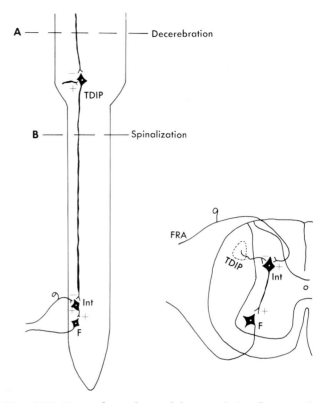

Fig. 4-27. Tonic descending inhibition of the flexion reflex pathway. The segmental pathway for the flexion reflex is diagrammed, using a single interneuron (*Int*) to represent the central component of the path. *FRA*, flexion reflex afferents entering through the dorsal root. In addition, the terminals of an axon belonging to a descending pathway (*TDIP*) are shown in synaptic relationship to the flexion reflex interneuron. The effect of nerve impulses in this descending pathway is to inhibit the interneurons mediating the flexion reflex. Because the activity of the descending pathway is normally continuous, this is called a tonic descending inhibitory pathway. The cells of origin of the pathway are located in the lower brainstem. It is presumed that these neurons receive a continuous excitatory drive, which is indicated by the synapse having a plus sign by it. In addition, the cells giving rise to the tonic descending inhibitory pathway are themselves subject to inhibition from higher levels of the nervous system, as indicated by the synapse having a minus sign by it. Transection of the upper brainstem (*A*) results in an increased activity in the tonic descending inhibitory pathway, because the neurons are released from the inhibitory control from higher centers. This increase in tonic inhibition of flexion reflex interneurons helps shift the reflex balance in the spinal cord in favor of the extensor motoneurons and contributes to decerebrate rigidity (the extensor hypertonus seen in animals having a transection of the upper brainstem). Transection of the spinal cord (*B*) eliminates the action of the tonic descending inhibitory pathway, allowing an increased activity of the flexion reflex interneurons. This contributes to the tendency for paraplegic individuals to display overly active flexion reflex responses and to develop a chronic posture of flexion.

Suppose that the extensor and flexor muscles about the knee joint are participating in the maintenance of a particular posture. If one set of muscles contracts too much, the opposing muscles are stretched. This will produce an afferent barrage that will tend to inhibit the contraction of the first set of muscles and to produce a further contraction of the second set. An excessive contraction of the second set of muscles will result in the reverse process. In this way the opposing muscles will produce a balance of tension that will keep the joint position fairly constant.

When the excitability of the alpha motoneurons is excessive, the alternation of contraction of the antago-nistic groups of muscles is not damped as it is normally. The sudden stretch of a muscle may then produce clonus, an alternating contraction of antagonistic muscles resulting in a series of extension and flexion movements. Clonus may last only a brief time (nonsustained), or it may continue for a long time (sustained).

Gamma loop. Because muscle spindles are located in parallel to extrafusal muscle fibers, the contraction of the latter will result in a reduction in the tension of the spindles. This in turn will reduce the afferent discharges of group Ia and II endings in the spindles. The impulses from the Ia fibers help maintain the

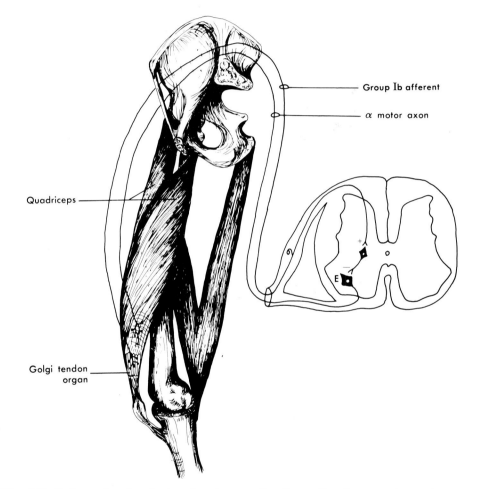

Fig. 4-28. Pathway for clasp knife reflex. A group Ib afferent fiber from a Golgi tendon organ is shown to connect synaptically with an interneuron in the intermediate region of the spinal cord gray matter. The interneuron is excited by the group Ib fiber, and it in turn inhibits an alpha motoneuron supplying the muscle containing the Golgi tendon organ. Golgi tendon organs from extensor muscles also tend to produce excitation of flexor muscles through interneuronal pathways. For this reason the pathway from group Ib afferents is sometimes called the inverse myotatic reflex. Group Ib afferents from flexor muscles do not have as powerful an action as do those from extensor muscles. Apparently the group Ib afferents from flexor muscles are primarily involved in presynaptic inhibitory pathways. The inhibition of an extensor muscle by a pathway from its own Golgi tendon organs has been thought to serve a protective function, because a dramatic increase in tension in a muscle can damage the muscle, the tendon, or the bone. Another function of the reflex pathway is as a tension servo.

excitability of the alpha motoneurons producing the contraction; thus the decrease in these impulses caused by the contraction serves as a negative feedback mechanism. However, the tension of muscle spindles may be maintained if the intrafusal fibers contract. This is accomplished by the discharge of gamma motoneurons. A muscle contraction may be continued effectively if both alpha and gamma motoneurons discharge during the same period of time.

Clasp knife reflex. Another example of a negative feedback mechanism is the clasp knife reflex (Fig. 4-28). When a muscle is stretched, the myotatic (stretch) reflex results in a contraction of the muscle. However, if a very great tension develops, which might damage the muscle or the bone to which it is attached, a reflex is set up that causes a sudden relaxation of the muscle. This reflex is caused by the activity of impulses in group Ib afferent fibers from Golgi tendon organs. These receptors are located within the tendinous insertions of the muscles. They are in series with the muscle fibers, and they are stimulated either by stretch or by contraction of the muscle (see Chapter 2); in other words, they are activated by an increase in tension of the muscle. However, they have a higher threshold than do muscle spindle afferents, so the tension must be high before they produce a large inhibitory effect.

Another way of interpreting the action of Golgi tendon organs in reflex control is that they may serve as a tension servo. Suppose that the stretch reflex is operative in maintaining the tension of a muscle at a particular level. If the muscle contracts in excess of the amount required to produce the desired tension, the Golgi tendon organs of the muscle will discharge at a higher rate and tend to inhibit the motoneurons to the muscle, thus relaxing the muscle and reducing the tension toward the appropriate level. Conversely, relaxation of a muscle will reduce the discharge rate of Golgi tendon organs, decreasing the amount of tonic inhibition of the motoneurons and allowing the motoneurons to produce a greater contraction of the muscle.

The group Ib fibers have other actions as well as the clasp knife reflex. Volleys in group Ib fibers from extensor muscles inhibit all extensor muscles postsynaptically, through a pathway involving at least one interneuron; they excite flexor muscles, also through at least one interneuron; and they presynaptically inhibit group Ib pathways. Volleys in group Ib afferent fibers from flexor muscles have little postsynaptic action on motoneurons, but they produce presynaptic inhibition of all group I pathways. The functional role of many of these group Ib effects is not yet clear.

In addition to these segmental effects, group Ib afferents send collaterals to end monosynaptically on the cells of origin of the dorsal and ventral spinocerebellar tracts, which they excite. Further information on the spinocerebellar tracts is presented in Chapter 8.

Renshaw cell system. As the axons of alpha motoneurons pass through the gray matter of the ventral horn toward the point of exit of the ventral root, they give off collaterals that innervate a group of interneurons located in lamina VII. These interneurons have been named after their discoverer, B. Renshaw. Renshaw cells are excited by several other pathways besides that involving motor axon collaterals; however, the latter is the best studied. When stimuli are applied to motor axons, whether in ventral roots or peripheral nerves, antidromically conducted volleys invade not only the appropriate motoneurons but also the recurrent axon collaterals, thus exciting Renshaw cells (Fig. 4-29, A). Each volley produces in a given Renshaw cell an EPSP lasting some 50 msec (Fig. 4-20, B). The action potentials generated by this EPSP lack much of an after-hyperpolarization, and the refractory period is very short. For these reasons, the Renshaw cells are able to fire repetitively at a very high rate throughout most of the duration of the EPSP (Fig. 4-20, A). The firing rate in response to large volleys may be up to 1,500 per sec for the first few spikes.

One of the sites of termination of Renshaw cell axons is on motoneurons. These endings produce a postsynaptic inhibition lasting some 50 msec (Fig. 4-11, B). Thus, the pathway from motoneurons to Renshaw cells to motoneurons is a negative feedback loop. The more actively motoneurons fire, the more actively Renshaw cells discharge and inhibit the motoneurons. The situation is, however, somewhat more complicated than this. Renshaw cell axons also terminate on interneurons and inhibit them. The particular interneurons inhibited by Renshaw cells are themselves inhibitory to motoneurons. Therefore, activation of Renshaw cells may decrease the amount of inhibition of some motoneurons, resulting in their disinhibition (Fig. 4-29, B). In anesthetized animals there is very little evidence of this type of disinhibition. This is probably caused by a low level of activity of the inhibitory interneurons. However, in unanesthetized preparations, disinhibition or a sequence of inhibition-disinhibition may occur in certain motoneurons when Renshaw cells are fired. In a series of elegant experiments, investigators in Lundberg's laboratory have shown that the inhibitory interneurons that are involved in recurrent facilitation are the group Ia interneurons responsible for reciprocal inhibition of the stretch reflex. Furthermore, the recurrent inhibition of these inhibitory interneurons is highly organized. Renshaw cells activated by discharges of motoneurons to a particular muscle inhibit the Ia interneurons that normally produce reciprocal inhibition of the motoneurons to the antagonistic muscles. Thus, the Renshaw cell path may serve to eliminate reciprocal inhibition. Such an action may be of particular value for actions that require the cocontraction of antagonistic sets of muscles. This would, for example, allow stabilization of a joint during a movement.

The Renshaw cell system is of special interest not only because it is a prototype for the study of the physiological role of recurrent collaterals, which are quite common in the central nervous system, but also because the pharmacology of the synapses of the motor axon collaterals on Renshaw cells is the best-documented pharmacology of the central nervous system. The pharmacology of this pathway is discussed later in this chapter.

Positive feedback. When the output of a system is fed back into the system to increase the output further, a positive feedback mechanism is involved. Many disease processes have a positive feedback linkage. For example, the vascular damage produced by hypertension may itself cause hypertension. However, there are several examples of a physiological role for positive feedback processes, including postactivation potentiation.

Postactivation potentiation (Fig. 4-30). Stimulation of the presynaptic element of a synapse may increase the ability of successive impulses to release the synaptic transmitter substance. Even a single presynaptic impulse may have this effect. However, a more striking effect is seen when a prolonged period of repetitive stimulation is employed. There are probably at least two mechanisms involved in this posttetanic potentiation. The potentiation following a single impulse may be caused by the activation of some mechanism used by the nerve terminal for mobilizing the transmitter substance; that is, stored transmitter is made ready for release, perhaps by the movement of synaptic vesicles nearer the presynaptic terminal membrane. The other type of potentiation, requiring repetitive stimulation, may be caused by the summed after-hyperpolarization that is produced by this type of stimulation. The after-hyperpolarization would result in a larger presynaptic action potential; this would trigger the release of more transmitter substance than would an ordinary-sized action potential.

The significance of posttetanic potentiation is that it makes most effective those synapses that are used the most. Pathways that are active have presynaptic terminals that may be in a state of potentiation; the postsynaptic potentials that are evoked by these terminals are thus larger than they would be if unpotentiated (see p. 102).

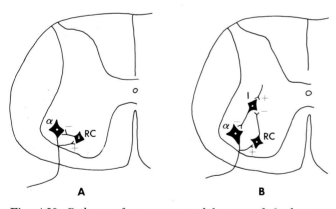

Fig. 4-29. Pathways for recurrent inhibition and facilitation. A, Recurrent inhibitory pathway. When alpha (α) motoneurons discharge, the activity invades the recurrent collaterals of the motor axons, as well as propagating to the periphery. The recurrent collaterals excite Renshaw cells (RC), which then inhibit the alpha motoneurons. The pattern of recurrent inhibition is complex, but in general the most effective recurrent inhibition is back onto the same motoneurons whose recurrent collaterals excite the Renshaw cells. B, Recurrent facilitatory pathway. Renshaw cells are excited by motor axon collaterals. The Renshaw cells then inhibit interneurons (I) that had previously been inhibiting alpha motoneurons. This type of recurrent facilitation is thus an example of disinhibition. The facilitation does not fire motoneurons, however. Recurrent facilitation is almost exclusively generated by recurrent collaterals of extensor motoneurons, and it affects only flexor motoneurons.

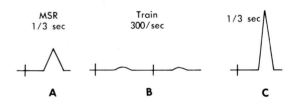

Fig. 4-30. Postactivation potentiation. The monosynaptic reflex is used here as a test of the synaptic efficacy of a central nervous system pathway. A, Reflex spike, as elicited once every 3 seconds. The rate is slow enough to allow replenishment of most of the transmitter stores between stimuli. B, Presynaptic terminals activated at a high rate, 300/sec, for 15 seconds. Each volley during the train evokes only a small reflex spike. The reasons for this are a temporary depletion of transmitter and the fact that the motoneurons are partially refractory. Following the train, low-rate stimulation of the monosynaptic reflex pathway evokes a much larger reflex spike than in the control period, C. The mechanisms for postactivation potential include an increase in the size of the presynaptic spike as a result of the summed after-hyperpolarization that would result from repetitive stimulation and a process called transmitter mobilization. The mobilization of transmitter implies a movement of synaptic vesicles within the terminal to a position near a release site, making the transmitter in the vesicles readily available for release.

Other normal somatic reflexes

Examples of normal somatic reflexes other than the stretch reflex, the clasp knife reflex, the flexion reflex, and the crossed extension reflex include the scratch reflex and the extensor thrust reflex. The classic studies on the scratch reflex and extensor thrust were done by Sherrington, using dogs that had undergone spinal transection. Gentle mechanical stimulation of the skin over the back and flanks evoked a rhythmic alternating movement of the hindlimbs, resembling the movement seen in the intact dog attempting to scratch. The accuracy of the scratching movement was much greater in the intact animal. The extensor thrust reflex was elicited by lightly stimulating the skin of the foot, either just behind the plantar cusion or between the cushion and the toe pads. The reflex consisted of a brief extensor movement of the hindlimb. Sherrington suggested that the extensor thrust reflex might serve to produce the main propelling force during locomotion. All of these reflexes have a basically segmental organization, although some (perhaps all) are under the control of supraspinal centers.

Another kind of reflex is the conditioned reflex. This usually involves primarily supraspinal structures, although there is some evidence that conditioned reflexes may be established in the spinal cord.

Reflexes involving respiratory and autonomic motoneurons

Respiratory reflexes. The motoneurons responsible for controlling the muscles of respiration are themselves controlled by the respiratory centers of the brainstem. However, they can also be affected by the pathways mediating voluntary actions, especially by the corticospinal tracts. In addition, their behavior is influenced by segmental reflex activity.

Respiratory motoneurons include those supplying the diaphragm, the intercostal muscles, and the accessory muscles of respiration. Most of the information available about respiratory motoneurons concerns the activity of intercostal motoneurons. Because the intercostal muscles contain muscle spindles, it is not surprising that the gamma loop apparatus is operative in the control of chest wall position and motion, just as it is for reflexes of the limbs. Respiratory gamma and alpha motoneuron discharges have been recorded from filaments of the intercostal nerves. The gamma motoneurons become active first during a respiratory movement; then the alpha motoneurons become active. Undoubtedly, the discharges of the gamma motoneurons increase the input from the muscle spindle afferents, including the group Ia fibers from primary endings, which in turn raises the level of excitability of the alpha motoneurons. Intracellular recordings from respiratory motoneurons have shown the presence of monosynaptic excitatory connections from group Ia fibers.

Although the pattern of respiration is generally set by pathways descending from the brainstem, information from peripheral receptor organs can modify the output of respiratory motoneurons. Part of this action is mediated by way of propriospinal pathways, although it is likely that part is also the result of the effects of ascending pathways on the activity of the respiratory centers.

Viscerosomatic reflexes. Stimulation of afferent fibers from visceral structures has been shown to produce marked effects on the activity of motoneurons to skeletal muscle. A variety of reflex actions of this type have been described. One is the production of a flexion reflex response when a hollow viscus is distended or when small afferent fibers from viscera are stimulated electrically. This type of response is of clinical significance because it accounts for the abdominal splinting seen in patients with disease affecting abdominal viscera. The exact reflex pattern varies considerably, according to the nature and distribution of the stimulus. This variation (local sign) is similar to that of the flexion reflex evoked by stimulation of afferent fibers from the skin of a limb.

Activity originating in the viscera causes many other reflex changes observed in skeletal muscle. For instance, muscles of the hindlimbs show alterations in tone as the urinary bladder becomes progressively distended.

The mechanisms underlying the viscerosomatic reflexes are under active investigation. Afferent fibers from the viscera have been found to excite interneurons that are also in pathways activated by cutaneous afferents. Thus, it is likely that such shared interneurons help mediate reflex activities of a similar nature triggered by afferent input from either viscera or the body surface. Afferents from the viscera have been found to cause a depolarization of the terminals of afferent fibers supplying the skin, thus presumably causing presynaptic inhibition of at least some cutaneous pathways. Recordings from alpha motoneurons to skeletal muscle of the hindlimb reveal excitatory and inhibitory postsynaptic potentials following stimulation of afferents from viscera. The pathways mediating these effects appear to include both propriospinal connections and long ascending and descending tracts.

Sympathetic reflexes. Although the sympathetic nervous system is predominantly under the control of pathways descending from the brain, it should be kept in mind that segmental reflex pathways also influence the discharges of sympathetic preganglionic neurons. Recordings can be made from the axons of preganglionic neurons dissected in the peripheral nervous system (for example, in a white ramus); or, with difficulty, recordings can be made, by the use of microelectrodes, from the cell bodies of preganglionic neurons in the intermediolateral cell column. The discharges of preganglionic neurons in the latter case are identified by antidromic invasion of action potentials when their axons are stimulated in the periphery. In such experiments it has been shown that sympathetic preganglionic neurons can be activated reflexly through segmental pathways. However, there is no evidence for a monosynaptic reflex pathway like that to alpha motoneurons supplying skeletal muscle. Apparently the segmental reflex pathways to sympathetic preganglionic neurons are all polysynaptic. Afferents that modify the activity of sympathetic preganglionic neurons arise both from receptors in the viscera and from receptors of the body wall. The sympathetic reflexes may thus be classified as both viscerovisceral and somatovisceral.

Parasympathetic reflexes. Parasympathetic preganglionic neurons have been studied in a fashion similar to that described above for the sympathetic preganglionic neurons. The parasympathetic motor nucleus is located in the sacral portion of the spinal cord (S2-3) in essentially the same position as the sympathetic motor nucleus, although there is not a distinct intermediolateral cell column in the sacral cord. Parasympathetic preganglionic neurons can be located with microelectrodes by stimulating their axons antidromically either in a ventral root or in the pelvic nerve. A recurrent inhibitory pathway from collaterals of preganglionic axons has been described. The pathway involves inhibitory interneurons, similar to Renshaw cells in some respects. As in the case of sympathetic preganglionic neurons, it appears that the primary control of parasympathetic preganglionic neuronal discharges comes from pathways descending from the brain. However, there are segmental reflex pathways to parasympathetic preganglionic neurons. These include both viscerovisceral and somatovisceral connections.

Pathological reflexes

Abnormal reflexes. Changes in normal reflex activity may be noted in certain pathological conditions. In some diseases, for instance, the activity of the stretch reflex pathway is increased, either because of an increased excitability of alpha motoneurons or an increased activity of gamma motoneurons. This may result in an increase in the number of motoneurons that will discharge in response to a tendon jerk; hence, the deep-tendon reflexes are said to be hyperactive.

The tonus of the muscles supplied by the overly active motoneurons may be increased; the patient is said to be spastic. Motoneurons of synergistic muscles may be discharged by an afferent volley in the nerve to a particular muscle; this will result in the contraction of muscles other than the one whose tendon is stretched, as in Hoffmann's reflex. This reflex, like any myotatic reflex, can be evoked in normal persons, but it may be hyperactive in those with disease. To evoke this reflex the hand is held in supination (palm up), and the slightly flexed index and small fingers are tapped, briefly extending them. The response is finger and thumb flexion. This is not a pathological reflex, nor is it the equivalent of Babinski's sign.

A sudden stretch of a muscle may cause it to contract violently, which may produce a sudden stretch of the antagonistic muscle; the two sets of muscles may then contract alternately, a condition known as clonus. In other diseases, reflexes may be hypoactive.

Patients having certain lesions in the brain develop reflex patterns that do not have a counterpart in the normal individual. These are called pathological reflexes, although the appearance of exaggerated or hypoactive normal reflexes may likewise signify a pathological condition. One of the most important of the pathological reflexes is Babinski's sign. A stimulus to the sole of the foot normally causes plantar flexion of the foot (physiological extension) in the adult human. Patients with certain brain lesions show a dorsiflexion of the great toe (physiological flexion) and often fanning of the other toes in response to stimulation of the sole, especially the lateral surface and ball of the foot. This response is actually a part of the flexion reflex and is suppressed in the adult, but it is normally present in the infant. Its presence in the adult signals the interruption of a supraspinal control system, the corticospinal tract (and possibly other tracts).

Spinal transection. When the spinal cord is completely transected, all voluntary motor activity below the transection is lost. In humans and other primates, the reflexes are hypoactive for a time, a condition called spinal shock. If the subject lives, the reflexes gradually return and become hyperactive. In humans, Babinski's sign is a prominent feature of the flexion reflex that may be elicited easily in the chronic spinal state. The flexion reflex can be evoked from a wide receptive field, and, accompanying it, there may be profuse autonomic reflex activity. Bladder and rectal contractions and sweating occur in response to stimulation and sometimes without obvious stimulation. The widespread responses, including flexion of one or both limbs and autonomic activity, are called mass reflexes. Stretch reflexes may also become hyperactive in subjects with spinal transection.

PHARMACOLOGY OF THE SPINAL CORD

The chemical transmitter substances responsible for the production of EPSPs are unknown for most central nervous system synapses. However, there is at least one pathway in which the transmitter substance is known and the pharmacology well documented. This is the pathway by which collaterals of motor axons excite the spinal cord interneurons called Renshaw cells.

Motor axons liberate acetylcholine at their peripheral terminals on skeletal muscle. According to a hypothesis of Dale, it can be predicted that other terminals made by branches of the same axons also liberate acetylcholine. It is now well accepted that recurrent collaterals from motor axons end on Renshaw cells, which are located in the ventral part of lamina VII in the spinal cord ventral horn. The axon collaterals excite the Renshaw cells by releasing acetylcholine. The receptors are nicotinic, and so the Renshaw cells may also be excited by nicotine as well as by other cholinergic drugs. Transmission is blocked by curarelike compounds, provided they can cross the blood-brain barrier if given systemically. Anticholinesterases prolong the excitation of Renshaw cells in response either to stimulation of motor axons or to acetylcholine. The Renshaw cells when excited produce IPSPs in motoneurons (see the section on spinal cord control mechanisms in this chapter).

There are probably other excitatory synapses in the brain and spinal cord that utilize acetylcholine as a transmitter substance. However, many excitatory synapses undoubtedly operate through the liberation of other substances. One candidate for this role is glutamic acid. This amino acid has been found to excite many types of neurons when it is liberated in their vicinity by the technique of microelectrophoresis. This technique involves the ejection of small quantities of a drug from a glass micropipette by the passage of a current through the pipette. An assemblage of several micropipettes fastened together can be used to give the experimenter the possibility of testing the actions of several drugs on the same neuron; one micropipette can be reserved as a recording electrode. However, a number of other substances are also very potent excitants of neurons. It will be very important for clinical practice when the transmitters at many central synapses are known. For instance, it would be helpful to have a specific drug to block pain without producing the undesirable side effects of narcotics.

Interneurons of the spinal cord may play an inhibi-

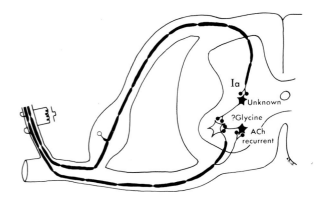

Fig. 4-31. Possible transmitters involved in spinal cord inhibitory pathways. The two inhibitory pathways illustrated are the group Ia reciprocal inhibitory pathway and the recurrent inhibitory pathway. The transmitter released by group Ia afferent fibers on inhibitory interneurons is not known (it may be glutamate). The transmitter at the synapse between recurrent collaterals and Renshaw cells is ACh. These two synapses involve excitatory transmitters. The synapses of the group Ia inhibitory interneurons and the Renshaw cell on motoneurons are likely to release the same transmitter. A strong candidate for this role is glycine.

tory role in certain pathways. Such interneurons are thought to release a special inhibitory transmitter substance (Fig. 4-31). Candidate transmitters include glycine and gamma-aminobutyric acid. Both of these substances have been shown to depress motoneurons when released from micropipettes by microelectrophoresis. However, some workers believe that glycine is more readily antagonized by strychnine than is gamma-aminobutyric acid, making glycine a more likely candidate for the transmitter producing IPSPs in the spinal cord. There is evidence that gamma-aminobutyric acid may be involved in presynaptic inhibition.

Besides the transmitters released by afferent fibers and by neurons intrinsic to the spinal cord, there are other transmitters associated with pathways descending into the spinal cord from the brain. It now appears that there are at least two pathways from the brainstem that utilize monoamines as transmitters. The monoamines are norepinephrine and 5-hydroxytryptamine. It is not yet clear whether these agents are primarily inhibitory or excitatory transmitters, because different neurons show either an increased or a decreased discharge rate during the action of monoamines applied by microelectrophoresis. It is conceivable that the sign of the action of these agents is determined by the nature of the postsynaptic receptors. The presence of these monoaminergic pathways is at least a partial explanation for the responses of spinal cord reflexes to agents that have actions on monoamine synapses peripherally but that also enter the central nervous system. In addition to spinal cord effects, however, such agents would also be expected to exert actions at monoamine synapses in the brain.

BIBLIOGRAPHY

Aitken, J. T., and Bridger, J. E.: Neuron size and neuron population density in the lumbosacral region of the cat's spinal cord, J. Anat. **95**:38-53, 1961.

Barron, D. H., and Matthews, B. H. C.: The interpretation of potential changes in the spinal cord, J. Physiol. (Lond.) **92**:276-321, 1938.

Bernhard, C. G.: The spinal cord potentials in leads from the cord dorsum in relation to peripheral source of afferent stimulation, Acta Physiol. Scand. [Suppl 106] **29**:1-29, 1953.

Blankenship, J. E., and Kuno, M.: Analysis of spontaneous subthreshold activity in spinal motoneurons of the cat, J. Neurophysiol. **31**:195-209, 1968.

Brock, L. G., Coombs, J. S., and Eccles, J. C.: The recording of potentials from motoneurons with an intracellular electrode, J. Physiol. (Lond.) **117**:431-460, 1952.

Burke, R. E.: Composite nature of the monosynaptic excitatory postsynaptic potential, J. Neurophysiol. **30**:1114-1137, 1967.

Burke, R. E.: Motor unit types of cat triceps surae muscle, J. Physiol. (Lond.) **193**:141-160, 1967.

Burke, R. E., Levine, D. N., Tsairis, P., and Zajac, F. E.: Physiological types and histochemical profiles in motor units of the cat gastrocnemius, J. Physiol. **234**:723-748, 1973.

Burke, R. E., and Tsairis, P.: Anatomy and innervation ratios in motor units of cat gastrocnemius, J. Physiol. **234**:749-765, 1973.

Clamann, H. P., Gillies, J. D., and Henneman, E.: Effects of inhibitory inputs on critical firing level and rank order of motoneurons, J. Neurophysiol. **37**:1350-1360, 1974.

Clamann, H. P., Gillies, J. E., Skinner, R. D., and Henneman, E.: Quantitative measures of output of a motoneuron pool during monosynaptic reflexes, J. Neurophysiol. **37**:1328-1337, 1974.

Coombs, J. S., Curtis, D. R., and Landgren, S.: Spinal cord potentials generated by impulses in muscle and cutaneous afferent fibres, J. Neurophysiol. **19**:452-467, 1956.

Curtis, D. R., and Eccles, J. C.: Synaptic action during and after repetitive stimulation, J. Physiol. **150**:374-398, 1960.

Eccles, J. C.: The physiology of nerve cells, Baltimore, 1957, The Johns Hopkins Press.

Eccles, J. C.: The mechanism of synaptic transmission, Ergeb. Physiol. **51**:367, 1961.

Eccles, J. C., Eccles, R. M., Iggo, A., and Lundberg, A.: Electrophysiological studies on gamma motoneurons, Acta Physiol. Scand. **50**:32-40, 1960.

Eccles, J. C., Eccles, R. M., and Lundberg, A.: Synaptic actions on motoneurons caused by impulses in Golgi tendon organ afferents, J. Physiol. (Lond.) **138**:227-252, 1957.

Eccles, J. C., Eccles, R. M., and Lundberg, A.: The action potentials of the alpha motoneurons supplying fast and slow muscles, J. Physiol. (Lond.) **142**:275-291, 1958.

Eccles, J. C., Eccles, R. M., and Lundberg, A.: Types of neurons in and around the intermediate nucleus of the lumbosacral cord, J. Physiol. (Lond.) **154**:89-114, 1960.

Eccles, J. C., Eccles, R. M., and Magni, F.: Central inhibitory action attributable to presynaptic depolarization produced by muscle afferent volleys, J. Physiol. (Lond.) **159**:147-166, 1961.

Eccles, J. C., Fatt, P., and Koketsu, K.: Cholinergic and inhibitory synapses in a pathway from motor-axon collaterals to motoneurons, J. Physiol. (Lond.) **126**:524-562, 1954.

Eccles, J. C., Kostyuk, P. G., and Schmidt, R. F.: The effect of electric polarization of the spinal cord on central afferent fibres and on their excitatory synaptic action, J. Physiol. (Lond.) **162**:138-150, 1962.

Eccles, J. C., Magni, F., and Willis, W. D.: Depolarization of central terminals of group I afferent fibres from muscle, J. Physiol. (Lond.) **160**:62-93, 1962.

Eccles, J. C., and Schade, J. P., editors: Organization of the spinal cord, New York, 1964, American Elsevier Publishing Co., Inc.

Eccles, J. C., Schmidt, R. F., and Willis, W. D.: Presynaptic inhibition of the spinal monosynaptic reflex pathway, J. Physiol. (Lond.) **161**:282-297, 1962.

Eccles, R. M., and Lundberg, A.: Integrative pattern of Ia synaptic actions on motoneurons of hip and knee muscles, J. Physiol. (Lond.) **144**:271-298, 1958.

Eccles, R. M., and Lundberg, A.: The synaptic linkage of "direct" inhibition, Acta Physiol. Scand. **43**:204-215, 1958.

Eccles, R. M., and Lundberg, A.: Synaptic actions in motoneurons by afferents which may evoke the flexion reflex, Arch. Ital. Biol. **97**:199-221, 1959.

Eldred, E., Granit, R., and Merton, P. A.: Supraspinal control of the muscle spindles and its significance, J. Physiol. (Lond.) **122**:498-523, 1953.

Frank, K., and Fuortes, M. G. F.: Potentials recorded from the spinal cord with microelectrodes, J. Physiol. (Lond.) **130**:625-654, 1955.

Frank, K., and Fuortes, M. G. F.: Presynaptic and postsynaptic inhibition of monosynaptic reflexes, Fed. Proc. **16**:39-40, 1957.

Gasser, H. S., and Graham, H. T.: Potentials produced in the spinal cord by stimulation of the dorsal roots, Am. J. Physiol. **103**:303-320, 1933.

Granit, R.: Reflexes to stretch and contraction of antagonists around the ankle joint, J. Neurophysiol. **15**:269-279, 1952.

Henneman, E., Clamann, H. P., Gillies, J. D., and Skinner, R. D.: Rank order of motoneurons within a pool: law of combination, J. Neurophysiol. **37**:1338-1349, 1974.

Henneman, E., Somjen, G., and Carpenter, D. O.: Functional significance of cell size in spinal motoneurons, J. Neurophysiol. **28**:560-580, 1965.

Henneman, E., Somjen, G., and Carpenter, D. O.: Excitability and inhibitability of motoneurons of different sizes, J. Neurophysiol. **28**:599-620, 1965.

Holmqvist, B., and Lundberg, A.: Differential supraspinal control of synaptic actions evoked by volleys in the flexion reflex afferents in alpha motoneurons, Acta Physiol. Scand. [Suppl. 186] **54**:1-67, 1961.

Hongo, T., Jankowska, E., and Lundberg, A.: Convergence of excitatory and inhibitory action on interneurons in the lumbosacral cord, Exp. Brain Res. **1**:338-359, 1966.

Hultborn, H., Jankowska, E., and Lindström, S.: Recurrent inhibition from motor axon collaterals of transmission in the Ia inhibitory pathway to motoneurones, J. Physiol. **215**:591-612, 1971.

Hultborn, H., Jankowska, E., and Lindström, S.: Recurrent inhibition of interneurones monosynoptically activated from group Ia afferents, J. Physiol. **215**:613-636, 1971.

Hultborn, H., Jankowska, E., and Lindström, S.: Relative contribution from different nerves to recurrent depression of Ia IPSPs in motoneurons, J. Physiol. **215**:637-664, 1971.

Kuno, M.: Quantal components of excitatory synaptic potentials in spinal motoneurons, J. Physiol. (Lond.) **175**:81-99, 1964.

Laporte, Y., and Lloyd, D. P. C.: Nature and significance of the reflex connections established by large afferent fibers of muscular origin, Am. J. Physiol. **169**:609-621, 1952.

Lloyd, D. P. C.: Reflex action in relation to pattern and peripheral source of afferent stimulation, J. Neurophysiol. **6**:111-119, 1943.

Lloyd, D. P. C.: Conduction and synaptic transmission of the reflex response to stretch in spinal cats, J. Neurophysiol. **6**: 317-326, 1943.

Lloyd, D. P. C.: Facilitation and inhibition of spinal motoneurons, J. Neurophysiol. **9**:421-438, 1946.

Lloyd, D. P. C.: Post-tetanic potentiation of response in monosynaptic reflex pathways of spinal cord, J. Gen. Physiol. **33**: 147-170, 1949.

Lloyd, D. P. C., and McIntyre, A. K.: Monosynaptic reflex responses of individual motoneurons, J. Gen. Physiol. **38**: 771-787, 1955.

Mendell, L. M., and Henneman, E.: Terminals of single Ia fibers; location, density and distribution within a pool of 300 homonymous motoneurons, J. Neurophysiol. **34**:171-187, 1971.

Nelson, P. G., and Lux, H. D.: Some electrical measurements of motoneuron parameters, Biophys. J. **10**:55-73, 1970.

Phillis, J. W.: The pharmacology of synapses, New York, 1970, Pergamon Press, Inc.

Rall, W., Smith, T. G., Frank, K., Burke, R. E., and Nelson, P. G.: Dendritic location of synapses and possible mechanisms for the monosynaptic EPSP in motoneurons, J. Neurophysiol. **30**:1169-1193, 1967.

Renshaw, B.: Influence of discharge of motoneurons upon excitation of neighboring motoneurons, J. Neurophysiol. **4**: 167-183, 1941.

Renshaw, B.: Central effects of centripetal impulses in axons of spinal ventral roots, J. Neurophysiol. **9**:191-204, 1946.

Rexed, B.: A cytoarchitectonic atlas of the spinal cord in the cat, J. Comp. Neurol. **100**:297-380, 1954.

Romanes, G. J.: The motor cell columns of the lumbosacral spinal cord of the cat, J. Comp. Neurol. **94**:313-364, 1951.

Schechter, M. M., and Zingesser, L. H.: The spinal arteries, Acta Radiol. (Stockh.) **5**:1124-1131, 1966.

Scheibel, M. D., and Scheibel, A. B.: Terminal axonal patterns in cat spinal cord. II. The dorsal horn, Brain Res. **9**:32-58, 1968.

Sherrington, C. S.: The integrative action of the nervous system, New Haven, 1906, Yale University Press.

Stuart, D. G., Mosher, C. G., and Reinking, R. M.: Properties and central connections of Golgi tendon organs with special reference to locomotion. In Banker, B., Pryzbylsky, R. J., Van Der Meulen, J., and Victor, M., editors: Research concepts on muscle development and the muscle spindle, Amsterdam, 1971, Excerpta Medica Foundation.

Szentagothai, J.: Neuronal and synaptic arrangement in the substantia gelatinosa Rolandi, J. Comp. Neurol. **122**:219-239, 1964.

Toennies, J. F.: Reflex discharge from the spinal cord over the dorsal roots, J. Neurophysiol. **1**:378-390, 1938.

Wall, P. D.: Excitability changes in afferent fibre terminals and their relation to slow potentials, J. Physiol. (Lond.) **142**:1-21, 1958.

Wall, P. D.: The laminar organization of dorsal horn and effects of descending impulses, J. Physiol. (Lond.) **188**: 403-424, 1967.

Wilson, V. J., and Burgess, P. R.: Disinhibition in the cat spinal cord, J. Neurophysiol. **25**:392-404, 1962.

CHAPTER 5

The brain and its environment

RELATIONSHIPS OF THE BRAIN TO THE SKULL AND MENINGES
Sutures, points, and lines of the skull

The brain is supported and covered by the three layers of the meninges within the cranial cavity. The calvarium, or skullcap, which makes up the vault or roof of the cavity, is composed of the superior parts of the frontal, the occipital, and the paired parietal and temporal bones (Fig. 5-1). The sutures (seams) between bones, and other points on the skull, are used as guides to the underlying parts of the brain. The coronal (curved) suture is formed by the junction of the posterior margin of the frontal bone with the anterior margins of the parietal bones, and passes from temple to temple. A slice made through the skull and brain along the coronal suture is a cut made in the coronal plane. Such cuts are also often called frontal sections. The sagittal (arrow) suture is the midline junction of the parietal bones. A cut made along or parallel to this suture produces a sagittal section of the brain. The lambdoidal (Greek letter lambda) suture is formed by the junction of the posterior margins of the parietal bone with the anterior margins of the occipital bone. The site of the junction of the sagittal and coronal sutures is called the bregma (front part of head). The junction of the sagittal and lambdoidal sutures is the lambda. At birth, the bones of the skull are separated at the sutures by 1 to 3 mm of peri-

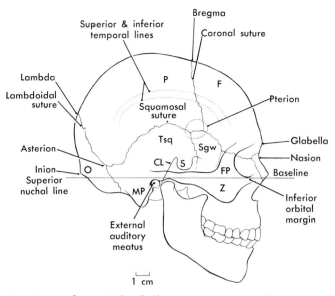

Fig. 5-1. Markings of the skull; sutures, points, and lines of the skull. *F*, frontal bone; *O*, occipital bone; *P*, parietal bone; *Sgw*, greater wing of sphenoid bone; *Tsq*, squamous portion of temporal bone; *Z*, zygoma; *CL*, clivus of occipital bone; *FP*, frontal process of zygoma; *MP*, mastoid process of temporal bone; *S*, sella turcica of sphenoid bone.

osteum, and the individual bones can be moved in relationship to each other. Increased intracranial pressure can separate the bones at the suture lines until about the age of 8, when growth of the skull by formation of bone at the suture lines binds the sutures together much more firmly, although growth still occurs until the late teens. At birth, the junction of the coronal and sagittal sutures at the bregma is incomplete, and there is a diamond-shaped space, the anterior fontanelle, between the bones. At the lambda there is a similar triangular space, the posterior fontanelle. The brain beneath the fontanelle is covered by extensions of the periosteum that fuse with the dura. The anterior fontanelle closes at 18 months of age and the posterior at 2 months.

The squamosal suture is formed by the junction of the inferior portion of the parietal bone with the superior margin of the squamous (scale) portion of the temporal bone. An important landmark of the skull is the pterion (wing, from the site of the wings on the helmet of the messenger of the gods, Mercury). The pterion is the half-dollar–sized area of the skull at the site of the H formed by the junctions of the frontal, parietal, temporal, and sphenoid bones. At birth the anterolateral fontanelle is present here, and it closes at 2 months. Another important point is the asterion (star) produced by the junction of the parietal, occipital, and temporal bones. At birth the postero-

lateral fontanelle is present here, and it closes at 2 years.

Muscle attachments make natural lines on the skull. The most important of these are the temporal lines that run along the frontal and parietal bones, and the nuchal lines of the occipital bone. The midpoint of the skull, called the inion (nape of the neck) or external occipital protuberance, along the superior nuchal line is prominent. At the frontal pole of the skull are two reference points often used in conjunction with the inion for making measurements: the nasion, the junction of the nasal and frontal bones, and the glabella (hairless), the point between the eyebrows.

Relationships of the brain to fossae and foramina of the skull

The calvarium covers the superior aspects of the frontal and temporal lobes, as well as the parietal and occipital lobes.

The floor of the cranial cavity conforms to the shape of the base of the brain and is divided into three step-like compartments: the anterior, middle, and posterior fossae (Fig. 5-2). The frontal lobes lie in the anterior fossa, which is made up of the frontal and sphenoid bones. The anterior portions of the temporal lobes and the base of the diencephalon lie in the middle fossa, which is made up of the sphenoid and temporal bones. The pituitary gland also lies in the middlle fossa in the sella turcica (turkish saddle) of the sphenoid bone. The posterior portions of the temporal lobes and the base of the occipital lobes lie on the tentorium, a shelf of dura (Fig. 5-8), that runs from the floor of the middle fossa to the internal protuberance of the occipital bone. The posterior fossa is the cavity of the skull below the tentorium and is made up of the posterior-medial-inferior faces of the temporal bones and the basilar portions of the occipital bone. The clivus (slope) is that part of the occipital bone rostral to the foramen magnum lying between the petrous portions of the temporal bone. The clivus is inclined at about 137° (123° to 152°) in the normal skull to the floor of the anterior fossa. This is one measurement of the basilar angle of the skull. The angle may be increased (that is, the clivus may be more horizontal) in some pathological states. The brainstem lies on the clivus, and the bases of the cerebellar hemispheres lie on the cerebellar fossae of the occipital bone.

All of the vascular and nervous communications of the brain enter and leave the base of the brain and pass through foramina in these fossae. These vessels and nerves are bilaterally paired structures (Figs. 5-3 to 5-5). Their foramina of passage can best be appreciated by examination of a skull. These foramina

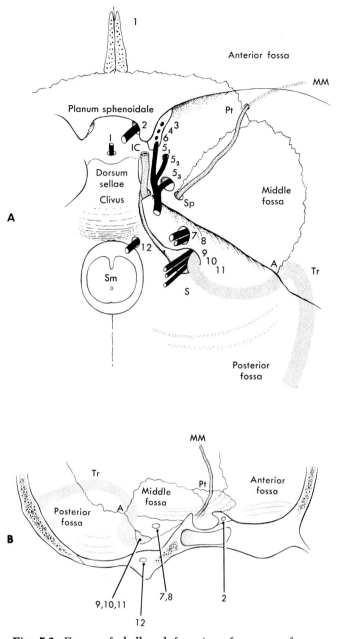

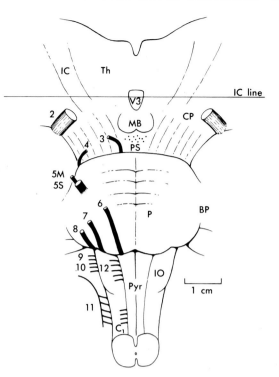

Fig. 5-3. Anterior-posterior view of the brainstem, with the sites of exit of the cranial nerves. The base of the brainstem is viewed along the anterior-posterior axis of the horizontal plane of the intercommissural line *(IC)* (see Figs. 5-4, 5-5, 5-8, 5-22, and 5-24 for orientation). Cranial nerves 2 to 12 and the motor roots of the first cervical *(C₁)* nerves are shown. Abbreviations: *BP*, brachium pontis; *CP*, cerebral peduncle; *IC*, internal capsule; *IO*, inferior olive; *MB*, mamillary bodies; *P*, pons; *PS*, posterior perforated substance; *Pyr*, pyramids; *Th*, thalamus; *V3*, third ventricle; *5M, 5S*, motor and sensory roots of cranial nerve V.

Fig. 5-2. Fossae of skull and foramina of passage of nerves and vessels. **A,** Interior of the base of the skull viewed from above. **B,** Interior of the left side of the skull in a lateral view. Foramina of exit of the cranial nerves indicated by the number of the nerve(s) passing through them: *1*, cribriform plate; *2*, optic foramen and canal; *3, 4, 6, 5₁*, superior orbital fissure; *5₂*, foramen rotundum; *5₃*, foramen ovale; *7, 8*, internal acoustic meatus; *9, 10, 11*, neural portion of jugular foramen; *12*, hypoglossal foramen. Foramina of exit of vessels and other structures: *I*, infundibulum passing through the dural diaphragm of the sella turcica; *IC*, internal carotid passing through carotid groove; *MM*, middle meningeal artery passing over pterion *(Pt)* and through foramen spinosum *(Sp)*; *Tr*, transverse sinus passing over asterion *(A)* and through vascular portion of jugular foramen; *S*, sigmoid sinus; *Sm*, spinomedullary junction, in foramen magnum.

are all visible on either standard lateral and anterior-posterior x-ray films of the skull or on special angled projections. Enlargement or erosion of the foramina suggests the presence of a tumor either locally in the skull or intracranially.

In the anterior fossa, the olfactory nerves (cranial nerve I) pass through the cribriform plate of the ethmoid bone.

In the middle fossa, the optic nerve (II) passes through the optic foramen of the sphenoid bone, which lies below and medial to the anterior clinoid (bedpost) process of the sella. The ophthalmic artery, which is the first intracranial branch of the carotid artery (Figs. 5-34 and 5-35), also passes through the optic foramen into the optic canal, which is about 10 mm in length. The artery lies below and lateral to the optic nerve, within the optic canal. The nerves to the extraocular muscles—the oculomotor (III), trochlear (IV), and abducens (VI) nerves—pass through the superior orbital fissure of the sphenoid

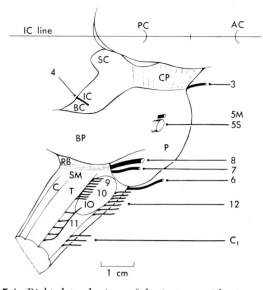

Fig. 5-4. Right lateral view of brainstem, with sites of exit of the cranial nerves. Cranial nerves 3 to 12 are shown (see Fig. 5-3). Abbreviations: *BC,* brachium conjunctivum; *BP,* branchium pontis; *C,* cuneate tubercle; *CP,* cerebral peduncle; *IC,* inferior colliculus; *IC* line, intercommissural line; *IO,* inferior olive; *P,* pons; *RB,* restiform body; *SC,* superior colliculus; *SM,* striae medullares; *T,* tuberculum cinereum (overlying spinal trigeminal tract and nucleus). A cross-sectional view of the spinomedullary junction seen obliquely has been added to aid in illustrating the columnar nature of the exit of nerves 9 to 12 and the spinal motor roots. The projection of the positions of the anterior *(AC)* and posterior *(PC)* commissures is shown.

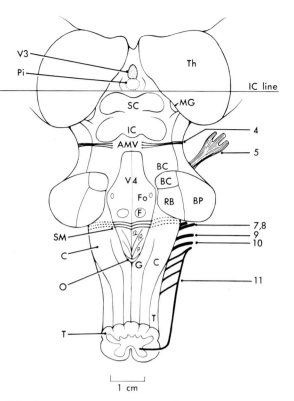

Fig. 5-5. Posterior-anterior view of brainstem. The site of origin of the fourth cranial nerve and the initial courses of the fifth sensory and seventh to eleventh nerves are shown. In the floor of the fourth ventricle the tubercles overlying the nuclei of the sixth nerve and the root of seventh nerve (*F,* facial colliculus), and the tubercles overlying the nuclei of the tenth and twelfth nerves and the area postrema *(P)* are shown. Abbreviations: *AMV,* anterior medullary velum; *BC,* brachium conjunctivum; *BP,* brachium pontis; *C,* cuneate tubercle; *Fo,* fovea superior; *G,* gracile tubercle; *IC,* inferior colliculus; *MG,* medial geniculate; *O,* obex; *P,* area postrema; *Pi,* pineal; *RB,* restiform body; *T,* tuberculum cinereum; *Th,* thalamus, *SC,* superior colliculus; *SM,* striae medullares; *V3,* third ventricle; *V4,* fourth ventricle. The level of the horizontal plane of the intercommissural line *(IC)* is indicated.

bone. Also passing into the orbit through the same fissure is the first, or ophthalmic, division of the sensory root of the trigeminal (V_1) nerve. The III, IV, VI, and V_1 nerves enter the fissure from the cavernous venous sinus of the dura. The cavernous sinus of the dura lies on either side of the sella turcica of the sphenoid bone, and the sinuses on each side are connected by the intercavernous (circular) sinuses (Fig. 5-8). The carotid artery enters the cranial cavity through the carotid groove, which lies in front of the foramen lacerum, a jagged opening between the posterior margin of the sphenoid bone and the anterior margin of the petrous portion of the temporal bone. The carotid artery then passes through the cavernous venous sinus and enters the cranial cavity just lateral to the anterior clinoid process of the sella turcica and the optic nerve. The second or maxillary division of the sensory root of the trigeminal nerve (V_2) passes through the foramen rotundum of the sphenoid bone. The third or mandibular division (V_3) of the sensory root, along with the motor root of V, passes through the foramen ovale of the sphenoid bone. The middle meningeal artery enters the skull through the foramen spinosum, which is slightly lateral and posterior to

the foramen ovale, and then runs in the dura with two venae comitantes on either side of it.

In the posterior fossa, the facial (VII) and statoacoustic nerves (vestibular and auditory components of the VIII) pass through the internal auditory meatus of the petrous portion of the temporal bone. The glossopharyngeal (IX), vagus (X), and spinal accessory (XI) nerves pass through the medial portion, or pars nervosa, of the jugular foramen, a large opening between the petrous temporal and the occipital bones. The sigmoid venous sinus, which carries the venous drainage of the brain to the internal jugular vein, exits through the posterolateral vascular portion of the jugular foramen. The hypoglossal (XII) nerve exits through the hypoglossal foramen of the occipital bone.

The spinal cord, the vertebral artery, and the ascending spinal portion of the spinal accessory (XI) nerve pass through the foramen magnum of the occipital bone.

Craniocerebral topography

In some species, such as the cat and to a lesser degree the monkey, there is a constant relationship between specific points on the skull and brain structures. This invariability is the basis of stereotaxis, the localization of brain structures by means of a coordinate system that takes certain skull landmarks as reference points. In humans, the relationship between skull landmarks and brain structures is too variable to allow for the very precise (±1 mm) localizations of structures that can be achieved in the cat. However, the approximate location (±1 cm) of the major fissures of the brain can be plotted on the scalp or on an x-ray film of the skull by a simple procedure, construction of Taylor-Haughton lines (Fig. 5-6). The distance from the nasion to the inion over the top of the calvarium is measured and divided into quarters. This can be done by using a tape and folding it into quarters. A line extending from the inferior orbital margin through the upper margin of the external auditory meatus is marked. This line is called the baseline, or the Frankfurt plane. A line drawn from the angle of the orbit to the ¾ point along the circumference of the skull marks the approximate location and direction of the lateral (sylvian) fissure separating the frontal and parietal lobes from the temporal lobe. A line (the posterior ear line) drawn perpendicular to the baseline through the mastoid (breast-shaped) process intersects the sylvian fissure line and marks the approximate posterior boundary of the temporal lobe. This vertical line extended to the circumference of the skull marks the upper end of the central (rolandic) fissure, which separates the frontal lobe and the parietal lobe. The course of the rolandic fissure is marked by a line drawn from the junction of a vertical line through the condyle of the mandible with the sylvian fissure to the circumference of the skull. The upper end of the rolandic fissure is about 1 cm posterior to the vertex of the skull and about 3 to 4 cm behind the coronal suture.

Puncture of the ventricular system for diagnostic and therapeutic purposes is carried out with reference to skull landmarks (Fig. 5-7). In the infant the lateral ventricles can be tapped by a needle introduced directly downward at the lateral margins of the anterior fontanelle. In the adult the lateral ventricles lie 4 to 5 cm beneath the outer surface of the skull. The anterior horns of the lateral ventricle extend 1 to 2 cm in front of the coronal suture. They can be tapped

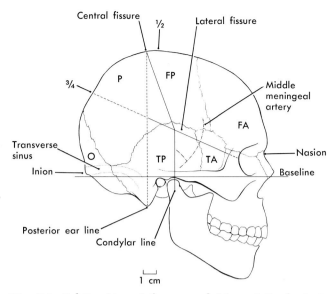

Fig. 5-6. Relationships of fissures and lobes of the brain to markings of the skull. Abbreviations: *FA,* anterior frontal lobe; *FP,* posterior frontal lobe (precentral gyrus); *O,* occipital lobe; *P,* parietal lobe; *TA,* anterior temporal lobe; *TP,* posterior temporal lobe.

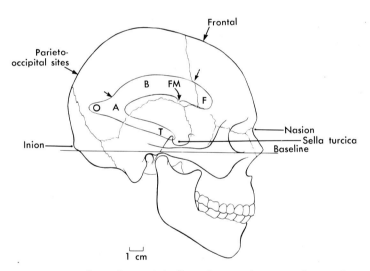

Fig. 5-7. Relationships of the lateral ventricles to markings of the skull. Note frontal and parieto-occipital sites for ventricular puncture (see Fig. 5-32). Abbreviations: *A,* atrium, *B,* body of ventricle; *F,* frontal, *O,* occipital, *T,* temporal horns; *FM,* site of foramina of Monro.

through a burr hole or small twist-drill hole 1 to 3 cm lateral to the midline and 1 cm in front of the coronal suture. The junction of the body and occipital horns is another commonly used site for ventricular tapping. The opening is made 3 cm lateral to the midline and 7 cm above the inion, a point that is usually about 1 cm anterior to the lambdoidal suture.

Cerebrospinal fluid may also be obtained by a midline puncture of the cisterna magna (cisternal tap) by a needle introduced through the atlanto-occipital membrane and under the posterior lip of the foramen magnum. The subarachnoid space may also be punctured easily by a needle, introduced into the side of the neck below the mastoid, that can be guided into the large neural foramen between C1 and 2 under fluoroscopic control (see Fig. 7-22), as well as by lumbar puncture (see Chapter 4).

Meningeal compartments

The inside of the skull is lined by the dura mater (hard mother-membrane), or pachymeninx (thick membrane), the outermost of the three layers of meninges. The dura is made up of tough collagenous fibers and at birth is attached to the skull, particularly at the suture lines. The dura functions as a periosteum in growth of the skull. It is less firmly adherent to the skull in the adult, and hemorrhage from lacerated dural vessels (middle meningeal artery, dural venous sinuses) or from diploic veins of the skull can dissect the dura away from the skull and form an epidural hematoma and compress the underlying brain.

Folds of the dura divide the space within the skull into two major compartments: the supratentorial and the infratentorial (Fig. 5-8). This division is formed by the tentorium (tent), a horizontal sheet of dura that originates from the floor of the middle fossa and from the clinoid processes and the medial tip of the petrous bone, where a dural thickening forms the petroclinoid ligament. The tentorium extends over the posterior cranial fossa to attach to the internal occipital protuberance. The midpoint of the tentorium is attached to the falx (see below) and is higher than the lateral margins of the tentorium, giving it the appearance of a tent. The semicircular opening in the center of the tentorium is called the tentorial notch, or incisura. The midbrain passes through this notch. The occipital and posterior temporal lobes lie on the tentorium, and the cerebellum lies under it in the infratentorial compartment that is the posterior fossa.

The supratentorial compartment is divided into right and left halves by the falx (sickle), a midline fold of the dura. The falx lies in the sagittal plane in the midline of the skull and dips into the longitudinal fissure of the cerebrum between the right and left hemispheres of the brain, extending inferiorly to about one half the depth of the supratentorial compartment. The falx extends from the floor of the anterior fossa to the internal occipital protuberance and in its posterior portion joins the midline of the tentorium. A similar but smaller falx cerebelli separates the cere-

bellar hemispheres and extends vertically to the inferior surface of the tentorium.

The margins and junctions of the falx and tentorium contain venous channels that receive veins from the surfaces of the brain (Fig. 5-8). The upper margin of the falx contains the superior sagittal sinus; the lower margin contains the inferior sagittal sinus, which is joined by the great vein of Galen at the point where the falx intersects the tentorium. The venous sinus in the midline of the tentorium is the straight sinus that joins the superior sagittal sinus at the outer margin of the tentorium just beneath the internal occipital protuberance. This point is approximately beneath the inion. The confluence of the sinuses, also called the torcular (wine press) of Herophilus, is drained by the right and left transverse sinuses running in the outer

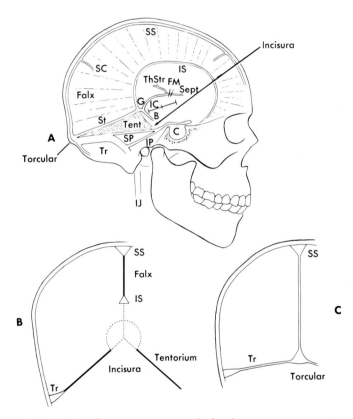

Fig. 5-8. Dural compartments and dural venous sinuses. **A,** Lateral view. **B** and **C,** Anterior-posterior views of frontal sections at the levels of the incisura and torcular. Abbreviations for sinuses: *C,* cavernous; *IS,* inferior sagittal; *IP,* inferior petrosal; *SC,* a superficial superior cerebral vein draining into the superior sagittal sinus; *SP,* superior petrosal; *SS,* superior sagittal; *St,* straight; *Tr,* transverse. Abbreviations for deep cerebral veins: *B,* basilar vein of Rosenthal; *IC,* internal cerebral vein; *Sept,* septal vein, *ThStr,* thalamostriate vein; *G,* great vein of Galen; *IJ,* internal jugular vein; *Tent,* tentorium; *FM,* site of foramen of Monro. The position of the thalamus is shown by the location of the intercommissural line, below the internal cerebral vein.

margins of the tentorium. The course of the sinuses takes them beneath the asterion, where they begin to turn sharply inferiorly and medially to pass into the jugular foramen.

If the dura is cut so that flaps of dura are made over the right and left cerebral hemispheres, and if the dural rings made by the falx and tentorium are also cut, the brain can be lifted out of the subdural space.

In the absence of a pathological condition, the subdural space is only a potential space, perhaps containing a very thin layer of fluid. However, hemorrhage from veins passing from the surface of the brain to the dura or from extensive bleeding from vessels on the surface of the brain can produce a subdural hematoma. Subdural hematomas are generally produced by trauma. The brain undergoes linear and rotatory movement within the skull and dura when the head is struck or when stopped abruptly, as in automobile-deceleration injuries. These movements can stretch and tear intracranial vessels, nerves, and fiber tracts within the brain.

Subarachnoid spaces and cisterns

The two inner surrounding membranes of the brain, the arachnoid (spiderweblike) and the pia (tender) mater, unlike the dura mater, are intimately attached to the brain and form an integral part of the surface-limiting membranes of the brain (Fig. 5-9). The surface of the brain itself is covered by an external limiting membrane composed of expansions of astroglial cells. This is capped by a single layer of cells that comprise the cells of the pia mater. A subpial space does not exist. Above the layer of pial cells, a meshwork of arachnoid cells makes a filmy membrane with a depth of up to a few millimeters. The arachnoid membrane is bounded by a layer of mesothelial cap cells. The cerebrospinal fluid is contained between

the trabeculations of the arachnoidal meshwork. Because of the intimate attachment of the pia and arachnoid, these two membranes are often referred to as the pia-arachnoid membrane, or the leptomeninx (delicate). In the living brain, the surface of the arachnoid membrane can be opened, and cerebrospinal fluid will then escape from the subarachnoid space. Large amounts of the membrane, however, may not be removed from the brain, because the blood vessels of the brain enter and leave the brain through this space and any large removal of this membrane will disrupt the vessels. Hemorrhage from vessels in the subarachnoid space will produce bloody cerebrospinal fluid. Subarachnoid hemorrhage is a clinically important condition, usually caused by the rupture of an aneurysm of one of the arteries of the circle of Willis. Large space-occupying hematomas equivalent to epidural or subdural hematomas do not form in the subarachnoid space. Blood from torn subarachnoid vessels flows into the cerebrospinal fluid. If the hemorrhage is violent, as in the case of rupture of an aneurysm, the hemorrhage can, in some cases, dissect through the arachnoid so that a hematoma is formed in the subdural (epiarachnoid) space.

In certain areas at the base of the brain, the subarachnoid space is much thicker than it is over the hemispheres. These fluid spaces, or cisterns, at the base of the brain appear to have the function of supporting the brain or cushioning the base of the brain against the bony ledges of the fossae of the base of the skull. The largest cistern is at the outflow of the fourth ventricle at the posterior margin of the foramen magnum of the skull and is called the cisterna magna. The interpeduncular cistern lies immediately superior to the clivus of the skull. Rostral to that cistern are the infrachiasmatic and suprachiasmatic cis-

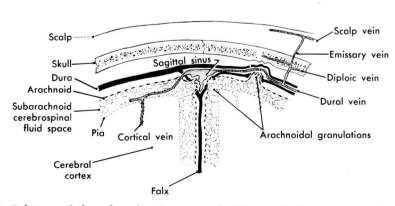

Fig 5-9. Relations of the subarachnoid space and of the cerebral veins to the dural venous sinuses. Diagram of a frontal section through the midline vertex of the head through the scalp, skull, meninges, and right and left hemispheres.

Table 5-1. Subarachnoid cisterns and their contents

Cistern	Location	Contents
Ventral cisterns		
Medullary	Between medulla and lower clivus	IX, X, XI, and XII; vertebral and posterior inferior cerebellar arteries
Pontine	Between pons and upper clivus	V and VI; basilar and anterior inferior cerebellar arteries
Interpeduncular	Between cerebral peduncles, posterior to dorsum sellae	III; basilar, superior cerebellar, posterior cerebral, and posterior communicating arteries
Chiasmatic	Anterior to optic chiasm, infundibulum, and anterior perforated substance; posterior to diaphragma sellae and anterior clinoid process	Internal carotid, anterior and middle cerebral, posterior communicating, and anterior choroidal arteries
Cerebellopontine	In front of cerebellar hemisphere and middle cerebellar peduncle; behind petrous ridges	VII, VIII, V, and VI; anterior inferior cerebellar artery (lateral aperture opens here)
Crural	Around cerebral peduncle	Posterior cerebral and anterior choroidal arteries
Sylvian fissure	From posterior part of orbital surface of frontal lobe to forward edge of medial aspect of temporal lobe and up sylvian fissure	Middle cerebral artery; basal vein of Rosenthal and middle cerebral veins
Dorsal cisterns		
Superior cerebellar	Under tentorium and over upper surface of cerebellum	
Quadrigeminal	Under splenium and over quadrigeminal plate; tentorial notch is behind	Pineal; great cerebral vein; terminal parts of basal veins; posterior cerebral artery
Pericallosal	Above corpus callosum and between and below cingulate gyri	
Wings of ambient cisterns	Surrounding pulvinar	May contain posterior cerebral artery, basal vein, anterior choroidal artery, and lateral posterior choroidal arteries
Intercommunicating cisterns		
Great cistern	Beneath cerebellar tonsils above and behind foramen magnum	Posterior inferior cerebellar arteries (medial aperture opens into part known as vallecula cerebelli)
Ambient	Lateral extensions of quadrigeminal cistern, continuous with crural and pontine cisterns; free edge of tentorial notch is lateral	IV; posterior cerebral, superior cerebellar, and choroidal arteries; basal vein
Lamina terminalis	In front of lamina terminalis; anterior to it is free edge of falx; roof is corpus callosum	Anterior cerebral and frontopolar arteries
General subarachnoid space	Over convexities of cerebrum and cerebellum	Distal branches of cerebral arteries; most large superficial cerebral veins; arachnoidal villi

terns surrounding the optic nerves and covering the sharp margins of the greater wing of the sphenoid bone. The cisterns and their contents are listed in Table 5-1.

STRUCTURE OF THE BRAIN
Development and general description

At birth, the brain weighs 300 to 400 g. The shape of the skull is largely determined by the rapid growth of the brain in the first year of life. The head circumference at birth averages 34 cm in males. The brain weight doubles to 800 to 900 g at the end of the first year of life, and the head circumference increases to 45 cm. The adult human brain weighs between 1,250 and 1,450 g. The brains of males are slightly heavier than the brains of females, but the brains of females are slightly heavier in proportion to body weight than the brains of males.

Gross inspection and consideration of the brain's embryological development show that the brain can be divided into four areas, although the boundaries between the areas are not distinct. During development, neural ectoderm forming the dorsal margin of the embryo invaginates and forms a tube in the third to fourth week of development. Germinal cells forming the inner margins of the tube proliferate and migrate outward, thickening the tube. The center of the tube is lined with ependymal cells and remains as the central canal of the spinal cord, which is only a potential space in the adult, and as the ventricular system of the brain, which is filled with cerebrospinal fluid. The divisions of the brain can also be made, there-

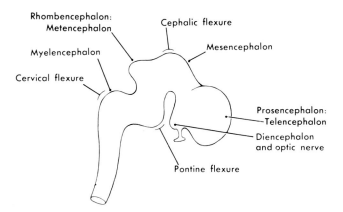

Rhombencephalon: Metencephalon
Myelencephalon
Cervical flexure
Cephalic flexure
Mesencephalon
Prosencephalon: Telencephalon
Diencephalon and optic nerve
Pontine flexure

Fig. 5-10. Flexures of the neural tube and development of major areas of the brain in a 6- to 7-week-old embryo.

fore, in terms of the anatomy of the ventricular system, the inner surface of the brain, which reflects brain development, as well as the outer surface.

In the fourth and fifth weeks of development, three expansions of the neural tube become evident: the rhombencephalon (hindbrain), the mesencephalon (midbrain), and the prosencephalon (forebrain). A flexure of the forebrain on the hindbrain is evident at this point. By the sixth week of development the rhombencephalon divides into the metencephalon (afterbrain) and myelencephalon (marrow brain), and the prosencephalon divides into the telencephalon (endbrain) and diencephalon (betweenbrain). The telencephalon divides into right and left cerebral hemispheres (Fig. 5-10).

The myelencephalon is synonymous with the medulla oblongata (bulb), generally referred to simply as the medulla. The metencephalon consists of the pons and the cerebellum. The term brainstem is used loosely to describe the medulla, pons, and midbrain and may also be used to include the diencephalon. The brainstem at a given level is composed of a roof, a portion of the ventricular system, a tegmentum, and a base. The word tectum is used in reference to the roof of the midbrain. The word tegmentum means covering and refers to the region of the brainstem below the ventricular cavity and covering the base.

The myelencephalon is the most caudal portion of the brain and is continuous with the spinal cord at the level of the foramen magnum. The medullary tegmentum contains numerous sensory, motor, and autonomic nuclei, including the nuclei of the glossopharyngeal (IX), vagus (X), and hypoglossal (XII) nerves, and the cranial part of the spinal accessory (XI) nerve. It also contains the supraspinal mechanisms that maintain respiration and blood pressure.

Destruction of the medulla, therefore, results in death from respiratory paralysis; destruction of the more rostral portions of the brain results in varying effects on consciousness without producing immediate death. A number of ascending and descending fiber tracts course through the medullary tegmentum. The base of the medulla consists of the descending corticospinal fibers, which travel in structures called the pyramids.

The metencephalon consists of the cerebellum (little brain) and the pons (bridge). The cerebellar hemispheres, like the cerebral hemispheres, consist of a cortex of gray matter, underlying projection axons, and deep nuclei that receive projections of the cortical cells. The tegmentum of the pons is analogous to that of the medulla. It contains the nuclei of the trigeminal (V), abducens (VI), facial (VII), and statoacoustic (VIII) nerves. The base of the pons includes longitudinally and transversely running fiber bundles and the pontine nuclei. The transverse fibers connect the pons with the cerebellum. It is this fiber system that gives the pons its name. The fourth ventricle is bounded inferiorly by the dorsal surface of the medullary and pontine tegmentum and superiorly by the cerebellum.

The mesencephalon is the shortest portion of the brain. It contains the roof plate, or tectum, which is composed of the colliculi, or corpora quadrigemina. Beneath the tectum is the cerebral aqueduct, the tegmentum, and the base. The superior and inferior colliculi (hills) are relay stations for vision and audition respectively. The tegmentum contains numerous nuclei, including the motor nuclei of the oculomotor (III) and the trochlear (IV) nerves. The base consists of the cerebral peduncles (foot, stalk), which are largely descending corticofugal fibers. The ventricular system of the midbrain, the aqueduct (of Sylvius), or iter, is the shortest and smallest in cross section of the ventricular cavities of the brain.

The diencephalon is attached to the telencephalon by stalks of axons and develops in relationship to the cortex. The optic vesicles and nerves (II) develop from the diencephalon. The diencephalon is composed of a superior portion, the thalamus (chamber), which contains the main afferent relay nuclei projecting to the cerebral cortex, and an inferior portion, the hypothalamus. The hypothalamus is a suprasegmental integrating area for autonomic and endocrine gland control. The hypophysis, or pituitary gland, is attached to the floor of the hypothalamus by the infundibulum (pituitary stalk). The diencephalon also contains the posterior-superiorly placed epithalamus, including the pineal gland and the habenular area, and the posterior-inferiorly located subthalamus, an area of cells and fibers lying between the diencephalon and mesencephalon. Structures in the subthalamus are principally related to motor systems, although many fiber systems pass through it. The diencephalon contains the midline third ventricle, the paired lateral ventricles being considered the first two ventricles.

The telencephalon includes the cerebral hemispheres. The term cerebrum is used loosely to describe the cerebral hemispheres or the supratentorial portion of the brain. The cerebral hemispheres consist of a cortex (bark) of gray matter and underlying white matter containing afferent and efferent axons. The olfactory nerves (I) are associated with telencephalic structures. The basal ganglia (the neostriatum [caudate and putamen] and the paleostriatum

[globus pallidus]) are subcortical nuclei that develop in relationship to the telencephalon. The cavity of the neural tube persists in the telencephalon as the lateral ventricles.

Brainstem

The term brainstem is generally used to refer to the medulla, pons, and midbrain. The external features of these structures will be described in this chapter; the internal features will be considered in Chapter 6.

Medulla oblongata (Figs. 5-3 to 5-5 and 5-11 to 5-13). The medulla oblongata is the most caudal part of the brain. It is derived from the fifth embryonic brain vesicle, the myelencephalon. The boundary between the medulla and the spinal cord lies just rostral

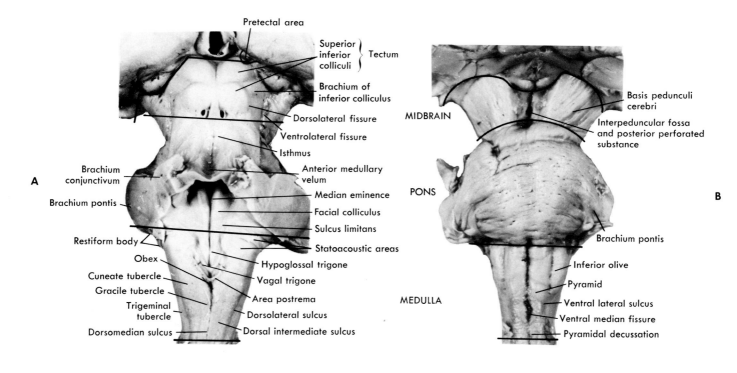

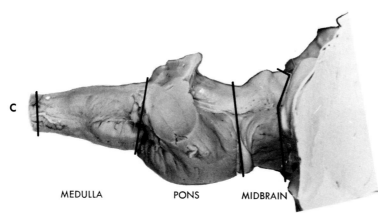

Fig. 5-11. Surface landmarks of the brainstem. The medulla, pons, and midbrain are shown. A, Dorsal view; B, ventral view; C, lateral view. The boundaries between each of these regions and between the medulla and spinal cord caudally and the midbrain and diencephalon rostrally are indicated by heavy lines.

to the first cervical nerve, or at the lowest level of the decussation (crossing) of the pyramids. The rostral boundary is at the level of the striae medullares dorsally and the lowest fibers of the pons ventrally; the widest part of the fourth ventricle is at the pontomedullary junction.

The medulla can be divided into a caudal and a rostral part on the basis of its relationship to the fourth ventricle. The central canal of the spinal cord continues through the caudal medulla, which therefore has a roof of brain tissue. In the rostral medulla, the central canal widens and comes to the surface to form the caudal part of the fourth ventricle.

The surface of the medulla has a number of features that can be used as landmarks. The dorsal median sulcus of the spinal cord continues along the dorsum of the medulla, crossing the obex, which is the V-shaped caudal end of the fourth ventricle. The ventral median fissure continues from the cord through the medulla to end at the pontomedullary junction; in the medulla it separates two structures known as the pyramids. On the lateral surface of the medulla is an oval-shaped prominence known as the inferior olive. The dorsolateral and the ventrolateral sulci of the spinal cord continue in the medulla, respectively dorsal and ventral to the inferior olive. The

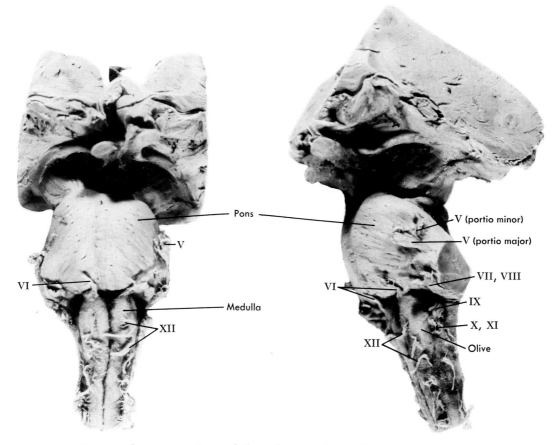

Fig. 5-12. Cranial nerves of the medulla and pons. The rootlets shown emerging from the preolivary sulcus of the medulla form the hypoglossal (XII) nerve. The rootlets exiting in the postolivary sulcus make up the glossopharyngeal (IX), vagus (X), and cranial portion of the accessory (XI) nerves; the spinal portion of the accessory is missing in the specimen, but would have ascended from the upper cervical spinal cord (C1 to C5 or C6) through the foramen magnum and then exited from the skull in company with the cranial accessory and vagus nerves through the jugular foramen. The facial (VII) and statoacoustic (VIII) nerves are found at the pontomedullary junction. The intermediate nerve is a part of the facial nerve situated between the main portion of the facial nerve and the more laterally placed statoacoustic nerve. The abducens (VI) nerve also exists at the pontomedullary junction, but it is near the midline. The trigeminal (V) nerve is attached to the lateral aspect of the rostral pons. It has a smaller motor root (portio minor) and a larger sensory root (portio major).

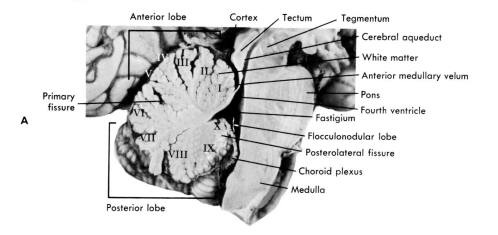

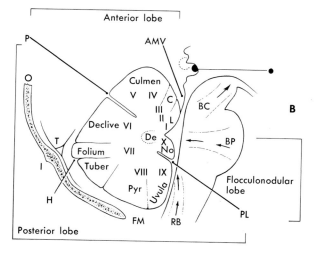

Fig. 5-13. A, Cerebellum in sagittal section. The lobular arrangement of the vermis is indicated in a fashion like that shown in B. Structures associated with the cerebellum, including the lower brainstem, are also shown. B, Major fissures and divisions of the human cerebellum. Sagittal section through the vermis. The relative position of the dentate nucleus *(De)*, which is actually lateral to the vermis, is shown. Note the position of the internal and external protuberances (*I,* inion) of the occipital bone *(O),* of the foramen magnum *(FM),* and of the torcular *(T).* Vermian lobules: *L,* lingula; *C,* central; *Pyr,* pyramis; *No,* nodulus. Major fissures: *P,* preclival or primary; *H,* horizontal; *PL,* posterolateral. Cerebellar peduncles: *BC,* brachium conjunctivum; *BP,* brachium pontis; *RB,* restiform body. *AMV,* anterior medullary velum. Subdivision of cerebellum following numerical designations proposed by Larsell. (After Dow, R. S.: J. Neurosurg. **18:**512-530, 1961.)

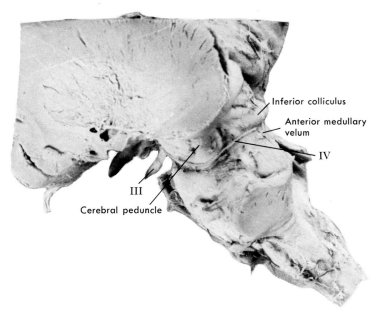

Fig. 5-14. Cranial nerves of the midbrain. The trochlear (IV) nerve is shown emerging from its decussation in the anterior medullary velum just caudal to the inferior colliculus. The trochlear nerve then passes around the midbrain and lies near the oculomotor (III), seen emerging from the interpeduncular fossa, to run forward into the orbit.

dorsal intermediate sulcus of the cord traverses the caudal medulla, where it separates two elongated elevations, the gracile tubercle dorsomedially and the cuneate tubercle laterally. The gracile fasciculus can be seen to terminate at the gracile tubercle, and the cuneate fasciculus at the cuneate tubercle. Just lateral to the cuneate fasciculus and cuneate tubercle is another prominence, the tuberculum cinereum, or trigeminal tubercle. A series of cranial nerve rootlets emerge from the lateral surface of the medulla between the trigeminal tubercle and the inferior olive. These form, from rostral to caudal, the glossopharyngeal (IX), vagus (X), and accessory (XI) cranial nerves. Ventral to the olive, between it and the pyramid, emerge the rootlets of the hypoglossal (XII) nerve.

The floor of the fourth ventricle is divided longitudinally by the dorsomedian sulcus. Near the midline on each side are prominences called the hypoglossal and the vagal trigones. Near the obex, in the lateral wall of the fourth ventricle, is the area postrema. In the lateral part of the fourth ventricle, at the pontomedullary junction, is part of the statoacoustic area, which continues into the pons. The statoacoustic area is crossed transversely by a number of fiber bundles known as the striae medullares, which are probably cerebellar afferent fibers.

The roof of the rostral medulla is formed by the tela choroidea. This is a connective tissue membrane lined by the ependyma. Blood vessels in the tela choroidea invaginate the ependyma to form the choroid plexus of the fourth ventricle. This is actually a paired structure. Each part is L-shaped, with a longitudinal limb extending from the pontomedullary junction along the midline to the obex and a transverse limb extending from the midline at the pontomedullary junction over the statoacoustic area. The tela choroidea is perforated at the midline near the obex and on each side at the lateral boundary of the medulla. These perforations are known as the median (of Magendie) and lateral (of Luschka) apertures and represent the only points of escape of the cerebrospinal fluid from the ventricular system into the subarachnoid spaces.

Pons (Figs. 5-3 to 5-5 and 5-11 to 5-14). The pons was named for the large bundle of fibers bridging its ventral surface. It is derived embryonically from the fourth brain expansion, the metencephalon, along with the cerebellum. The rostral boundary of the pons is the decussation of the trochlear nerves just caudal to the inferior colliculi of the midbrain for the dorsal surface and the rostral limits of the crossing fibers of the pons for the ventral surface. The point of separation between the pons and the cerebellum lies just lateral to the roots of the trigeminal nerve.

The landmarks on the surface of the pons include the following structures. On the dorsal aspect of the pons is the rostral portion of the fourth ventricle. The dorsomedian sulcus continues along the midline from the medullary fourth ventricle. Next to the midline in the caudal pons is a swelling known as the facial colliculus. More laterally at the same level is the statoacoustic area. In the rostral portion of the floor of the fourth ventricle, there is a ridge of tissue called the median eminence along the midline. Lateral to this is a groove known as the sulcus limitans, derived from the embryonic structure of the same name. The roof of the fourth ventricle of the pons is formed by the anterior medullary velum. The fourth ventricle narrows at the level of the rostral pons, merging at the isthmus region (junction of pons and midbrain) with the cerebral aqueduct.

The most prominent feature of the lateral and ventral surfaces of the pons is the collection of pontocerebellar fibers, which pass transversely to form the middle cerebellar peduncle (brachium pontis). In the junction region between the pons and medulla, the restiform body, or inferior cerebellar peduncle, is seen entering the cerebellum; at the isthmus the superior cerebellar peduncle (brachium conjunctivum) exits from the cerebellum. A number of cranial nerves are associated with the pons. At the pontomedullary junction, the abducens (VI) nerve exits in line with the row of hypoglossal (XII) rootlets in the medulla; both are purely motor nerves. The facial (VII) and statoacoustic (VIII) nerves also leave the brainstem at the pontomedullary junction, but in line with the rootlets of nerves IX, X, and XI of the medulla. The facial nerve is just medial to the statoacoustic nerve. At midpons the trigeminal nerve may be seen emerging in line with the facial nerve. The trigeminal nerve has two roots: a sensory portio major, attached to the trigeminal ganglion, and a motor portio minor, without a ganglion.

A region of clinical importance is the cerebellopontine angle. This is located at the lateral junction of the pons and medulla with the cerebellum. Important structures in the cerebellopontine angle include the facial (VII) and statoacoustic (VIII) cranial nerves. The lateral aperture of the fourth ventricle opens into the cerebellopontine subarachnoid cistern.

Midbrain (Figs. 5-3 to 5-5, 5-11, and 5-14). The midbrain is derived from the embryonic mesencephalon and is often known by that name in the adult. The rostral boundary is made with the diencephalon. Dorsally, the boundary passes through the posterior commissure; ventrally, it is at the caudal border of the mamillary bodies. The region of junction between the midbrain and the pons is often referred to as the isthmus. The cerebral aqueduct traverses the midbrain. The portion of the midbrain forming a roof over the cerebral aqueduct is called the tectum. The portion below the aqueduct is the tegmentum; the same name is often applied to the parts of the pons and medulla that are located in a similar position with respect to the ventricular system. Below the tegmentum the midbrain has a basal portion called the basis pedunculi or cerebral peduncle.

The surface of the midbrain tectum is characterized by two pairs of swellings known as the inferior and superior colliculi. The four structures together are often referred to as the corpora quadrigemina. Just rostral to the superior colliculi is the pretectal area. A band of fibers runs rostrally from each inferior colliculus just lateral to the superior colliculus on the same side; this fiber bundle is the brachium of the inferior colliculus. A dorsolateral fissure separates the tectum from the tegmentum. The ventrolateral fissure demarcates the tegmentum from the basis pedunculi. On the ventral surface of the midbrain the basis pedunculi can be seen to consist of two large fiber bundles, the cerebral peduncles. These are separated by the interpeduncular fossa. The cranial nerves associated externally with the midbrain are the trochlear (IV) and oculomotor (III) nerves. The former decussate in the anterior medullary velum, exit caudal to the inferior colliculi, and pass around the lateral aspect of the midbrain to accompany the oculomotor and abducens nerves in their passage to the orbit. The oculomotor nerves leave the brainstem in the interpeduncular fossa. The surface of the interpeduncular fossa is called the posterior perforated substance because of the numerous perforations made by the passage of blood vessels into the brain substance.

Cerebellum

The cerebellum is composed of three major lobes: the anterior, posterior, and flocculonodular (Figs. 5-13 and 5-15). The anterior and posterior lobes are readily demarcated by the primary fissure, which can be seen to run transversely across the dorsal surface of the cerebellum. The flocculonodular lobe is found ventral to the cerebellum and is separated from the posterior lobe by the posterolateral fissure. The inferior cerebellar peduncles (restiform body) join the cerebellum to the medulla and spinal cord. The middle cerebellar peduncles (brachium pontis) connect the cerebellum and pons. The anterior medullary velum and the superior cerebellar peduncles (brachium conjunctivum) connect the cerebellum with the midbrain and diencephalon.

The vermis is a ridgelike structure that runs longitudinally along the midline of the cerebellum. The expansions of cerebellum on each side of the vermis are the hemispheres. The zones of juncture between the vermis and the hemispheres are known as the intermediate regions.

The cerebellar lobes can be further subdivided into lobules. Each lobule contains a number of folia (transversely running ridges). The lobules have acquired a multitude of esoteric names over the years, but only a few are used in the present discussion. Some of the terms that have been applied to cerebellar lobules in the past and are still in frequent use are as follows: Lobule I of the vermis is often called the lingula. The last two lobules of the vermis of the posterior lobe are the pyramis and the uvula. The hemisphere adjacent to the uvula is the tonsil.

Table 5-2. Human cerebellar divisions

| Lobes | Vermis | | Hemisphere | |
	Division	Name	Division	Name
Anterior	I, II	Lingula	H I, II	Viniculum lingula
	III	Central	H III	Central lobule
	IV, V	Culmen	H IV, V	Anterior quadrangular lobule
Primary fissure				
Posterior	VI	Declive	H VI	Posterior quadrangular lobule
	VIIA	Folium, anterior tuber	H VIIA	Superior and inferior semilunar lobules
	VIIB	Posterior tuber	H VIIB	Gracile lobule
	VIIIA,B	Pyramis	H VIIIA,B	Biventer lobules
Posterolateral fissure	IX	Uvula	H IX	Tonsil
Flocculonodular	X	Nodulus	H X	Flocculus

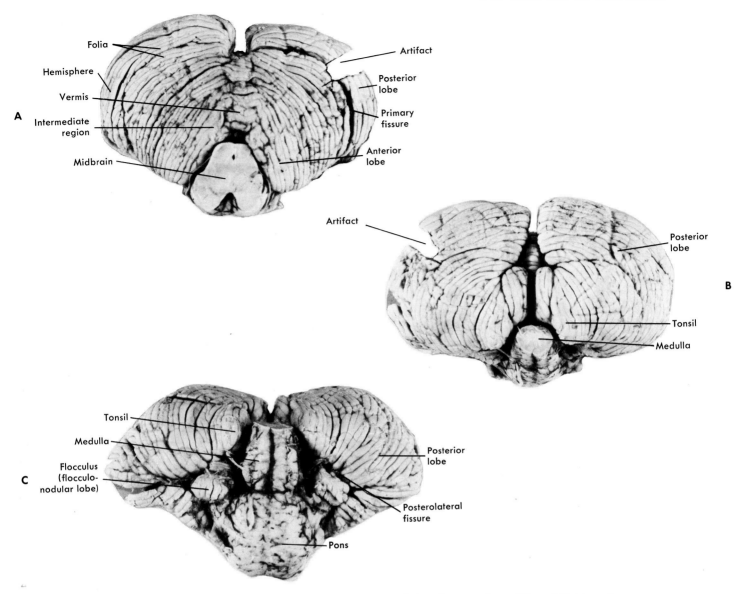

Fig. 5-15. Cerebellum. **A,** Superior; **B,** posterior; and **C,** inferior surfaces. The subdivision of the cerebellum into lobes is indicated: the primary fissure is between the anterior and posterior lobes; the posterolateral fissure is between the posterior and flocculonodular lobes. The sagittal organization into vermis, intermediate region, and hemisphere is also shown. The relationship between the tonsil and the medulla can be seen.

Lobule X of the vermis is the nodulus, and its corresponding hemispheric lobule is the flocculus. These relationships are indicated in Table 5-2.

Separate terms have been used for the subdivisions of the vermis and those of the intermediate region or hemispheres; however, there is a correspondence between lobules of the vermis and those of the intermediate region and hemisphere, because the grooves dividing the cerebellum into lobules run transversely across the entire structure.

The simplest terminology for the lobules of the cerebellum is that of Larsell (Fig. 5-13). For mammals in general, the vermis can be divided into lobules I through X, beginning with the most rostral. The intermediate and hemispheric lobules are numbered H I through H X. The first five lobules are in the anterior lobe; the next four are in the posterior lobe; the tenth is the flocculonodular lobe. The organization in humans is essentially the same as in other mammals, although the intermediate and hemispheric components have names rather than numerical designations.

An interesting historical treatment of the terminology that has been applied to the subdivisions of the cerebellum may be found in an atlas of the human cerebellum by Angevine, Mancall, and Yakovlev (1961).

Another way in which the cerebellum may be subdivided is based on its phylogenetic development. The most primitive part of the cerebellum seems to be the flocculonodular lobe. This region is thus often referred to as the archicerebellum. A somewhat less primitive part of the cerebellum is the vermis, which, along with some of the intermediate region, is called the paleocerebellum. The most recently evolved part of the cerebellum is the neocerebellum, composed of the hemispheres and the rest of the intermediate regions.

If the cerebellum is sectioned, the cortex can readily be distinguished from the underlying white matter. If the section is sagittal (Fig. 5-13) along the midline, the lobular organization is seen to depend on the branching pattern of the white matter and the folding of the cortex into groups of folia. The tree-like branching pattern of the white matter gave rise to the term arbor vitae in the days of the early anatomists, when it was thought that the cerebellum was vital to life.

Diencephalon

The diencephalon is composed of the thalamus, the hypothalamus and associated hypophysis (pituitary gland), the epithalamus and associated epiphysis (pineal gland), and the subthalamus. Each of these areas consists of groups of nuclei and their associated projections. The dorsally placed thalamus can be regarded as largely a sensory structure with a group of lateral nuclei, each projecting to a specific sector of the cortex, and a group of medial nuclei that have afferent and intrathalamic connections. The ventrally placed hypothalamus can be regarded as largely a segment of the autonomic motor system, which can integrate complex patterns of somatic, motor, endocrine, and autonomic activity. The epithalamus is functionally related to the subcortical projections of the limbic cortex. The subthalamus is largely functionally related to the basal ganglia.

Thalamus (Figs. 5-16 to 5-19). The thalamus consists of two oval masses that lie between the internal capsule laterally and the lateral and third ventricles medially. The rostrocaudal axes of the ovals are directed so that the caudal portions of the thalami, which lie at the level of the posterior commissure, diverge. The thalami widen caudally as they follow the lateral-going course of the posterior limb of the internal capsule. The taenia, or line of attachment, of the choroid plexus runs along the dorsomedial border of the thalamus. The lateral ventricles lie above this line, on the superior surface of the thalami, which make a convex bulge into the lateral walls of the bodies of the ventricles. The third ventricle lies beneath this point and lines the medial wall of the thalamus. The choroid plexuses can be visualized as trefoil, or cloverleaf, structures expanding superiorly and laterally into each lateral ventricle and inferiorly into the third ventricle from this point. They lie in the tela choroidea, a membranous invagination that extends through the choroid fissure of the ventricles. The massa intermedia, or interthalamic adhesion, a round plaque of tissue of variable size, bridges the third ventricle above the hypothalamic sulcus. The hypothalamic sulcus of the wall of the third ventricle is the border between the thalamus and hypothalamus.

Hypothalamus (Figs. 5-17 to 5-20). An initial orientation to the structure of the hypothalamus can be obtained by inspection of the ventral surface of the brain. Five rostrocaudal areas that are related to underlying hypothalamic nuclei can be distinguished on the basilar surface of the brain: the preoptic, chiasmal, infundibular, median eminence, and mamillary areas. In addition to this rostrocaudal division, the hypothalamus can be divided into three parasagittal zones: the periventricular, medial, and lateral areas (see Chapter 6). The preoptic area, which is a telencephalic structure functionally related to the hypothalamus, lies rostral to the optic chiasm. The anterior perforated substance is the basilar surface of the preoptic area. Many small perforating vessels of the anterior and middle cerebral arteries penetrate the anterior perforated substance. Occlusion of these arteries or those of the posterior perforating substance can be produced by ruptured aneurysms of the circle of Willis or by surgical treatment of aneurysms. Such occlusions can produce brainstem infarction, coma, or severe hypothalamopituitary dysfunction.

The hypothalamus has its rostral boundary at the lamina terminalis of the third ventricle at the level of the anterior commisure. The optic chiasm lies just behind this level. The third ventricle dips ventrally here to form the optic recess of the ventricle, with the chiasm lying just beneath the floor of the recess. The infundibulum, or stalk, of the pituitary gland comes from the floor of the third ventricle at the level of the infundibular recess of the ventricle, just behind the chiasm. The median eminence, or tuber cinereum, lies just caudal to the infundibulum. The

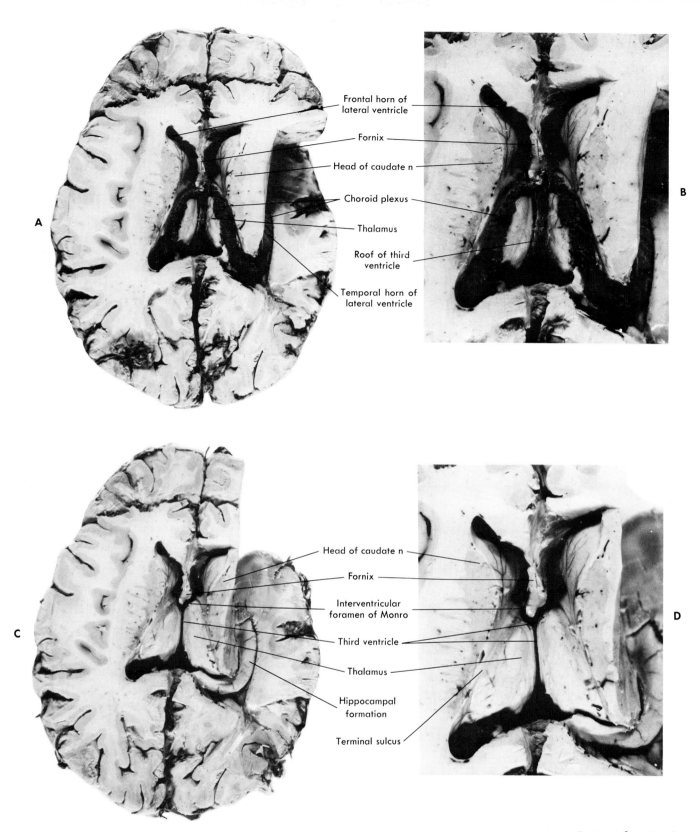

Frontal horn of
lateral ventricle

Fornix

Head of caudate n

Choroid plexus

Thalamus

Roof of third
ventricle

Temporal horn of
lateral ventricle

Head of caudate n

Fornix

Interventricular
foramen of Monro

Third ventricle

Thalamus

Hippocampal
formation

Terminal sulcus

Fig. 5-16. Structures of the diencephalon and telencephalon in horizontal section. The brain has been cut in horizontal section just beneath the level of the corpus callosum. In **A** and **B,** the choroid plexuses of both lateral ventricles were left intact, and the course of the choroid plexus into the temporal horn of the right lateral ventricle was exposed by a dissection into the temporal lobe. The roof of the third ventricle is intact. The relationship between the caudate nucleus and the thalamus is better shown in **C** and **D.** In these photographs, the choroid plexus and the roof of the third ventricle have been removed. The terminal sulcus (containing the thalamostriate vein) separates the caudate nucleus and thalamus. The floor of the temporal horn is seen to be the hippocampal formation.

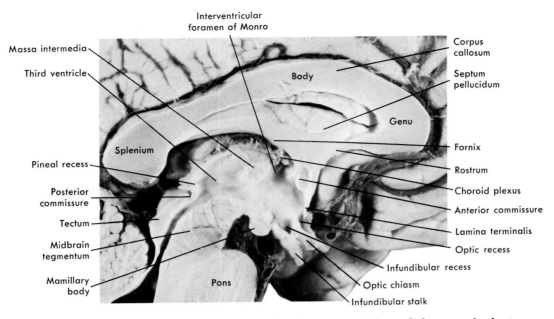

Fig. 5-17. Structures around the third ventricle. The view is of the medial aspect of a brain that has been sectioned in the sagittal plane. The section passes through the third ventricle and the cerebral aqueduct. The recesses of the third ventricle are indicated, as well as structures belonging to the epithalamus and hypothalamus.

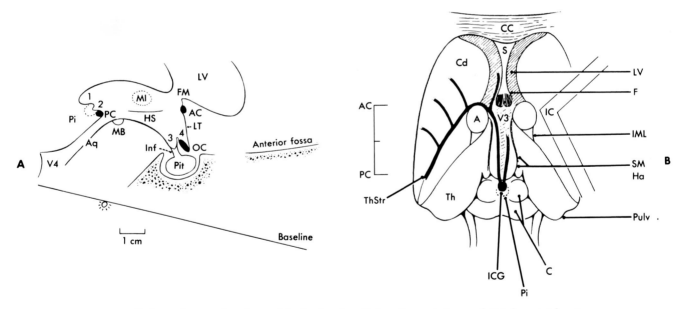

Fig. 5-18. Surface and radiographic landmarks of the diencephalon and third ventricle. **A,** Midline sagittal aspect. **B,** Dorsal aspect viewed from above from within the lateral ventricles. The position of the internal capsule *(IC)* has been indicated on the right and the levels of the anterior and posterior commissures on the left. Ventricular system landmarks: *AC,* anterior commissure; *Aq,* aqueduct; *FM,* foramen of Monro; *HS,* hypothalamic sulcus; *LT,* lamina terminalis; *LV,* lateral ventricle; *MI,* massa intermedia; *PC,* posterior commissure; *V3* and *V4,* third and fourth ventricles. Third ventricle recesses: *1,* suprapineal; *2,* pineal; *3,* infundibular; *4,* optic. Other abbreviations: *A,* anterior nucleus of thalamus; *C,* colliculi; *CC,* corpus callosum; *Cd,* caudate; *F,* fornix; *Ha,* habenular trigone; *Inf,* infundibulum; *IML,* internal medullary lamina; *MB,* mamillary body; *OC,* optic chiasm; *Pi,* pineal; *Pit,* pituitary; *Pulv,* pulvinar; *S,* septum pellucidum; *SM,* stria medullaris; *Th,* thalamus; *ICG,* internal cerebral vein draining into vein of Galen; *ThStr,* thalamostriate vein.

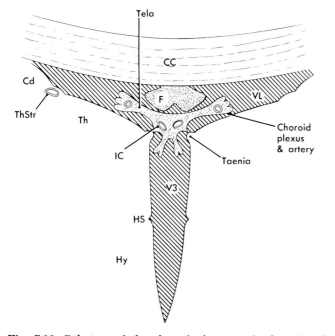

Fig. 5-19. Relations of the choroid plexus to the lateral and third ventricles. The tela choroidea (velum interpositum) is attached to the taenia. The choroid plexus invaginates into each lateral ventricle through the choroid fissure and into the roof of the third ventricle. Abbreviations: *CC*, corpus callosum; *Cd*, caudate; *F*, fornix; *Hy*, hypothalamus; *HS*, hypothalamic sulcus; *IC*, internal cerebral vein; *VL*, lateral ventricle; *ThStr*, thalamostriate vein; *Th*, thalamus; *V3*, third ventricle.

paired mamillary bodies mark the caudal extent of the hypothalamus, which lies at the transverse level of the posterior commissure. The posterior perforated substance lies between and caudal to the maxillary bodies and transmits many fine branches of the posterior cerebral arteries.

Epithalamus (Fig. 5-21). Included in the epithalamus are the pineal body, the posterior commissure, the habenular trigone and habenular commissure, and the stria medullaris.

The pineal body is attached by a stalk to the habenular and posterior commissures. There is good evidence that it is an endocrine gland. A function ascribed to it, which may be mediated by the hormone melatonin, is an inhibition of the gonads. One feature of clinical interest is its tendency to calcify with age; thus it is visible on x-ray films of the skull in about 70% of adults, giving a landmark that is of value in the x-ray diagnosis of lateral shifts of the brain caused by mass lesions.

The posterior commissure contains fibers interconnecting the superior colliculi and also the pretectal areas.

The habenular nucleus is located in the habenular trigone. Fibers in the stria medullaris connect septal,

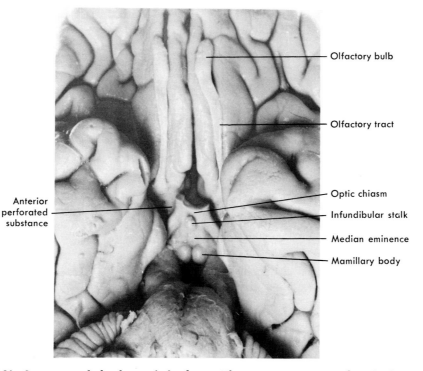

Fig. 5-20. Structures of the base of the brain. The structures associated with the ventral aspect of the hypothalamus include the mamillary body, median eminence, infundibular stalk, and the optic chiasm. Other structures indicated are elements of the olfactory system, including the olfactory bulb, olfactory tract, and the anterior perforated substance.

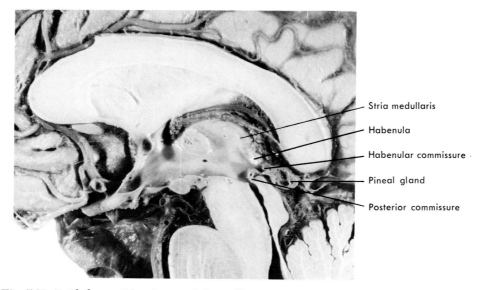

Fig. 5-21. Epithalamus. The view is of the midline structures of a brain cut in sagittal section.

lateral preoptic, and anterior thalamic areas with the habenular nucleus of each side; crossing fibers pass through the habenular commissure. Efferent fibers of the habenular nucleus enter the habenulo-peduncular tract and end in the interpeduncular nucleus, located between the cerebral peduncles of the midbrain (see Chapter 6).

Subthalamus. Because the subthalamus cannot be seen from the exterior surface of the brain or from the ventricular surface, its description will be deferred to Chapter 6.

Cerebral hemispheres

During the course of evolution, the surface of the cerebral cortex has undergone a progressive increase in size in relation to body size and has become increasingly folded. The increase in telencephalic size in higher as compared with lower mammals is much greater than the increase in the size of the brainstem. The brains of lower mammals, such as the rodent, have a smooth surface. Such brains are called lissencephalic. The cat and dog have a moderate degree of fissuring of the brain. The monkey brain has a more complex pattern of fissures, which resembles that of the human brain, but the fissures are not very deep. The great apes, such as the chimpanzee, have brains with a fissural pattern rather similar to that of the human brain, although their brains are smaller in proportion to body size. The porpoise, on the other hand, has a larger brain in proportion to body size and a very complex fissural pattern.

The fissural pattern of the cortex is the key to the anatomy of the cortical convolutions, or gyri (rings). The fissures divide the cortex into four fairly obvious lobes that can be seen from the lateral surface of the brain—the frontal, temporal, parietal, and occipital lobes—and two additional lobes that are less obvious—the insular area seen by spreading the lateral fissure and the limbic lobe, a series of gyri of the central medial surface of the hemisphere (Figs. 5-22 to 5-26). Portions of the limbic lobe are structurally distinct (paleocortex and archicortex) and are considered phylogenetically older than the cortex of the other lobes, which can be called neocortex. This subject is discussed in more detail in Chapter 10.

The fissures of the cortex can be divided into the primary, or major, fissures and the sulci (furrows), or minor fissures. The terms fissure and sulcus are often interchanged, but the distinction is useful. The designation of a fissure as major or minor is in some cases arbitrary, as is a good deal of the terminology of the gross anatomy of the brain, which is often more useful as a guide to denoting areas than in signifying function.

Most of the major fissures are present early in development and are quite deep, extending almost to the ventricles. Their position in some cases can be seen from the ventricular side of the brain as indentations in the ventricular wall, such as the calcar avis (cock's spur) produced by the calcarine fissure. The divisions between the lobes of the brain have been made on the basis of these fissures. There is some functional significance in the fissural pattern of the brain, because the cortical mechanisms involved

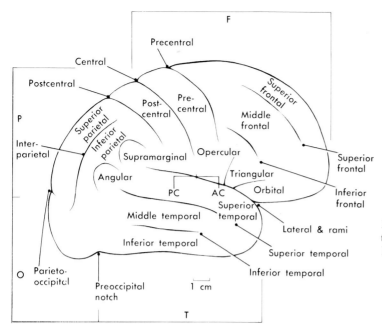

Fig. 5-22. Right lateral view of the fissures, sulci, and gyri of the lateral aspect of the cerebral hemisphere. Abbreviations of lobes of the brain: *F,* frontal; *O,* occipital; *P,* parietal; *T,* temporal. The position of the diencephalon is shown by the projection of the intercommissural line: *AC,* anterior commissure; *PC,* posterior commissure. Fissures and sulci indicated by labels with lead lines; gyri indicated on brain.

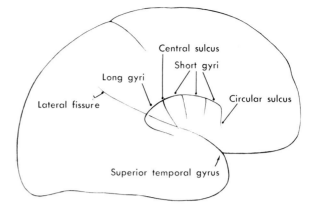

Fig. 5-23. Insular lobe. Lateral aspect shown in position under the frontal, parietal, and temporal opercula bordering the lateral fissure.

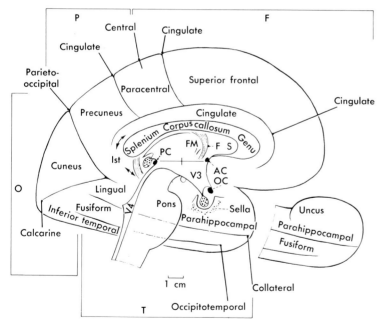

Fig. 5-24. Right lateral view of the fissures, sulci, and gyri of the medial aspect of the cerebral hemisphere and of the brainstem. The position of the intercommissural line is shown. The medial tip of the temporal lobe is shown in outline on the figure and in more detail at the right. Conventions and abbreviations as in Fig. 5-22. Other abbreviations: *F,* fornix; *FM,* foramen of Monro; *Ist,* isthmus of limbic lobe; *OC,* optic chiasm; *S,* septum; *V3* and *V4,* third and fourth ventricles.

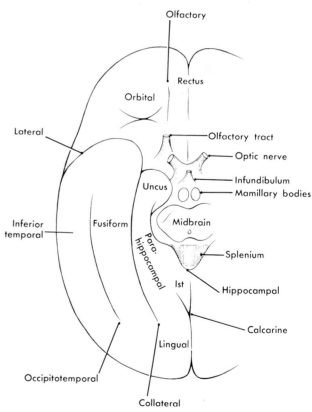

Fig. 5-25. View of the basilar aspect of the right cerebral hemisphere and of the base of the diencephalon. The temporal lobe sulci are complex, and their terminology varies. The superior temporal sulcus can be numbered t1. Sulcus t2 is designated here as the inferior temporal sulcus. Sulcus t3 is designated here as the occipitotemporal sulcus; some authors term it the inferior temporal sulcus. *Ist,* isthmus of limbic lobe. Conventions as in Fig. 5-22.

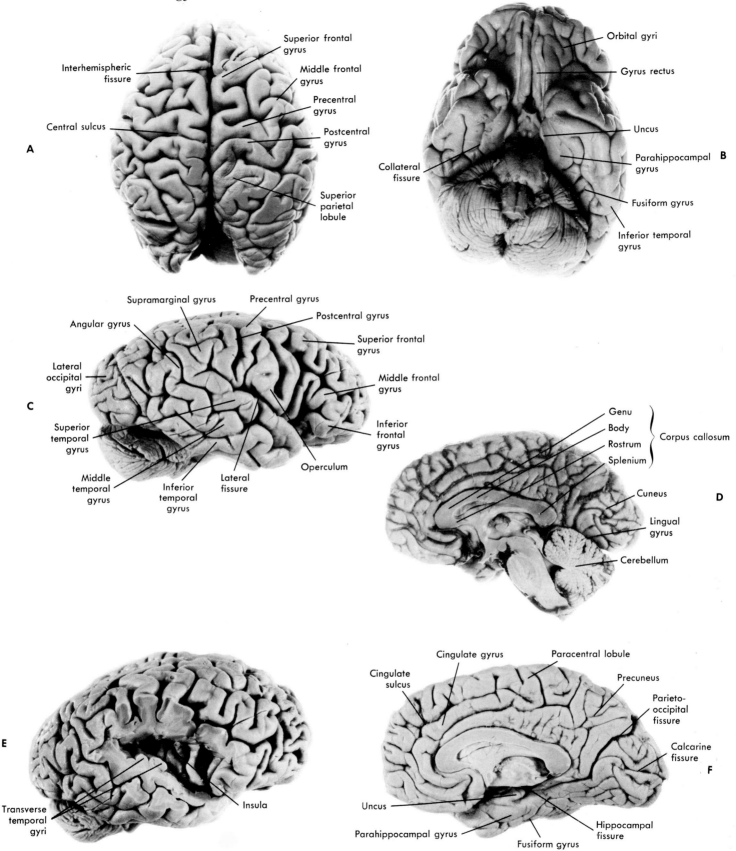

Fig. 5-26. Cerebral hemispheres. The principal fissures, sulci, and gyri are shown.

in specific neurological functions, such as vision and audition, are localized in particular lobes of the brain. However, specific functional areas are not necessarily bounded by fissures or sulci, and the reverse is also true.

The major fissures of the hemisphere are the lateral (sylvian), central (rolandic), parieto-occipital, collateral, hippocampal, cingulate, and calcarine (Figs. 5-22 to 5-26). The lateral and central fissures are the principal major fissures. The lateral fissure has a stem between the frontal and temporal lobes. The cortex forming the lips of the fissure is called the operculum (cover); there are frontal, parietal, and temporal opercula. The central fissure is the border of the frontal and parietal lobes. The parieto-occipital fissure on the mesial surface of the hemisphere is the mesial border of the parietal and occipital lobes. Their border on the lateral surface of the hemisphere is an arbitrary line extending from this fissure down to the preoccipital notch on the lateral inferior margin of the cortex. The collateral fissure is the border of the mesial basilar temporal lobe and the parahippocampal gyrus portion of the limbic lobe. The hippocampal (choroidal) fissure divides the parahippocampal cortex of the limbic lobe from the phylogenetically older portion of the limbic lobe, the dentate gyrus and the hippocampus proper, together called the hippocampal formation. The cingulate fissure on the mesial surface of the hemisphere separates the frontal and parietal lobes from the cingulate gyrus portion of the limbic lobe. The calcarine fissure does not demarcate a lobe, but horizontally divides the mesial surface of the occipital lobe.

The lobes are then divided into lobules or gyri by the sulci, which are shallower and more branched than the major fissures. Certain lobules and gyri generally can be distinguished; however, the patterns in individual brains are variable, and the diagrams shown here are highly schematic. Without examining the complete fissural pattern, it can be difficult to identify fissures of one area of the brain. During a craniotomy the only reliable method of identifying the motor and sensory cortices is by electrical stimulation and recording.

The frontal lobe, which is the largest, is divided into six major gyri (Figs. 5-22 and 5-26). The rostral part of the lateral surface of the lobe is divided by two horizontal sulci, the superior and inferior frontal sulci, into three gyri, the superior, middle, and inferior frontal gyri. The inferior gyrus is further subdivided into three parts, the orbital, triangular, and opercular regions, by two branches of the lateral fissure, the anterior horizontal and ascending rami of the fissure. The caudal boundary of the rostral por-

tion of the lobe is the precentral sulcus; and caudal to this is the precentral gyrus, which is a part of the motor cortex. It is bounded caudally by the central fissure. The inferior surface of the frontal lobe, which rests in the anterior fossa, is divided by the olfactory sulcus medially into the gyrus rectus (straight) and laterally into the orbital gyri.

The temporal lobe is divided by three horizontal sulci, the superior, inferior, and occipitotemporal sulci, into four gyri, the superior, middle, and inferior temporal gyri, and the fusiform, or lateral occipitotemporal, gyrus. The caudal border of the superior temporal gyrus runs caudally and medially into the lateral fissure and breaks into two transverse temporal gyri, or Heschl's gyri, which form the auditory cortex.

The mesial occipital lobe is divided by the calcarine fissure superiorly into a cuneate (wedge-shaped) lobule and inferiorly into a lingual, or medial occipitotemporal, gyrus. The calcarine cortex, also called striate cortex, is the visual cortex.

On its lateral surface, the parietal lobe is divided into three main areas. The vertical postcentral sulcus is the caudal boundary of the postcentral gyrus, or the somatic sensory cortex. The cortex of the caudal portion of the lobe is divided by the horizontal interparietal sulcus into the superior and inferior parietal lobules.

The inferior parietal lobule area can be considered for descriptive purposes to include the anteriorly located supramarginal gyrus, capping the end of the lateral fissure, and the posteriorly placed angular gyrus, capping the superior temporal sulcus. These two gyri are involved in language function and other complex processes.

The mesial surface of the parietal lobe is divided into two portions, the paracentral lobule and the precuneate lobule, by a branch of the cingulate fissure. The central fissure cuts the edge of the hemisphere in a variable manner and appears at the upper margin of the middle of the paracentral lobule.

The insular (island) lobe, or the isle of Reil, lies beneath the lips of the opercula, bounded by the circular sulcus. The insula is divided by the more or less vertically placed central sulcus. The anterior insula is composed of a number of short gyri, and the posterior portion consists of two long gyri.

The limbic lobe is an anatomical construct, a "synthetic" lobe consisting of the mesial central portions of the cortex, which form a ring around the ventricular system. The gyri of this lobe can also be grouped with the major lobes overlying them. Starting at the rostral portion of the brain and following the limbic lobe caudally and then inferiorly are the cingulate gyrus, the isthmus, the parahippocampal gyrus and its rostral medial pole, the uncus (hook), and the medially placed hippocampal formation (see Chapter 10).

The right and left hemispheres are not strictly symmetrical; the left sylvian fissure is generally slightly longer than the right, and the sulcal pattern of the superior temporal gyrus is more complex. These differences may reflect the fact that language functions are represented or controlled in the left hemisphere in most persons: left-sided language dominance is the rule in left-handed as well as in right-handed persons (see Chapter 11).

Each lateral ventricle contains a part of the choroid plexus (Fig. 5-16). Actually, the choroid plexuses of the lateral ventricles are continuous with that of the roof of the third ventricle, the connections being made through the interventricular foramina (of Monro). The taenia of each choroid plexus runs along the floor of the body and trigone of the lateral ventricle and then the roof of the inferior horn.

Subcortical nuclei of the hemispheres: basal ganglia

The term basal ganglia is often used in reference not only to the nuclear masses deep within the telencephalon, but also to structures in the diencephalon and midbrain that are functionally related to these nuclei, such as the subthalamic nucleus and the substantia nigra. In a more restricted sense, the telencephalic basal ganglia include the caudate nucleus, the putamen, and the globus pallidus, which are related to the neocortex. The amygdaloid nucleus should be considered a telencephalic nucleus related to the limbic cortex. During the course of evolutionary development of the cortex, the basal ganglia have also increased in size relative to the brainstem. In some primates the basal ganglia are larger in relation to the rest of the brain than they are in humans.

The only portion of the basal ganglia that can be seen from the ventricular surface of the brain is the caudate nucleus, which forms a part of the floor of the lateral ventricle (Fig. 5-16). The relationship between the caudate nucleus, the putamen, the globus pallidus, and the substantia nigra will be discussed in Chapters 6 and 8.

White matter of the hemispheres

The subcortical white matter can be divided into the commissures that connect the hemispheres, the ascending and descending projection fibers that connect the hemispheres with subcortical areas, and the intracortical projection fibers, often called association fibers. The projection and the association fiber systems will be discussed in Chapter 6.

The major commissures are the corpus callosum, the anterior commissures, and the commissure of the fornix. They tend to connect homologous points in each hemisphere. The rostral portion of the corpus callosum (Figs. 5-17, 5-24, and 5-26) is the genu (knee), and the caudal portion is the splenium (having a bandaged appearance). The callosal fibers penetrating the rostral portion of the hemisphere from the genu are the forceps minor; the caudally directed fibers of the splenium are the forceps major; and a stratum of these fibers running over the lateral ventricle is the tapetum. The anterior commissure interconnects the temporal lobes.

The fornix, which lies under the corpus callosum for part of its course (Fig. 5-17), can be considered to be largely a descending projection system of the hippocampal formation of the limbic cortex, although it also has commissural and intracortical components.

The mass of the white matter under the surface of the frontal and parietal lobes on either side of the corpus callosum is called the centrum semiovale. This mass of white matter can become quite swollen following various types of injury to the brain, resulting in herniation of the cingulate gyrus laterally under the falx and the parahippocampal gyrus and uncus downward through the incisura of the tentorium.

VENTRICULAR SYSTEM

The lateral ventricles are C-shaped cavities within the substance of each hemisphere (Figs. 5-7 and 5-27 to 5-32). They can be thought of as having horns radiating from a center, the atrium (trigone) of the ventricle, which lies under the parietotemporo-occipital junction. The glomus of the choroid plexus lies here. The glomus may calcify and appear on x-ray films. It is important not to confuse it with a calcified pineal gland, as the glomus is about 2 cm lateral to the midline and can be misinterpreted as a pineal gland displaced by a mass. From the atrium the horns radiate to the frontal lobe (frontal horn), the temporal lobe (temporal horn), and the occipital lobe (occipital horn). The body of the lateral ventricular system lies in the precentral area and in the parietal lobe. At the junction of the frontal horn and the body of the ventricle is the foramen of Monro, through which the lateral ventricle communicates with the third ventricle, which lies between the two halves of the diencephalon. The site of the foramen of Monro can be located on a venous phase angiogram as just rostral to the junction of the thalamostriate and internal cerebral veins (Fig. 5-41). The third ventricle terminates at the end of the diencephalon by narrowing into a short aqueduct, the narrowest point in the ventricular system. The aqueduct runs through the mesencephalon and then expands into a diamond-shaped cavity, the fourth ventricle, which lies between the medulla ventrally and the cerebellum superiorly. The ventricular system then communicates with the subarachnoid space of the brain by way of a medially placed aperture (the foramen of Magendie) at the level of the obex and two laterally placed apertures of the left and right sides of the fourth ventricle (the foramina of Luschka), which lie approximately at the level of the eighth nerve bilaterally. The central canal of the spinal cord is probably not patent in adults. The total volume of ventricular cavities is about 35 ml. Each lateral ventricle contains about 7 to 10 ml of ventricular fluid.

Lateral ventricles

The rostral part and roof of the frontal horn are formed by the rostrum, genu, and body of the corpus callosum. The floor and lateral wall are the head of the caudate nucleus; the medial wall is the rostral part of the septum pellucidum. The interventricular foramen is situated posterior to the region where the rostrum of the corpus callosum becomes continuous with the lamina terminalis.

The body of the lateral ventricle lies posterior to the interventricular foramen and anterior to the trigone. Its roof is formed by the midportion of the body of the corpus callosum. The floor of the body is divided by the terminal sulcus, or striothalamic groove, into a lateral part and a medial part, formed by the body of the caudate nucleus and by the thalamus respectively. The medial wall is the posterior part of the septum pellucidum above and the fornix below.

The trigone is the juncture of the body and the occipital and temporal horns. The floor of the trigone has a bulge, the collateral eminence, caused by the collateral fissure. The medial wall has another bulge, the calcar avis, produced by the calcarine fissure. The roof has still another bulge, the bulb, caused by the radiating fibers of the splenium of the corpus callosum. The lateral wall is formed by the tapetum and contains the tail of the caudate nucleus.

Near the junction of the trigone and the temporal horn, the optic radiation arches laterally over the temporal horn (Meyer's loop). The floor of the temporal horn is formed by the hippocampus and laterally by a bulge produced either by the occipitotemporal sulcus or the collateral fissure. The rostral end of the temporal horn becomes spoon-shaped as it fans out over the pes hippocampi. The roof of the temporal horn is the tail of the caudate and laterally part of the internal capsule. In the tip of the horn the roof contains the amygdaloid nucleus. The temporal horn has a slitlike shape; the medial superior part is called the supracornual cleft, and the lateral inferior segment is the lateral cleft.

The occipital horn is quite variable in size and shape. The lateral wall contains the optic radiation. The other walls are formed by the white matter of the occipital lobe and by the radiating fibers of the corpus callosum.

Third ventricle

The third ventricle is a small midline structure. The interventricular foramen enters it near its anterosuperior margins, anterior to the thalamus and behind the pillars of the fornix. Each side of the third ventricle consists of the thalamus above and posteriorly and the hypothalamus below and anteriorly. The thalamus and hypothalamus are divided by a shallow crease, the hypothalamic sulcus, which extends from the interventricular foramen to the beginning of the cerebral aqueduct. The thalami of the two sides may be fused over a variable area, the massa intermedia.

The anterior wall of the third ventricle contains the anterior commissure, the anterior pillars of the fornix, and the lamina terminalis, which slopes anteriorly and downward to the optic recess. The floor of the third ventricle is produced by the hypothalamus anteriorly and the subthalamus posteriorly. Behind the optic chiasm is the infundibulum of the hypophysis, with the infundibular recess. Posterior to these are the tuber cinereum and the mamillary bodies.

The roof of the third ventricle is composed of the velum interpositum, which is invaginated by the choroid plexus. At the posterior end of the roof is the suprapineal recess. Below this in the posterior wall of the third ventricle is the habenular commissure. The pineal body is attached below the habenular commissure, and the pineal recess projects into it. Beneath the pineal body is the posterior commissure.

Cerebral aqueduct

Beneath the posterior commissure is the opening of the cerebral aqueduct, which passes through the periaqueductal gray matter of the mesencephalon. Ventral to the aqueduct is the tegmentum of the mesencephalon and rostral pons; dorsal to it is the tectum.

Fourth ventricle

The aqueduct opens into the fourth ventricle. The floor of the fourth ventricle is the tegmentum of the caudal pons and the medulla. The roof is formed by the anterior medullary velum rostrally and the posterior medullary velum and tela choroidea caudally. The latter contains the median aperture, or the foramen of Magendie. At the lateral aspect of the fourth ventricle is the middle cerebellar peduncle; medial and caudal to this is the inferior cerebellar peduncle. The lateral recesses of the fourth ventricle sweep around the medulla and contain the lateral apertures, or the foramina of Luschka. Cerebrospinal fluid passes from the fourth ventricle to the subarachnoid cisterns of the posterior fossa through the median and lateral apertures. The lumen of the fourth ventricle rises to an apex dorsally, called the fastigium.

Choroid plexuses

The covering of certain parts of the brain is very thin, consisting only of ependymal epithelium and pia mater. In some of these regions a rich capillary plexus develops and invaginates the ependymal layer into the ventricular system. These invaginations are called choroid plexuses. A choroid plexus is present in each lateral ventricle, the third ventricle, and the fourth ventricle (Figs. 5-13, *A*, and 5-16). The line of attachment of a choroid plexus is called a taenia.

The choroid plexus of each lateral ventricle is continuous with that of the third ventricle through the interventricular foramen. The taeniae in the lateral ventricle pass along the thalamus in the body of the ventricle, the thalamus and posterior column of the fornix in the trigone, and in the supracornual cleft of the temporal horn. The choroid plexus is largest in the trigone; this part of it is called the glomus. No choroid plexus is found in the frontal horn. The taeniae of the choroid plexus of the third ventricle pass along the stria medullaris to the region of the habenular commissure. A separate choroid plexus develops in the fourth ventricle. The taeniae of this plexus pass along the ependymal roof of the fourth ventricle near the obex in a rostrolateral direction into the lateral recesses.

Pneumoventriculography and radionuclide encephalography

Replacing the fluid within the subarachnoid space and ventricular system with a contrast medium of differing density to x-rays was a procedure developed by the neurosurgeon, Walter Dandy. Air injected into the spaces fills and outlines these cavities, and being less opaque on the x-ray films, the cavities appear as more intensely exposed, darker areas on radiographs (Figs. 5-27 and 5-32, *A*). Although the early investigators attempted to replace the entire content of the ventricular system with air, at the present time so-called fractional pneumoencephalography (PEG) is

done. A total amount of about 35 ml of air is slowly injected into the lumbar subarachnoid space, with the patient sitting upright. The air is injected in 10- to 15-ml increments while the patient's head is flexed and extended in a manner so as to fill the different portions of the subarachnoid cisterns and ventricular system sequentially. By maneuvering of the head, the air bubble can be kept in different portions of the ventricular system and the outlines of the system can be seen. If the intracranial pressure is raised, it is generally safer to inject the air (or a positive contrast medium, such as an iodinated oil) into one lateral ventricle (ventriculography) (Fig. 5-32). This method is of great value in diagnosing the size of the ventricu-

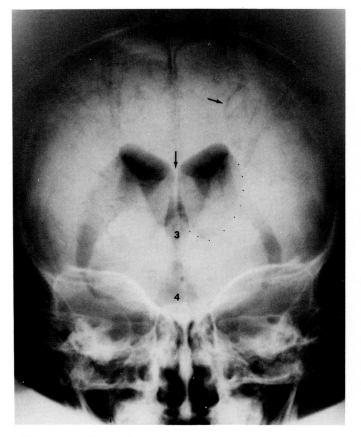

Fig. 5-27. Ventricular system. Anterior-posterior pneumoencephalogram, supine (brow-up) position. Air has filled the fourth ventricle *(4)*, aqueduct, third ventricle *(3)*, and the lateral ventricles. For each lateral ventricle note the frontal horn, which is outlined by the dots on the patient's left side, the body of the ventricle, and the trigone. These parts of the ventricle appear as areas of different density because of varying amounts of air contained in the different portions of the ventricle. The blacker areas contain more air. The temporal horns can be seen curving downward. The tips of the temporal horns are seen through the orbits. Also note the septum pellucidum *(midline arrow)* and air in the subarachnoid spaces of the sulci of the convexity of the hemisphere *(upper arrow)*. (Courtesy Dr. Lawrence H. Zingesser.)

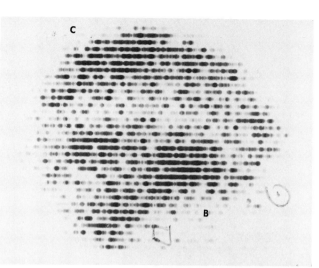

Fig. 5-28. Intracranial subarachnoid cisterns. Isotope cistern-ography. Right lateral scan of head. Normal pattern of cerebro-spinal fluid flow. Radioactive-iodinated serum albumin was in-jected in the lumbar subarachnoid space, and the brain was subsequently scanned. The isotope has entered the basilar cisterns (B) and has passed into the subarachnoid spaces over the convexities of the hemisphere (C) around the sagittal sinus. Note that there is less radioactivity in the area of the ventricu-lar system, which appears as a light area. Compare with Fig. 5-29. The circle marks the position of the eye, and the square the position of the external acoustic meatus. (Courtesy Dr. Lawrence H. Zingesser.)

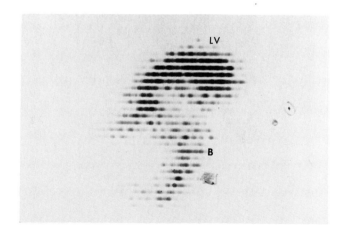

Fig. 5-29. Ventricular system. Isotope cisternography. Right lateral scan of head. Abnormal pattern of cerebrospinal fluid flow. The isotope has entered the basilar cisterns (B) but has failed to pass over the cerebral convexities. Instead, the isotope has entered the ventricular system, which is dilated. The frontal and occipital horns and the bodies of the lateral ven-tricles (LV) are delineated clearly. In this case the basilar cisterns were obstructed by a chronic inflammatory process caused by tuberculous meningitis. Compare with Fig. 5-28. (Courtesy Dr. Lawrence H. Zingesser.)

lar system and in studying possible obstructions of or encroachments on the ventricular system by intra-cranial masses.

Radionuclide encephalography can reveal the pat-tern of flow in the cerebrospinal fluid pathways. Fol-lowing the injection of a radioactive isotope into the lumbar subarachnoid space the brain is scanned at intervals over 24 to 48 hours. If the cerebrospinal fluid flow is normal, most of the isotope will pass into the basilar cisterns and over the convexities of the hemispheres (Fig. 5-28). If there is obstruction along this pathway, the isotope refluxes into the ven-tricles (Fig. 5-29).

Computer tomography

A recently introduced noninvasive procedure has already proved remarkably useful and seems destined to increase in value as its resolution improves with further technical advances. This is the application of computer data processing to x-ray tomography. The basis of computer tomography is that soft tissues have slightly different absorption coefficients. By taking a number of measurements of the amount of x-ray absorption and systematically changing the angle of passage of the x-ray beam through the body, it is possible to calculate absorption coefficients for small blocks of tissue and then to assemble an image of the tissue under examination.

For neuroradiological applications, the following procedure is now widely utilized. A narrowly focused x-ray beam is rotated around the head many times. The amount of radiation emitted is known, and that which passes through the skull and brain is recorded, using scintillation crystals. In effect, slices of the head are scanned in this manner. By varying the position of the slice, the brain can be progressively scanned from the base to the vertex. The data from the scans is processed by computer, which then dis-plays the absorption coefficients of the blocks of tissue making up each slice on a cathode ray tube. The intensity of the cathode ray beam is proportional to the absorption coefficient. Examples of five to-mographic slices taken at progressively more super-ficial levels in a normal individual are shown in Fig. 5-30. Structures that can be recognized are indicated and include the fourth ventricle, the basilar and carotid arteries and the optic chiasm, the third ven-tricle and tectum, the frontal horns and trigones of the lateral ventricles and the pineal gland, and the lateral ventricles. One difficulty with the displays is that the anatomy of the brain is viewed from above, a perspective unfamiliar to many because neuro-pathological specimens are often sectioned in the coronal rather than the horizontal plane.

Computer tomography can be helpful in demonstrating some structures that are difficult to visualize by other means. For example, the retrobulbar tissues are shown to advantage in Fig. 5-30, *F*. The optic nerves and lateral and medial rectus muscles are all readily seen. Pathological conditions affecting the configuration of the ventricular system are easily recognized. For instance, the enormous increase in the size of the ventricles in a case of normal pressure hydrocephalus is seen in three slices in Fig. 5-31. Mass lesions, including brain tumors and hemorrhages, can often been seen by computer tomography,

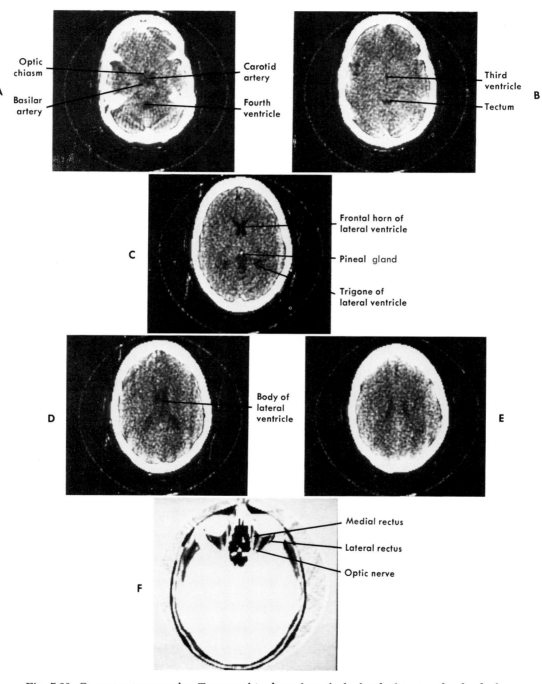

Fig. 5-30. Computer tomography. Tomographic slices through the head of a normal individual. The slice in **A** is at a level near the base of the brain; the slices in **B** through **E** are progressively more superficial. Some of the structures visualized are indicated. The tomograph in **F** was made with different parameters and shows the retrobulbar region of the orbits. (Courtesy Dr. M. Sarwar.)

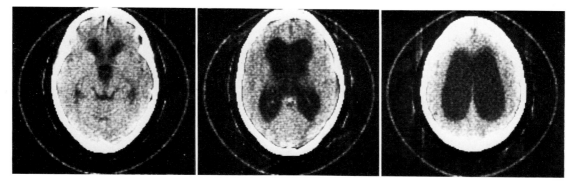

Fig. 5-31. Computer tomography. Three tomographs taken through the head of an individual with normal pressure hydrocephalus. The massive dilatation of the ventricular system is obvious. (Courtesy Dr. M. Sarwar.)

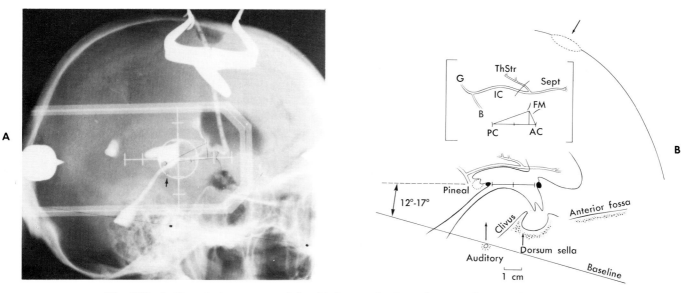

Fig. 5-32. A, Stereotaxic anatomy of the third ventricle. Lateral ventriculogram after injection of air and radiopaque contrast medium into the ventricular system. The patient was in a supine position. Note the cannula inserted into the lateral ventricle through a frontal burr hole at the level of the coronal suture. The position of the anterior and posterior commissures, the intercommissural line, and a line from the posterior margin of the foramina of Monro to the posterior commissure have been constructed on a film. The Frankfurt plane (baseline) is indicated by dots on the inferior orbital margin and on the external acoustic meatus. The arrow marks the site of the target constructed on the film. The target was the medial portion of the spinothalamic tract at the mesencephalodiencephalic border. The procedure was performed for relief of intractable pain. **B,** Landmarks used in stereotaxic surgery. Lateral view of third ventricle. See Fig. 5-32, **A,** for comparison. The intercommissural line between the anterior *(AC)* and posterior *(PC)* commissures and the midpoint of the line (the anterior-posterior zero point) are shown. The *FM-PC* line is also shown. This line and the *FM-pineal* line have also been used as landmarks for stereotaxis. Note that the foramen of Monro *(FM)* is about 2 cm above the dorsum sella, and the posterior commissure is about 3 cm above the external acoustic meatus, when the intercommissural line is in a horizontal position. The position of the deep venous drainage of the cerebrum with respect to the third ventricle is shown. The venous angle made by the thalamostriate vein lying on the floor of the lateral ventricle and the internal cerebral vein in the roof of the third ventricle are also shown. Abbreviations: *G,* great vein of Galen; *B,* basilar vein of Rosenthal; *IC,* internal cerebral vein; *ThStr,* thalamostriate vein; *Sept,* septal vein.

although there are problems with visualization of lesions near bone.

STEREOTAXIC ANATOMY

In animals in which the skull shape is quite similar among individual members of the species, brain structures can be located by reference to a three-dimensional coordinate system in which the zero reference lines pass through certain skull structures. In the system devised by Victor Horsley and Robert Clarke, the horizontal plane is defined by the baseline, the inferior orbital-external acoustic meatus plane. This plane is kept parallel to the horizontal plane of the sterotaxic head holder by bars placed on the orbital margins and into the external acoustic canals (see Appendix I). The zero horizontal plane for cat and monkey brain atlases using this system is taken as a plane 10 mm above the baseline. Distances above this are measured in millimeters and are designated positive or dorsal; those below are negative or ventral. The zero reference for the frontal plane is the interaural line. Areas rostral to this are designated as positive or anterior; those behind, which would be in the cerebellum and caudal brainstem, are negative or posterior. The zero reference for the sagittal plane is the sagittal midline plane of the brain, and distances from the midlines are designated as left or right.

This system is not accurate in the human brain because of the variability of skull shapes. However, structures in the periventricular areas of the brain can be localized with reference to ventricular landmarks. Because the structures that are of surgical interest, the basal ganglia and the thalamus, are adjacent to the ventricular system, this has proved to be a useful and practical development. The most widely used coordinate system was devised by J. Talairach. The ventricle is punctured; the ventricular system is filled with a contrast material, such as air or an iodinated oil that is opaque to x-rays; and the third ventricle is outlined (Fig. 5-32). A line is then constructed connecting the anterior and posterior commissures. In the majority of human brains, this line measures 25 ± 2 mm. This line is taken as the horizontal axis of the brain. It is of interest that this line is not parallel to the baseline; the front of the line is tilted upward an average of 12° to the baseline. The frontal plane of the brain is defined as a line perpendicular to this line, and the midpoint of the anterior-posterior (A-P) line is taken as the A-P zero reference point. The horizontal and lateral zeros are also based on the intercommissural line.

To take into account the variability caused by different sizes of the thalamus, Talairach devised a method of dividing the height of the thalamus into quarters and the intercommissural line into thirds. By reference to various detailed stereotaxic atlases, the structures lying within these areas in different sagittal, frontal, or horizontal planes can be found. The sections of the human brainstem illustrated in Appendix III (B and C) were cut along the axes of the intercommissural line. The position of the sections with reference to the intercommissural line zero reference points and the projection of this line on each section also are shown.

In the animal stereotaxic technique described in Appendix I, the head and reference frame are rigidly fixed together, and the electrode moves in rectilinear coordinates with respect to the head. The newest human stereotaxic machines work on the ingenious principle of having electrode holders fixed on arcs of a sphere whose center is the center of the machine. This center is shown by cross hairs that are superimposed on the x-ray film. The patient's head is held by a ring with four pins that pierce the skull above the orbits and mastoid processes. The projection of the center of the machine (the point on which the electrodes are centered) is shown on the film on which the intercommissural line is constructed (Fig. 5-32). The ring holding the head is then moved in three axes with respect to the center of the machine to superimpose the center on the center of the intercommissural line or on any other target point that is desired. Inasmuch as the electrode can enter the skull from any point on the surface of a sphere, the most favorable approach can be chosen for inserting the electrode to the target, avoiding vessels or areas it would not be safe to puncture.

VASCULAR SUPPLY OF THE BRAIN
Carotid and vertebral origins at the aortic arch

The functional anatomy of the vascular system of the brain as revealed by angiography presents quite a different appearance from the anatomy of the vessels shown in drawings made from anatomical specimens. This difference is in part caused by the angle of projection in which the angiograms are obtained and in part by the patterns of filling of vessels. The general anatomical plan of the major arteries of the brain is considered first, followed by discussion of their course and appearance in angiograms. The physiological effects of occlusions of vessels are discussed on pp. 169-171.

The brain receives its blood supply from four vessels, the paired carotid and vertebral arteries. Branches of the vertebral arteries supply the posterior portions of the cerebrum, the cerebellum, and the brainstem. Branches of the carotid artery supply the

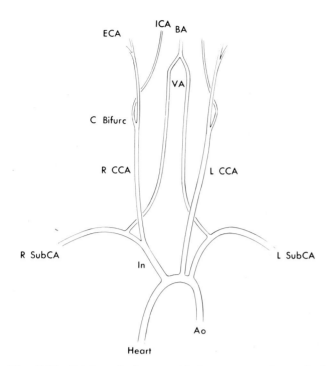

Fig. 5-33. Origins of the carotid (anterior) and vertebral (posterior) circulations from the aortic arch. Abbreviations: *Ao,* aorta; *In,* innominate artery; *R* and *L SubCA,* right and left subclavian arteries; *R* and *L CCA,* right and left common carotid arteries; *C Bifurc,* carotid bifurcation; *ECA,* external carotid artery; *ICA,* internal carotid artery; *VA,* vertebral arteries; *BA,* basilar artery.

anterior and middle portions of the cerebrum and diencephalon. The vertebral arteries supply about 20% of the total cerebral blood flow, and the carotid arteries 80%.

The carotid and vertebral arteries fill from the aortic arch (Fig. 5-33). The origins of the right and left carotids are not symmetrical. On the right side the aortic arch gives off the innominate artery, which divides at the level of the right sternoclavicular joint to form the right carotid artery and the right subclavian artery. On the left side, the left carotid artery arises directly from the aortic arch in the superior mediastinum.

The origins of the vertebral arteries are symmetrical. They arise as the first branch of the right and left subclavian arteries. They then ascend in the root of the neck over the transverse processes of the C7 vertebral body. This point is lateral to the location of the stellate (lowest cervical and first thoracic) sympathetic ganglion. The vertebral artery may have an ansa (loop) of the sympathetic chain around it at this point.

The carotid and vertebral arteries may have anomalous origins. The left carotid arises from the innomi-

nate in 10% to 20% of cases; the left vertebral arises from the aortic arch in 6% of cases; one vertebral may be absent, although this is rare.

The common carotid arteries ascend in the neck deep to the sternocleidomastoid muscles. The artery lies in the carotid sheath of cervical fascia with the vagus nerve and internal jugular vein. The artery lies medial and deep to the vein. The common carotid artery divides into internal and external branches at the level of the upper border of the thyroid cartilage, which is at the level of the third or fourth cervical vertebral bodies. The internal carotid is given off deep and lateral to the external carotid and goes medially as it ascends. The external carotid gives off numerous branches in the neck that supply the neck, face and scalp, and part of the dura by way of the middle meningeal artery, which originates from the maxillary branch of the external carotid artery. The internal carotid artery gives off no branches until it enters the skull, where branches are given off in the temporal bone (caroticotympanic branch) and in the cavernous sinus (meningohypophyseal branches). After entering the cranial cavity the internal carotid gives off three branches, the ophthalmic, posterior communicating, and anterior choroidal arteries, and then terminates by dividing into the anterior cerebral and middle cerebral arteries. The posterior communicating and the anterior cerebral and internal carotid arteries make up the rostral part of the circle of Willis (Figs. 5-34 and 5-35).

The vertebral artery ascends to the brain by entering the transverse foramina of the cervical vertebrae at C6. The prominent tubercle of the C6 transverse process, known interestingly enough as the carotid tubercle because the carotid artery can be compressed against it, can be palpated at the root of the neck. The vertebral artery ascends in the transverse foramina of C6 to C1, surrounded by a plexus of veins and sympathetic nerve fibers. When exposing the spine from the anterior approach, one should remember that the vertebral artery lies anterior or superficial to the cervical nerve roots exiting from the spinal cord in the intervertebral foramina. The vertebral artery gives off muscular branches that anastomose with branches of the external carotid artery. After passing out of the transverse foramen of the C1, the vertebral artery turns medially and enters the dura in front of the first dural attachment of the dentate ligament of the spinal cord and passes along the lateral and then the ventral aspect of the brainstem (Figs. 5-34, 5-36, and 5-37). Here the vertebral artery gives off the posterior inferior cerebellar artery. The two vertebral arteries then come together at the level of the pontomedullary junction and join to form the basilar artery.

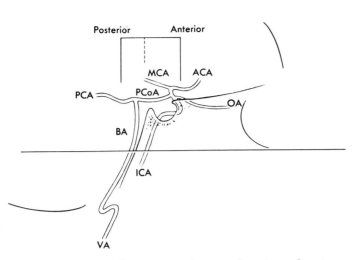

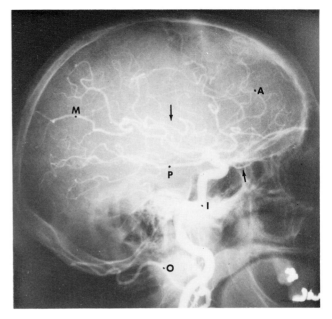

Fig. 5-34. Course of entry into the cranial cavity and major intracranial terminal branches of the carotid and vertebral arteries. Anterior circulation: *ICA,* internal carotid artery; *OA,* ophthalmic artery; *PCoA,* posterior communicating artery; *ACA,* anterior cerebral artery; *MCA,* middle cerebral artery. Posterior circulation: *VA,* vertebral artery; *BA,* basilar artery; *PCA,* posterior cerebral artery. See Figs. 5-35 and 5-36 for the pattern of filling of these vessels from the internal carotid artery and the vertebral artery respectively. In about one third of cases there is a significant amount of filling of the posterior cerebral artery from the carotid circulation, as shown in Fig. 5-35.

Fig. 5-35. Carotid circulation. Right carotid angiogram, lateral projection, arterial phase. The main trunks and terminal branches of the anterior cerebral *(A),* middle cerebral *(M),* and, in this case, the posterior communicating artery and posterior cerebral artery *(P)* have been filled after injection of contrast medium into the common carotid artery in the neck. Note the ophthalmic artery *(lower arrow)* filling from the internal carotid artery; the branches of the middle cerebral artery draping over the insula and the parietal and temporal opercula *(upper arrow)* that comprise the vessels of the sylvian triangle; the course of the internal carotid artery *(I)* in the petrous bone and in the sphenoid bone (carotid siphon); the occipital artery *(O)* branch of the external carotid artery in the suboccipital muscles and scalp. (Courtesy Dr. Lawrence H. Zingesser.)

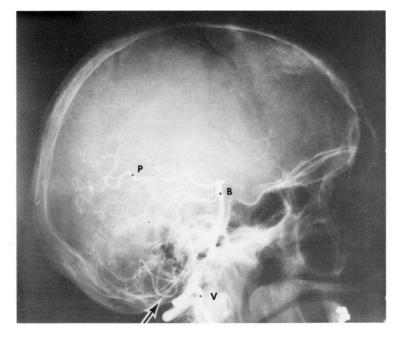

Fig. 5-36. Vertebral-basilar circulation (same patient as in Fig. 5-35). Right vertebral angiogram, lateral projection, arterial phase. The right and left vertebral arteries *(V)* are both filled, and the loops made by each vertebral artery at the C_1 vertebra can be seen. The left vertebral artery is visualized because contrast medium that fills the basilar artery *(B)* after injection in one vertebral artery often runs into the opposite vertebral artery for a variable distance. The right and left superior cerebellar arteries fill from the basilar artery at the point marked by the dot opposite *B,* and the basilar artery terminates in the posterior cerebral arteries *(P);* only the right posterior cerebral is seen clearly. Note the anterior medullary segment (caudal loop) of the posterior inferior cerebellar artery *(arrow).* (Courtesy Dr. Lawrence H. Zingesser.)

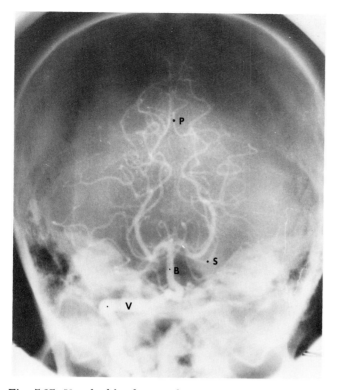

Fig. 5-37. Vertebral-basilar circulation. Right vertebral angiogram, anterior-posterior half-axial (Towne) projection, arterial phase. Note the loop made by the vertebral artery *(V)* at C₁ and the basilar artery *(B)*, which appears rather short in this projection, which is a view on a line approximately from the forehead to the foramen magnum. Note the superior cerebellar arteries *(S)* and the W-shaped configuration of the posterior cerebral arteries *(P)* as they loop around the brainstem. Note the medial terminal calcarine cortex branches along the midline of the hemispheres, marked with a dot. (Courtesy Dr. Lawrence H. Zingesser.)

The basilar artery extends the length of the pons and then bifurcates beneath the mesencephalon to form the posterior cerebral arteries, which make up the caudal part of the circle of Willis.

In case of occlusion in the neck of any of the vessels to the brain, collateral circulation can bypass the block to varying degrees in different individuals. Within the neck there are anastomoses of the muscular branches of the thyrocervical trunk, the deep ascending cervical artery and vertebral artery (all branches of the subclavian artery), and between the external carotid artery and vertebral artery. An obstruction of the internal carotid artery in the neck can be bypassed to some degree by the intracranial anastomosis between branches of the internal and external carotid arteries that is formed by the ophthalmic artery branch of the internal carotid. The intracranial internal carotid circulation can receive blood from terminal vessels of the internal maxillary branch of the external carotid artery by way of the ophthalmic artery.

Cerebral angiography

The vascular system can be visualized on x-ray films by the injection of iodinated water-soluble contrast medium into vessels. In cerebral angiography, which was first described by the Portuguese neurologist Egas Moniz, the injection is made into one of the arteries supplying the brain, and a series of ten consecutive anteroposterior and ten lateral films are taken. These films are taken during the cerebral transit time of the medium over a period of about 10 seconds. They show the arterial, intermediate, and venous phases of the circulation. To visualize right and left sides of the anterior circulation, the right and left common carotid arteries can be punctured percutaneously in the neck. Various approaches can be used to visualize the posterior circulation. The right or left brachial arteries can be punctured and contrast medium injected against the direction of blood flow with sufficient pressure to reach the origin of the vertebral artery. Medium flowing up one vertebral artery will enter the basilar artery and opacify the posterior circulation. On the right side a brachial artery injection will also fill the right carotid artery. The vertebral arteries can also be punctured in the neck percutaneously. Finally, a catheter can be introduced into the origins of each of the four vessels supplying the brain by threading a catheter from the femoral artery up the aorta to the aortic arch, and this technique is now widely used.

Intracranial vascular supply of the brain: circle of Willis

The anterior part of the brain receives its blood supply from the internal carotid arteries; the brainstem, cerebellum, and parts of the temporal and occipital lobes are supplied by the vertebral arteries. There are anatomical connections between the vessels of the two systems at the circle of Willis, but functionally the systems usually are almost completely separate.

A key structure for understanding the relations of the branches of the internal carotid arteries and the vertebral system to the brain is the circle of Willis. This is a ring composed of vessels located beneath the hypothalamus and surrounding the optic chiasm and the pituitary stalk. The components of the circle are the single anterior communicating artery and the paired anterior cerebral, internal carotid, posterior communicating, and posterior cerebral arteries (Fig. 5-38). The structure of the circle of Willis most easily can be grasped and remem-

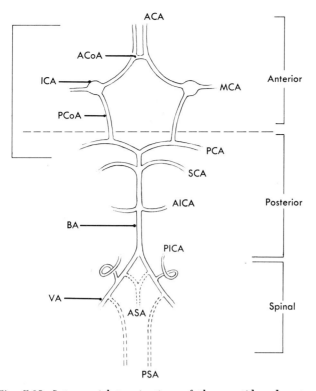

Fig. 5-38. Intracranial terminations of the carotid and vertebral arteries. Circle of Willis. View looking downward into the cranial fossae with the brain removed. Anterior circulation: *ACA,* anterior cerebral artery; *ACoA,* anterior communicating artery; *ICA,* internal carotid artery; *MCA,* middle cerebral artery; *PCoA,* posterior communicating artery. Posterior circulation: *PCA,* posterior cerebral artery; *SCA,* superior cerebellar artery; *AICA,* anterior inferior cerebellar artery; *BA,* basilar artery; *VA,* vertebral artery; *PICA,* posterior inferior cerebellar artery. Spinal circulation: *ASA,* anterior spinal artery; *PSA,* posterior spinal arteries. There are usually two posterior spinal arteries on the dorsal surface of the cervical spinal cord.

bered if it is thought of as a hexagon. The anterior half of the hexagon supplies blood to the anterior circulation fed from the internal carotid arteries through the anterior cerebral arteries and the middle cerebral arteries. The posterior half of the hexagon supplies blood to the posterior circulation fed from the basilar artery by way of the posterior cerebral arteries. The vessels that provide the anastomoses that make up the circle, the single anterior communicating artery, which connects the right and left anterior circulations, and the two posterior communicating arteries, which connect the anterior and posterior circulations, are rather inconsistent in their development, and variations in the size and patency of these vessels are almost the rule rather than the exception.

Aneurysms of intracranial arteries are most commonly found at the junctions of the vessels of the circle of Willis. The neck of the aneurysmal sac arises at the junction of arteries. The media of the arteries is greatly thinned or absent at the point where the neck of the sac bulges from the artery. In addition to the defect of the media, the internal elastic membrane is deficient in the sac as well. The cerebral arteries have no external elastic membrane and have a thin adventitial coat. The commonest aneurysms are of the carotid artery at the junction of the posterior communicating artery, of the anterior cerebral artery at the junction of the anterior communicating artery, and of the middle cerebral artery where it trifurcates in the sylvian fissure.

Intracranial arteries

Anterior circulation. The internal carotid artery enters the skull through the carotid canal in the petrous part of the temporal bone, passing along the carotid groove in front of the foramen lacerum to cross through the cavernous sinus (Figs. 5-34, 5-35, and 5-39). The artery has an S-shaped course within the sinus, which has been named the carotid siphon. As it pierces the dura, the carotid artery gives off its first major branch, the ophthalmic artery, then the posterior communicating artery, and then the anterior choroidal artery. The artery then bifurcates into the anterior cerebral and middle cerebral arteries.

The anterior cerebral artery runs horizontally and medially to enter the ventral part of the longitudinal fissure between the cerebral hemispheres. It connects with the contralateral anterior cerebral artery by way of the anterior communicating artery. The anterior cerebral artery gives off ganglionic branches near its juncture with the anterior communicating artery; these pass through the anterior perforated substance and help supply the basal ganglia, the internal capsule, and the anterior hypothalamus. Beyond the anterior communicating artery, the anterior cerebral artery gives off the frontopolar artery to the undersurface of the frontal lobe and small branches to the midline structures, such as the rostral corpus callosum. The anterior cerebral artery then curves around the genu of the corpus callosum as the pericallosal artery, giving off the callosomarginal artery, which runs parallel to it but above the cingulate gyrus. These arteries branch further and supply the medial and dorsal surface of the frontal and parietal lobes, including the medial part of the motor and somatosensory cortex (Fig. 5-40).

The middle cerebral artery runs along the lateral (sylvian) fissure. It gives off two groups of ganglionic branches, the medial and lateral striate arteries, which enter the brain through the anterior perforated substance and help supply the internal capsule, basal

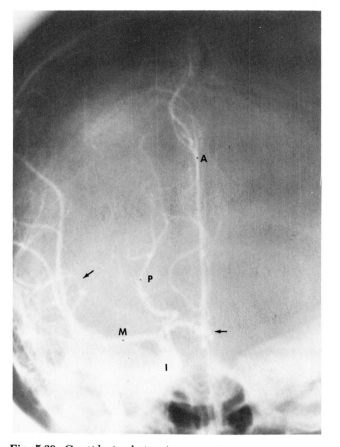

Fig. 5-39. Carotid circulation (same patient as in Fig. 5-35). Right carotid angiogram, anterior-posterior half-axial (Towne) projection, inclined to baseline so that the orbits and petrous bones are superimposed, arterial phase. The anterior *(A)*, middle *(M)*, and, in this case, the posterior *(P)* cerebral arteries have been filled from the internal carotid artery *(I)*. Note the insular branches of the middle cerebral artery (*left arrow;* compare with Fig. 5-35). The position of the anterior communicating artery has been indicated by the *right arrow.* (Courtesy Dr. Lawrence H. Zingesser.)

ganglia, and thalamus. The largest of the medial striate arteries are known as lenticulo-optic arteries, and the largest of the lateral striates are the lenticulostriate arteries. The middle cerebral artery distributes a number of cortical branches to the lateral surface of the frontal, parietal, and temporal lobes. The area of cortex nourished by these vessels includes the premotor, motor, and somatosensory cortices of the cerebral convexities (Fig. 5-40).

The anterior choroidal artery enters the temporal horn of the lateral ventricle and ends in the glomus of the choroid plexus of the lateral ventricle. It supplies the internal capsule, parts of the basal ganglia and thalamus, and part of the midbrain.

The posterior communicating artery connects the anterior with the posterior part of the circle of Willis. It also gives off ganglionic branches that help supply the hypothalamus, thalamus, and subthalamus.

Posterior circulation. The other major vascular channel of the brain, besides the internal carotid system, is the vertebral-basilar system (Figs. 5-34 and 5-36). The vertebral arteries pass up the neck through foramina in the transverse processes of cervical vertebrae 6 to 1. After making a loop between the atlas and the occipital bone, each vertebral artery enters the skull through the foramen magnum. The two vertebral arteries merge at the pontomedullary junction to form the basilar artery. The left vertebral artery is generally larger than the right. The basilar artery passes in the midline ventral sulcus of the pons to end just posterior to the posterior clinoid process. The vertebral-basilar system supplies the posterior cerebrum, midbrain, pons, medulla, and cerebellum. The major branches of the basilar artery are the posterior cerebral, superior cerebellar, and paramedian, lateral, and anterior inferior cerebellar arteries. The

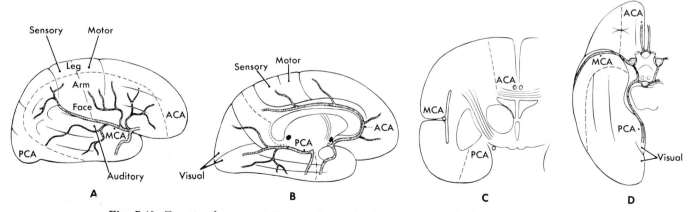

Fig. 5-40. Functional representation in the cerebral territories supplied by terminal cerebral branches of the anterior and posterior circulations. **A,** Lateral aspect of hemisphere; **B,** medial aspect; **C,** frontal section; **D,** inferior aspect. Abbreviations: *ACA,* anterior cerebral artery; *MCA,* middle cerebral artery; *PCA,* posterior cerebral artery.

main branches of the vertebral arteries are the posterior inferior cerebellar, paramedian, and anterior and posterior spinal arteries.

Each posterior cerebral artery passes around the midbrain in the cisterna ambiens, then passes through the incisura of the tentorium to pass along the medial surface of the temporal and occipital lobes, and ends in the calcarine fissure to supply the visual cortex (Fig. 5-40). Posteromedial ganglionic branches of the posterior cerebral artery supply the posterior hypothalamus, parts of the thalamus, and parts of the midbrain; one of these branches is the medial choroidal artery, which ends in the choroid plexus of the third ventricle. Posterior choroidal branches help supply the posterior thalamus, subthalamus, and internal capsule. Cortical branches pass to much of the inferior surface of the temporal lobe and the occipital lobe.

The superior cerebellar artery divides into medial and lateral branches. The medial division supplies the mesencephalon, pons, medial cerebellum, and deep cerebellar nuclei. Lateral branches go to the lateral part of the superior cerebellar cortex.

Paramedian and lateral pontine arteries supply the respective parts of the pons.

The anterior inferior cerebellar artery runs along the pontomedullary border and supplies the brainstem, the superior and middle cerebellar peduncles, and the anterior part of the undersurface of the cerebellum. It often gives rise to the internal auditory artery, which supplies the internal ear.

The posterior inferior cerebellar artery supplies the choroid plexus of the fourth ventricle, the lateral medulla, the inferior cerebellar peduncle, and part of the cerebellum.

The relationships of the different cerebellar arteries can be most easily grasped if one remembers that there are *one* pair of *superior* cerebellar arteries and *two* pairs of *inferior* cerebellar arteries. Of the *inferior* cerebellar arteries, the rostral pair coming off the basilar artery goes anteriorly around the brainstem; so they are the *anterior inferior* cerebellars. The caudal pair, coming off the vertebrals, goes posteriorly along the side of the medulla and then posteriorly around the tonsils and vermis of the cerebellum, and they are therefore the *posterior inferior* cerebellars. Displacement of this vessel from its normal position on angiograms is a sensitive indicator of tumors or other masses in the posterior fossa. Therefore this vessel is important enough to have its own abbreviation (PICA).

The paramedian arteries supply the medial part of the medulla.

Pattern of blood supply to brain tissue

The blood vessels entering the brain penetrate it generally at right angles to the surface and then branch and ramify in the gray and white matter. The capillary network of the cortex is very dense; it has been estimated that neurons are rarely more than 50 μm away from a capillary. The cerebral arteries are often considered to be end-arteries in the sense that large anastomoses are not formed between the branches of the large parent arteries of the circle of Willis. The arterial supplies of the three major arterial trunks (anterior, middle, and posterior cerebral arteries) have definite borders. Because of the poor overlap of arterial supplies, the borders between major territories are known as "watershed areas" or the "last meadows"; if prolonged systemic hypotension occurs, as in surgical shock, these areas develop infarcts before other cerebral areas (Fig. 5-40). However, after the occlusion of a major arterial trunk, a collateral circulation will develop in some cases. In these cases the distal branches of an intact vessel will supply the distal branches of a proximally occluded vessel, and there may even be some backflow down the occluded vessel to the point of occlusion.

Venous drainage

The capillary network of the brain drains into superficial veins and deep veins. The superficial veins ascend to the surface of the cerebrum and cerebellum. They then run over the surface to enter the venous sinuses in the margins of the dura. The deep veins, which arise largely in the basal ganglia and thalamus, drain into a set of deep veins that are periventricular in location. The deep veins also eventually drain into the dural venous sinuses (Fig. 5-8).

There are a set of superficial and deep veins that drain the anterior circulation (Fig. 5-41) and another set of superficial and deep veins that drain the posterior circulation (Fig. 5-42). In both cases the ultimate direction of the venous flow is largely the same, toward the confluence of the sinuses and then through the transverse and sigmoid sinuses to the internal jugular vein.

The superficial cerebral veins include the superior cerebral veins, which carry blood from the convexity of the hemispheres to the superior sagittal sinus; the middle cerebral veins, which drain the cerebral hemispheres around the insula into the sinuses of the base of the skull; and the inferior cerebral veins, draining the orbital and inferior temporal and occipital cortex into the sphenoparietal, cavernous, petrosal, and transverse sinuses of the base of the skull. The great anastomotic vein of Trolard connects the middle cerebral

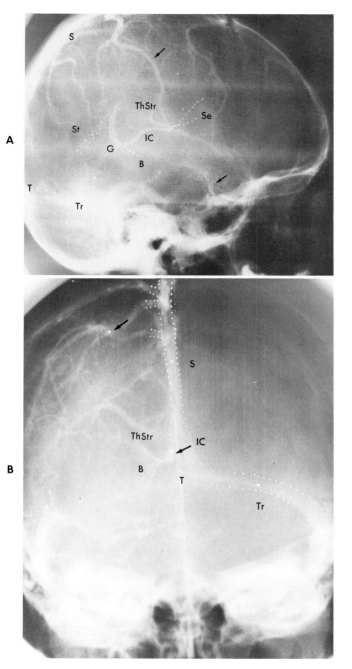

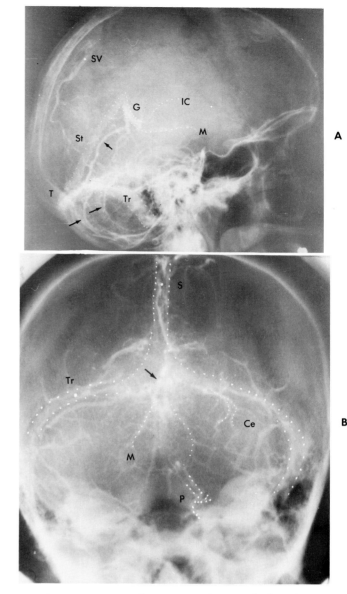

Fig. 5-41. A, Venous drainage of the carotid circulation. Right carotid angiogram, lateral projection, venous phase. Superior veins *(upper arrow)* and inferior veins *(lower arrow)* of the superficial venous system are seen draining into the superior sagittal dural sinus *(S)* and the sphenoparietal dural sinus respectively. The septal vein *(Se)*, the thalamostriate vein *(ThStr)*, the internal cerebral vein *(IC)*, the basilar vein of Rosenthal *(B)*, and the great vein of Galen *(G)* of the deep venous system are dotted. The vein of Galen drains into the straight sinus *(St)*, which drains into the torcular *(T)*, which drains into the transverse *(Tr)* dural sinuses. B, Venous drainage of the carotid circulation. Right carotid angiogram, anterior-posterior half-axial (Towne) projection, venous phase. Superior veins *(upper arrow)* are seen draining into the superior sagittal dural sinus *(S)*. The right thalamostriate *(ThStr)* and the basilar vein of Rosenthal *(B)* of the deep venous system are seen draining into the right internal cerebral vein *(IC)*. (Courtesy Dr. Lawrence H. Zingesser.)

Fig. 5-42. A, Venous drainage of the vertebral-basilar circulation. Vertebral angiogram, lateral projection, venous phase. Superior superficial veins *(SV)* are seen in the parieto-occipital area. The portions of the deep venous system that are filled are the internal cerebral vein *(IC)*, the posterior mesencephalic vein *(M)*, and the vein of Galen *(G)* draining into the straight sinus *(St)*, the torcular *(T)*, and the transverse *(Tr)* dural sinus. The *upper arrow* indicates a superior cerebellar vein draining into the vein of Galen. The *lower arrows* indicate inferior cerebellar veins draining into the transverse dural sinus. (Same patient as shown in Fig. 5-35.) B, Venous drainage of the vertebral-basilar circulation. Vertebral angiogram, anterior-posterior half-axial (Towne) projection, venous phase. A few superior superficial veins (unmarked) are seen draining into the parieto-occipital portion of the superior sagittal dural sinus *(S)*. The internal cerebral veins and vein of Galen are seen end-on *(arrow)*, superimposed on the torcular. Cerebellar hemispheric veins *(Ce)* are seen draining into the transverse dural sinus *(Tr)*. The posterior mesencephalic vein *(M)* is seen draining into the vein of Galen. The petrosal complex of veins *(P)* is draining into the superior petrosal dural sinus. (Courtesy Dr. Lawrence H. Zingesser.)

veins with the superior sagittal sinus; it is one of the veins draining the motor cortex. The lesser anastomotic vein of Labbé connects the middle cerebral veins with the transverse sinus. It rather inconstantly marks the posterior limit of the anterior, surgically resectable portion of the temporal lobe.

The deep cerebral veins include the paired internal cerebral veins, the great vein of Galen, and the basal veins of Rosenthal. The internal cerebral veins lie in the roof of the third ventricle and merge with the basal veins to enter the great vein of Galen (Figs. 5-8 and 5-32). The vein of Galen enters the straight sinus. The basal veins of Rosenthal originate in the anterior perforated space. They curve around the cerebral peduncles and join the internal cerebral veins over the pineal gland. Tributaries enter the basal veins, draining parts of the diencephalon and upper brainstem.

The cerebellar veins and some of the veins of the brainstem connect with the dural sinuses of the base of the skull.

The dural sinuses were discussed with the meninges. They include the superior sagittal, inferior sagittal, straight, occipital, sphenoparietal, cavernous, superior petrosal, inferior petrosal, and transverse sinuses (Fig. 5-8).

Collateral venous drainage occurs by way of veins that are termed emissary veins, which connect the venous sinuses to veins outside the skull. The mastoid and parietal emissary veins are large emissary veins that pass from the diploic space of the skull to the scalp (Fig. 5-9).

Other channels of collateral drainage are the connections between the cavernous sinus and the veins of the orbit, the nose, and the pterygoid plexus of veins, and between the veins of the posterior fossa and the vertebral plexus of veins.

The vascular supply to the brain is summarized in the following outline, which gives the origins of the major branches of the vessels.

I. Arterial supply
  A. Aortic arch
    1. Right
      a. Innominate (brachiocephalic)
        (1) Right common carotid
        (2) Right subclavian
          (a) Vertebral
          (b) Thyrocervical
          (c) Internal mammary
          (d) Costocervical
          (e) Axillary
            i) Brachial
    2. Left
      a. Left common carotid
      b. Left subclavian
        (1) Vertebral
        (2) Thyrocervical
        (3) Internal mammary
        (4) Costocervical
        (5) Axillary
          (a) Brachial
  B. Common carotid artery
    1. Internal carotid
    2. External carotid
      a. Superior thyroid
      b. Lingual
      c. Facial (external maxillary)
      d. Occipital
      e. Posterior auricular
      f. Superficial temporal
      g. Maxillary (internal maxillary)
        (1) Middle meningeal
  C. Arteries of anterior circulation
    1. Internal carotid artery
      a. Ophthalmic
      b. Posterior communicating
      c. Anterior choroidal
      d. Anterior cerebral
      e. Middle cerebral
    2. Anterior cerebral artery
      a. Penetrating branches: anterior perforating branches; Heubner's artery (not constant) is largest branch
      b. Cortical branches
        (1) Anterior communicating
        (2) Frontopolar
        (3) Callosomarginal
        (4) Pericallosal
    3. Middle cerebral artery
      a. Penetrating branches: perforating branches or medial and lateral striate arteries
      b. Cortical branches
        (1) Frontal
        (2) Anterior temporal
        (3) Parietal
        (4) Angular
        (5) Posterior temporal
  D. Arteries of posterior circulation
    1. Vertebral artery
      a. Posterior spinal
      b. Anterior spinal
      c. Posterior inferior cerebellar
      d. Basilar
    2. Basilar artery
      a. Paramedian
      b. Lateral (circumferential)
      c. Anterior inferior cerebellar
      d. Superior cerebellar
      e. Posterior cerebral artery
    3. Posterior cerebral artery
      a. Penetrating branches
        (1) Medial choroidal
        (2) Lateral choroidal
        (3) Posterior pericallosal
      b. Cortical branches
        (1) Anterior temporal
        (2) Posterior temporal
        (3) Calcarine
        (4) Parieto-occipital

II. Venous drainage
  A. Veins of anterior circulation
    1. Superficial (external) cerebral veins
      a. Superior cerebral to superior sagittal sinus
      b. Middle cerebral to sphenoparietal and cavernous sinuses, and to Trolard's vein to superior sagittal sinus and Labbé's vein to transverse sinus
      c. Inferior cerebral veins to basilar vein of Rosenthal and sinuses of base of skull
    2. Deep (internal) cerebral veins
      a. Septal to internal cerebral vein to vein of Galen
      b. Thalamostriate to internal cerebral vein to vein of Galen
      c. Basilar vein of Rosenthal to vein of Galen
      d. Vein of Galen to straight sinus
  B. Veins of posterior circulation
    1. Occipital, choroidal, and superior cerebellar veins to vein of Galen
    2. Lateral, inferior, and posterior cerebellar veins to transverse sinus
  C. Dural venous sinuses
    1. Along calvarium
      a. Superior sagittal to torcular (confluence of the sinuses)
      b. Inferior sagittal to straight
      c. Torcular to transverse to sigmoid to internal jugular vein
    2. Along base of skull
      a. Sphenoparietal to cavernous to superior and inferior petrosal to transverse

SURGICAL EXPOSURE OF THE BRAIN

The convexities of the cerebral cortex are easily accessible to the surgeon; however, structures at the base of the brain are less accessible. The carotid arteries, the optic nerves, and the brainstem, with nerves III through XII, bind the base of the brain to the base of the skull. These structures can be approached by subfrontal, subtemporal, and suboccipital routes. Surgical openings in the skull are either trephinations (burr holes, circular drill openings), craniotomies (removal of a flap of calvarium, frequently crossing suture lines, which is usually replaced at the end of the procedure), or craniectomies (piecemeal removal of bone, which is not replaced). In a typical frontotemporal craniotomy, a coronal incision is made in the scalp, and the scalp is reflected forward. The periosteum is incised along the midline of the frontal bone up to about the coronal suture. The periosteum and the temporal muscle are incised along the coronal suture to the pterion and along the superciliary arch above the orbit to the frontal process of the zygomatic bone. Burr holes are then made with a perforator drill and a burr drill in the skull at the glabella, the bregma, the pterion, and the frontal process of the zygoma. A twisted wire (Gigli's saw) is passed under the skull, above the dura, and between two burr holes, and the bone is sawed through from the inside to the outside. The flap of bone, which is attached to the temporal muscle, is then reflected laterally, exposing the dura. The middle meningeal artery is seen running in the dura at the pterion. The dura is then incised in a horseshoe fashion so that the flap of dura has its base along the sagittal venous sinus, exposing the junction of the veins entering the sinus from the surface of the brain and exposing the interhemispheric fissure. The lateral (sylvian) fissure lies at the lateral margin of the dural opening. When the frontal lobe is gently retracted slightly from the floor of the anterior fossa, the olfactory tract is visible. The arachnoid over the optic nerves is opened and cerebrospinal fluid is drained from the subarachnoid spaces and the ventricles, making the brain slightly more movable; with slight further retraction the carotid artery, the oculomotor nerve, the pituitary stalk, and the optic chiasm are visible. This approach is used for surgery of the pituitary gland and for most aneurysms of the circle of Willis.

A subtemporal approach involves making a frontoparietotemporal craniotomy hinged on the temporalis muscle or making a vertical incision of the temporalis muscle and a smaller craniectomy. At the end of the procedure, the muscle is sutured over the craniectomy defect in the skull, providing protection for the underlying dura. When the dura is opened, the anterior margin of the temporal lobe is seen. When the temporal lobe is elevated away from the floor of the middle fossa, the dura covering the trigeminal nerve and the middle meningeal artery in the foramen spinosum are seen. On further elevation of the temporal lobe, the rim of the tentorium is seen. The trochlear (IV) nerve and the cerebral peduncle can be seen passing through the tentorial notch, as well as the posterior cerebral artery arising from the basilar artery. Surgery of the roots of nerves V and VIII and of aneurysms at the junction of the basilar artery and the circle of Willis can be performed through this approach.

In the suboccipital approach, a craniectomy of the suboccipital bone below the level of the inion is carried out. When the dura is opened, the cisterna magna, and beneath it the posterior aspect of the cerebellar hemispheres, can be seen. If the arachnoid is opened and the cerebellar tonsils are lifted, the obex of the medulla, and above it the foramen of Magendie leading to the fourth ventricle, are seen. If the cerebellar hemispheres are elevated and retracted medially on either side, the vertebral arteries entering through the foramen magnum can be seen, with nerves IX through XI going into the jugular foramen. Superiorly the cerebellopontine angle and nerves VII and VIII can be seen in the internal acoustic meatus, and most superiorly nerve V and the tentorial notch can be seen. Surgery of aneurysms of the posterior inferior cerebellar artery, of the cerebellum, and of cranial nerves V and VII to XI can be performed through this approach. At the end of the operation the skull defect produced by the craniectomy is covered by suturing together the thick suboccipital muscles that attach to the nuchal lines.

CELLULAR ENVIRONMENT OF THE BRAIN
Intracranial compartments

To understand the mechanisms that control the cellular environment of the brain, it is important to consider the relative volumes of the functional compartments within the cranial cavity. The total volume of the intracranial compartment is about 1,400 ml in normal individuals. The extracellular compartment consists of the blood, the cerebrospinal fluid (CSF), and the extracellular fluid (ECF). The intracellular compartment consists mostly of the neurons and glia. Exact measurement of the volumes of these compartments has proved to be quite difficult, but approximate figures can be given. The intracranial blood volume is about 10% of the average brain weight of 1,350 gm, or about 100 to 150 ml. The CSF volume amounts to another 100 to 150 ml. The volume of ECF cannot be stated with certainty, for the controversy about the size of the extracellular space of the brain is not completely resolved. However, the most recent evidence indicates that the volume of the extracellular space of the brain is somewhat smaller than that of other organs and is about 15% of the total volume of the tissue. This indicates an extracellular volume of about 200 ml. The total volume of the extracellular compartment is therefore about 400 to 500 ml. The intracellular compartment is occupied by neurons and glia in about equal volumes; however, the glia, which are smaller than neurons, are more numerous. The ratio of glial cells to neurons increases in brains of increasing size. In rat cortex there are more neurons than glia, whereas in the human cortex it has been estimated that there are at least twice as many glia as neurons. Therefore, the relative volumes of neurons and glia differ in various species as well as in different parts of the brain in the same species.

Regulation of the extracellular fluid of the brain

In a famous aphorism the French physiologist Claude Bernard declared that the maintenance of an internal environment of fixed composition was the necessary condition for a freely mobile life. Probably in no other organ is the regulation of the extracellular environment as important as in the brain, because

neuronal functioning depends on the ratio of the concentration of ions across the cell membrane. The chemical composition and pressure of the extracellular fluid of the brain appears to be regulated and buffered against changes in its composition by a series of mechanisms: (1) by the buffering capabilities of the blood; (2) by regulatory mechanisms at the blood-brain interface; (3) by glial and neuronal uptake of ions; and (4) by stimulation of central chemoreceptors that evoke renal or respiratory responses that regulate the blood and ultimately the environment of the brain.

The buffering and excretory mechanisms of the blood are the first line of defense of the brain's extracellular fluid against changes to which the organism is subjected. The second line of defense appears to be the endothelial cell lining of the cerebral capillaries. The endothelial cells of cerebral capillaries are joined by tight junctions through which many classes of small molecules cannot pass. In this respect the capillary endothelium of the brain differs from that of other organs. The tight endothelial junctions are at least one structural correlate of the so-called blood-brain barrier. The barrier is an operational definition and indicates that many substances penetrate the brain slowly or not at all after injection into the bloodstream. Some substances are completely excluded, particularly large protein molecules and highly charged molecules. Other molecules, particularly those with a high lipid solubility such as anesthetics (ether, cyclopropane), pass easily from the blood to the brain. The common cations and anions (Na^+, K^+, Cl^-) are maintained at different concentrations in the CSF and in the blood. Some of these ions and other substances, such as urea, pass more slowly than others from the blood to the brain.

In addition, some substances enter the brain water more rapidly than they enter the CSF. These substances then tend to pass from the brain to the CSF, with the CSF acting as a sink.

It is not known if the endothelial cell is the barrier to all of these substances. The perivascular glia limitans, the sheets of astrocytic processes that ensheath the basement membranes of brain capillaries, may contribute to barrier functions. However, the astroglial ensheathment of brain capillaries is not complete, with about 15% of many capillaries being in contact with oligodendroglia or neuronal processes. Mechanisms that transport substances out of the CSF, although poorly understood and localized anatomically, must also contribute to a functional barrier.

The relative impermeability of cerebral capillaries breaks down in areas of infarction, tumor growth, or infection. The breakdown of the barrier in chronic tuberculous meningitis results in a CSF with a chemical composition that resembles a dialysate of blood plasma more closely than normal CSF resembles plasma (Table 5-3). This appears to be the basis of the decreased Cl⁻ concentration of the CSF in tuberculous meningitis. Another effect of bacterial meningitis is that the barrier to penetration of many antibiotics into the brain, such as the penicillins, is lowered. This is advantageous in the treatment of meningitis. The local increase in permeability in and around tumors or abscesses can be made use of diagnostically. Intravenously administered radioactive compounds, labeled with mercury 203 or technetium 99m, will enter areas of increased permeability, and the abnormal areas can then be localized by scintillation scanning of the brain.

A third ECF regulatory mechanism for which evidence has recently been found is the apparent ability of glial cells, probably the astrocytes, to take up K^+ and perhaps other ions. This appears to be a mechanism for buffering against changes in ionic concentration around neurons. These changes are produced by high levels of neuronal activity that can release large amounts of K^+ and CO_2 into the ECF.

The fourth class of regulatory mechanisms is the stimulation of central chemoreceptors and possibly osmoreceptors by substances in the blood. The anatomical structure and physiological activity of these central receptors are not known in any detail. The hypothalamic-pituitary axis and the pontomedullary respiratory centers are the main sites of these activities. The hypothalamic-pituitary axis responds to increase in blood osmolality with secretion of the antidiuretic hormone that promotes water retention by the kidney. Pontomedullary neurons respond to changes of blood pH. Acidosis evokes increased depth and frequency of inspiration.

It is not known if the blood-brain barrier is particularly permeable to the relevant blood substances at the sites of these actions. However, it is known that in certain areas, in particular the median eminence of the hypothalamus and the area postrema of the medulla, the usual barrier does not exist. The area postrema is a chemoreceptor trigger zone for vomiting, and substances, such as apomorphine, that evoke emesis by central action act on neurons at this point.

In addition to being bathed in fluid of constant chemical composition, neurons are maintained in an environment that is under a certain degree of pressure. In normal adults this varies from about 120 to 180 mm of water when the individual is in a recumbent position. This is equivalent to an average pressure of 12 mm Hg, or one tenth of the systolic blood pressure. The intracranial CSF pressure is lower when the individual is erect.

Finally, the cerebral blood flow, which amounts to 15% to 20% of the cardiac output, is regulated to maintain a constant flow despite variations in systemic (aortic) blood pressure.

The interrelationships of the ECF and the CSF and the relationships of the production and absorption of these fluids to cerebral blood flow and to the intracranial pressure are complex and still poorly understood. However, certain relationships have been partially clarified, as discussed on the following pages.

CEREBROSPINAL FLUID
Composition

The ventricular system and subarachnoid spaces are filled with CSF. The fluid is normally colorless and crystal clear, and when a test tube of CSF is held up to the light its appearance is like that of water. Each lateral ventricle contains about 7 ml of fluid, the entire ventricular system about 35 ml of fluid, and the subarachnoid spaces including the spinal space about 100 to 125 ml. The CSF differs from the blood in that it contains virtually no cells (0 to 5 white blood cells, usually lymphocytes, per mm^3 of CSF) or protein (15 mg/100 ml in the ventricular fluid and 45 mg/100 ml in the spinal subarachnoid fluid). Increased numbers of white cells or red cells in disease states will give the CSF a cloudy appearance, and protein concentrations greater than 200 mg/100 ml give the CSF a xanthochromic (yellowish orange) color. Breakdown of hemoglobin pigment from red cells following subarachnoid hemorrhage can also produce xanthochromia. The osmotic pressure of the blood varies with the state of hydration of the individual, but in general the lumbar CSF appears to be very nearly isotonic with the blood plasma, which has an average osmolality of 300 mOsm/kg of water. To maintain near isotonicity of the CSF and blood, the CSF in the absence of protein would have to have more of the major cations and anions of the body fluids than blood has. In fact, CSF freshly secreted from the choroid plexus has a higher concentration of Na^+ and Cl^- than blood plasma. The composition of the CSF is modified slightly during its circulation (see below).

Some of the major constituents of the CSF and the blood are listed in Table 5-3. This table gives average ranges of constituents in lumbar CSF and in venous blood in general, but it does not give the exact ratios of chemical distribution between newly secreted CSF and blood entering the brain. These ratios can vary with the blood concentration of the chemical constituents.

Table 5-3. Major constituents of the CSF and the blood

	Lumbar CSF	Blood
Na mEq per liter	148†, ‖	136-145‡
K mEq per liter	2.88†	3.5-5.0‡
Cl mEq per liter	120-130‡	100-106‡
Glucose* (fasting) mg/100 ml	50-75‡, ‖	70-100‡, ‖
Protein mg per 100 ml	15-45‡	6,000-8,000‡
Albumin	80%	50%-60%
Gamma globulin	6%-10%	13%-23%
Cells per mm³		
White	0-5‡	4,800-10,800‡
Red	0‡	4.2-5.9 million‡
pH	7.3§	7.41§
HCO₃ mEq per liter	22.9§	23.4§

*Glucose is generally 20 mg/100 ml less in CSF than is blood.
†Bradbury, M. W. B., and others: Clin. Sci. **25**:97-105, 1963.
‡Blood chemical analysis, MGH case records (normal values), N. Engl. J. Med. **283**:1276-1285, 1970.
§Posner, J. B., and others: Arch. Neurol. **12**:479-496, 1965.
‖CSF: blood Na ratio varies with blood concentration.

The fact that the composition of the CSF does not resemble that of an ultrafiltrate of blood indicates that it is not formed by simple diffusion across membranes that are selectively permeable to cations and anions and impermeable to protein molecules. The composition of CSF suggests that active secretion and possibly absorption of ions is involved in its production.

Formation

The CSF is formed at least in part by the choroid plexuses. They can be partially lifted from the ventricles, and CSF can be seen to form on and drip from their surfaces. However, after choroid plexectomy CSF production is still about 40% of normal. It is therefore thought that CSF can also be formed at sites other than the choroid plexus, perhaps by vessels in the subarachnoid space.

Knowledge of CSF formation and absorption was greatly advanced by the experimental technique of ventriculocisternal perfusion, in which solutions of known concentrations are perfused into one lateral ventricle and collected in the cisterna magna. Changes in the fluid can be analyzed to see what substances have been added to or taken from the fluid by the choroid plexus and ventricular lining. This technique is methodologically similar to that used to study renal glomerular filtration. These studies have shown that the CSF is formed at a rate of 0.3 to 0.4 ml/min, so that the total volume of the CSF is probably replaced every 6 hours. An important point is that the formation of CSF is relatively independent of the pressure within the ventricles and subarachnoid space, although the rate of formation does decrease at very high back pressures. The rate of formation is also probably relatively independent of the systemic blood pressure. In contrast, the absorption of CSF is directly related to the CSF pressure, being equal to the rate of formation at normal pressures and increasing almost tenfold at 600 mm CSF.

There are probably a number of different processes involved in the formation of the CSF, with different mechanisms involved in the movement of water, ions, and large molecules. It is probable that water enters to some extent by filtration, inasmuch as the pressure within the choroid plexus capillaries is higher than that of the CSF. Water might also move in relationship to osmotic gradients determined by ion movements. Ions probably enter in part by diffusion along concentration gradients and also are probably actively transported. Larger molecules may enter by diffusion or by mediated transport dependent on carrier systems.

The secretory or active transport processes of the choroid plexus epithelial cells are not well understood. Vesicles are found in the cytoplasm of these cells, and it has been suggested that these vesicles are involved in pinocytosis, the transport of substance in vesicle form through the epithelial cells to the CSF.

The choroid epithelium contains high concentrations of carbonic anhydrase, the enzyme that catalyzes the reactions $CO_2 + H_2O = H_2CO_3$. On the basis of what is known of this system in renal tubular cells it is probable that this system is involved in movements of H^+, HCO_3^-, Na^+, Cl^-, and H_2O. Inhibition of carbonic anhydrase by intravenous administration of acetazolamide (Diamox) reduces CSF formation.

The choroid epithelium is also capable of actively concentrating chemicals in the iodide series in the atomic table. The choroid plexus therefore takes up the sodium pertechnetate technetium 99m (^{99m}Tc) administered intravenously for brain scanning. Technetium is an isotope derived from the decay of molybdenum 99. Technetium has a half-life of 6 hours and emits 140 kev gamma radiation. Choroid plexus uptake can be blocked by the prior administration of perchlorate (ClO_4^-) ions. Iodine (Lugol's solution) will also block the uptake, but less effectively.

The composition of the CSF is modified after secretion by the choroid plexus during its circulation through the ventricular system. CSF secreted by the choroid plexus is higher in K^+ than the CSF in the cisterna magna, and if ventriculocisternal perfusion is carried out with solutions higher or lower than the K^+ concentration normally found in the ventricles, the efflux fluid is closer in concentration to the correct value than the perfusion fluid is. This means that the brain tissue surrounding the ventricles has a modifying effect on the ionic content of the CSF.

Circulation

The CSF has a slow but definite circulation, which was first demonstrated by Blackfan and Dandy. They injected dyes into the lateral ventricles and observed their passage through the ventricular system and out the foramina of the fourth ventricle into the subarachnoid space. They also demonstrated that if the ventricular system were occluded, for instance at the aqueduct, there would be a progressive dilatation of the proximal ventricular system, suggesting that fluid normally is largely absorbed distally to the ventricular system itself. A large portion of the CSF formed in the ventricular system enters the subarachnoid space, then passes forward through the basilar cisterns of the brain and up over the cerebral convexities to be absorbed into the blood at the site of the pacchionian granulations, fingers of arachnoid that invaginate lateral expansions of the superior sagittal dural venous sinus (Fig. 5-9).

In recent years the proof of the slow circulation of the CSF has been well demonstrated by the technique of radionuclide encephalography, which involves injection of radioactive isotopes into the lateral ventricles of the brain or into the spinal subarachnoid space (Figs. 5-28 and 5-29). The brain is then scanned by a scintillation counter, and successive scannings over 24 hours reveal the slow passage of the radioactive material through the ventricular system, into the basilar cisterns, and out over the hemispheres of the brain. That all of the absorption of the CSF is not through the arachnoid villi is strongly suggested by the fact that the pacchionian granulations are not developed at birth and do not become well developed until several years of age. In addition, ventriculocisternal perfusion studies show that fluid can be absorbed in the ventricular system and in the subarachnoid space.

Absorption

As in the case of the formation of the CSF, there are probably a number of active and passive mechanisms for the absorption of water, electrolytes, and large molecules. The pressure-dependence of CSF absorption has been mentioned above. It is probable that a considerable amount of CSF is removed by bulk flow across the membranes of the arachnoid villi. It is thought that the membranes have pores in them that are large enough to pass small protein molecules but are smaller in size than the diameter of a red blood cell (7 μm). Obstruction of the villi by red blood cells can occur following a subarachnoid hemorrhage and lead to impaired CSF absorption.

Hydrocephalus

Mechanical obstruction of the ventricular outflow either within the ventricular system or in the basilar cisterns leads to a raised CSF pressure and to progressive dilatation of the ventricular system. If the obstruction is acute, the dilatation of the ventricular system, which is termed hydrocephalus, can occur within 12 hours. This produces stretching of the ventricular ependyma, and breaks occur at the tight junctions between ependymal cells. If the hydrocephalus develops more slowly because of partial obstruction of the ventricular outflow, the ventricles grow in size largely at the expense of the white matter of the cortex, which becomes compressed. Dandy distinguished between noncommunicating and communicating hydrocephalus. Noncommunicating hydrocephalus is an operational definition. It is the condition in which dye that is placed in the lateral ventricle does not appear in the lumbar subarachnoid space. This clearly would be caused by an obstruction either in the ventricular system or in the fourth ventricular outflow. In communicating hydrocephalus, the dye does appear. In this case blockage of the absorption of CSF is either in the basilar cisterns or at the pacchionian granulations, or blockage might represent some disparity between CSF production and formation. Therefore, the terms communicating and noncommunicating hydrocephalus really do not distinguish different physiological mechanisms and should probably be replaced with the terms obstructive hydrocephalus, with the site of the obstruction defined as clearly as possible in each clinical situation, and hydrocephalus caused by unknown mechanisms. Hydrocephalus that develops in the adult is generally caused by some mechanical obstruction in the circulation of CSF, either by tumor or by subarachnoid hemorrhage and subsequent scarring of the basilar CSF pathways, or by gliosis and obstruction of the aqueduct. Hydrocephalus in infants is more common that in adults. In some cases the same mechanisms of mechanical obstruction of fluid outflow are present. However, in the majority of cases no definite cause can be found. Infants with so-called communicating hydrocephalus, in which there is no obstruction of fluid flow from the lateral ventricles to the lumbar subarachnoid space, comprise the largest group of neonatal hydrocephalics. The dynamics of CSF production and absorption by means of ventriculocisternal perfusion have not been extensively studied in this group of children. The available data suggest defective CSF absorption mechanisms.

The relationship of the CSF pressure to ventricular dilatation is not clear in all cases of hydrocephalus. A condition has been described in elderly patients with dementia in which there is normal CSF pressure and marked enlargement of the ventricles. There is no obvious degenerative disease of brain tissue in these patients with normal-pressure hydrocephalus, and the mechanism of ventricular enlargement has not been definitely determined.

CEREBRAL BLOOD FLOW
Methods of measurement

The brain has an extremely high blood flow, receiving 15% to 20% of the cardiac output, or about 750 ml of blood per minute. The total flow to the brain through the ascending arteries can be measured with electromagnetic flowmeter probes placed around the arteries. However, major clinical interest centers on measurement of blood flow in particular regions of the brain, employing nontraumatic techniques that can be repeated at frequent intervals. Measurement of cerebral blood flow (CBF) based on the Fick principle is the most clinically useful method yet devised to accomplish this. Substances that diffuse freely from the blood into brain tissue but are not metabolized by the tissue, such as N_2O or xenon 133, are used as indicators or tracers in the CBF measurements based on this principle. The Fick principles states that the amount of a substance *(Q)* that passes from the blood into a tissue in a unit of time is proportional to the difference in the concentration of the substance in the arterial blood *(QA)* and in the venous blood *(QV)* and to the rate of blood flow *(F)*. This can be expressed as

$$Q = F(QA - QV)$$

or

$$F = \frac{Q}{QA - QV}$$

If *Q* is introduced at a particular time *(T)*, *Q* will vary over time until the substance is saturated in the tissue at a concentration that is proportional to its concentration in the blood. The ratio of brain to blood concentration is called the blood-brain partition coefficient of the substance. The expression can be rearranged and integrated over time so that flow can be calculated from the A-V concentration differences of the tracer substance that is sampled by means of catheters placed in the carotid artery and in the jugular vein. The partition coefficient for the substance, which is a constant, and the times at which the samples are drawn must also be known. Total flow through the brain can be measured in this manner.

The principle can also be applied to a situation in which a substance such as ^{133}Xe is introduced into the brain by a single rapid injection into the carotid artery. After the diffusion of the substance into the brain tissue, the rate of removal of the substance, which is proportional to blood flow, can be followed by recording the decay of radioactivity with detectors placed over the scalp. Using this technique, one can calculate flow rates from the decay curves for individual cortical regions.

Measurements of total flow have shown correlations with the functional state of the brain. Flow may be reduced by as much as one half in anesthetized patients and may be reduced in elderly and in demented individuals. Through the use of these methods and autoradiographic techniques, regional flow studies have shown quite high flows of 1 to 2 ml/g of tissue per minute in the gray matter of the cortex and in some subcortical areas, such as the colliculi of the midbrain. Flow values in white matter are one fifth to one third the values in gray matter.

Autoregulation of cerebral blood flow and the effects of CO_2 and O_2

One of the most important functional properties of the cerebral circulation is its ability to maintain a constant flow despite wide changes of systemic blood pressure. When systemic blood pressure is slowly changed, as by hemorrhage, the CBF remains fairly constant until a blood pressure of about 60 mm Hg is reached. Then the flow decreases rather rapidly as the blood pressure is decreased further (Fig. 5-43). The mechanism by which this occurs is not clear, although it is probable that some phe-

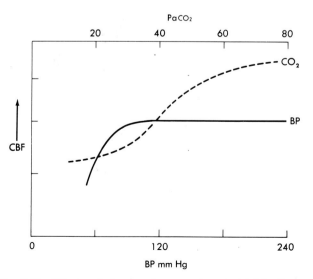

Fig. 5-43. Effects of changes in systemic arterial blood pressure and of changes of arterial P_{CO_2} on cerebral blood flow.

nomenon akin to the Bayliss effect occurs in cerebral blood vessels. The Bayliss effect, in which vessels respond to an increase in pressure by contracting and to a decrease in pressure by relaxing, appears to be an intrinsic property of the vessel wall. Changes in the level of systemic blood pressure itself are opposed by the action of the carotid sinus baroceptor reflexes, which further tends to stabilize the CBF.

The other important regulator of the CBF is the concentration of CO_2 in the blood and brain tissue. Increasing the arterial Pco_2 above the normal level of 40 mm Hg produces dilatation of cerebral vessels and an increased CBF. The response follows a skewed sigmoid curve, with a greater response at higher than at lower than normal Pco_2 levels. The change in flow is about 2.5% for each change of 1 mm Hg of Pco_2, with the greatest response around the normal level of Pco_2. The cellular mechanism of action of CO_2 on the cerebral vessels is not known. CO_2 may relax the smooth muscle of the arterial walls. The importance of the diameter of the cerebral vessels in controlling CBF can be appreciated by considering the equation describing flow in tubes:

$$F = \frac{(\text{Inflow pressure} - \text{Outflow pressure}) \; \text{Radius}^4}{\text{Length} \times \text{Viscosity of fluid}}$$

It can be seen that small changes in the radius of the vessels can have a very large effect on flow.

Local increases of CO_2 within the brain tissue, produced by neuronal metabolic activity, can produce increased blood flow. Increases in local flow can be measured after a single evoked response in the cortex. Following a seizure, local acidosis, vascular dilatation, and increased blood flow can occur in the cortex. Detailed descriptions of the relationships between changes in cellular metabolism, CBF, and electrical activity in individual brain regions are only now being obtained. In general, an independent change in any of these parameters of tissue function will evoke changes in the other parameters.

Increasing the Po_2 above the normal levels of 90 to 95 mm Hg generally reduces the CBF, and lowering it raises the CBF. Consciousness is lost at Po_2 levels below 20 mm Hg. Markedly lowering the Po_2 produces changes in Pco_2 and evokes carotid and aortic O_2 chemoreceptor vasopressor reflexes, so it has been difficult to determine how much of the effect of O_2 is directly on the cerebral vessels. The level of blood glucose also affects cerebral metabolism, and changes in consciousness are generally noted as the blood glucose level falls to about 50 mg/100 ml, or to below one half of its normal level.

Cerebral arteries, particularly those of the pia-arachnoid, the circle of Willis, and cerebral arterioles,

have plexuses of noradrenalin containing nerve fibers in their walls. The fine structural relationship of the terminations of these axons to the smooth muscle fibers of the vessels has not yet been well defined. Some of these fibers arise in the superior cervical ganglion and enter the skull as a plexus around the carotid arteries. It is not definitely known if parasympathetic fibers innervate intracranial vessels. The functional significance of the sympathetic innervation is unclear. Some studies have shown a small to moderate increase of CBF with sympathetic block or cutting of the sympathetic trunks, and other studies have shown no effect.

The relationships between the factors that control the CBF are particularly important in patients with head injuries, intracranial tumor, and during and after intracranial surgery. The autoregulation of the CBF in response to changing systemic blood pressure is impaired at high CO_2 tensions. In addition, autoregulation is impaired following local brain injury caused by direct mechanical insult or following an infarction. This type of situation can occur, for example, in a patient who incurs head and chest injury in an automobile accident and is hypovolemic and hypoventilating. One effect of the loss of autoregulation can be to produce a relative hyperemia in damaged brain tissue. In this situation the surface veins draining the injured area may be bright red in color (red cerebral veins) rather than blue, because of the shunting of arterial blood through the dilated vessels of the injured area.

Cerebral ischemia

The functions of the cerebral cortex and subcortical areas that have high blood flows, such as the thalamus and colliculi, are highly sensitive to ischemia, anoxia, and hypoglycemia. The human cortex will not generally recover normal function if subjected to more than 3 to 5 minutes of complete ischemia. Subcortical fiber tracts and peripheral nerve fibers will continue to function for up to perhaps 10 minutes of total ischemia, and will recover after longer periods of ischemia if blood flow is restored. Total occlusion of flow to the brain generally occurs as a result of cardiac arrest. Following occlusion of one carotid or one vertebral artery, there generally is enough collateral circulation to the brain in children and in young adults, who generally do not have atheromatous plaques in the carotid arteries or in the vessels of the circle of Willis, to prevent cerebral ischemia. However, perhaps half of elderly individuals cannot tolerate an abrupt occlusion of one of the major arteries to the brain and will exhibit neurological dysfunction. The functional effects of occlusion of the major venous drainage of the brain are rather similar to those of arterial occlusion, although the stasis produced by venous occlusion may lead to abrupt rises in intracranial pressure and hemorrhage from the capillaries of the brain. Usually one transverse venous sinus or one jugular vein can be occluded safely. However, the superior sagittal venous sinus usually cannot be occluded without compromising cortical function, although some young persons can tolerate this. Some of the specific neurological deficits produced by occlusion of intracranial arteries, the so-called stroke syndromes, are described in Chapter 12.

An important factor in the vulnerability of the brain to ischemia is the differential sensitivity of different portions of the neuron. The synaptic regions of the neuron are more sensitive than the soma. Synaptic transmission fails after about 45 to 90 seconds of cerebral ischemia, and this abolishes the spontaneous waves of the electroencephalogram (EEG) (Fig. 5-44). At this time the membrane potential of cortical neurons and presynaptic terminals is not greatly affected, and normal synaptic transmission will recover if blood flow is restored. However, as ischemia progresses, the dendrites and soma of the neurons depolarize, although subcortical portions of the axon will conduct for about 10 minutes. The inhibitory pathways in the cortex and spinal cord are more

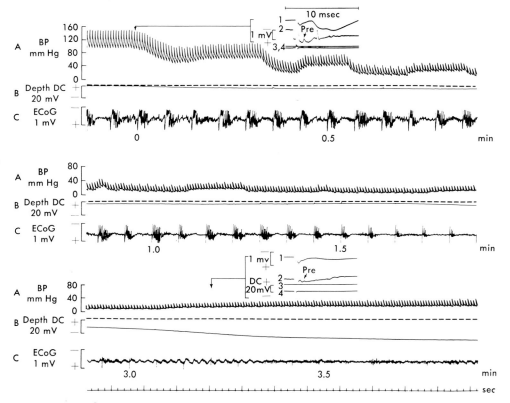

Fig. 5-44. Failure of synaptic transmission and spontaneous and evoked electrocortical potentials in cerebral ischemia produced by arterial hypotention. Recordings of aortic blood pressure on line *A*, transcortical potential between layer 4 of the cortex and underlying axons, recorded with a micropipette in layer 4, on line *B*, and the electrocorticogram from the surface of the sensorimotor cortex on line *C*. Recordings in cat, anesthetized with sodium pentobarbital. Starting at time 0, one third of the total blood volume was withdrawn from the aorta over a 3-minute period, producing severe hypotension. The thalamocortical afferent fibers to the cortex were stimulated every 4 seconds, producing a primary evoked potential and rhythmic after-potentials (spindle bursts). Note the failure of spontaneous activity between the bursts of evoked activity and the failure of electrocortical activity 3 minutes after the start of hypotension. Also note the development of a large negative shift of transcortical potential of about 30 mV caused by the relative depolarization of the somata and dendrites of cortical neurons and of intracortical axon terminals with respect to the subcortical portions of their axons. The inserts show, on a fast oscilloscope sweep, the cortical-evoked potential on line 1, the activity of presynaptic fibers (*Pre*) and a postsynaptic neuronal spike response on line 2, and the transcortical potential as the distance between lines 3 and 4.

sensitive to ischemia than the motoneurons are; and following a period of ischemia, cortical epileptic activity and marked hyperactivity of the spinal motoneurons can occur when flow is restored.

The metabolic demands of neurons for oxygen and glucose are high, and little of these substances is stored within the brain. Some degree of protection against cerebral ischemia can be provided by reducing cerebral metabolism. Hypothermia and some types of anesthetic reduce cerebral metabolism and therefore cerebral blood flow. Hypothermia is the more powerful of these methods, which are generally used together. If the temperature of the body and the brain are reduced to 30°C by surface cooling of the body, the brain can withstand about twice the normal period of ischemia. This is useful during some intrathoracic and intracranial vascular surgical procedures. Spontaneous respiration ceases at body temperatures below about 33°C, and a respirator must be used. The heartbeat slows during cooling, and at about 27°C ventricular fibrillation and cardiac arrest occur. The circulation must be maintained with a pump if profound hypothermia of 15° to 20°C is produced.

INTRACRANIAL PRESSURE
Methods of measurement

The intracranial pressure (ICP) and the pressure within the lumbar subarachnoid space, the cerebral subarachnoid space, and the ventricular system are approximately equal when the patient is lying in a horizontal position. In most persons the pressure is between 120 and 180 mm of CSF, or about 9 to 14 mm Hg. The pressure is the sum of the secretory pressure of the CSF, the tissue turgor pressure of the brain, and the intravascular pressure within brain tissue.

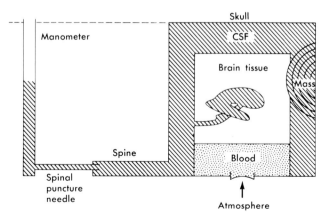

Fig. 5-45. Relationships between brain tissue, intravascular, and cerebrospinal fluid compartments that influence the intracranial and intraspinal pressure.

If the pressure is measured with a water manometer attached to a needle in the lumbar subarachnoid space, with the patient in a sitting position, the column of water in the manometer will rise, not to the level of the top of the cerebral subarachnoid space as might be expected, but only to the level of the cisterna magna (Fig. 5-45). The pressure in the lumbar space is about 550 mm of CSF at this time. A simple explanation for the fact that the CSF runs out into the manometer but does not rise to the level of the CSF in the subarachnoid space over the convexities of the brain is that the CSF does not lie within a closed container, nor in a container that is freely open to the atmosphere, but in a container that is partially vented to the atmosphere by the vasculature, particularly by the venous system returning to the thorax. This venting can be thought of as an elastic membrane placed across an opening in the container formed by the skull.

The effects of this venting to the vascular system can be seen by observation of the CSF column in the manometer, which fluctuates slightly with quiet respiration but can rise to 600 to 800 mm CSF with forced expiration against a closed glottis (Valsalva's maneuver). Direct occlusion of the venous outflow by manual compression of the jugular veins will also produce a sharp rise of CSF pressure. This procedure, referred to as the Queckenstedt maneuver, can be used to test the patency of the subarachnoid space in the spinal cord. The test is of value only in confirming the presence of an almost complete block of the space, such as produced by a large tumor. Myelography is a more accurate method of demonstrating blockage of the spinal subarachnoid space. The arterial pulse also produces a brief pressure wave within the ventricles and cranial cavity.

The effects of venting by the elastic vasculature can also be seen when removing CSF. Removal of a small amount of fluid that has been under pressure in a closed box produces a rapid fall of pressure within the box. In contrast, following a lumbar puncture about 10% of the CSF, or 15 ml, will flow freely from the spinal subarachnoid space when it is tapped. This drainage of fluid normally reduces the pressure roughly by less than one half.

Increased intracranial pressure

The brain can function normally when subjected to transient increases of pressure of up to 1,000 mm of CSF (75 mm Hg). However, if the intracranial pressure remains chronically elevated at 250 mm CSF or higher, headache will generally develop. This is thought to be caused by traction on the dura, which is largely innervated by branches of the trigeminal nerve. Chronically increased pressure in the range of 250 to 500 mm CSF interferes with neural functioning. This disturbance is expressed by impairment of consciousness and by centrally evoked abnormal respiratory and vasomotor responses. Ophthalmoscopic examination of the optic nerve head may reveal edema of the nerve, called papilledema, or a choked disk. There is no simple or linear relationship that can be applied to all individuals to relate the magnitude of the intracranial pressure to the neurophysiological disturbances produced. Torsion of the brain produced by intracranial masses, dilatation of the ventricular system, and cerebral edema—all related to the specific cause of the raised intracranial pressure in individual cases—can each contribute to the disturbances of neurological function.

When increasing intracranial pressure is caused by expansion of a mass, such as tumor or hematoma, the intracranial pressure rises slowly at first because of the elasticity of the venous system, and the increased volume of the mass is compensated for by a decrease in the size of the venous and CSF compartments. Cerebral blood flow tends to remain constant because of increased blood pressure. However, at CSF pressure ranges of about 400 to 500 mm, compensation fails and the pressure rises rapidly as the mass expands. Chronic recording of intracranial pressure in patients with intracranial masses has shown that, in addition to respiratory and cardiac pulsations transmitted to the brain by the vascular system, the intracranial pressure can undergo large increases of pressure of up to 100 mm Hg. During these plateau waves, which last 10 to 15 minutes and may occur several times per hour, the patient's neurological function worsens. The plateau waves are accompanied by an increase in cerebral blood volume that appears to be caused by a compensatory dilatation of cerebral arterioles in an attempt to maintain flow.

Emergency therapeutic measures for the relief of raised intracranial pressure are based on the concept of reducing the volume of the extracellular compartment. The methods most commonly employed are drainage of CSF, which is most safely accomplished in the presence of an intracranial mass lesion by ventricular drainage, and the intravenous administration of hypertonic solutions of mannitol or urea, which reduce brain water by osmotic dehydration. These solutions increase the osmotic pressure of the blood and enter the brain slowly; thus an osmotic gradient is produced that removes water from the brain.

Decreased tissue blood flow is probably the major cause of neural dysfunction when the intracranial pressure is elevated. The effect of increased pressure in itself on neuronal function is not known. If the in-

tracranial pressure reaches arterial systolic pressure, there can be no flow through the intracranial arteries, a condition seen on angiography in some very severe cases of head injury. The initial systemic vasomotor and respiratory responses produced by rising intracranial pressure are a rise of systolic arterial pressure, bradycardia, and bradypnea. The rise in blood pressure is called the Cushing reflex, and it appears to be a compensatory mechanism to maintain the cerebral perfusion pressure. The reflex can be evoked by mechanical deformation of the medullary tegmentum. A rise of blood pressure can also be evoked by increasing the pressure in the subarachnoid space around a segment of thoracic spinal cord isolated from the brain. The initial effect of the increase in pressure is to increase the discharge of spinal cord sympathetic neurons. In the intact nervous system, neurons involved in the control of vasomotor and respiratory function at all levels of the neuraxis appear to be affected by increased intracranial pressure, which probably accounts for some of the variability of the responses seen in patients with increased intracranial pressure. When the mechanisms that can compensate for increasing intracranial pressure fail, the compensatory hypertension of the Cushing reflex also fails, and hypotension and tachycardia are generally seen as a preterminal event. In this case the graph of the patient's vital signs (blood pressure, pulse, respiration, and temperature) will show a crossing of the descending blood pressure line and of the ascending pulse line when plotted on the same scale of 0 to 200. This may not always be the cross of death, as it has been called, but it generally does indicate a poor prognosis.

BIBLIOGRAPHY
The brain

Angevine, J. B., Mancall, E. L., and Yakovlev, P. I.: The human cerebellum, Boston, 1961, Little, Brown and Co.

Ariëns Kappers, C. U., Huber, G. C., and Crosby, E. C.: The comparative anatomy of the nervous system of vertebrates, including man, New York, 1936, The Macmillan Co.

Bailey, P., and von Bonin, G.: The isocortex of man, Urbana, Ill., 1951, University of Illinois Press.

Clarke, E., and O'Malley, C. D.: The human brain and spinal cord; a historical study illustrated by writings from antiquity to the twentieth century, Berkeley, 1968, University of California Press.

Connolly, C. J.: External morphology of the primate brain, Springfield, Ill., 1950, Charles C Thomas, Publisher.

Cunningham, D. J.: Manual of practical anatomy, vol. 3, ed. 13. Revised by Romanes, G. J., London, 1968, Oxford University Press, Inc.

Delmas, A., and Pertuiset, B.: Cranio-cerebral topometry in man, Springfield, Ill., 1959, Charles C Thomas, Publisher.

Ford, D. H., and Schadé, J. P.: Atlas of the human brain, Amsterdam, 1966, Elsevier Publishing Co.

Haymaker, W., Anderson, E., and Nauta, W. J. H.: The hypothalamus, Springfield, Ill., 1969, Charles C Thomas, Publisher.

Noback, C. R., and Montagna, W.: The primate brain, vol. 1. Advances in primatology, New York, 1970, Appleton-Century-Crofts.

Olszewski, J., and Baxter, D.: Cytoarchitecture of the human brain stem, Philadelphia, 1954, J. B. Lippincott Co.

Pernkopf, E.: Topographische und Stratigraphische Anatomie des Kopfes, 2 vols. Topographische Anatomie des Menchen, Munich, 1957, 1960, Verlag Urban & Schwarzenberg.

Riley, H. A.: Atlas of the basal ganglia, brain stem and spinal cord, Baltimore, 1943, The Williams & Wilkins Co.

Singer, M., and Yakovlev, P. I.: The human brain in sagittal section, Springfield, Ill., 1954, Charles C Thomas, Publisher.

Sobotta, J.: Atlas of descriptive human anatomy, vols. 1 to 3. In Uhlenhuth, E., editor. New York, 1954, Hafner Publishing Co., Inc.

Truex, R. C., and Carpenter, M. B.: Human neuroanatomy, Baltimore, 1969, The Williams & Wilkins Co.

Walker, A. E.: The primate thalamus, Chicago, 1938, The University of Chicago Press.

Stereotaxic anatomy

Andrew, J., and Watkins, E. S.: A stereotaxic atlas of the human thalamus and adjacent structures; a variability study, Baltimore, 1969, The Williams & Wilkins Co.

Horsley, V., and Clarke, R. H.: The structure and functions of the cerebellum examined by a new method, Brain 31:45-124, 1908.

Schaltenbrand, G., and Bailey, P.: Introduction to stereotaxis with an atlas of the human brain, Stuttgart, 1959, Georg Thieme Verlag.

Talairach, J., David, M., Tournoux, P., Corredor, H., and Kvasina, T.: Atlas d'anatomie stereotaxique, Paris, 1957, Masson & Cie, Editeurs.

Ventricular and vascular anatomy

Dandy, W. E.: Ventriculography following the injection of air into the cerebral ventricles, Ann. Surg. 68:5-11, 1918.

Davidoff, L. M., and Dyke, C. G.: The normal encephalogram, Philadelphia, 1937, Lea & Febiger.

Davis, D. O., and Pressman, B. D.: Computerized tomography of the brain, Radiol. Clin. North Am. 12:297-313, 1974.

Di Chiro, G.: An atlas of detailed normal pneumoencephalographic anatomy, Springfield, Ill., 1961, Charles C Thomas, Publisher.

Huang, Y. P., Wolf, B. S., Antin S. P., and others: The veins of the posterior fossa; anterior or petrosal draining groups, Am. J. Roentgenol. Radium Ther. Nucl. Med. 104:36-56, 1968.

Kaplan, H. A., and Ford, D. H.: The brain vascular system, Amsterdam, 1966, Elsevier Publishing Co.

Nelson, E., and Rennels, M.: Innervation of intracranial arteries, Brain 93:475-490, 1970.

Padget, D. H.: The cranial venous system in man in reference to development, adult configuration and relation to the arteries, Am. J. Anat. 98:307-355, 1956.

Stephens, R. B., and Stilwell, D. L.: Arteries and veins of the human brain, Springfield, Ill., 1969, Charles C Thomas, Publisher.

Weibel, J., and Fields, W. S.: Atlas of arteriography in occlusive cerebrovascular disease, Philadelphia, 1969, W. B. Saunders Co.

Cellular environment of the brain

Caley, D. W., and Maxwell, D. S.: Development of the blood vessels and extracellular spaces during postnatal maturation of rat cerebral cortex, J. Comp. Neurol. 138:31-48, 1970.

Dempsey, E. W., and Wislocki, G. B.: An electron microsopic study of the blood-brain barrier in the rat, employing silver nitrate as a vital stain, J. Biophys. Biochem. Cytol. 1:245-256, 1955.

Pappas, G. D.: Some morphological considerations of the blood-brain barrier, J. Neurol. Sci. 10:241-246, 1970.

Rosomoff, H. L.: Methods for simultaneous quantitative estimation of intracranial contents, J. Appl. Physiol. 16:395-396, 1961.

Van Harreveld, A., and Malhotra, S. K.: Extracellular space in the cerebral cortex of the mouse, J. Anat. 101:197-207, 1967.

Woodward, D. L., Reed, D. J., and Woodbury, D. M.: Extracellular space of rat cerebral cortex, Am. J. Physiol. 212:367-370, 1967.

Cerebrospinal fluid

Brooks, C. McC., Kao, F. F., and Lloyd, B. B.: Cerebrospinal fluid and the regulation of ventilation, Philadelphia, 1965, F. A. Davis Co.

Coben, L. A.: Uptake of iodide by choroid plexus in vivo and location of the iodide pump, Am. J. Physiol. 217:89-97, 1969.

Dandy, W. E.: Experimental hydrocephalus, Ann. Surg. 70:129-142, 1919.

Davson, H.: Physiology of the cerebrospinal fluid, Boston, 1967, Little, Brown and Co.

Davson, H., Hollingsworth, G., and Segal, M. B.: The mechanism of drainage of the cerebrospinal fluid, Brain 93:665-678, 1970.

Fishman, R. A.: Blood-brain and CSF barriers to penicillin and related organic acids, Arch. Neurol. 15:113-124, 1966.

Katzman, R., Graziani, L., Kaplan, R., and Escriva, A.: Exchange of cerebrospinal fluid potassium with blood and brain, Arch. Neurol. 13:513-524, 1965.

Lorenzo, A. V., Page, L. K., and Watters, G. V.: Relationship between cerebrospinal fluid formation, absorption and pressure in human hydrocephalus, Brain 93:679-692, 1970.

Millen, J. W., and Woolam, D. H. M.: The anatomy of the cerebrospinal fluid, London, 1962, Oxford University Press, Inc.

Moir, A. T. B., Ashcroft, G. W., and others: Cerebral metabolites in the cerebrospinal fluid as a biochemical approach to the brain, Brain 93:357-368, 1970.

Pollay, M., and Davson, H.: The passage of certain substances out of the cerebrospinal fluid, Brain 86:137-150, 1963.

Welch, K., Sadler, K., and Gold, G.: Volume flow across choroidal ependyma of the rabbit, Am. J. Physiol. 210:232-236, 1966.

Cerebral blood flow

Collewijn, H., and Van Harreveld, A.: Intracellular recording from cat spinal motoneurones during acute asphyxia, J. Physiol. (Lond.) 185:1-15, 1966.

Eccles, R., Løyning, Y., and Oshima, T.: Effects of hypoxia on monosynaptic reflex pathway in the cat spinal cord, J. Neurophysiol. 29:315-332, 1966.

Gelfan, S.: Altered spinal motoneurons in dogs with experimental hind-limb rigidity, J. Neurophysiol. 29:583-611, 1966.

Harper, A. M.: Autoregulation of cerebral blood flow; influence of the arterial blood pressure on the blood flow through the cerebral cortex, J. Neurol. Neurosurg. Psychiatr. **29**:398-403, 1966.

Kety, S. S., and Schmidt, C. F.: The determination of cerebral blood flow in man by the use of nitrous oxide in low concentrations, Am. J. Physiol. **143**:53-66, 1945.

Lassen, N. A.: Cerebral blood flow and oxygen consumption in man, Physiol. Rev. **39**:183-238, 1959.

Lassen, N. A.: The luxury-perfusion syndrome and its possible relation to acute metabolic acidosis localized within the brain, Lancet **2**:1113-1115, 1966.

Lewis, B. M., Sokoloff, L., Wechsler, R. L., Wentz, W. B., and Kety, S. S.: A method for the continuous measurement of cerebral blood flow in man by means of radioactive krypton, J. Clin. Invest. **39**:707-716, 1960.

Meyer, J. S., Yoshid, K., and Sakamoto, K.: Autonomic control cerebral blood flow measured by electromagnetic flowmeters, Neurology (Minneap.) **17**:638-648, 1967.

Moniz, E.: L'angiographie cérébrale ses applications et résultats en anatomie, physiologie et clinique, Paris, 1934, Masson & Cie, Editeurs.

Niechaj, A., and Van Harreveld, A.: The nature of postasphyxial rigidity examined by intracellular recording from motoneurons, Exp. Neurol. **18**:67-78, 1967.

Reivich, M., Isaacs, G., Evarts, E., and Kety, S. S.: The effect of slow wave sleep and REM sleep on regional cerebral blood flow in cats, J. Neurochem. **15**:301-306, 1968.

Rosomoff, H. L., and Holaday, D. A.: Cerebral blood flow and cerebral oxygen consumption during hypothermia, Am. J. Physiol. **179**:85-88, 1954.

Russell, R. W. R., Simcock, J. P., Wilkinson, I. M. S., and Frears, C. C.: The effect of blood pressure changes on the leptomeningeal circulation of the rabbit, Brain **93**:491-504, 1970.

Siesjo, B. K., and Zwetnow, N. N.: The effect of hypovolemic hypotension on extra- and intracellular acid-base parameters and energy metabolites in the rat brain, Acta Physiol. Scand. **79**:114-124, 1970.

Taveras, J. M., Fischgold, H., and Dilenge, D., editors: Recent advances in the study of cerebral circulation, Springfield, Ill., 1970, Charles C Thomas, Publisher.

Williams, V., and Grossman, R. G.: Ultrastructure of cortical synapses after failure of presynaptic activity in ischemia, Anat. Rec. **166**:131-141, 1970.

Zingesser, L. H., Schechter, M. M., Dexter, J., Katzman, R., and Scheinberg, L. C.: Regional cerebral blood flow in patients with subarachnoid hemorrhage, Acta Radiol. [Diagn.] (Stockh.) **9**:573-588, 1969.

Intracranial pressure

Cushing, H.: Concerning a definite regulatory mechanism of the vasomotor centre which controls blood pressure during cerebral compression, Johns Hopkins Hosp. Bull. **12**:290-292, 1901.

Langfitt, T. W.: Increased intracranial pressure. In Ojemann, R. G., editor: Clinical neurosurgery, vol. 16, Baltimore, 1969, The Williams & Wilkins Co.

Lundberg, N.: Continuous recording and control of ventricular fluid pressure in neurosurgical practice, Acta Psychiatr. Neurol. Scand. (Suppl. 149) **36**:1-193, 1960.

Meyer, G. A., and Winter, D. L.: Spinal cord participation in the Cushing reflex in the dog, J. Neurosurg. **33**:662-675, 1970.

Risberg, J., Lundberg, N., and Ingvar, D. H.: Regional cerebral blood volume during acute transient rises of the intracranial pressure (plateau waves), J. Neurosurg. **31**:303-310, 1969.

Shulman, K., and Verdier, G. R.: Cerebral vascular resistance changes in response to cerebrospinal fluid pressure, Am. J. Physiol. **213**:1084-1088, 1967.

Zwetnow, N. N.: The influence of an increased intracranial pressure on the lactate, pyruvate, bicarbonate, phosphocreatine, ATP, ADP and AMP concentrations of the cerebral cortex of dogs, Acta Physiol. Scand. **79**:158-166, 1970.

CHAPTER 6

Internal structure of the brain and thalamocortical interactions

A survey of the internal structures of the brain is presented in this chapter. Emphasis will be placed on the nuclei and tracts that are known to be of clinical significance. Further details about many brain structures will be given in later chapters concerned with various systems. After a description of the main structures found within the brainstem, the cerebellum, the diencephalon, and the deep regions of the telencepha-

lon, the organization of the cerebral cortex and its connections will be considered. The interactions between the thalamus and the cerebral cortex will be discussed at the end of this chapter.

The objective of this chapter is to orient students to the organization of the brain so that they will have minimal difficulty in assimilating the material in later chapters on the various systems. The topic of thalamocortical interactions is introduced prior to the consideration of the sensory and motor pathways. These pathways can be regarded as providing the input and output channels of the thalamocortical circuits.

INTERNAL STRUCTURE OF THE BRAIN
Brainstem

The brainstem will be considered here to consist of the medulla, pons, and midbrain. The brainstem resembles the spinal cord in many ways. However, there are special nuclei in the brainstem that do not have homologues in the spinal cord; and the long ascending and descending pathways, which are common to both the brainstem and the spinal cord, change their relative positions at different levels. A knowledge of the main features of brainstem organization is essential for neurological diagnosis, because many brain diseases affect the brainstem. The external features of brainstem anatomy are described in Chapter 5.

Organization of the brainstem

The brainstem can be considered to have a more complex elaboration of the basic structure of the spinal cord. Sensory cranial nerve nuclei are placed dorsally in the brainstem; motor cranial nerve nuclei are ventrally situated. The ascending and descending tracts tend to be located peripheral to a central core of gray matter. In addition to the cranial nerve nuclei, there are a number of special nuclei that have developed in relationship to sensory pathways ascend-

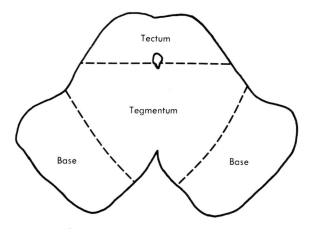

Fig. 6-1. Outline of cross section through the brainstem, showing the locations of the main subdivisions: the tectum, the tegmentum, and the base. The tectum lies dorsal to the ventricular system. The tegmentum is just ventral to the ventricular system. The base forms the ventralmost part of the brainstem. The section is through the midbrain.

ing to cortical structures (cerebral and cerebellar cortex and tectum) or motor pathways descending from the cerebral cortex or from subcortical nuclei.

Three terms are commonly used to describe sectors of the brainstem: the tectum, the tegmentum, and the base. These terms all apply to the midbrain, so they will be introduced with reference to this level of the brainstem. (The pons and medulla also have a tegmentum and base, but no tectum.) An outline of the midbrain is shown in Fig. 6-1. The component of the ventricular system located in the midbrain is the cerebral aqueduct. That part of the midbrain which is dorsal to the aqueduct is called the tectum (roof). The portion of the midbrain just ventral to the aqueduct is the tegmentum (covering). Appended to the ventral side of the tegmentum are fiber tracts and associated nuclei in a zone called the base.

Five major types of nuclei can be distinguished in the brainstem:

1. Cranial nerve nuclei (The sensory and motor nuclei of cranial nerves III to XII resemble the dorsal and ventral horns of the spinal cord in many ways.)
2. Sensory relay nuclei
3. Motor relay nuclei
4. Cerebellar relay nuclei
5. Nuclei whose connections and functions are as yet incompletely known (Many of the cell groups in the reticular formation fall into this category.)

Although this classification is somewhat arbitrary in that some nuclei have several functions, it can serve as an orientation to the nuclei of the brainstem.

Five major types of fiber systems can be distinguished within the brainstem:

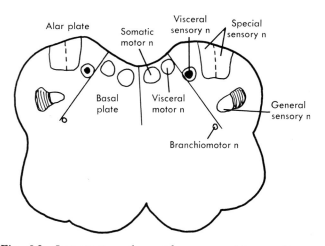

Fig. 6-2. Organization of cranial nerve nuclei according to embryological derivation. The brainstem, like the spinal cord, is derived from the neural tube. The alar and basal plate regions develop into sensory and motor regions respectively. The cranial nerve nuclei in the area derived from the alar plate can be classified as special sensory, general sensory, and visceral sensory. The nuclei of basal plate origin include visceral motor (parasympathetic), branchiomotor (to branchial arch musculature), and somatic motor nuclei. The locations of cranial nerve nuclei having these functions are shown on a drawing of a cross section through the medulla.

1. Cranial nerves
2. Sensory tracts
3. Motor tracts
4. Cerebellar projections
5. Intrinsic projections

The major brainstem nuclei and tracts are summarized in Tables 6-1 and 6-2. They are described and illustrated at each level of the brainstem in the following sections on the medulla, pons, and midbrain.

Before describing the composition of the brainstem, it will be useful to consider the general pattern of organization of the cranial nerve nuclei. As in the spinal cord, the brainstem forms from the alar and basal plates of the neural tube. The alar plate region has a sensory function, and that of the basal plate is motor. An intermediate region between the alar and basal plates may develop visceral functions, like those of the sympathetic cell column in the intermediolateral gray matter of the spinal cord. In the brainstem, the neural tube may be modified by the separation of the alar plate derivatives as the ventricular system expands laterally (Figs. 6-2 and 6-3). The sensory nuclei, which are derived from the alar plate, thus take a dorsolateral rather than dorsal position in much of the brainstem. The sensory nuclei can be further subdivided into special sensory, general sensory, and visceral sensory nuclei, and these are located progressively more medially in the alar plate

Table 6-1. Brainstem nuclei

		Brainstem level	Major function
Cranial nerve nuclei			
XII	Hypoglossal	Medulla	Tongue muscles
X	Dorsal motor of vagus	Medulla	Parasympathetic preganglionics to viscera of neck, thorax, and upper abdomen
VII,IX,X	Ambiguus	Medulla	Muscles of pharynx and larynx
	Solitary	Medulla	Taste and other visceral afferents
IX	Inferior salivatory	Medulla	Parasympathetic preganglionics to parotid gland
VIII	Superior, lateral, medial, and inferior vestibular	Medulla, pons	Vestibular
	Dorsal and ventral cochlear	Pontomedullary junction	Hearing
VII	Superior salivatory	Pons	Parasympathetic preganglionics to submaxillary, sublingual, lacrimal, and other glands
	Facial	Pons	Muscles of facial expression
VI	Abducens	Pons	Lateral rectus muscle
V	Spinal	Pons to cervical spinal cord	Faciocranial sensation
	Principal sensory	Pons	Faciocranial sensation
	Motor	Pons	Muscles of mastication
	Mesencephalic	Pons, midbrain	Jaw and eye muscle proprioception
IV	Trochlear	Midbrain	Superior oblique muscle
III	Oculomotor	Midbrain	Several extraocular muscles
	Edinger-Westphal	Midbrain	Parasympathetic preganglionics to intrinsic eye muscles
Sensory relay nuclei			
	Cuneate	Medulla	Somatic sensory
	Gracile	Medulla	Somatic sensory
	Superior olivary	Pons	Auditory
	Trapezoid	Pons	Auditory
	Lateral lemniscus	Pons	Auditory
	Inferior colliculus	Midbrain	Auditory
	Superior colliculus	Midbrain	Visual
Motor relay nuclei			Output to:
	Reticular formation	Medulla, pons, midbrain	Cerebral cortex, cerebellum, spinal cord
	Red	Midbrain	Spinal cord
	Pretectal area	Midbrain	Oculomotor system
Cerebellar relay nuclei			
	Arcuate	Medulla	Probably displaced cells of pontine nuclei
			Input from:
	Inferior olivary	Medulla	Spinal cord, tegmentum
	Lateral (external) cuneate	Medulla	Spinal cord
	Reticular (lateral, paramedian)	Medulla	Spinal cord
	Pontine	Pons	Cerebral cortex
Nuclei with incompletely known functions			
	Reticular formation	Medulla, pons, midbrain	Various brain structures
	Raphe	Medulla, pons, midbrain	Limbic system, spinal cord
	Locus ceruleus	Pons (isthmus)	Cerebral cortex, cerebellum, spinal cord
	Substantia nigra	Midbrain	Basal ganglia, thalamus
	Periaqueductal gray	Midbrain	Various brain structures
	Interpeduncular	Midbrain	Limbic system

region. Medial to the visceral sensory column is the visceral motor (parasympathetic) column. Ventral to this is a special visceral efferent (branchiomotor) column, which consists of motoneurons that supply muscles associated with structures derived from the branchial arches. The most medial cranial nerve nuclei are the somatic motor nuclei, which innervate muscles derived from the somites of the embryonic head.

Section orientation

Most of the sections through the brain illustrated in this and the following chapters are oriented in one of two ways. For the medulla, pons, and midbrain, it

Table 6-2. Brainstem fiber systems

		Brainstem level	Major function
Brainstem cranial nerves			
XII	Hypoglossal	Medulla (exits in preolivary sulcus)	Tongue muscles
XI	Accessory cranial root	Medulla (exits in postolivary sulcus)	Muscles of pharynx
X	Vagus	Medulla (exits in postolivary sulcus)	Pharyngeal and laryngeal muscles; parasympathetic innervation of thoracic and upper abdominal viscera
	Solitary tract (related to VII,IX,X)	Medulla	Visceral afferents, including taste
IX	Glossopharyngeal	Medulla (exits in postolivary sulcus)	Pharyngeal sensation; stylopharyngeus muscle
VIII	Statoacoustic nerve	Pontomedullary junction	
	Vestibular nerve		Vestibular functions
	Cochlear nerve		Hearing
VII	Facial	Pons (exits at pontomedullary junction)	
	Motor root		Muscles of facial expression
	Intermediate root (nervus intermedius of Wrisberg)	Pons (exits at pontomedullary junction)	Parasympathetic innervation of glands of face; visceral afferents, including taste
V	Trigeminal		
	Sensory root (portio major)	Pons	Faciocranial sensation
	Motor root (portio minor)	Pons	Muscles of mastication
	Mesencephalic tract	Pons, midbrain	Jaw and eye muscle proprioception
	Spinal (descending) tract	Pons, medulla, upper cervical spinal cord	Faciocranial sensation
VI	Abducens	Pons (exits at pontomedullary junction)	Extraocular muscle (lateral rectus)
IV	Trochlear	Midbrain (near isthmus)	Extraocular muscle (superior oblique)
III	Oculomotor	Midbrain	Extraocular muscles; intrinsic eye muscles
Sensory pathways (excluding afferents to cerebellum)			
Medial lemniscus		Medulla, pons, midbrain	Somatic sensory fibers
Spinothalamic		Medulla, pons, midbrain	Somatic and visceral pain and temperature
Trapezoid body		Pons	Auditory
Lateral lemniscus		Pons, midbrain	Auditory
Brachium of inferior colliculus		Midbrain	Auditory
Motor pathways (excluding efferent projections of cerebellum)			
Reticulospinal		Medulla, pons	Somatic and autonomic motor control
Vestibulospinal		Medulla	Balance and posture
Rubrospinal		Midbrain, pons, medulla	Somatic motor control
Tectospinal		Midbrain, pons, medulla	Neck motor control
Corticospinal (pyramids)		Midbrain, pons, medulla	Voluntary movement of extremities
Corticobulbar		Midbrain, pons, medulla	Voluntary movement of head musculature
Corticopontine		Midbrain, pons	Feedback loop between cerebral cortex and cerebellum
Cerebellar projections			
Afferent			
Inferior cerebellar peduncle		Medulla	Input from:
Dorsal spinocerebellar		Medulla	Spinal cord
Cuneocerebellar		Medulla	Spinal cord
Rostral spinocerebellar (in part)		Medulla	Spinal cord
Reticulocerebellar		Medulla	Reticular formation
Vestibulocerebellar		Medulla	Vestibular nuclei and nerve
Olivocerebellar		Medulla	Inferior olivary nucleus
Middle cerebellar peduncle		Pons	
Pontocerebellar		Pons	Cerebral cortex
Superior cerebellar peduncle		Isthmus	
Ventral spinocerebellar		Isthmus	Spinal cord
Efferent			Output to:
Juxtarestiform body		Medulla	Brainstem
Superior cerebellar peduncle		Midbrain	Red nucleus; thalamus; brainstem
Intrinsic fiber systems			
Central tegmental tract		Medulla, pons, midbrain	Projections to inferior olivary nucleus and from reticular formation
Habenulopeduncular tract		Midbrain	Limbic system
Medial longitudinal fasciculus		Medulla, pons, midbrain	Oculomotor system

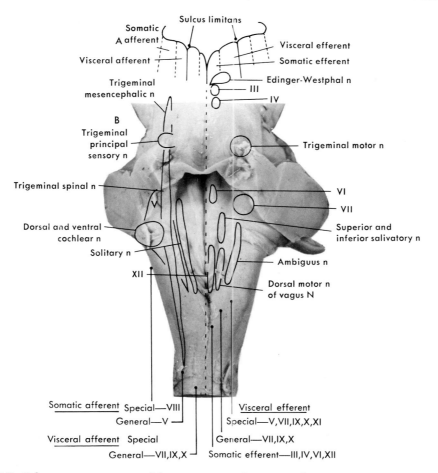

Fig. 6-3. Columnar arrangement of brainstem cranial nerve nuclei. **A,** Transverse section of the rostral medulla, showing the fourth ventricular surface. The positions of the different functional columns are indicated. **B,** Approximate loci of cranial nerve nuclei superimposed on a photograph of the dorsal surface of the lower brainstem. Note that the positions of the Edinger-Westphal nucleus and of the third and fourth cranial nuclei have been indicated only schematically. Review figure in conjunction with Table 6-3. *V,* vestibular n; *III,* oculomotor n; *IV,* trochlear n; *VI,* abducens n; *VII,* facial motor n; *XII,* hypoglossal n; *X,* dorsal motor nucleus of vagus nerve.

is convenient to cut sections at right angles to the long axis of the brainstem. Examples of such sections can be seen in Figs. 6-4, 6-6, and 6-7. However, for the diencephalon and the telencephalon, it is usual to cut sections in an orientation more like the stereotaxic plane (see discussion of stereotaxis in Chapter 5 and in Appendix I), because the human brain undergoes a bend between the brainstem and higher levels. Sections in the stereotaxic plane may include the brainstem, but the angle of section in this event may result in a given section including structures in several levels. An example of such a section can be seen in Fig. 6-12. A few illustrations in this and later chapters show horizontal sections. These are particularly useful to demonstrate the internal capsule and surrounding nuclei (Fig. 6-9, *B*).

Medulla (Fig. 6-4)

The medulla can be subdivided into a caudal part, which resembles the spinal cord in having a central canal covered dorsally by nervous tissue, and a rostral part that forms the caudal floor of the fourth ventricle.

The cranial nerve nuclei of the medulla (Table 6-3) can be classified according to function as follows:

Somatic motor: Hypoglossal nucleus
Branchiomotor: Ambiguus nucleus
Visceral motor: Dorsal motor nucleus of vagus; inferior salivatory nucleus
Visceral sensory: Solitary nucleus
General sensory: Spinal nucleus of trigeminal
Special sensory: Medial and inferior vestibular nuclei; dorsal and ventral cochlear nuclei

The hypoglossal nucleus is found near the midline

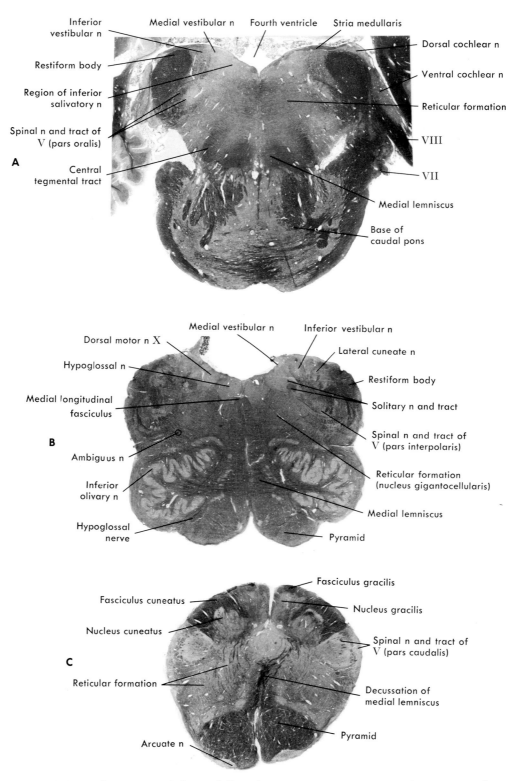

Inferior vestibular n
Medial vestibular n
Fourth ventricle
Stria medullaris
Dorsal cochlear n
Restiform body
Ventral cochlear n
Region of inferior salivatory n
Reticular formation
Spinal n and tract of V (pars oralis)
VIII
Central tegmental tract
VII
Medial lemniscus
Base of caudal pons

A

Dorsal motor n X
Medial vestibular n
Inferior vestibular n
Hypoglossal n
Lateral cuneate n
Medial longitudinal fasciculus
Restiform body
Solitary n and tract
Spinal n and tract of V (pars interpolaris)
Ambiguus n
Reticular formation (nucleus gigantocellularis)
Inferior olivary n
Medial lemniscus
Hypoglossal nerve
Pyramid

B

Fasciculus gracilis
Fasciculus cuneatus
Nucleus gracilis
Nucleus cuneatus
Spinal n and tract of V (pars caudalis)
Reticular formation
Decussation of medial lemniscus
Arcuate n
Pyramid

C

Fig. 6-4. Internal structure of the medulla. The sections in **A** to **D** are taken transversely through different levels of the medulla. The levels correspond to those indicated on the illustrations of the brainstem in **E** and **F**. The level in *A* is at the pontomedullary junction; that in *B* is in the rostral medulla; the level in *C* is at the caudal medulla; and that in *D* is at the decussation of the pyramid at the junction between medulla and spinal cord.

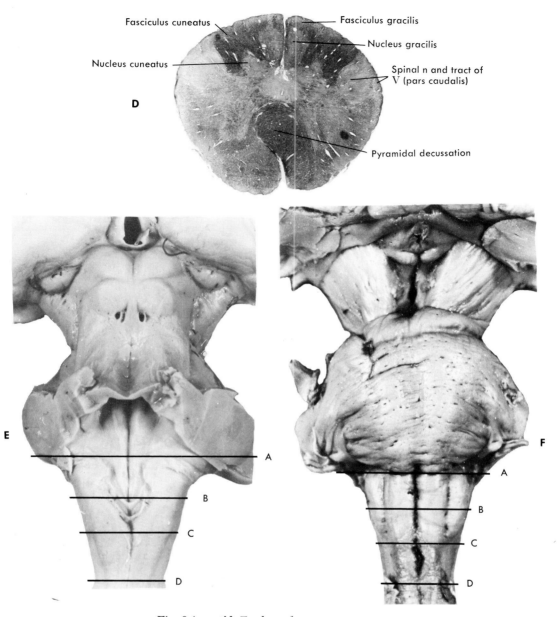

Fasciculus cuneatus

Fasciculus gracilis

Nucleus cuneatus

Nucleus gracilis

Spinal n and tract of V (pars caudalis)

D

Pyramidal decussation

E   A   B   C   D

F   A   B   C   D

Fig. 6-4, cont'd. For legend see opposite page.

just ventral to the central canal in the caudal medulla and to the fourth ventricle in the rostral medulla. The axons of hypoglossal motoneurons collect into bundles, which can be seen coursing ventrally between the medial lemniscus and the inferior olivary nucleus, to exit from the brainstem between the pyramid and the inferior olivary nucleus. The hypoglossal nerve innervates the intrinsic muscles, the genioglossus, and several other extrinsic muscles of the ipsilateral half of the tongue. It should be noted that the genioglossus muscles protrude the tongue. However, protrusion is along the midline only if both genioglossus muscles act in concert; if one genioglossus muscle is

paralyzed, the other protrudes the tongue past the midline and toward the paralyzed side.

The nucleus ambiguus is located about midway between the spinal nucleus of the trigeminal and the inferior olivary nucleus. It extends over much of the length of the medulla. The axons of the motoneurons course dorsomedially and then turn laterally to leave the medulla in the postolivary sulcus. The fibers distribute to muscles of the pharynx, larynx, and upper esophagus through the IX, X, and XI cranial nerves. Interruption of these fibers will result in hoarseness (unilateral vocal cord paralysis) or aphonia (bilateral paralysis) and difficulty in swallowing, often with

Table 6-3. Brainstem cranial nerve components: columnar arrangement of first-order sensory receptive nuclei and of motoneurons of brainstem cranial nerves

Component	Dorsolateral to ventromedial nuclei	Nerves	Major innervation
Sensory			
Somatic sensory			
Special somatic sensory (inner ear)	Superior, lateral, medial, and inferior vestibular	VIII, vestibular portion	Vestibular ganglion
	Dorsal and ventral cochlear	VIII, auditory portion	Spiral ganglion
General somatic sensory (facial skin and mucosa, muscle spindles)	Trigeminal sensory nuclei		
	Principal sensory nucleus	V	Scalp and facial skin and mucosa
	Nucleus of the spinal trigeminal tract	V, VII, IX, X	
	Mesencephalic nucleus	V	Muscle spindles
Visceral sensory			
Special visceral sensory (taste, cardiopulmonary reflexes)	Solitary	VII, IX, X	Tongue; baroceptors and chemoceptors
General visceral sensory (internal organs)	Solitary	VII, IX, X	Deep face, pharynx, viscera
	(Sulcus limitans)		
Visceral motor			
Special visceral motor* (branchiomotor)	Trigeminal motor	V	Muscles of mastication
	Facial motor	VII	Muscles of facial expression
	Ambiguous	IX, X, XI	Pharyngeal muscles
General visceral motor (parasympathetic)	Edinger-Westphal	III	Pupilloconstrictor and ciliary muscles
	Superior salivatory	VII	Salivary and lacrimal glands
	Inferior salivatory	IX	Salivary (parotid) gland
	Dorsal vagal	X	Visceral parasympathetic
Somatic motor (myomeric)	Oculomotor	III	Extraocular muscles
	Trochlear	IV	Extraocular muscles
	Abducens	VI	Extraocular muscles
	Hypoglossal	XII	Tongue muscles

*Alternately classified as special somatic motor.

regurgitation into the nasopharynx because of paralysis of the soft palate. If one side of the palate is paralyzed, the uvula deviates toward the normal side.

The dorsal motor nucleus of the vagus is located just dorsolaterally to the hypoglossal nucleus. It extends longitudinally much of the length of the medulla, merging rostrally with the inferior salivatory nucleus. The axons of the parasympathetic preganglionic neurons of the dorsal motor nucleus course ventrolaterally, joining fibers from the nucleus ambiguus to leave the medulla in the postolivary sulcus. The preganglionic fibers distribute through the vagus nerve to viscera of the neck, thorax, and abdomen, where the fibers terminate on parasympathetic postganglionic neurons located in ganglia near or in plexuses within the walls of the viscera (see p. 80). Interruption of the parasympathetic fibers of the vagus nerve on one side has little consequence. However, a bilateral lesion may result in severe tachycardia.

The inferior salivatory nucleus is located just rostral to the dorsal motor nucleus of the vagus and in a comparable position. This nucleus is adjacent to the pontomedullary junction. The axons of its parasympathetic preganglionic neurons pass ventrolaterally and exit the brainstem in the postolivary sulcus to distribute with the glossopharyngeal nerve. The fibers synapse in the otic ganglion, from which arise postganglionic fibers supplying the parotid gland. Interruption of these fibers unilaterally is of little consequence.

The solitary nucleus is a visceral sensory nucleus in which afferents of the VII, IX, and X cranial nerves synapse. These afferents enter the brainstem through the respective nerves and then collect in the solitary tract. The solitary nucleus has several subdivisions located around the rim of the solitary tract. The afferents projecting to this nucleus arise from a variety of sensory receptors, including taste buds, the baroreceptors and chemoreceptors of the carotid sinus and aortic arch regions, and receptors responsible for triggering the cough reflex and the gag reflex. Unilateral lesions of the glossopharyngeal nerve will produce a sensory deficit of the posterior part of the tongue (including loss of taste there) and pharynx (with loss of the gag reflex).

The spinal nucleus of the trigeminal nerve is a general sensory nucleus that extends from the rostral third of the pons to the upper cervical spinal cord (Fig. 6-3). The nucleus can be subdivided into several components: the pars oralis, pars interpolaris, and pars caudalis (Fig. 6-4). The pars oralis extends from the pons to the level of the rostral end of the hypoglossal nucleus; the pars interpolaris extends from this level to the obex; and the pars caudalis extends at least to the second cervical segment of the spinal cord. Afferents entering the brainstem through the trigeminal nerve descend in the spinal tract of the trigeminal, which runs caudally parallel and just lateral to the spinal nucleus. The afferents terminate at various levels of the nucleus. They supply sensory receptors in the skin of the face and in the mucous membranes of the nasal (including sinuses) and oral cavities and the meninges. There are also afferent projections to the spinal nucleus of the trigeminal from cutaneous receptors around the external ear; these enter the brainstem through cranial nerves VII, IX, and X, and they descend in the spinal tract before synapsing in the spinal nucleus. The sensory functions of the spinal nucleus are discussed at greater length in Chapter 7. Lesions interrupting the spinal tract will produce a loss of pain and temperature sensibility over the region of the face innervated by the fibers. Trigeminal neuralgia is an important clinical problem, the cause of which is still unclear. This is a severe, spontaneous pain in the distribution of the trigeminal nerve (one or more divisions); it occurs intermittently and lasts for seconds. There is often a trigger zone that when stimulated induces a paroxysm of pain.

The medial and inferior vestibular nuclei are located just medial to the restiform body. These nuclei extend the length of the medulla and into the caudal pons. They receive afferent connections from the sensory epithelia of the labyrinth and are involved in vestibular functions, including control of head and eye movements and postural adjustments. Damage to the vestibular nerve or the vestibular nuclei may produce the abnormal eye movements of nystagmus and disturbances of posture and balance.

The dorsal and ventral cochlear nuclei are located, respectively, dorsal and lateral to the restiform body. The afferent connections to these nuclei are from the organ of Corti of the inner ear, and they serve as relay nuclei in the auditory pathway. Damage to the cochlear nuclei produces a sensorineural type of deafness.

The sensory relay nuclei of the medulla are the cuneate and gracile nuclei, or dorsal column nuclei. These are located in the caudal medulla. The axons of the dorsal column sensory pathways, the fasciculi cuneatus and gracilis, terminate in these nuclei (see Chapter 7), and the neurons of the cuneate and gracile nuclei give rise to a major ascending tract of the brainstem, the medial lemniscus. The axons of the cuneate and gracile nuclei cross the midline in the decussation of the medial lemniscus. The medial lemniscus ascends next to the midline just medial to the inferior olivary nucleus. Rostral to the inferior olivary nucleus, the medial lemniscus begins to shift laterally. The medial lemniscus carries discriminative tactile information and is responsible for vibratory and position sensation. Lesions interrupting the medial lemniscus or the cuneate and gracile fasciculi or nuclei produce deficits in these sensations over the parts of the body supplied by them. Because the medial lemniscus is a crossed pathway, the sensory deficit would be contralateral, whereas a lesion of the dorsal column or the dorsal column nuclei would produce an ipsilateral deficit.

Another major sensory pathway passes through the medulla from the spinal cord en route to the thalamus. This is the spinothalamic tract, which lies just dorsal to the inferior olivary nucleus in the middle portion of the medulla. The spinothalamic tract is responsible for pain and temperature sensations (see Chapter 7). An interruption of the spinothalamic tract in the brainstem causes a loss of pain and temperature sensations of the contralateral side of the body, because the pathway is crossed.

The motor relay nuclei of the medulla include some of the reticular formation nuclei, including the nucleus gigantocellularis. The reticular formation of the medulla occupies the central part of the tegmentum. The nucleus gigantocellularis contains numerous very large neurons, many of which give rise to axons that descend into the spinal cord as the medullary reticulospinal tract (see Chapter 8). The medial vestibulospinal tract originates in the medial vestibular nucleus. Other descending motor pathways that pass through the medulla include the lateral vestibulospinal, rubrospinal, tectospinal, and corticospinal tracts. Most of these are difficult to locate on sections of the medulla, but the corticospinal tract occupies the prominent pyramid of the medulla. The bulk of the corticospinal tract crosses at the caudal end of the medulla in a structure known as the pyramidal decussation. Destruction of the corticospinal tract above its decussation results in weakness of the contralateral arm and leg, accompanied by spasticity and a positive sign of Babinski.

Several of the nuclei of the medulla serve to relay information to the cerebellum. These include the arcuate, the inferior olivary, the lateral cuneate, and several of the reticular nuclei. The arcuate nuclei are minor nuclei located just ventral to the pyramids and probably can be considered displaced cells of the pontine nuclei. The inferior olivary nucleus is a striking, irregularly shaped nucleus that extends much of the length of the rostral medulla. It gives rise to the climbing fiber projection to the contralateral cerebellum by way of the inferior cerebellar peduncle. The lateral cuneate nucleus is found at levels near the rostral end of the cuneate nucleus. It relays information to the cerebellum from the spinal cord, which ascends in the cuneate fasciculus; the cuneocerebellar tracts enters the cerebellum through the ipsilateral inferior cerebellar peduncle. Several nuclei of the reticular formation project to the cerebellum (lateral and paramedian reticular nuclei), as do some of the

vestibular nuclei (medial and inferior). Other cerebellar inputs in the medulla include the dorsal, ventral, and rostral spinocerebellar tracts and direct vestibular afferent projections. Most of these enter the cerebellum through the inferior cerebellar peduncle, although the ventral and part of the rostral spinocerebellar tracts ascend through the brainstem to the isthmus region and turn back into the cerebellum through the superior cerebellar peduncle. The inferior cerebellar peduncle also contains efferents from some of the deep cerebellar nuclei, which project to the vestibular nuclei and the reticular formation. Damage to the brainstem structures that interconnect with the cerebellum produces cerebellar signs (see Chapter 8).

Because the inferior cerebellar peduncle is such an important structure, its contents will be summarized here. This peduncle is often subdivided into a larger and more laterally placed restiform body and a smaller, medially placed juxtarestiform body (Fig. 6-5). The restiform body contains cerebellar afferents, including the dorsal spinocerebellar tract, the cuneocerebellar tract, part of the rostral spinocerebellar tract, reticulocerebellar fibers, and the olivocerebellar projection. The juxtarestiform body is largely concerned with interconnections of the vestib-

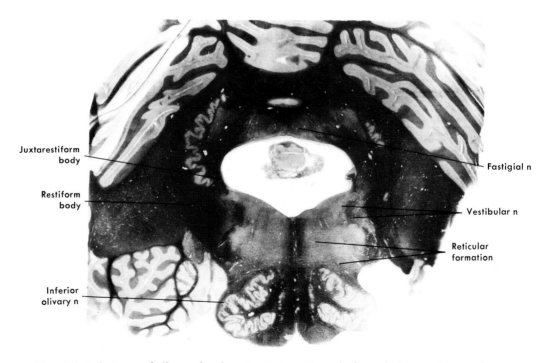

Fig. 6-5. Inferior cerebellar peduncle. The juxtarestiform body and the restiform body are shown, as well as a number of brainstem structures that are connected with the cerebellum through the inferior cerebellar peduncle: vestibular nuclei, reticular formation, and inferior olivary nucleus. One of the deep cerebellar nuclei, the fastigial nucleus, projects to the brainstem in part through the inferior cerebellar peduncle.

ular system and the cerebellum, and it contains directly projecting vestibular afferents and second-order vestibulocerebellar fibers, as well as efferents from the fastigial nucleus to the vestibular nuclei and the reticular formation. All of the cerebellar projections in the inferior cerebellar peduncle are largely uncrossed, except for the olivocerebellar projection.

Some of the nuclei of the medulla have incompletely known functions. These include some of the nuclei of the reticular formation and also the nuclei of the raphe. The reticular formation has a diversity of functions, including regulation of autonomic as well as somatic motor activity and modification of sensory input to the brain (see Chapter 8 and 9). The reticular formation also plays a major role in regulating higher functions of the nervous system, including the state of consciousness (see Chapter 11). The raphe nuclei are also thought to play a part in descending motor control and in the modulation of the states of consciousness. An important observation about the raphe nuclei of the medulla, pons, and midbrain is that many of the neurons contain high concentrations of 5-hydroxytryptamine (serotonin); thus these cells are believed to give rise to the serotonergic pathways of the brain and spinal cord.

The central tegmental tract and the medial longitudinal fasciculus, two important intrinsic fiber pathways of the brain, should be mentioned. Both are found throughout the length of the brainstem. The central tegmental tract is located, as its name suggests, within the tegmentum. An important component of the central tegmental tract in the medulla are fibers descending from the midbrain to end in the inferior olivary nucleus. The medial longitudinal fasciculus in the medulla is largely a descending bundle of fibers projecting to the spinal cord. These include the medial vestibulospinal tract, but also tectospinal and reticulospinal fibers.

Pons (Fig. 6-6)

The pons can be usefully subdivided into three parts: the caudal pons, the rostral pons, and the isthmus region. The caudal pons is associated with the facial motor nucleus and nerve and with the abducens nucleus and nerve. The abducens nucleus and the genu of the facial nerve form the facial colliculus, a surface landmark on the floor of the fourth ventricle. The rostral pons is associated with the trigeminal nerve and several trigeminal nuclei. The isthmus region is the junction between the pons and the midbrain.

The cranial nerve nuclei of the pons (Table 6-3) can be classified as follows:

Somatic motor: Abducens nucleus

Branchiomotor: Facial motor nucleus; trigeminal motor nucleus
Visceral motor: Superior salivatory nucleus
General sensory: Principal sensory nucleus of trigeminal; mesencephalic nucleus of trigeminal; spinal nucleus of trigeminal, pars oralis
Special sensory: Lateral and superior vestibular nuclei

The abducens nucleus is located near the midline in the caudal pons and helps form the facial colliculus. The axons of the motoneurons pass in a ventral direction and exit the brainstem at the junction of the pons and medulla lateral to the midline. The abducens nerve supplies the lateral rectus muscle in the ipsilateral orbit. Damage to the abducens nucleus or nerve results in a paralysis of lateral gaze in one eye.

The facial motor nucleus is also found in the caudal pons. It is located in a position in the tegmentum comparable to that occupied by the nucleus ambiguus in the medulla, which is appropriate because both supply muscles derived from branchial arch tissue. Also like the nucleus ambiguus, the axons of the facial motor nucleus take an initially dorsomedial course before turning ventrolaterally to leave the brainstem. The facial nerve fibers initially run dorsomedially and approach the floor of the fourth ventricle, where they are found dorsal to the abducens nucleus. At the rostral end of the abducens nucleus, the facial nerve fibers turn in the genu of the facial nerve, and then they pass ventrolaterally, running between the facial motor nucleus and the spinal nucleus of the trigeminal, and finally exit in the cerebellopontine angle just medial to the VIII nerve. The facial nerve branchiomotor fibers supply the muscles of facial expression and the stapedius muscle. Interruption of the fibers causes paralysis of these muscles; the facial weakness encompasses the upper as well as the lower face, as typically seen in Bell's palsy.

The trigeminal motor nucleus is another branchiomotor nucleus. It is in the rostral pons, occupying a position comparable to that of the facial motor nucleus. The axons of the motoneurons of the trigeminal motor nucleus leave the pons in the motor root (portio minor) of the trigeminal nerve. They distribute through the mandibular branch of the trigeminal and supply the muscles of mastication, the tensor tympani, and a few other muscles of the head. Damage to the motor nucleus of the trigeminal nerve or of the motor axons will cause a paralysis of the muscles of mastication.

The superior salivatory nucleus is the only autonomic or visceral motor nucleus of the pons. The cells of this nucleus are difficult to locate, but appear to

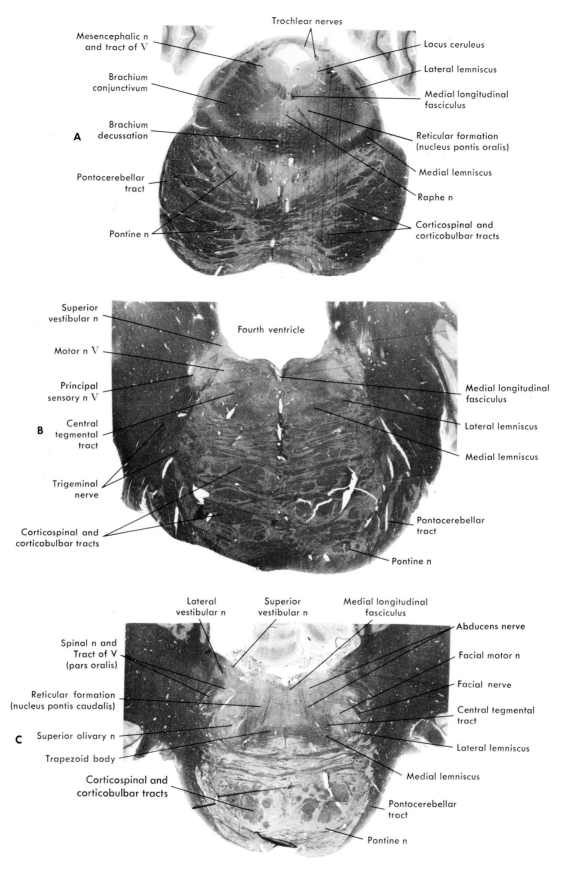

Fig. 6-6. Internal structure of the pons. The sections in **A** to **C** are taken transversely through different levels of the pons. The corresponding levels are indicated in **D** and **E. A**, Isthmus region; **B**, rostral pons; and **C**, caudal pons.

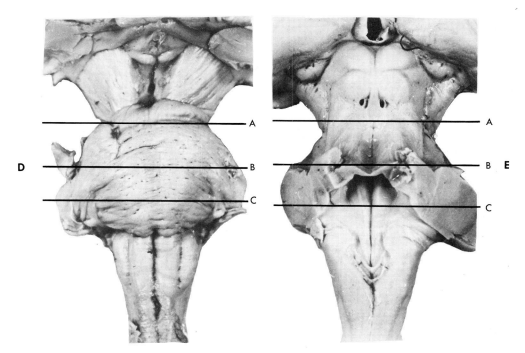

Fig 6-6, cont'd. For legend see opposite page.

occupy a similar region to that of the dorsal motor nucleus and the inferior salivatory nucleus, but in the caudal pons. The efferent fibers leave the brainstem in the intermediate nerve, a small branch of the facial nerve situated between the facial and VIII cranial nerves. The fibers are parasympathetic autonomic preganglionics, and they pass through the chorda tympani nerve to end in the submandibular ganglion or through the greater petrosal nerve to synapse in the sphenopalatine ganglion. The postganglionic fibers from the submandibular ganglion innervate the submandibular and sublingual salivary glands; those from the sphenopalatine ganglion supply the lacrimal gland and glands of the mucous membranes of the nose and palate. Interruption of these causes loss of tearing and a dry cornea.

The visceral afferents of the facial nerve enter through the intermediate nerve, and then they turn caudally in the solitary tract to terminate in the solitary nucleus of the medulla. There is no visceral afferent nucleus in the pons.

The general sensory nuclei of the pons belong to the trigeminal nerve. The spinal nucleus of the trigeminal has already been discussed. The principal sensory nucleus of the trigeminal is located in the rostral pons just lateral to the trigeminal motor nucleus. Fibers carrying sensory information from the face and the oral and nasal cavities have their cell bodies in the trigeminal ganglion, and the central processes enter the pons through the sensory root (portio major) of the trigeminal. Some of the afferents terminate in the principal sensory nucleus; the same afferents may send a descending collateral by way of the spinal tract to synapse in the spinal nucleus of the trigeminal. Damage to the principal sensory nucleus presumably interferes with the transmission of tactile information from the face, but this is of no clinical significance, presumably because touch is also a function of the spinal nucleus.

The mesencephalic nucleus of the trigeminal is actually a sensory ganglion and is located within the central nervous system. Other centrally located sensory ganglia have been described in lower vertebrates (notably in the lamprey by Sigmund Freud), but the mesencephalic nucleus is the exception in mammals. The neurons of the mesencephalic nucleus are pseudounipolar cells that closely resemble dorsal root ganglion cells. They are found in a column that extends from the rostral level of the principal sensory nucleus of the trigeminal rostrally to the level of the superior colliculus. The location within the pons is lateral to the rostral fourth ventricle, and that within the midbrain is lateral to the aqueduct. The mesencephalic tract of the trigeminal consists of the peripheral processes of these cells. These processes are large myelinated axons that leave the pons in the portio minor of the trigeminal nerve and innervate stretch receptors in the muscles of mastication. The central processes of the cells make reflex connections within the brainstem, including monosynaptic connections with motoneurons of the trigeminal motor nucleus. Interruption of the mesencephalic tract of the trigeminal would eliminate the stretch reflexes of such muscles as the masseter.

The lateral and superior vestibular nuclei are located in the lateral wall of the fourth ventricle. The lateral vestibular nucleus extends from the pontomedullary junction to about the level of the abducens nucleus, and the superior vestibular nucleus extends well rostrally in the pons and is adjacent to the principal and mesencephalic nuclei of the trigeminal over part of its length. Like the inferior and medial vestibular nuclei, the lateral and superior nuclei are involved in postural control and in the regulation of eye movements (see Chapter 7). Damage would produce abnormalities in these functions.

The sensory relay nuclei of the pons belong to the auditory pathway. These include the superior olivary nucleus, the nucleus of the trapezoid body, and the nucleus of the lateral lemniscus. The superior olivary nucleus is found at levels from that of the facial motor nucleus to that of the trigeminal motor nucleus. In the caudal pons, it is ventromedial to the facial motor nucleus. The nucleus of the trapezoid body is a collection of scattered cells within the trapezoid body medial to the superior olivary nuclei. The trapezoid body is a fiber bundle in the ventral tegmentum of the caudal pons. The fibers consist chiefly of a projection from the ventral cochlear nucleus, which decussates and then ascends as the lateral lemniscus. There are also ipsilateral ascending fibers from the cochlear nuclei in the lateral lemniscus, as well as fibers that originate from the superior olivary nuclei and the nuclei of the trapezoid body. In the rostral pons, the lateral lemniscus contains the nucleus of the lateral lemniscus. All of these structures belong to the auditory pathway. Interruption of the pathway on one side produces diminished audition in both ears, rather than deafness in one ear, because of the crossed and uncrossed pattern of ascending connections. Other sensory pathways ascend through the pons, including the medial lemniscus and the spinothalamic tract.

The motor relay nuclei of the pons include the nucleus pontis caudalis and the nucleus pontis oralis of the reticular formation. The nucleus pontis caudalis extends from the caudal pons to the level of the trigeminal motor nucleus, and the nucleus pontis oralis extends rostrally from this level to the midbrain. These reticular nuclei are the origin of the pontine reticulospinal tract. Another major descending pathway that originates in the pons is the lateral

vestibulospinal tract; this is a projection from the lateral vestibular nucleus. The rubrospinal, tectospinal, and corticospinal tracts pass through the pons, and part of the corticobulbar tract ends in the pons; the corticopontine tracts end in the pontine nuclei.

The cerebellar relay nuclei of the pons are the pontine nuclei. These are a mass of neurons in the base of the pons, separated into clusters by the longitudinally coursing corticospinal, corticobulbar, and corticopontine tracts and by the transversely running pontocerebellar fibers. The pontocerebellar fibers originate from the cells of the pontine nuclei and decussate to enter the cerebellum through the contralateral middle cerebellar peduncle (brachium pontis). This is the massive collection of pontocerebellar fibers that gives the bridgelike appearance to the ventral surface of the pons and hence its name (bridge). An efferent pathway reaches the pons from the cerebellum through the uncinate fasciculus; this exits the cerebellum through the superior cerebellar peduncle and then turns caudally into the pons and medulla to terminate in the reticular formation and the vestibular nuclei.

Nuclei of the pons with poorly understood functions include the nuclei of the raphe and the nucleus locus ceruleus. Many of the neurons of the raphe nuclei contain 5-hydroxytryptamine, as mentioned in the discussion of the medulla. The cells of the nucleus locus ceruleus and adjacent nuclei contain norepinephrine. These monoamine-containing neurons have been the subject of intensive investigations in recent years. The pathways of projection of these cells have been mapped with the aid of the fluorescence histochemistry technique (see Appendix I). There are projections to rostral levels of the central nervous system, including the cerebral cortex, the hypothalamus, and limbic structures, and there are also projections to the cerebellum and to the spinal cord. It appears that a relatively small number of monoaminergic neurons exert an influence on an unusually wide territory of central nervous system structures. The monoamine pathways from these nuclei appear to play a role in the regulation of the sleep cycle and may take part in a diversity of other activities as well.

Two fiber systems present in the pons and the medulla are the central tegmental tract and the medial longitudinal fasciculus (MLF). The central tegmental tract includes an important descending pathway from the midbrain to the inferior olivary nucleus; in addition, it contains a major ascending projection from the reticular formation to the diencephalon. The MLF also contains both descending and ascending fibers. The descending pathways include some reticulospinal fibers and the tectospinal tract. Ascending fibers of the MLF in the pons are chiefly vestibular projections to the motor nuclei controlling eye movements.

Midbrain (Fig. 6-7)

The two levels of the midbrain that will be considered are a caudal level through the inferior colliculus and a rostral level through the superior colliculus.

The cranial nerve nuclei of the midbrain (Table 6-3) are as follows:

Somatic motor: Trochlear; oculomotor

Visceral motor: Edinger-Westphal

General somatic: Mesencephalic nucleus of trigeminal

The trochlear nucleus (Table 6-1) is located near the midline just ventral to the periaqueductal gray matter; the nucleus is circular in outline and appears to nest among fibers of the MLF. The trochlear nerve encircles the periaqueductal gray, coursing in a caudal direction. The fibers decussate in the anterior medullary velum (Fig. 6-6, A), and then exit the brainstem just caudal to the inferior colliculus. The trochlear nerve innervates the superior oblique muscle, which assists in downward, medial eye movements. Interruption of the nerve or damage to the nucleus would interfere with such eye movements on one side.

The oculomotor nucleus is also near the midline just ventral to the periaqueductal gray, but at the level of the superior colliculus. The nuclei of the two sides form a wedge, or heart-shaped structure. The nerve fibers run ventrally and caudally to leave the brainstem in the interpeduncular fossa. Some of the fibers are crossed, and some are uncrossed. The muscles innervated include the levator palpebrae, the superior, inferior, and medial rectus muscles, and the inferior oblique. The movements produced by various components of the oculomotor nerve include lid elevation and upward, medial, and downward eye movements. Damage to the nucleus or the nerve results in ptosis and a laterally deviated eye on one side.

The Edinger-Westphal nucleus consists of cells dorsal and dorsomedial to the somatic motoneurons of the oculomotor nucleus. The neurons of the Edinger-Westphal nucleus are parasympathetic preganglionic cells that project through the oculomotor nerve to the ciliary ganglion of the same side. Postganglionic fibers from the ciliary ganglion enter the eye and supply the smooth muscle of the pupillary sphincter and the ciliary body. Their activity causes pupillary constriction (miosis) and contraction of the ciliary muscle, with a resultant relaxation of the suspensory ligaments of the lens and passive rounding of the lens. Damage to the parasympathetic supply to the

eye will cause pupillary dilatation (mydriasis) due to the loss of activity in the sphincter and to unbalanced activity in the sympathetics that supply the pupillary dilator muscles. There is also a loss of the ability to accommodate for near vision.

The mesencephalic nucleus of the trigeminal has already been discussed.

The sensory relay nuclei of the midbrain include the inferior and the superior colliculi. The inferior colliculus contains a prominent nucleus and receives a major input from the lateral lemniscus. The output of the inferior colliculus is largely through the brachium of the inferior colliculus to the medial geniculate body of the thalamus. There is also a decussation of the inferior colliculus, serving in interactions between the two sides. The inferior colliculus functions as a part of the auditory pathway (see Chapter 7). The superior colliculus has a cortical structure, with a number of fiber and cellular layers. The input to the superior colliculus includes a prominent projection from the optic nerve through the brachium of the superior colliculus (Fig. 6-11). There are also corticotectal and spinotectal connections. Efferents include brainstem connections and the tectospinal tract. The superior colliculus serves as a center for reflex activity related to visual function. An important aspect includes the control of eye movements, especially vertical eye movements.

In addition to auditory and visual pathways, the sensory pathways that pass through the midbrain include the medial lemniscus and the spinothalamic tract.

Motor relay nuclei of the midbrain include the reticular formation, the red nucleus, and the pretectal area. Although the reticular formation of the midbrain does not have direct spinal projections, it undoubtedly has important indirect connections with lower levels of the nervous system. The red nucleus gives rise to the rubrospinal tract, a pathway that crosses just ventral to the red nuclei and then descends into the spinal cord. The pretectal area is located just rostral to the superior colliculus. It receives connections from the optic tract through the brachium of the superior colliculus, and projections are made from each pretectal region to the Edinger-Westphal nuclei of both sides. This system serves to organize the pupillary reflex to light. Interruption of this system is characteristic of the Argyll-Robertson pupil, which is seen in central nervous system syphilis. Although the pupil is small and fails to respond to light, it can still constrict during accommodation. The pathway for accommodation does not utilize the brachium of the superior colliculus or the pretectal area; thus the lesion may be in one of these sites.

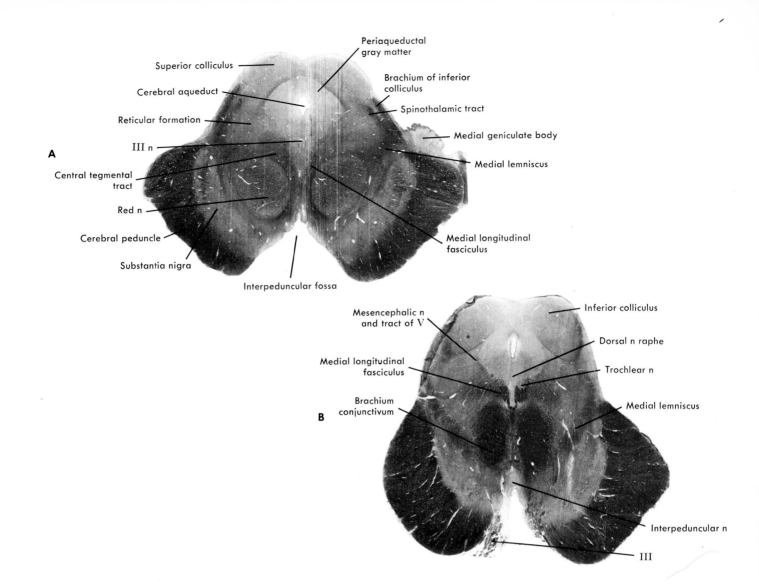

A

Superior colliculus

Cerebral aqueduct

Reticular formation

III n

Central tegmental tract

Red n

Cerebral peduncle

Substantia nigra

Interpeduncular fossa

Periaqueductal gray matter

Brachium of inferior colliculus

Spinothalamic tract

Medial geniculate body

Medial lemniscus

Medial longitudinal fasciculus

B

Mesencephalic n and tract of V

Medial longitudinal fasciculus

Brachium conjunctivum

Inferior colliculus

Dorsal n raphe

Trochlear n

Medial lemniscus

Interpeduncular n

III

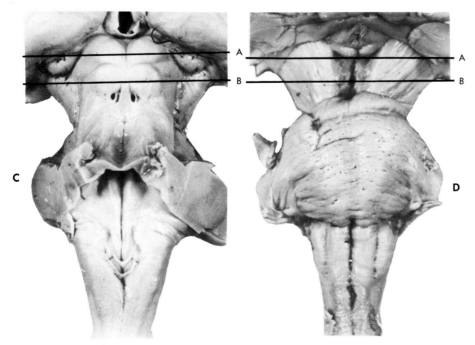

C

D

A

B

A

B

Fig. 6-7. Internal structure of the midbrain. The sections in **A** and **B** are taken transversely through two different levels of the midbrain. The corresponding levels are indicated in **C** and **D**. The level in *A* is through the superior colliculus; that in *B* is through the inferior colliculus.

Motor pathways that pass through the midbrain include the corticospinal, corticobulbar, and corticopontine tracts, located in the cerebral peduncle.

The cerebellar relay nucleus found in the midbrain is the red nucleus. This nucleus receives a projection from the contralateral globose and emboliform nuclei by way of the brachium conjunctivum (superior cerebellum peduncle) and its decussation. Some of the fibers of the brachium conjunctivum descend into the lower brainstem (hook fasciculus), and a major projection continues rostrally past the red nucleus to end in the thalamus (dentatothalamic projection).

Some of the midbrain structures with incompletely defined functions include the substantia nigra, the central gray, and the interpeduncular nucleus. The substantia nigra has reciprocal connections with the caudate nucleus and putamen. Lesions of the substantia nigra have been implicated in parkinsonism. Neurons of the substantia nigra utilize dopamine as a neurotransmitter. These cells contain melanin pigment, which apparently is a by-product of catecholamine metabolism. The melanin-containing neurons give the black coloration to the nucleus and thus its name. The periaqueductal gray of the midbrain has been thought to play a role in reaction to painful stimulation. It receives collaterals from the spinothalamic tract. Recently it has been shown that electrical stimulation within the periaqueductal gray can result in analgesia. The interpeduncular nucleus receives a prominent projection from the habenular nucleus of the epithalamus, the habenulopeduncular tract. These structures form a part of the limbic system and are believed to be involved in visceral activities. The central tegmental tract and the MLF in the midbrain have a similar composition to that described for them in the section on the pons.

Cerebellum (Fig. 6-8)

The cerebellum, along with the pons, is a component of the metencephalon. A section through the cerebellum shows its basic organization, which consists of an outer coating of gray matter, the cortex, and an interior core of white matter. Within the white matter are a series of deep cerebellar nuclei, which have a lateral to medial arrangement. The lateralmost nucleus is an irregular structure that resembles closely the inferior olivary nucleus. This is called the dentate nucleus (in lower mammals it may be called the lateral nucleus). In the hilus of the dentate nucleus is an elongated structure called the emboliform nucleus, and medial to this are several subdivisions of the globose nucleus (the equivalent structures in the cat are referred to as the interposed nuclei). The most medial deep cerebellar nucleus is

called the fastigial nucleus. It is adjacent to the tent-like dorsal extension of the fourth ventricle, the fastigium (tent).

Afferent fibers enter the cerebellar white matter by way of the three cerebellar peduncles (inferior, middle, and superior), and efferents from the deep cerebellar nuclei and a few Purkinje cells leave the cerebellar white matter in the inferior or superior cerebellar peduncles.

Diencephalon (Fig. 6-9)

The diencephalon can be subdivided into four major regions: the thalamus (or dorsal thalamus), the epithalamus, the subthalamus, and the hypothalamus. The thalamus is an oval mass of gray matter that lies between the internal capsule and the third ventricle. It can be subdivided into several regions, each with a number of nuclei, as will be discussed below. The epithalamus consists of the habenular nucleus, the stria medullaris, and the pineal gland. The subthalamus includes the subthalamic nucleus, the zona incerta, and the fields of Forel. The hypothalamus contains a number of nuclei in the walls of the third ventricle below the hypothalamic sulcus, the floor of the third ventricle, and the mammillary bodies. Associated with the hypothalamus is the pituitary gland.

Thalamus (Figs. 6-10 to 6-14 and 6-15, *B*). The caudal end of the thalamus includes the prominent pulvinar and the lateral and medial geniculate bodies. The latter are ventral to the pulvinar and sometimes are called the metathalamus. These structures are seen in sections through the junction between the midbrain and the diencephalon.

A section taken more rostrally shows that the middle region of the thalamus is split into lateral and medial parts by a sheet of white matter called the internal medullary lamina. There is also an external medullary lamina, which separates the lateral thalamic region from the reticular nucleus of the thalamus.

The lateral mass of the thalamus is further subdivided into the dorsal tier of nuclei and a ventral tier. The dorsal tier of nuclei includes the pulvinar caudally, the lateral posterior nucleus, and the lateral dorsal nucleus. The ventral tier consists of the ventral posterior nucleus caudally and the ventral lateral and ventral anterior nuclei at progressively more rostral levels. The ventral posterior nucleus has two parts, the ventral posterior lateral (VPL) and the ventral posterior medial (VPM) nuclei.

The medial thalamic mass contains several nuclei, but the most prominent are the medial dorsal nucleus and the midline nuclei. There are several nuclei, including the centromedian nucleus, within the internal medullary lamina, and thus are classed as the intra-

Text continued on p. 198.

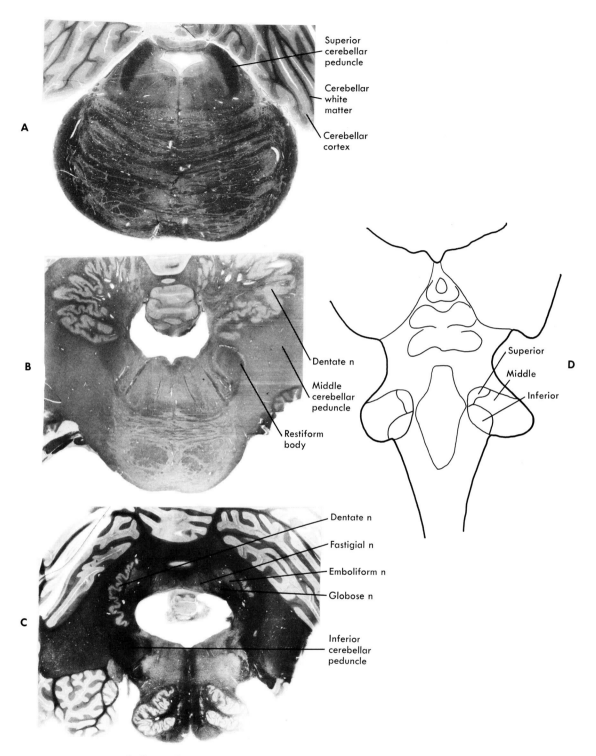

Fig. 6-8. Cerebellar peduncles and deep nuclei. The sections in **A** to **C** show the cerebellar peduncles and the deep nuclei of the cerebellum. The drawing in **D** shows the approximate locations of the cut edges of the cerebellar peduncles in a specimen of the brainstem from which the cerebellum has been removed.

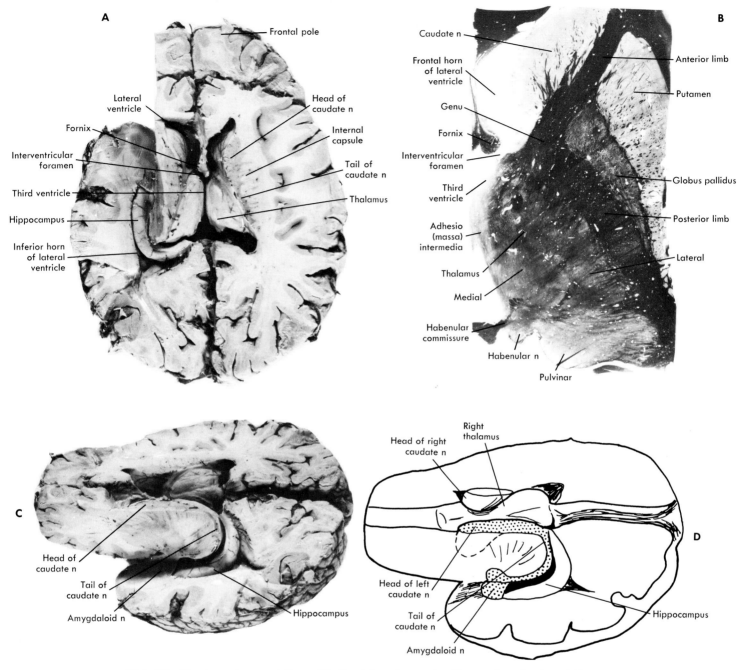

Fig. 6-9. Structures in association with the internal capsule. The sections in **A** and **B** are taken horizontally. The gross specimen in **A** is dissected further on the left to demonstrate the hippocampus in the floor of the temporal horn of the lateral ventricle; to do this, a vertical cut was made through the internal capsule. The head and tail of the caudate nucleus are seen just medial to the cut on the left and to the internal capsule on the right. The thalamus on each side protrudes into the third ventricle, and the interventricular foramen of Monro is seen just behind the columns of the fornix. The stained horizontal section in **B** shows the V-shaped internal capsule in a plane somewhat more inferior than that in **A**. The anterior limb, genu, and posterior limb of the internal capsule are indicated. The anterior limb separates the head of the caudate nucleus from the lentiform nucleus (putamen and globus pallidus). The genu is at the level of the interventricular foramen. The posterior limb of the internal capsule separates the thalamus from the lentiform nucleus. The specimen in **C** is the same as that in **A**, but viewed from the left side. **D** shows the course of the caudate nucleus as it curves into the temporal lobe, where it helps form the roof of the temporal horn of the lateral ventricle. The caudate nucleus terminates at the amygdaloid nucleus.

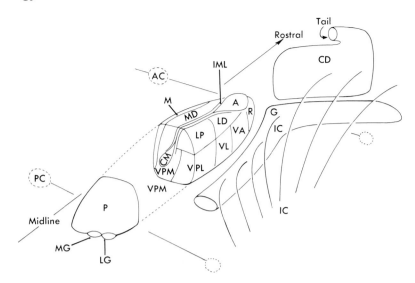

Fig. 6-10. Nuclei of the thalamus and relationships of the thalamus to the intercommissural line, to the head of the caudate nucleus, and to the internal capsule. The right thalamus is shown from a posterolateral view in an "exploded" drawing, in which the pulvinar is shown as detached by a frontal cut to show a frontal section of the thalamus. Specific nuclei, anterior group: *A*, anterior. Lateral group, dorsal tier: *LD*, lateral dorsal; *LP*, lateral posterior; *P*, pulvinar. Lateral group, ventral tier: *VA*, ventral anterior; *VL*, ventral lateral; *VPM* and *VPL*, ventral posterior medial and lateral. Medial group: *MD*, medial dorsal. Metathalamic group: *LG*, lateral geniculate; *MG*, medial geniculate. Nonspecific nuclei: *CM*, centromedian; *M*, midline groups. *R*, reticular. The internal medullary lamina, *IML*, encloses *CM* and other nonspecific nuclei *(not shown)*. Other abbreviations: *AC*, *PC*, anterior and posterior commissures; *Cd*, head of caudate; *IC*, internal capsule; *G*, genu of capsule.

Table 6-4. Thalamic nuclei and projections

Thalamic divisions and nuclei	Extrathalamic afferent input	Cortical projection	Function
Specific (cortical relay) nuclei			
Metathalamic			
Medial geniculate (MG)	Auditory pathway	Temporal	Auditory
Lateral geniculate (LG)	Optic tract	Occipital	Visual
Lateral (ventral tier)			
Ventral posterior lateral (VPL)	Medial lemniscus	Postcentral parietal	Sensory (body)
Ventral posterior medial (VPM)	Trigeminothalamic	Postcentral parietal	Sensory (face)
Ventral lateral (VL)	Dentate nucleus	Precentral frontal	Motor
Ventral anterior (VA)	Globus pallidus	Frontal	Motor
Medial			
Medial dorsal (MD)	Amygdaloid, hypothalamus	Orbitofrontal, frontal	Limbic
Anterior			
Anterior ventral (AV)	Mamillary body	Cingulate	Limbic
Anterior medial (AM)			
Anterior dorsal (AD)			
Association nuclei			
Lateral (dorsal tier)			
Pulvinar (Pul)	Parieto-occipital-temporal	Parieto-occipital-temporal	Higher functions
Lateral posterior (LP)	Parieto-occipital-temporal	Parieto-occipital temporal	
Lateral dorsal (LD)	Cingulate	Cingulate	Limbic
Nonspecific (diffusely projecting) nuclei			
Intralaminar			
Centromedian (CM)	Reticular formation, globus pallidus	Putamen	
Centrolateral (CL)	Reticular formation, spinothalamic tract		
Nuclei with subcortical connections			Modulation of thalamocortical activity
Reticular	Thalamus	Thalamus	

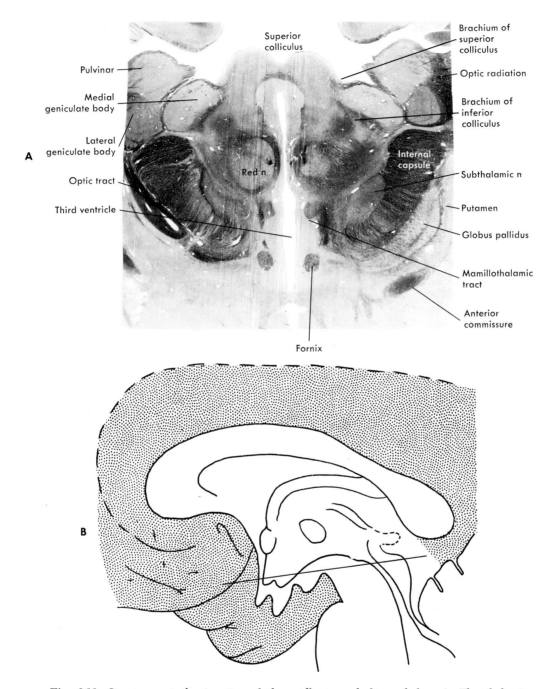

Fig. 6-11. Structures at the junction of the midbrain and diencephalon. **A,** The thalamic nuclei of the metathalamus—the lateral and medial geniculate bodies—and the pulvinar. The terminations of the optic tract and of the brachium of the inferior colliculus in these thalamic relay nuclei are indicated, as is the initial portion of the optic radiation. The orientation of the section is shown in **B.**

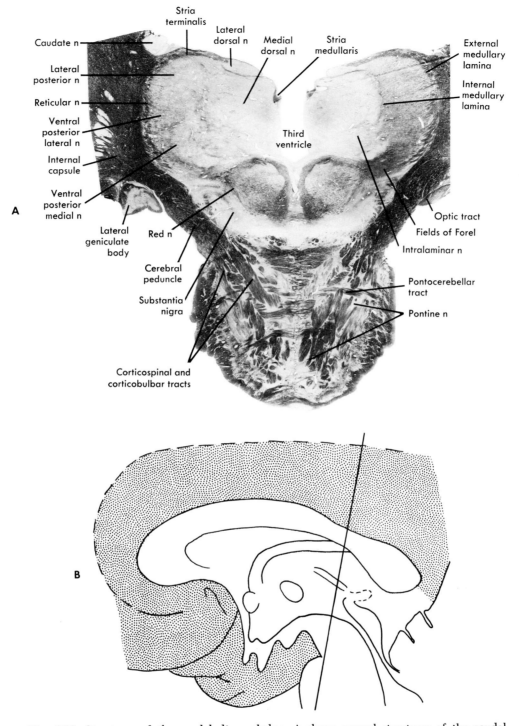

Fig. 6-12. Structures of the caudal diencephalon. **A** shows several structures of the caudal thalamus, as well as structures of the neighboring telencephalon, midbrain, and pons. The orientation of the section is indicated in **B**. At this level the lateral thalamic region contains the lateral posterior and lateral dorsal nuclei of the dorsal tier and the ventral posterior lateral and ventral posterior medial nuclei of the ventral tier. The lateral geniculate body is present on the left, the optic tract on the right. The medial thalamic region contains the medial dorsal nucleus. The reticular nucleus is separated from the lateral thalamic area by the external medullary lamina, and the medial thalamic area is demarcated by the internal medullary lamina. The intralaminar nuclei are within the internal medullary lamina. The stria medullaris of the epithalamus is along the medial edge of the thalamus. Ventral to the thalamus are the fields of Forel in the subthalamus.

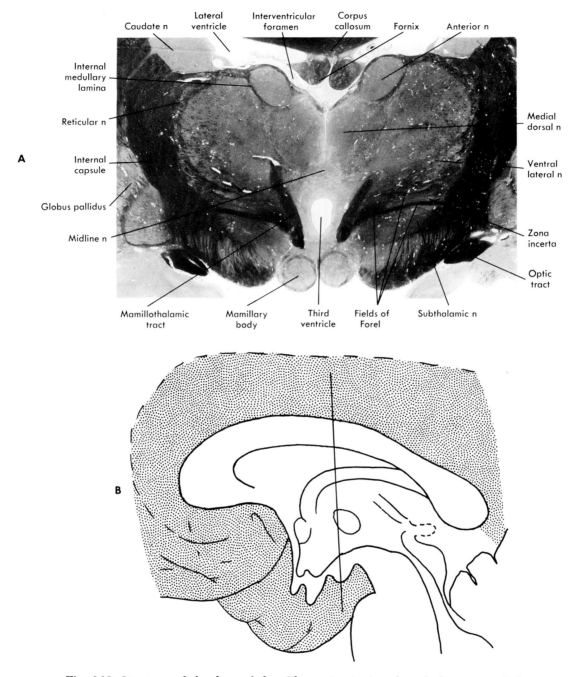

Fig. 6-13. Structures of the diencephalon. The section in **A** is through the anterior thalamic nuclei dorsally and the mamillary bodies ventrally. The orientation of the section is indicated in **B**. The thalamic nuclei present, in addition to the anterior nuclei, include the reticular nucleus, the ventral lateral nucleus, and the medial dorsal and midline nuclei. The internal medullary lamina splits to separate from the anterior nuclei, in addition to dividing the lateral from the medial groups. Subthalamic structures present include the subthalamic nucleus, zona incerta, and the fields of Forel. The hypothalamic structures include the mamillary nuclei. The mamillothalamic tracts are shown interconnecting the mamillary nuclei and the anterior thalamic nuclei.

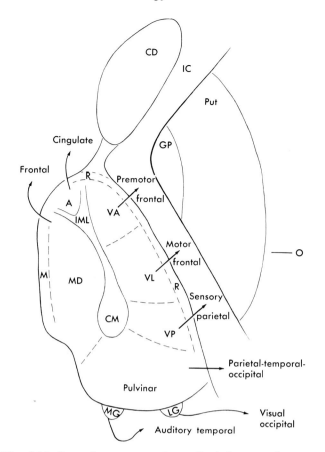

Fig. 6-14. Cortical projections of specific thalamic nuclei, composite of several horizontal sections 2 to 5 mm dorsal to the intercommissural line. Specific nuclei, anterior group: *A*, anterior. Lateral group, ventral tier: *VA*, ventral anterior; *VL*, ventral lateral; *VP*, ventral posterior. Lateral group, dorsal tier: pulvinar. Medial group: *MD*, medial dorsal. Metathalamic group: *MG*, medial geniculate; *LG*, lateral geniculate. Nonspecific nuclei: *CM*, centromedian; *M*, midline group; *R*, reticular. Other abbreviations: *CD*, caudate; *GP*, globus pallidus; *IC*, internal capsule; *IML*, internal medullary lamina; *Put*, putamen; *O*, intercommissural anterior-posterior zero point.

laminar nuclei. In the rostral thalamus, the internal medullary lamina splits to enclose the anterior thalamic nuclei.

The thalamic nuclei are best understood in terms of their connections. Thalamic nuclei that receive a specific input and project to localized areas of the cerebral cortex are called specific nuclei. There are specific thalamic nuclei in the lateral, medial, and anterior regions of the thalamus. Nuclei that affect the cortex diffusely are called nonspecific thalamic nuclei. These include several intralaminar nuclei. Some thalamic nuclei connect with the association areas of the cerebral cortex and so are called association nuclei. The thalamic nuclei will be described briefly here; somewhat more detailed descriptions will be found in later chapters concerned with brain systems.

The metathalamic nuclei are the lateral and medial geniculate bodies. The most important input to the lateral geniculate body is through the optic tract, and the lateral geniculate body functions as a relay nucleus in the visual pathway (see Chapter 7). The output is through the optic radiations to the visual receiving area of the occipital lobe. The medial geniculate body receives its major input from the inferior colliculus by way of the brachium of the inferior colliculus and thus is a relay nucleus in the auditory pathway (see Chapter 7). The output of the medial geniculate body is through the auditory radiation to the auditory receiving area in the transverse temporal gyri.

The ventral tier nuclei of the lateral thalamus are also specific nuclei. The VPL and VPM nuclei receive connections from the somatic sensory pathways, including the medial lemniscus and spinothalamic tracts (to VPL) and the trigeminothalamic tract (to VPM). These nuclei are sensory relay nuclei in the somatic sensory pathways (see Chapter 7). The output from the VPL and VPM nuclei ascends to the somatic sensory region of the cerebral cortex in the postcentral gyrus of the parietal lobe.

The ventral lateral nucleus, a cerebellar relay nucleus (see Chapter 8), receives a major projection from the contralateral dentate nucleus of the cerebellum through the fields of Forel. The ventral lateral nucleus in turn projects to the motor cortex in the precentral gyrus of the frontal lobe.

The ventral anterior nucleus is the termination point of a projection from the globus pallidus through the fields of Forel, so it is a part of the basal ganglion circuit (see Chapter 8). The ventral anterior nucleus connects to the premotor regions of the frontal lobe.

The medial dorsal nucleus is a specific nucleus of the medial thalamus. It receives inputs from the amygdaloid nucleus and the hypothalamus, and it projects among other places to the orbitofrontal and prefrontal regions of the cerebral cortex. The medial dorsal nucleus is part of the limbic system (see Chapter 10).

The anterior thalamic nuclei are also a part of the limbic system. A major projection to the anterior nuclei is from the mamillary body by way of the mamillothalamic tract. The anterior nuclei connect with the cingulate gyrus.

The nonspecific thalamic nuclei include the several intralaminar nuclei. They receive inputs from a variety of sources, including the reticular formation, basal ganglia, cerebellum, and other thalamic nuclei, and they project diffusely to the cortex or to the basal ganglia.

The association nuclei include the dorsal tier of the

lateral thalamic nuclei: the pulvinar, lateral posterior and lateral dorsal nuclei. These nuclei are most importantly interconnected with association areas of the parietal, temporal, and occipital lobes of the cerebral cortex.

Some thalamic nuclei also project to subcortical structures and so can be classified as subcortical thalamic nuclei. One example is the reticular nucleus, which receives connections from various thalamic nuclei and from the cerebral cortex and projects back to thalamic nuclei. The intralaminar nuclei also have intrathalamic projections.

Precise and comprehensive descriptions of the thalamus are made difficult by the fact that many of the thalamic nuclei have indistinct cytoarchitectural boundaries. This has led to their being classified in different ways and with different terminology. Walker's Anglo-American terminology is the most widely used; it has been followed by most anatomists and is used in this text. Hassler has made a more extensive parcellation of thalamic nuclei in humans and has considerably modified the Anglo-American terminology. In some cases the nuclei of these two classifications are identical, but many of them are not. In particular, in Hassler's classification the lateral thalamic motor and sensory relay nuclei are divided somewhat differently than in the Anglo-American terminology. Hassler's parcellation correlates well with functional effects of stimulation and destruction of the different lateral nuclei carried out for the treatment of move-

Table 6-5. Probable identities of some nuclei of the lateral thalamus.

Hassler's terminology	Anglo-American terminology
LPO (lateropolaris)	VA (ventral anterior)
VOA (ventralis oralis anterior)	VL (anterior basal part of ventral lateral)
VOP (ventralis oralis posterior)	VL (posterior basal part of ventral lateral)
DO (dorsalis oralis)	VL (dorsal part of ventral lateral)
VIM (ventralis intermedius)	VP or VIM (possibly vestibular and reticular projections)
VC (ventralis caudalis)	VP (ventral posterior)

ment disorders and for pain relief in humans. Table 6-5 shows the probable identities of clinically important nuclei of the Anglo-American and Hassler's classifications. However, much of the work on which the Anglo-American terminology is based was carried out in monkeys; therefore, the homologies of these nuclei with nuclei in humans as described by Hassler is uncertain.

Epithalamus (Figs. 6-7, 6-12, and 6-15). Included in the epithalamus are the stria medullaris, the habenular trigone, the habenular commissure, the posterior commissure, and the pineal gland.

The habenular nucleus is located in the habenular trigone. Fibers in the stria medullaris connect septal, preoptic, and anterior thalamic areas with the

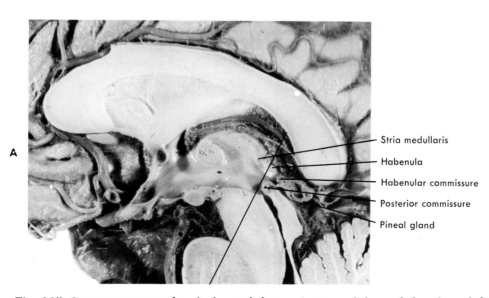

Fig. 6-15. Structures associated with the epithalamus. **A,** View of the medial surface of the brain, cut in sagittal section. The epithalamic structures shown are the stria medullaris, habenular area, habenular commissure, posterior commissure, and pineal gland. Note the cysts in the pineal gland. The line indicates the orientation of the section in **B,** which shows the stria medullaris and the habenular nucleus.   *Continued.*

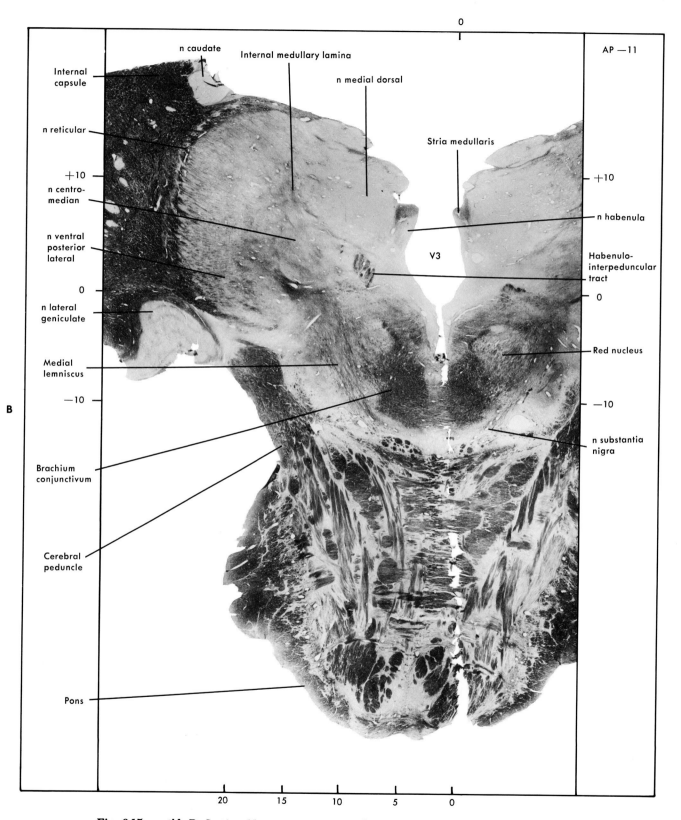

Fig. 6-15, cont'd. B, Section 11 mm posterior to midpoint of anteroposterior commissure line.

habenular nucleus of each side; the crossing fibers pass through the habenular commissure. Efferent fibers from the habenular nucleus enter the habenulopeduncular tract and end in the interpeduncular nucleus located between the cerebral peduncles of the midbrain.

The posterior commissure contains fibers interconnecting the superior colliculi and the pretectal areas.

The pineal gland is attached by a stalk to the habenular and posterior commissures. The endocrine functions of the pineal gland include inhibition of the gonads by secretion of a hormone called melatonin. One feature of clinical interest is the tendency of the pineal gland to calcify with age so that it is visible on x-ray films of the skull in about 70% of adults. This provides a landmark of value in the radiologic diagnosis of lateral shifts of the brain due to mass lesions.

Subthalamus (Figs. 6-11 and 6-13). The subthalamus is a part of the diencephalon that is buried within the substance of the brain and therefore cannot be seen from the external surface. Its components include the subthalamic nucleus, the zona incerta, and the fields of Forel. The subthalamic nucleus is an almond-shaped nucleus found adjacent to the internal capsule in a position just rostral to the substantia nigra. The connections of the subthalamic nucleus are with the basal ganglia and are described in Chapter 8. The zona incerta and other nuclear areas within the subthalamus are sometimes regarded as a diencephalic continuation of the reticular formation. The fields of Forel are the white matter of the subthalamus. Fiber tracts passing through the fields of Forel include the projections to the thalamus from the cerebellum and the basal ganglia. These will also be discussed in Chapter 8.

Hypothalamus (Figs. 6-13 and 6-16 to 6-19). The hypothalamus is located ventral to the hypothalamic sulcus of the third ventricle. The caudal boundary of the hypothalamus is the mamillary body, and the rostral boundary is the lamina terminalis. The optic chiasm and the anterior commissure are landmarks associated with the rostral boundary of the hypothalamus. The hypothalamus can be subdivided into four caudorostral zones: the mamillary, median eminence, infundibular, and chiasmal zones. In addition, the preoptic area of the telencephalon is closely related in function and connectivity to the hypothalamus; this is just rostral to the chiasmal area. The hypothalamus can also be subdivided in the transverse plane into lateral and medial areas; the fornix serves as a landmark for this subdivision in the middle region of the hypothalamus.

The paired mamillary bodies mark the caudal extent of the hypothalamus. The posterior nucleus of the hypothalamus lies dorsally and medially at this level.

The medial eminence, or tuber cinereum, lies just rostrally, and the tuberal, dorsomedial, and ventromedial nuclei lie above the median eminence.

The infundibulum, or stalk, of the pituitary gland arises from the floor of the fourth ventricle just rostral to the median eminence.

The optic chiasm is just ventral to the lamina terminalis; above it are the supraoptic, paraventricular, and anterior nuclei of the hypothalamus.

Some of the major fiber systems that connect with the hypothalamus will be mentioned here; further discussion of the connections and functions of the hypothalamus can be found in Chapters 9 and 10.

The hypothalamic nuclei include neurosecretory neurons that are related to the pituitary gland. Some of these nuclei include the supraoptic, paraventricular, and the tuberal nuclei. The supraoptic and paraventricular nuclei project by way of the hypothalamo-hypophyseal tract to the posterior lobe of the pituitary gland (neurohypophysis), where the axons release the antidiuretic and oxytoxic hormones into the circulation. The tuberal nuclei send axons to the median eminence region and infundibular stalk, where the axons liberate releasing factors and inhibitory factors into the pituitary portal circulation to act on cells of the anterior pituitary gland (adenohypophysis).

The projection system of the lateral preoptic and

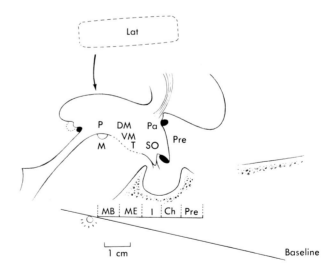

Fig. 6-16. Hypothalamic areas and nuclei. Diagram of major nuclei projected on a midline sagittal section through the third ventricle. Areas: *MB,* mamillary body; *ME,* median eminence; *I,* infundibular; *Ch,* chiasmatic; *Pre,* preoptic. Nuclei: *P,* posterior; *M,* nuclei of mamillary body; *DM,* dorsomedial; *VM,* ventromedial; *T,* tuberal; *Pa,* paraventricular; *SO,* supraoptic; *Pre,* preoptic; *Lat,* lateral area of hypothalamus. Compare with Figs. 5-18, 5-24, 5-25, and 6-18.

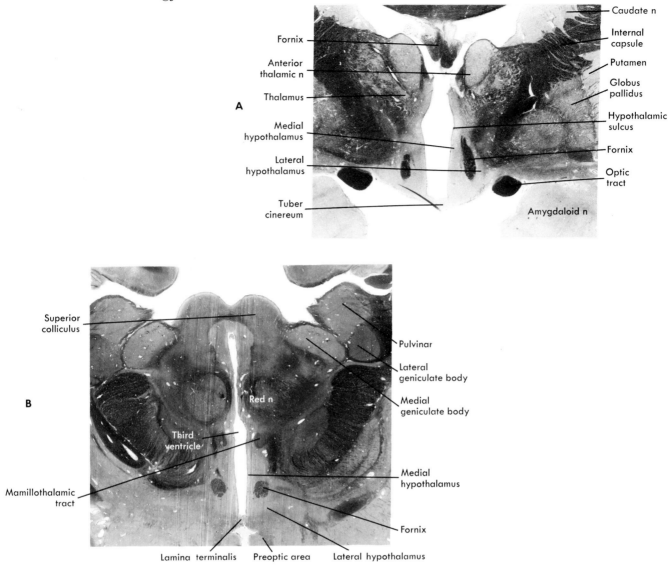

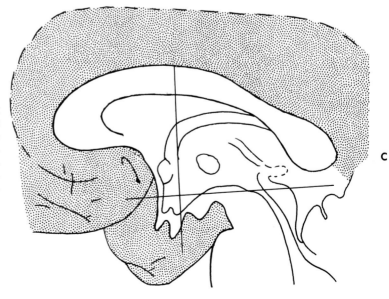

Fig. 6-17. Hypothalamus. Two sections are shown that pass through the hypothalamus. The section in **A** is in the stereotaxic plane, and the one in **B** is in the horizontal plane; the orientation of the sections is shown in **C**. The fornix provides a landmark that subdivides the hypothalamus into lateral and medial regions. The hypothalamic sulcus indicates the boundary between the hypothalamus and the thalamus.

lateral hypothalamic areas is the medial forebrain bundle. Its fibers arise from a number of limbic structures at the base of the frontal lobe surrounding the termination of the olfactory tract. The bundle passes through the lateral preoptic and hypothalamic nuclei,

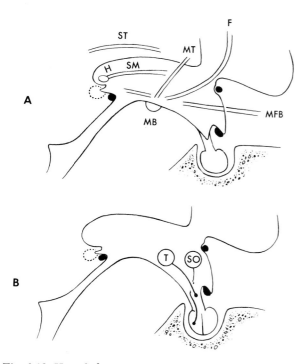

Fig. 6-18. Hypothalamic tracts. **A,** Projection systems: *F,* fornix; *H,* habenular nucleus; *SM,* stria medullaris; *MB,* nuclei of mamillary body; *MT,* mamillothalamic tract (the mamillotegmental tract is not shown); *MFB,* medial forebrain bundle; *ST,* stria terminalis. **B,** Hypothalamic-hypophyseal tracts: *T,* tubero-infundibular tract; *SO,* supraoptic-hypophyseal tract.

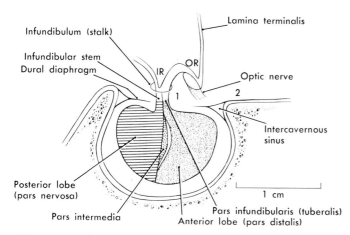

Fig. 6-19. Lobes of the hypophysis and of the infundibulum, sagittal section. Abbreviations: *IR,* infundibular recess; *OR,* optic recess of the third ventricle; *1,* postchiasmatic subarachnoid cistern; *2,* prechiasmatic subarachnoid cistern.

and many fibers ascend, descend, enter, and leave at all levels of the bundle, which appears to extend to the level of the midbrain. Some of the descending connections of the lateral hypothalamic area are in the periaqueductal gray.

The projection systems of the medial preoptic and hypothalamic nuclei are also related to the limbic system. The fornix, mamillothalamic, and mamillotegmental tracts are the most prominent fiber bundles of the medial hypothalamus. The fornix is a dense bundle of fibers that arises in the hippocampal formation. The pair of fornices arch over the third ventricle, just below the corpus callosum, to enter the preoptic area and the hypothalamus by splitting around the anterior commissure. The precommissural fornix projects to the preoptic nuclei and, in lower mammals, to septal nuclei. The postcommissural fornix descends through the medial hypothalamus to end in the mamillary nuclei. The mamillothalamic tract has already been described; it connects the mamillary nuclei with the anterior nuclei of the thalamus and is often seen in the same sections with the fornix. The mamillotegmental tract projects to the midbrain.

Telencephalon

The telencephalon consists of the two cerebral hemispheres and the corpus callosum, which interconnects them. Each cerebral hemisphere consists of an outer zone of gray matter, the cerebral cortex, subjacent white matter, and deep nuclei called the basal ganglia. The neurons within the cerebral hemisphere are connected with the diencephalon, brainstem, and spinal cord through fiber tracts that are contained in the internal capsule, the fornix, the medial forebrain bundle, and other structures.

Basal ganglia (Figs. 6-9 and 6-20)

The term basal ganglia is often used with reference not only to the nuclear masses deep within the telencephalon, but also to structures in the diencephalon and midbrain that are functionally related to the telencephalic nuclei, such as the subthalamic nucleus and the substantia nigra. In a more restricted sense, the basal ganglia are just the telencephalic nuclei, including the caudate nucleus, putamen, and globus pallidus (pallidum), which are related to the neocortex (see below). The claustrum should probably be included among the basal ganglia, presuming that it relates to the insular cortex. The amygdaloid nucleus can also be considered a basal ganglion, but related to the limbic cortex. From a phylogenetic standpoint, the amygdaloid nucleus would be regarded as the archistriatum, the pallidum

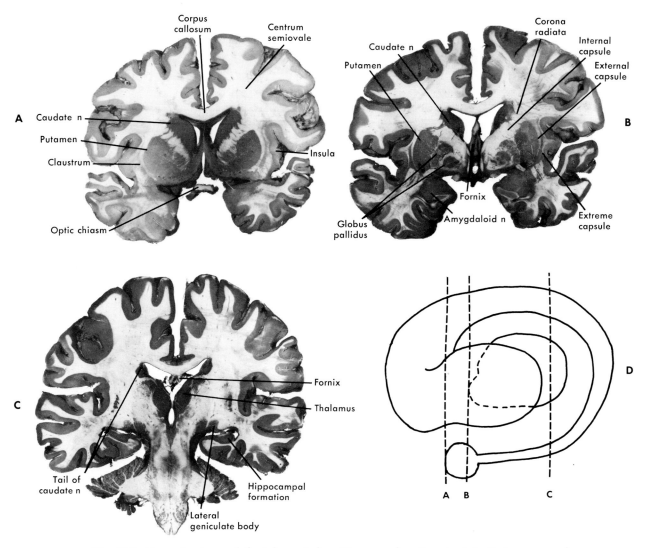

Fig. 6-20. Deep structures of the telencephalon. The coronal sections in **A** to **C** show some of the deep structures of the telencephalon, including the basal ganglia. The approximate levels of the sections are indicated on the drawing of the basal ganglia in **D**. The basal ganglia include the caudate nucleus, putamen, globus pallidus, and claustrum. Telencephalic white matter includes the centrum semiovale, the corpus callosum, the corona radiata, the internal, external, and extreme capsules, and the fornix.

as the paleostriatum, and the caudate and putamen as the neostriatum.

The connections of the basal ganglia associated with the neocortex are discussed in Chapter 8; those of the amygdaloid nucleus are considered in Chapter 10. What follows is a general description of the topography of the basal ganglia.

The caudate nucleus derives its name from the fact that it has a tail in addition to a head. The head of the caudate nucleus is rostral to the foramen of Monro and bulges into the lateral ventricle, forming the lateral wall of the ventricle and the medial boundary of the anterior limb of the internal capsule. The caudate narrows to a taillike structure that runs dorsolateral to the thalamus and then curves ven-

trally and then rostrally again to course in the roof of the inferior horn of the lateral ventricle. The tail of the caudate nucleus terminates at the amygdaloid nucleus.

The putamen is a large nucleus that, along with the pallidum, is located along the lateral margin of the internal capsule. The putamen resembles the caudate in cytoarchitecture, and in fact the two are continuous rostrally by way of cellular bridges across and under the anterior limb of the internal capsule. These cellular bridges give the basal ganglia at this level a striated appearance; hence the name striatum is often applied to the combination of caudate nucleus and putamen. The term corpus striatum includes these two nuclei and also the pallidum.

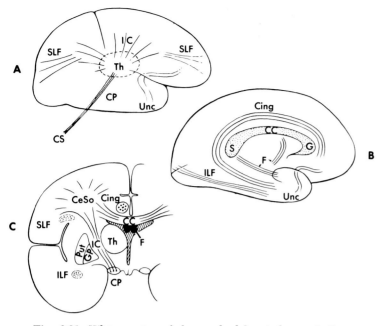

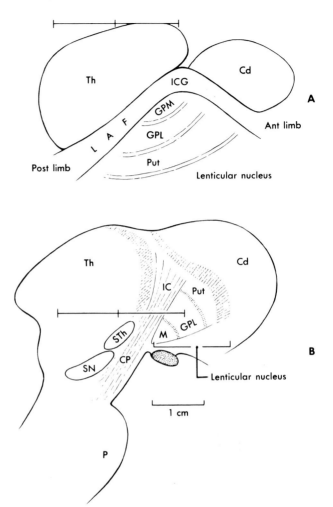

Fig. 6-21. White matter of the cerebral hemispheres. **A,** Lateral; **B,** medial aspects of the cerebral hemisphere; **C,** frontal section of the cerebrum near the anterior-posterior midpoint of the intercommissural line. Projection fibers: *IC,* internal capsule; *CP,* cerebral peduncle; *CS,* corticospinal tract; *F,* fornix. Long intracortical (association) fibers: *Cing,* cingulum; *ILF,* inferior longitudinal fasciculus; *SLF,* superior longitudinal fasciculus; *Unc,* uncinate fasciculus. Commissural fibers; *CC,* corpus callosum; *G,* genu; *S,* splenium. Other abbreviations: *CeSo,* centrum semiovale; *GP,* globus pallidus; *Put,* putamen; *Th,* thalamus.

The globus pallidus is located just medial to the putamen. It is subdivided into two parts, an outer segment and an inner segment. The combined putamen and pallidum is often called the lentiform (lens-shaped) nucleus.

The claustrum is a sheet of gray matter located just lateral to the putamen. The layer of white matter between the claustrum and the putamen is called the external capsule, whereas that superficial to the claustrum is the extreme capsule. The extreme capsule is just subjacent to the cortex of the insula.

The amygdaloid nucleus is in the temporal lobe and is located at the tip of the inferior horn of the lateral ventricle. In this position, it is directly ventral to the lentiform nucleus.

White matter of hemispheres

The subcortical white matter can be divided into the commissures that connect the hemispheres, the ascending and descending projection fibers that connect the hemispheres with subcortical areas, and the intracortical projection fibers, often called association fibers (Fig. 6-21).

Fig. 6-22. Relationships of the limbs of the internal capsule to the thalamus and the caudate and lenticular nucleus. **A,** Composite diagram of several sections of the periventricular area of the right cerebrum cut in the horizontal plane around the level of the intercommissural line, viewed from above. See **B** and Fig. 5-18 for orientation. The position of the intercommissural line is shown along the midline of the brain. Composite diagram of sagittal sections at various distances lateral to the midline of the brain. Nuclei: *Cd,* caudate; *P,* pons; *Put,* putamen; *GPM, GPL,* globus pallidus, medial and lateral segments; *M,* globus pallidus medial segment; *SN,* substantia nigra; *STh,* subthalamic nucleus; *Th,* thalamus. Fibers: *IC,* internal capsule; *G,* genu; *CP,* cerebral peduncle; *F, A, L,* location of motor fibers for facial, arm, and leg movement found on the basis of stimulation during stereotaxic surgery (Bertrand, G., Blundell, J., and Musella, R.: J. Neurosurg. **22:**333-343, 1965). The motor fibers found in such studies are located more posteriorly in the posterior limb of the internal capsule than had previously been described on the basis of neuropathological studies.

The major commissures are the corpus callosum, the anterior commissure, and the commissure of the fornix. They tend to connect homologous points in each hemisphere. The rostral portion of the corpus callosum is the genu (knee), and the caudal portion is the splenium (having a bandaged appearance). The callosal fibers penetrating the rostral portion of the hemisphere from the genu are the forceps minor; the caudally directed fibers of the splenium are the forceps major, and a stratum of these fibers running over the lateral ventricle is the tapetum.

The ascending and descending projection fibers form a raylike pattern, which can be appreciated when the overlying gray matter is removed. These fibers are called the corona radiata. The internal capsule is the funnel of these fibers, which passes downward between the caudate nucleus and thalamus medially and the lentiform nucleus of the basal ganglia laterally (Fig. 6-22). When cut in a horizontal section, the funnel of internal capsular fibers can be seen to be bent into a V shape by the laterally placed mass of the lenticular nucleus (Figs. 6-9 and 6-22, A). The medially directed point of the V is the genu. The anterior limb of the internal capsule lies between the lentiform nucleus (putamen and globus pallidus) and the caudate nucleus of the basal ganglia. The posterior limb lies between the lentiform nucleus and the thalamus. The posterior limb contains ascending projections to the sensory cortex and descending projections from the motor cortex. The structure of the corona radiata and internal capsule is complex. The main fiber bundles are the thalamic peduncles of reciprocal thalamocortical projections composed of corticopetal sensory pathways and the descending corticofugal projections to the thalamus. Fibers projecting to the brainstem and spinal cord also descend in the internal capsule and funnel into the cerebral peduncles.

The fornix, which lies under the corpus callosum for part of its course, can be considered to be largely a descending projection system of the hippocampal formation of the limbic cortex, although it also has commissural and intracortical components (see Chapter 10).

The intracortical projection fibers consist of long fasciculi and short arcuate (U-shaped) fibers. The terminal anatomy and function of the long tracts have not been studied as extensively in humans as perhaps they should be, considering the probable functional importance of these tracts. The major long tracts are the superior longitudinal fibers that extend from the frontal to occipital poles of the hemisphere, the inferior longitudinal fibers from the temporal to occipital pole, the uncinate fibers from the frontal to

temporal poles, and the cingulum, a tract within the cingulate cortex. The short arcuate fibers run beneath sulci to connect adjacent gyri.

The mass of the white matter under the surface of the frontal and parietal lobes on either side of the corpus callosum is called the centrum semiovale. This mass of white matter can become quite swollen following various types of injury to the brain, resulting in herniation of the cingulate gyrus laterally under the falx and of the parahippocampal gyrus and uncus downward through the incisura of the tentorium.

CEREBRAL CORTEX
Structure

The cortex is characterized by its laminar structure and by its vertical and horizontal fiber organization. The cells of the cortex lie in horizontal laminae, or strata (Fig. 6-23). The cells within the laminae are of at least two types, pyramidal and stellate. The pyramidal and stellate cells in a lamina tend to be similar to others of that lamina in terms of size and structure;

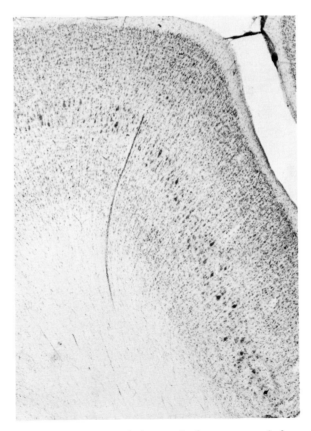

Fig. 6-23. Lamination of the cerebral neocortex of the cat. Sagittal section through the motor cortex (the anterior sigmoid gyrus) and the cruciate sulcus (right side of figure) of the cat. Nissl stain. Note the paucity of neurons in lamina I and the large pyramidal neurons of the motor cortex (Betz cells) of lamina V. Compare with Fig. 6-26.

Table 6-6. Cellular and fiber structure of the cortical laminae

Layer	Main constituents	
	Cells	Fibers
1	Few; horizontal cell somata and dendrites; apical dendrites of pyramidal cells of deeper layers	Tangential plexus of axons of cells in deeper layers; commissural, nonspecific, and specific axons
2, 3	Pyramidal—small, medium, and a few large pyramidal cells Stellate—basket and double bouquet cells	Stripe of Kaes-Bechterew; nonspecific axonal plexus; some specific afferent fibers
4	Stellate—basket and double dendritic bouquet cells	Outer stripe of Baillarger; specific axonal plexus
5	Pyramidal—giant and large pyramidal cells with recurrent ascending axons	Inner band of Baillarger
6	Fusiform cells with recurrent ascending axons	Deep plexus

so there are laminae in which the predominant cells are small, medium, or large-sized pyramids and stellate cells (Table 6-6). The apical dendrites of the pyramidal cells extend vertically through adjacent laminae, bringing them into contact with axons of cells of several laminae and with extrinsic axons ending in adjacent laminae. Vertically projecting axons, particularly of stellate cells, appear to be associated with the apical dendrites of pyramidal neurons. Groups of pyramidal cells of different laminae, lying within the same vertical slab of cortex, and vertically ascending axons appear to form cell columns that are functionally related to a peripheral receptive field or a group of muscles. Horizontally projecting axons of stellate cells and horizontally running afferent fibers traverse these vertical cell columns.

The structure of the cortex appears to be designed for obtaining multiple access to the efferent pyramidal neurons through a variety of pathways ending on different portions of their somata and dendrites, with a wide variety of spatial and temporal interactions of these inputs being possible.

Cortical neurons

The cortical neurons can be divided most simply into pyramidal cells and stellate cells on the basis of the structure of their somata and dendrites on silver stains (Fig. 6-24). The pyramidal cells are vertically oriented cells. They have a pyramidal soma and a vertically oriented apical dendrite that ascends toward the pia for a variable distance before branching. Several basilar dendrites are given off more or less

horizontally near the basilar axon hillock region of the cell. Dendrites may also arise from almost any point on the perikaryon. The dendrites have prominent spines. The dendritic field (the area encompassed by the dendrites of a pyramidal cell) is usually circular or oval when regarded in a horizontal section parallel to the pial surface. The pyramidal cells vary greatly in size from the giant cells of layer 5 of the motor cortex (often referred to as Betz cells, after the Russian anatomist V. A. Betz) to small pyramidal cells.

The stellate cells have a spherical soma and a number of moderately branched dendrites, which are often devoid of spines. These cells have also been called granule cells. The appearance of these cells is illustrated in Figs. 6-24 and 6-25. These two basic types of cells can be subclassified, according to the projections of their axons, into those cells with axons that descend into the white matter, which can be considered efferent cells, and into those with axons that project intracortically, either in a horizontal or an ascending fashion, which can be considered interneurons. Some cells have both types of projection, with descending axons giving off a recurrent collateral. In general, the cells with efferent axons are largely pyramidal cells, and those with purely intracortical projections are stellate cells.

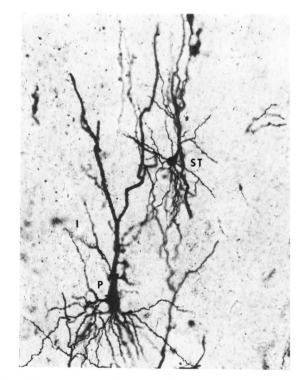

Fig. 6-24. Pyramidal *(P)* and stellate *(ST)* cells of the neocortex. Motor cortex of the cat. Golgi-Cox stain. Vertical calibration bar, 10 μm.

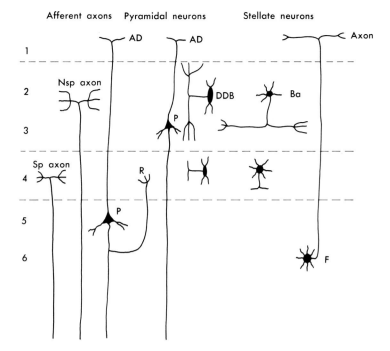

Fig. 6-25. Major patterns of distribution of afferent axons, pyramidal neurons, and stellate neurons in neocortical laminae. Abbreviations: *Sp, Nsp,* specific and nonspecific axons; *P,* pyramidal neuron; *AD,* apical dendrite; *R,* recurrent axon collateral. Types of stellate neurons; *DDB,* double dendritic bouquet neuron; *Ba,* basket neuron; *F,* fusiform neuron. Nonspecific and specific axons are actually distributed more widely throughout the layers of the cortex than is shown in this simplified diagram.

Certain subgroups of cells can be distinguished in the stellate cell category on the basis of their structure, their axonal projections, and their tendency to lie largely in a particular cortical lamina. The cells with double dendritic bouquets, sprays of dendrites at their upper and lower poles, lie largely in the second and third cortical layers. The predominant cells of the sixth layer, which are fusiform in shape and appear to have many ascending axons, may be stellate cells. Other authors consider them to be inverted pyramidal cells.

Cortical glial cells

Glial cells appear to participate in the electrical activity of all parts of the central nervous system. A complete description of the functional anatomy of any area should include a description of the glia. However, a discussion of the anatomy and physiology of glia as related to neuronal activity is given only for the cortex, because most investigations of mammalian glial electrophysiology have been carried out on the cortex. There is also reason to believe that the role of glia may be relatively more important for cortical neuronal functioning because of the high metabolic rate of the cortex and the complexity of the cortical neuropil as compared with some other areas of the nervous system.

There are more glial cells than neurons in the human cortex, although in less complex brains, such as those of rodents, the reverse is thought to be the case. Glia develop in large numbers in the ontogeny of the cortex after the basic neural architecture has developed. The increased numbers of glia appear to be particularly associated with the growth of the dendritic and axonal processes of neurons and with the onset of myelination, which is a function of oligodendrocytes. The ratio of glia to neurons in the human cortex has been estimated as about 2:1 or even higher. Detailed data about the structure of human glial cells are not available. In the cat cortex there are slightly greater numbers of oligodendrocytes than astrocytes. The oligodendrocytes are found as intrafascicular cells, lying between bundles of nerve fibers in the white matter, and as perineuronal satellite cells. There are no specializations of the membranes between the somata of oligodendrocytes and neurons or between the somata of astrocytes and neurons. The function of the oligodendrocytes as satellite cells of neuronal perikarya is unknown. The myelin wrappings of axons are formed of spirally wound, compacted oligodendroglial membranes. Whether satellite oligodendroglia are related to axons adjacent to neuronal somata, or whether they have functions directly related to the neuronal soma, is unknown.

The astrocytes are slightly larger than the oligodendroglia but are still quite small cells. In the cat cortex they have a diameter of about 8 to 10 μm, with about six main processes coming off the soma. Astrocytes are fairly evenly distributed in the different cortical layers. A layer of glial processes bounds the surface of the cortex beneath the layer of pial cells. Cortical capillaries are largely, but not completely, ensheathed by glial processes, the perivascular glia limitans. Neuronal processes and oligodendroglia can be in contact with the areas of basement membrane of cortical capillaries not covered by astrocytic processes.

The microglia comprise about 10% of the cortical glia and tend to be found in perivascular and subpial locations.

Cortical laminae

Despite its clearly laminated appearance on Nissl staining, the exact number of laminae in individual cortical areas is not always obvious. The laminae tend to blend into each other, especially on silver stains. Most investigators have distinguished six layers (Fig. 6-26). However, five to seven and even more layers have been proposed. Their cellular and fiber structure are summarized in Table 6-6.

The afferent input to the cortex appears to ramify in axonal plexuses largely in the middle and upper layers of the cortex. The nonspecific afferents are distributed more superficially than the specific afferents and appear to be in part the fibers from the nonspecific thalamic nuclei. The specific afferents are the axons of the efferent neurons of the specific thalamic nuclei. However, there is insufficient information concerning both the cells of origin and the sites of termination of axons designated as specific and nonspecific. Another set of cortical afferents arises from neurons in layer 3 of the comparable cortical area on the contralateral side. These commissural fibers cross in the corpus callosum and terminate in layers 1 to 4. Similar connections are made by cortical association fibers, which connect cortical neurons within the same hemisphere. The terminals of these commissural and corticocortical fibers are distributed in sprays that appear to relate to the columnar organization of the cortex. Interneurons with horizontally ramifying axons also lie in the middle and upper layers. The efferent output of the cortex appears to come largely from the middle and deep layers. Recurrent ascending axons also come from cells in the deep layers.

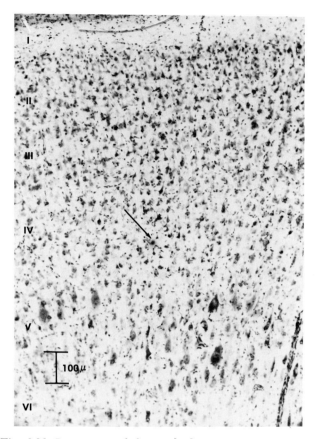

Fig. 6-26. Lamination of the cerebral neocortex. Motor cortex of the cat. Nissl stain. Lamina IV has been marked with a spot of fast green dye *(arrow)*, which was iontophoretically ejected from a micropipette tip (see Techniques, Appendix I).

Intracortical and afferent axon terminations

Axons of many intracortical neurons appear to end on somata and proximal dendritic trunks of pyramidal cells and to form synapses of the symmetrical type.

Many of the afferent axons end on spines of pyramidal neurons. These form asymmetric synapses with a wide synaptic cleft and a dense postsynaptic membrane. These are the type I of Gray's classification. It has been suggested that the intracortical axons that have synaptic terminals with flattened vesicles that end on somata of pyramidal cells are inhibitory interneurons, and the afferent axons that end on spines of dendrites are excitatory afferents.

The basic circuit of the cerebral cortex, the sequence in which cortical cells are involved by afferent activity entering the cortex, cannot be specified yet. In this respect the analysis of the cerebellar and hippocampal cortices is far more advanced than that of the cerebral cortex. However, it appears likely that specific afferent fibers can make monosynaptic contacts with the somata and dendrites of pyramidal cells in layers 3 and 4. Specific afferent fibers also influence pyramidal cells by way of stellate interneurons. Nonspecific afferents are probably related to pyramidal cells and stellate cells in a similar manner. The electrophysiological effects thought to be produced by these connections are discussed later in this chapter.

It must be remembered that detailed investigation of cortical cell types and of the fine structure of the cortex has been made in comparatively few species, largely in the rodent and the cat, and in only a few areas of the cortex. The sensory-motor and visual cortices have been the most intensively studied areas. The extent to which these findings are applicable to the human cortex is not clear, because the fine structure of the human cortex has not been studied in as much detail.

Cortical cytoarchitectonic areas

The layers of the cortex are of different thicknesses and have different cytological appearances in different parts of the cortex. Numerous attempts have been made to classify cortical areas on the basis of these differences, usually using Nissl-stained sections of the cortex (cytoarchitectonics) and in some cases myelin-stained sections (myeloarchitectonics). Several different terminologies, such as those of Brodmann and Vogt, have been used to express these differences.

The greater portion of the cortex, which can be considered to have six layers, is called the isocortex (equal cortex) in Vogt's terminology. The largest portion of the isocortex is called the eulaminate (well-layered) cortex in the terminology of Bailey and von Bonin. This is essentially the cortex of the frontal, temporal, and parietal lobes, which has layers of fairly balanced thickness and which is neither specific sensory nor

motor. The sensory cortices have thick second and fourth layers that contain many stellate (granular) cells. The second and fourth layers are also known as the outer and inner granular layers respectively. The appearance of the small cells in these layers when viewed through a lower power light microscope suggested the name koniocortex (dust cortex) for the sensory cortices. Axonal plexuses of afferent fibers make prominent horizontal stripes of fibers in the second and fourth layers of the sensory cortices. The axonal plexus of lateral geniculate fibers in the fourth layer of the visual cortex is quite prominent. It appears as a distinct white band in the gray matter of the calcarine cortex. This stripe is known in the visual cortex as the line of Gennari or of Vicq d'Azyr. It is homologous with the outer stripe of Baillarger of other areas. This stripe can be used to identify the calcarine cortex when the brain is sectioned grossly, as is often done in the first stage of a neuropathological examination of a brain.

The motor cortex has less prominent second and fourth granular layers and has large pyramidal cells in the fifth layer. The motor cortex is called the agranular cortex.

The cortex of the medial border of the temporal lobe, the area of the parahippocampal gyrus and the hippocampal formation (dentate gyrus and Ammon's horn, or the hippocampus proper), which are part of the synthetic limbic lobe, and the orbitofrontal cortex around the olfactory tract differ from the isocortex in a number of ways. These cortices were designated allocortex (other cortex) by Vogt. The allocortex is characterized in part by having a superficial layer of myelinated fibers. There is a gradation in laminar

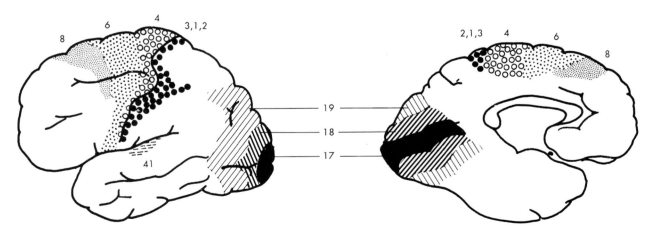

Fig. 6-27. Brodmann areas. Some of the more commonly referred to Brodmann areas are shown on the lateral and medial views of the cerebral hemisphere. Area 4 is in the precentral gyrus; area 3,1,2 is in the postcentral gyrus. Area 17 is the cortex above and below the calcarine fissure, and areas 18 and 19 surround area 17. Area 41 consists of the transverse temporal gyri.

Table 6-7. Areas often designated by Brodmann's numbers

Cortical area	Brodmann number
Motor-precentral frontal	4
Premotor frontal	6
Rostral frontal	8, 9, 10
Sensory-postcentral parietal	1, 2, 3
Visual-occipital	17
Paravisual-occipital	18, 19
Auditory-temporal	41

structure of the allocortex, from the lateral portions to the most medial portion, which is the hippocampal formation. The dentate gyrus and hippocampus proper (Ammon's horn) can be regarded as having only three layers, only one of which is a layer of large pyramidal cells. The allocortex of the parahippocampal gyrus and the hippocampal formation are regarded as phylogenetically older than the isocortex. In Kappers' terminology the parahippocampal gyrus cortex is the paleocortex (old, ancient cortex); the hippocampal formation is called the archicortex (first cortex); and the isocortex is the neocortex.

Types of cortex intermediate in structure between those described here can also be distinguished. The cytoarchitectural maps made in the earlier part of this century subdivided the major types of cortex into many areas. Brodmann's map, which is the most widely reproduced, contains 52 areas. This map provides a convenient way of referring to parts of the cortex. Cortical areas and the Brodmann numbers frequently used to designate them are given in Table 6-7. Although some correlations of cytoarchitecture and function can be drawn, further analysis of the cortex appears to require other methods of study.

Localization of function in the cortex

The presence of different cytoarchitectural areas of the cortex, which in the cases of at least the sensory cortices and the motor cortex can be correlated with specific thalamocortical projection systems and specific functions, has led to the concept of the localization of different functions in different cortical areas. The concept of localization of function is extremely old and must have been held even in ancient times by physicians who cared for the wounded. The Edwin Smith surgical papyrus, circa 1600 BC, contains descriptions of paralysis following head and spinal cord injuries. The manuscript contains a series of rules to guide the surgeon, leading him to the conclusions: "Thou shouldst say . . . 'an ailment I will treat,' or 'an ailment not to be treated'." However, it is interesting that, despite the vivid descriptions of

wounds in the *Iliad*, a persuasive argument can be made that the ancient Greeks regarded the thoracic cavity, which contained the vital pneuma, or air, as the site of the phrenos, rather than the brain, perhaps because most persons tend to localize their emotional sensations to the area of the chest cavity.

In the early nineteenth century the concept of localization of function in the cortex was developed in detail by the German anatomist Gall to include localization of complex, or higher, functions. The doctrine that the mental faculties are located in distinct cortical areas is the essence of the doctrine of phrenology (phrenos, mind; logos, discourse). Inasmuch as the development of the shape of the skull is largely caused by molding by the developing brain, it was not at all illogical to consider that an individual's mental faculties could be estimated by palpation and measurement of the size of the prominences of the skull. This concept was popularized by Gall's student Spurzheim.

In operational terms localization of function means that during the occurrence of a function, related cellular activity can be recorded in a particular brain area, or that ablation of the area uniquely disrupts that function, or that stimulation of the area uniquely evokes that function. When the experimental data on which the concept of localization of function is based are regarded in terms of this definition, it is apparent that the localizations of many functions are not unique to specific brain areas. Instead there are multiple areas of representation, which perhaps were developed to provide safety factors, and there is also considerable overlap of functional areas.

Multiple representation can be seen clearly in the somatic sensory system. If the skin is stimulated and recording is carried out in the postcentral cortex, specific groups of cells will be found to be most responsive to stimulation of specific parts of the body. There is a topographic, or point-to-point, correspondence of the body surface, of the retina, and of the cochlea, with the respective primary sensory cortices. There is a distortion of the area of the receptive field in these topographic projections, because certain parts of the body, such as the lips, fingers, and macula, have greater areal representation in the cortex than do other parts of the receptive surface. A figure called a homunculus (little man) can be drawn whose bodily parts are in proportion to the size of the cortical area related to that part. The homunculus can be used to illustrate the relative areal representation of parts of the body in the cortex (Fig. 7-12). A similar motor homunculus can be constructed, showing the parts of the body that move when the precentral cortex is stimulated. These homunculi in the precentral and postcentral cortex are dangling upside down, with their feet on the mesial side of the hemisphere, their arms in midconvexity, and their faces just above the lateral (sylvian) fissure. However, if the procedures of cortical sensory and motor mapping are carried out over the entire cortex, other areas are found that also respond to appropriate stimulation. In the case of the somatic sensory system a second receptive area can be mapped out. In humans this area lies in the parietal operculum bordering the sylvian fissure. It receives input from the ipsilateral as well as from the contralateral side of the body and has intracortical connections with the primary sensory cortex. The auditory and visual cortices have not been investigated as intensively as the somatic sensory cortex in humans, because they are less accessible. However, in animals, click-evoked responses can be recorded with a short latency from a large area of the temporal lobe besides the primary auditory cortex, in which there is a tonotopic representation of the cochlea. The visual system appears to have two cortical topographic representations of the retina. From this brief discussion it can be seen that although there are primary receptive cortical areas, sensory systems also involve wide areas of the cortex.

In an analogous manner, movement of the same muscle can be produced by stimulation of several cortical areas. In addition to the precentral motor homunculus, there are secondary and supplementary motor areas. Eye muscle movements can be evoked not only from the premotor cortex but also from the occipital cortex. This is not to say that the primary and secondary somatic sensory areas are equivalent in function, for there are differences in the responsiveness of the cells in the primary and secondary sensory areas to peripheral sensory stimuli, and in the type of motor activity evoked from different motor areas (see Chapter 7 and 8).

The other aspect of the question of the uniqueness of representation of function is that of overlap of representation. Detailed maps of sensory, motor, and autonomic representation in the human cortex are largely the result of studies of Penfield and his collaborators in Canada. These studies were carried out during the course of craniotomies performed with the patient under local anesthetic for the localization and excision of cortical epileptic foci. The maps of localization of sensory and motor function in the great apes and monkeys are rather similar to those in humans. Many of the studies on nonhuman primates and lower species were carried out by Woolsey and his collaborators. Their work has provided a picture of the evolutionary development of cortical representation in many species. In the lower species there

is considerable overlap of the areas from which movement can be evoked and in which sensory potentials are recorded. These species are often said to have a sensory-motor cortex. Even in humans, stimulation of the precentral cortex evokes a considerable number of subjective sensory responses as well as movement; stimulation of the postcentral cortex evokes movement, although not as frequently as it evokes sensation. Therefore, although the concept of localization of function is valid, the widespread activity of many cortical and subcortical areas in the performance of sensory motor and complex functions must be stressed.

Despite the reservations expressed above, it should be emphasized that certain cortical areas do participate in specific functions, such as the production of volitional activity or the receipt of sensory data. The areas that are known to have such relationships are outlined on the drawing of the cerebral hemisphere in Fig. 6-28. The difficulty is that other areas may have similar roles.

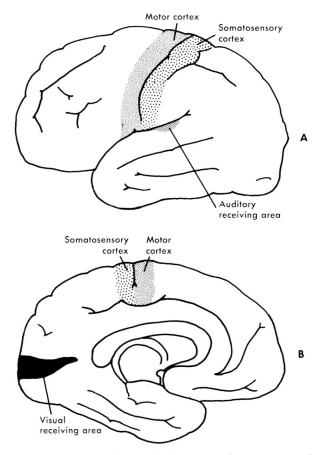

Fig. 6-28. Regions of the cerebral cortex, indicating some of the areas known to have specific functions. **A** shows the functional areas of the lateral aspect of the cerebral hemisphere; **B** shows the medial aspect.

THALAMOCORTICAL ELECTROPHYSIOLOGY
Characteristics of electrocortical activity

Cells of the cerebral cortex exhibit continual fluctuations of membrane potential, which are frequently in synchrony with the potentials of large numbers of adjacent cells, resulting in large extracellular potentials of varying frequency. The electrocorticogram (ECoG) records this activity with a gross electrode. Such an electrode records the summed extracellular postsynaptic and spike potentials generated by aggregates of neuronal somata, dendrites, and axons. The recording, however, reflects largely postsynaptic potentials (PSPs).

The term electrocorticogram should be reserved for recordings made from the surface of the brain, and the term electroencephalogram (EEG) should be used for the conventional clinical recordings made from the scalp. The frequency spectrum of the potentials of the EEG and ECoG are the same, but the amplitude of the EEG is about one tenth that of the ECoG because of attenuation of current produced by recording through the skull and scalp.

The ECoG potentials range from 0.2 to 1 mV in amplitude and have their predominant frequency in the 6- to 20-Hz. range. The individual waves are largely negative-going and wax and wane in amplitude and frequency. Slower potential shifts lasting from seconds to minutes can also be recorded from the cortex. These potential shifts are about the same amplitude as the predominant ECoG waves and are usually associated with changes of the amplitude and frequency of the faster ECoG waves (Fig. 6-29). In addition to fast and slow potentials that can be

recorded from the cortex, a standing, or steady, potential of about 2 mV exists between the cortical surface and the underlying white matter, with the potential from the surface of the cortex recorded as negative. Therefore, cortical electrical activity can be considered to be the spectrum of activity ranging from transcortical steady potential differences to rhythmic potentials of moderate frequency. A similar spectrum of potentials can be recorded from the spinal cord, brainstem, and cerebellar cortex; but electrocortical activity is marked by much greater amplitude, synchrony, and rhythmicity. Large rhythmic electrocortical potentials also occur in sleep and during surgical anesthesia. Rhythmic potentials can be recorded from other parts of the nervous system during sleep and anesthesia, but much of this activity is driven by thalamocortical activity. This type of activity is often called spontaneous because it is present when there are no obvious external stimuli to evoke it. The amplitude and rhythms of electrocortical potentials, however, change with varying states of alertness, and sensory stimulation will evoke specific patterns of electrocortical activity.

Far more is known about basic circuits of the cerebellar cortex and the way in which information is processed in the cerebellum than is known about the cerebral cortex (see Chapter 8). Present research on the cortex is largely directed toward understanding the sequence of activities produced by activation of different afferent pathways to the cortex and toward discovering the neural connections that are involved in generating rhythmic activity. The investigation of the electrophysiology of both individual cells and of aggregates of cells (ECoG activity) is useful in this study. The analysis of the relationship of individual cellular activities in generating ECoG waves is also of considerable practical and theoretical importance.

Properties of cortical neurons

The electrical properties of only one class of cortical neurons have been studied in detail. These are the pyramidal cells with corticofugal axons that project into the cerebral peduncle or medullary pyramid or both. It is possible to identify these cells electrophysiologically when they are penetrated by a micropipette by stimulating their axons in the peduncle or pyramid and antidromically discharging them (Fig. 6-30). Recordings have also been made in other types of cortical cells; but until anatomical marking techniques are more widely used to identify the cells penetrated, and methods are developed to characterize them physiologically, the properties of stellate cells and of the pyramidal cells without descending axons will be less fully known.

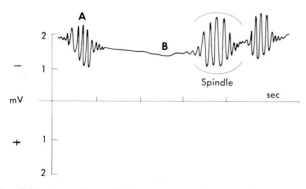

Fig. 6-29. A portion of the spectrum of potentials that can be recorded from the cortical surface with gross electrodes. **A,** Rhythmic potentials generally varying in frequency from about 6 to 20 cycles per second (illustrated here at 10 cycles per second) that wax and wane in amplitude. **B,** A slow potential shift, in a positive direction, of the transcortical potential. The potential shift is shown occurring in association with a decrease in the rhythmic potentials.

The pyramidal cells can be divided into large cells, with large efferent axons, and smaller cells. The largest cells have somata measuring about 20 × 70 μm. Their axons, which descend in the pyramids, conduct impulses with velocities of up to 80 m/sec.

The following discussion of the electrical properties of cortical neurons is confined to the properties of the large pyramidal cells. The membrane potentials of these neurons may be as large as –75 mV in deeply anesthetized animals. The average membrane potential during normal activity is probably lower, about –60 to –65 mV, because of the depolarizing synaptic input that impinges on the cell during normal electrocortical activity. The average input (total) resistance of these neurons is about 7 megohms, and the specific resistance of the membrane has been calculated as about 2,000 ohm-cm². The time constant of the membrane is about 8 msec.

These passive electrical properties of pyramidal cells are qualitatively similar to those of spinal motoneurons (see Chapter 4), although the specific resistance of the membrane is generally higher in pyramidal cells. Therefore the time constant of the membrane is longer.

The generation of action potentials appears to occur at the axon hillock and to spread to the soma and proximal dendrites, generating a spike with an inflection on the rising phase (Fig. 6-30). The action potential is thought to spread into only the proximal portions of the dendrites. It is thought that this accounts for the after-depolarization that often follows the spike. Therefore, generation of spikes in the dendritic membrane, or in portions of the soma other than the axon hillock, does not appear to occur in normal neocortical neurons. However, generation of spikes in dendrites does appear to occur in injured cortical neurons.

The action potential generally reverses polarity, reaching a value of 12 to 20 mV at the peak of the overshoot. The falling phase of the action potential

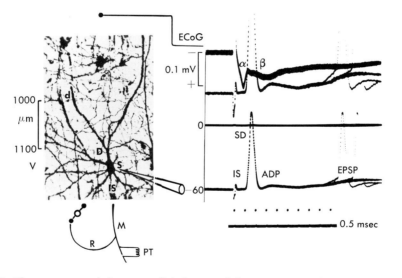

Fig. 6-30. Characteristics of the intracellularly recorded action potentials of a large pyramidal neuron of the motor cortex, following antidromic stimulation of the pyramidal tract, and relationships to the ECoG response recorded from the cortical surface. The morphological structure of the pyramidal neurons is illustrated in the Golgi-Cox–impregnated section of layer V of the cat motor cortex. The depth of the section from the pial surface is indicated by the scale. Note the vertical orientation of the cell soma *(S)*, apical dendrite *(D)*, distant dendritic branches *(d)*, and axon hillock and initial segment *(IS)* of the myelinated axon *(M)*, which descends in the cerebral peduncle and pyramidal tract *(PT)*. The ECoG response evoked by stimulation of the axons of these cells, displayed in the upper trace, consists of two brief positive deflections, α and β. The action potential of the pyramidal neuron is evoked with a latency of 0.8 msec from the baseline resting membrane potential of the cell of –60 mV, without a prepotential. An IS phase and a slightly more rapidly rising SD phase caused by spread of the action potential from the initial segment of the neuron to the soma and proximal dendritic tree can be distinguished. Note the positive-going overshoot of the action potential. A small after-depolarizing potential *(ADP)* follows the action potential. A depolarizing potential *(EPSP)* that evokes an action potential follows the antidromically evoked spike with a latency of 3 msec. A recurrent axon collateral *(R)* and an excitatory interneuron are the minimal circuit that can be involved in generating the EPSP.

can exhibit an after-hyperpolarization that tends to go to the K+ equilibrium potential. These electrophysiological properties of cortical neurons are also similar to those of spinal motoneurons. Many cortical neurons exhibit very little accommodation of their firing when they are depolarized by intracellularly injected currents.

Properties of cortical glia

Intracellular recordings have been made in cortical glial cells, but the types of cells penetrated have not been definitely identified as oligodendrocytes or astrocytes. There are reasons, however, to think that the cells that have very high membrane potentials of –85 to –95 mV are astrocytes. Oligodendrocytes in tissue culture have membrane potentials of –60 to –70 mV, and it is likely that they have high membrane potentials in vivo, too. The membranes of cortical glia, which have high membrane potentials, behave passively during the passage of depolarizing currents through the glial cell, in contrast to the membranes of neurons in which the depolarization produced by the current evokes action potentials (Fig. 6-31). The high membrane potential glia appear to be much more permeable to ions, probably K+ ions, than cortical neurons are. The specific resistance of the membranes of the high membrane potential glia appears to be much less than that of neurons, and the time constant of the membrane is therefore also considerably shorter, being about 0.4 msec.

The dependence of the membrane potential of mammalian glia on the transmembrane concentration

of K+ has been tested by varying the concentration of K+ around glia in optic nerves and in the cortex. A change of potential of about 40 mV for a tenfold change in extracellular K+ concentration was found, which is less than that predicted by the Nernst equation. Whether their membrane potential is determined in part by permeability to other ions, whether mammalian glia are therefore different from invertebrate and amphibian glia in this respect, or whether these results are caused by technical difficulties is not known.

A phenomenon that may be of importance in the functioning of astrocytes is the electrical coupling of cells by the presence of gap junctions of low resistance between them. The muscle cells of the heart are coupled together in a functional syncytium by gap junctions. Gap junctions exist between cortical astrocytes, but the extent to which they electrically couple the cells is unknown. In the optic nerves of amphibia such coupling exists and appears to be functionally important in carrying currents, which can be recorded as slow potentials on the surface of the nerve.

Some of the electrical properties of cortical neurons and glia, as well as their probable ionic content, are illustrated and contrasted in Fig. 6-32.

Activation of cortical neurons

The cortex is normally activated by the afferent fiber systems entering it. These are thalamocortical specific and nonspecific fibers, short and long intracortical fibers, and commissural fibers. The pattern of afferent fiber systems terminating on cortical neurons appears to be much more complex than the climbing-fiber Purkinje cell and the mossy-fiber granule cell glomerulus pattern of termination found in the cerebellum (see Chapter 8); thus, the patterns

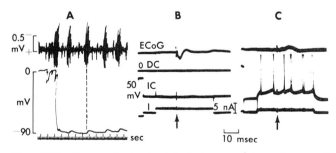

Fig. 6-31. Some electrophysiological properties of cortical neurons and glia. **A**, Glial cell of the cat motor cortex. Small irregular potentials were recorded as the micropipette was advanced for several hundred micra through the cortex, and then a very large membrane potential was recorded as a glial cell was penetrated. The cell exhibited characteristic slow depolarizing potentials in synchrony with spindle-burst activity of the ECoG (upper line). **B**, lack of spikes or PSP response of the glial membrane to the intracellular passage of depolarizing current (I) of about 3 nanoamperes (nA) (fourth line) and to the discharge of thalamocortical afferents (arrow), which evoke a primary ECoG response (first line). **C**, Spike and EPSP responses evoked in a pyramidal tract neuron by intracellular and thalamocortical stimulation.

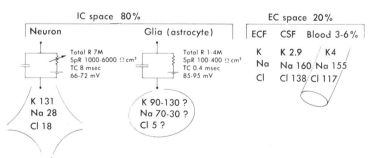

Fig. 6-32. Schematic representation of ranges of values (in mEq/l) for the distribution of some major cations and anions in brain compartments and average values for electrical properties of neurons and glial cells. Data from cat motor cortex. Abbreviations: M, megohms; R, resistance; SpR, specific resistance; TC, time constant.

of activity evoked in cortical neurons following afferent stimulation are correspondingly more variable.

Several types of responses can be recorded from the surface of the cerebral cortex when different afferent pathways to the cortex are stimulated. The most frequently studied response is called the cortical evoked potential. This is produced by stimulation of a sensory pathway or by stimulation of a specific thalamic relay nucleus. The cortical evoked potentials that result from the activation of the visual, auditory, and somatosensory systems are termed visual, auditory, and somatosensory evoked potentials. These are very useful clinically for the study of sensory transmission in patients who cannot describe their sensory experience (for example, infants). The evoked potential consists of an initial primary response, and

there may be a later secondary response. A different type of response is seen when the nonspecific thalamic nuclei are stimulated (see below). Stimulation of the surface of the cerebral cortex results in still another kind of activity called the direct cortical response. Evoked potentials are often used as indicators of cortical function. They undergo complex changes in different states of consciousness and during different stages of anesthesia. Furthermore, they are altered during selective attention and also during habituation to repeated stimulation.

The cortical evoked potentials produced by specific thalamocortical fibers have been studied most thoroughly in the case of the activation of pyramidal tract neurons of the motor cortex activated by stimulation of the cerebellar-dentatothalamic pathway.

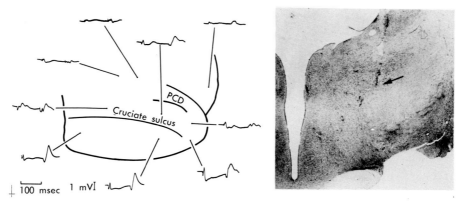

Fig. 6-33. Cortical distribution of primary and augmented response evoked by the first and second stimuli of a train of stimuli delivered at 10/sec to a specific thalamic nucleus in the cat. Note the changes in morphological structure of both the primary response to the first shock and the augmented response to the second shock when recorded from different points on the anterior and posterior sigmoid gyri. *PCD,* postcruciate dimple. The cortex caudal to this point does not contain giant pyramidal cells typical of motor cortex. The site of the stimulating electrode, which was in the ventral lateral nucleus, is shown in the photomicrograph of a frontal section of the thalamus.

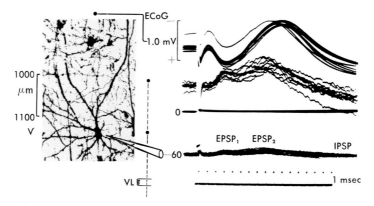

Fig. 6-34. The primary response PSP pattern, evoked in a large pyramidal neuron of the motor cortex, and the primary ECoG response, evoked by stimulation of a specific thalamic nucleus (ventral lateral).

Similar studies have been carried out on visual cortex neurons activated by stimulation of the lateral geniculate body. The results are generally similar, although there are differences in latencies of the potentials evoked in cortical neurons of specific areas following stimulation of the specific thalamic nucleus projecting to it. The majority of these studies have been carried out in the cat, and the results are described here. Studies done with the primate, and the few done with patients with implanted electrodes (see Appendix I) or during the course of neurosurgical procedures, have shown a similar sequence of activities, although the latencies are different and the pattern of potentials evoked can be more complex.

Following stimulation of the cerebellocortical projection in the cat, with single shocks delivered to the ventral lateral (VL) nucleus or to its ascending axons in the internal capsule, cortical neurons are activated with a short latency in the sigmoid gyri, the cortical area corresponding to the motor-sensory cortex of humans (Fig. 6-33). The areas in which responses are evoked by stimulation of the VL nucleus can be mapped by recording activity at successive points over the hemisphere. Short-latency responses of large amplitude are confined to the margins of the sigmoid gyri bordering the cruciate sulcus. The response is maximal, for a particular point of stimulation within the thalamus, in a corresponding small area of the pericruciate cortex. The response becomes smaller toward the boundaries of the pericruciate area. This finding is the functional correlate of a certain degree of topographic, or point-to-point, axonal projections from the specific relay nucleus to the cortex.

The afferent volley evoked by stimulation of the VL nucleus arrives in the cortex after a latency of about 0.7 msec and is signalled by a brief small positive potential recorded extracellularly from the cortical surface (Fig. 6-34). Intracellular recording in large pyramidal tract neurons reveals a series of EPSPs that occur concurrently with the initial large positive and subsequent large negative waves of the evoked potential recorded from the surface of the cortex.

The initial excitatory potential appears to be a monosynaptic EPSP evoked by activity of thalamic axons, for it has a latency of 0.5 to 1.0 msec after the arrival of the thalamocortical afferent volley. A second group of EPSPs has a latency of 3 to 10 msec. These slightly slower EPSPs may be monosynaptically evoked by activity of smaller, slower, thalamocortical fibers, or may be caused by excitation through interneurons. Presumably the different types of stellate cells are the interneurons involved.

The short latency EPSPs are followed by a large,

prolonged IPSP. The sequence of evoked EPSPs followed by IPSPs is the commonest sequence of potentials seen in cortical neurons and in many subcortical nuclei following synchronous activation of their afferent projections by single-shock stimuli. These potentials underlie the primary response of the cortical evoked potential. Stimulation of the afferent projections with shocks of increasing strength evokes progressively larger IPSPs. The shortest latency at which this IPSP can be evoked is 2 msec, although it generally has a latency of about 5 msec. Therefore it is possible that the IPSP is mediated at least in part by a direct thalamocortical inhibitory projection.

An analysis of the role of the different types of axons that project from the VL nucleus to the cortex and that might mediate different portions of the PSP pattern has not been carried out. In the case of spinal motoneurons it has been possible to determine which effects are mediated by afferents of different size by dissecting out and stimulating different peripheral

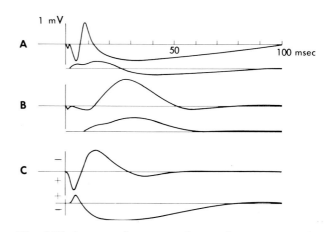

Fig. 6-35. Patterns of response of cortical neurons to thalamocortical and direct cortical stimulation. The upper line of each set of tracings is the ECoG response, and the lower line is a typical PSP pattern recorded in a large pyramidal cell. Action potential (spike) responses that frequently occur at the peaks of the EPSPs have been omitted. **A,** Primary response evoked by stimulation of a specific thalamic nucleus, recorded in the projection area of the nucleus. **B,** Response evoked by nonspecific thalamic stimulation. **C,** Direct cortical response (DCR) evoked by a strong shock to the cortex. The negative wave of the ECoG response is a prominent feature of the DCR. The negative wave appears to be a PSP evoked in superficial dendrites and somata following excitation of presynaptic axons produced by the shock. Only the negative wave is evoked by weak direct cortical stimulation. With stronger stimulation, late positive and then early positive components of the response appear. The intracellular response recorded in the soma of a deep, large pyramidal neuron to a strong cortical shock is a prominent IPSP or an EPSP-IPSP sequence. The vertical scales, as shown in **C,** represent 1 mV for the ECoG response and 5mV for the intracellular potentials.

nerves supplying skin and muscle, or by stimulating the whole nerve and blocking the activity of some fibers. Equivalent techniques have not been perfected for the central nervous system.

Stimulation of the nonspecific thalamic nuclei evokes EPSPs in cortical pyramidal neurons that are of longer latency and are larger than those evoked by stimulation of the specific afferent axons. The latency of the response is generally between 30 and 50 msec. IPSP's are not prominently evoked by nonspecific stimulation (Fig. 6-35, *B*).

Direct cortical stimulation evokes very large, prolonged IPSPs in almost every cortical neuron penetrated. Short-latency EPSPs can precede the IPSP (Fig. 6-35, *C*).

The basic excitatory circuits within the cortex appear to be monosynaptic and polysynaptic connections from afferent axons to pyramidal tract cells and recurrent excitatory pathways. Long-latency EPSPs evoked by specific or nonspecific stimulation might also be caused by polysynaptic pathways within the thalamus that terminate in a projection to the cortex (Fig. 6-36).

The basic inhibitory circuits within the cortex probably engage inhibitory interneurons that lie within the cortex, because IPSPs can be evoked in cortical neurons by direct stimulation of slabs of cortex that have been chronically isolated from afferent input. The inhibitory interneurons appear to be excited to some degree by axon collaterals of pyramidal tract neurons (Fig. 6-37). In addition, there is a possibility of direct inhibitory projections entering a local cortical area either from subcortical loci or from other cortical areas.

Activation of cortical glia

Some glial cells exhibit slow depolarizing and late, slow hyperpolarizing potentials during the course of and following periods of increased activity of adjacent neurons (Fig. 6-38). The glia whose membrane potential levels are responsive to the level of activity

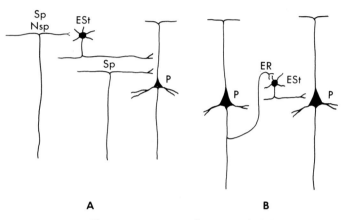

Fig. 6-36. Possible excitatory cortical circuits. **A,** Monosynaptic excitation of pyramidal neurons (*P*) by specific thalamocortical axons (*Sp*), and disynaptic (or polysynaptic) excitation by excitatory stellate neurons (*ESt*). The stellate neurons are probably excited by specific and nonspecific axons. **B,** Recurrent excitation of a pyramidal neuron by a disynaptic pathway involving a recurrent axon collateral (*ER*) and an excitatory stellate neuron (*ESt*). See Fig. 6-30.

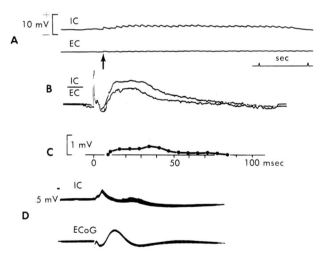

Fig. 6-38. Cortical glial cell potentials evoked by neuronal activity. **A,** Summation of slow glial depolarizations. *IC,* intracellular recording in a glial cell. Steplike depolarizations that summated were evoked in response to each shock of a train of stimuli delivered to the ventrolateral nucleus at a frequency of 8/sec. *EC,* Extracellular recording immediately adjacent to the glial cell. **B,** Intracellularly and extracellularly recorded depolarizations compared. **C,** Algebraic subtraction of IC and EC records shown in **B,** giving the time course of glial depolarization after a single thalamic volley. **D,** Time course of intracellular potentials evoked in a pyramidal tract neuron of the same area (IC) and the ECoG response evoked by a similar single thalamic volley to the ventrolateral nucleus.

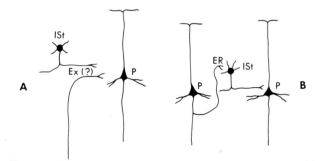

Fig. 6-37. Possible inhibitory cortical circuits. **A,** Inhibition of a pyramidal neuron (*P*) by an inhibitory stellate neuron (*ISt*), and possible inhibition of a pyramidal neuron by extrinsic fibers (*Ex*) entering the cortical area. **B,** Recurrent inhibition of a pyramidal neuron by a disynaptic pathway involving an excitatory recurrent axon collateral (*ER*) and an inhibitory stellate neuron (*ISt*).

of adjacent neurons are probably astrocytes; possibly oligodendrocytes have similar activity. At the present time the activity of these cells can be discussed only in general, in terms of the glia. Glial cells depolarize during the spontaneous increases in cortical activity that generate the waves of the EEG (Fig. 6-31). Such natural glial depolarization have an amplitude of several millivolts. However, during a seizure, glial cells may become quite depolarized, with a decrease of membrane potential from –85 mV to –60 mV. Some glial cells that depolarize during periods of increased neuronal activity exhibit a subsequent slow hyperpolarization of several millivolts.

It is currently thought that glial depolarization is mediated by a substance, probably K$^+$, released from neurons during their activity. It is possible that glia take up K$^+$ during periods of intense neuronal activity and help to buffer the extracellular space. One way in which glia could passively take up K$^+$ is shown in Fig. 6-39. If a glial process enveloping a synaptic junction is depolarized by K$^+$ released at that site, current will flow both extracellularly and intracellularly between the depolarized portion of the membrane and normally charged portions of the membrane. This current flow will be carried into and out of the cell by K$^+$, the ion to which the membrane is most permeable. The effect of the current flow will be to transport K$^+$ passively from a site of high extracellular concentration to a site of lower concentration. Glial uptake of K$^+$ might occur by means of passive uptake or diffusion or might be caused by an active process dependent on glial metabolism. Metabolic interaction of neurons and glia is also likely but unproved. Their most likely metabolic interaction

is to function as a buffering system for removing by-products of neuronal activity. If so, the glia would not be essential for neuronal function, but their activity would allow a higher level of neuronal activity. The major substances released by neural activity are probably the neurotransmitters and CO_2 and K$^+$. There is now also evidence that glia function in transmitter metabolism.

Glia do contain high concentrations of carbonic anhydrase, although the type of glia containing this enzyme has not been identified with certainty. It is possible that some glia may be involved in CO_2 metabolism in the brain.

Glial potential changes mediated by neuronal activity may play a role in or be a sign of K$^+$ uptake by glia. It is not known if the late, slow hyperpolarizing potentials observed in cortical glia are a passive response of the glial membrane to decreases in extracellular K$^+$ or whether they are a sign of active transport of ions, possibly K$^+$ or Cl$^-$ into glia.

Generation of rhythmic activity

The ongoing PSP patterns of thalamic and cortical neurons are characterized by rhythmicity, incrementing activity, synchrony, and characteristic shifts in frequency of rhythms and degree of synchronization. The rhythmicity of PSPs is seen as a regular recurrence of PSPs at a fixed frequency. There frequently is a regular alteration of EPSPs and IPSPs. Incrementing activity refers to increase in amplitude of successive PSPs; this usually occurs for three to five PSPs (waxing), and then the amplitude of the PSPs decreases (waning). Synchrony of the PSPs of many adjacent cortical neurons has been mentioned above. An exact measurement of the number of cells whose PSPs are in synchrony in various states of cortical activity has not been made, but it is clear that a considerable degree of synchrony of pyramidal cell activity must exist during the recording of rhythmic ECoG potentials.

The degree of rhythmicity and synchrony of PSPs in a thalamocortical sector at any one time can be inversely correlated, in general, with the degree of afferent input to the sector at that time. The greatest rhythmicity in parietotemporo-occipital areas is generally seen when afferent sensory-evoked activity to the thalamus is minimal. Widespread cortical rhythmicity is produced by general anesthesia and in particular by barbiturate-produced anesthesia. However, local rhythmic activity can be seen in the motor cortex immediately preceding movement. Therefore, the relationship of rhythms of individual cortical areas to levels of thalamic activity and to states of arousal is quite complex. Much more will have to be learned

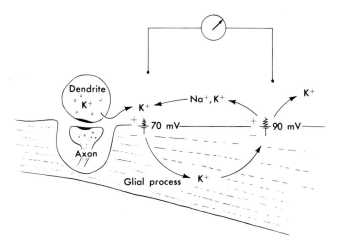

Fig. 6-39. Diagrammatic representation of the hypothesis of glial uptake and passive transport of K$^+$ released from neurons as a result of currents generated by differential depolarization of portions of the glial cell membrane.

about the activity in individual thalamocortical sectors before a general description of rhythmic cortical activity can be given and before its role in the functioning of the cortex is understood.

The PSP activity of thalamocortical neurons can be regarded as a result of an oscillator network in which intracortical and subcortical elements provide positive and negative feedback. The historical sequence of development of knowledge of this network is instructive in understanding the mechanisms involved. Important findings were the changes in EEG rhythms in different states of arousal (H. Berger, 1929; E. D. Adrian and B. H. C. Matthews, 1934), the EEG-synchronizing effect of transecting the upper brainstem (F. Bremer, 1938), the localized primary and diffuse secondary cortical responses evoked by peripheral sensory stimulation (A. Forbes and B. Morison, 1939), the localized primary and augmenting cortical responses evoked by stimulation of specific thalamic relay nuclei (E. W. Dempsey and R. S. Morison, 1943), the diffuse cortical recruiting responses evoked by stimulation of the nonspecific thalamic nuclei (H. Jasper and J. Droogleever-Fortuyn, 1947), the EEG-desynchronizing effect of stimulation of the brainstem reticular formation (G. Moruzzi and H. W. Magoun, 1949), the PSP patterns found in cortical neurons during antidromic and orthodromic stimulation (C. G. Phillips, 1956; C. L. Li, 1961), and the PSP patterns of thalamic neurons during rhythmic activity (D. P. Purpura and B. Cohen, 1962).

In this section the activity of reticular, thalamic, and cortical neurons is discussed in terms of their interactions in producing synchronized or desynchronized thalamocortical activity. The more complex relationships of the states of activity of particular subcortical nuclei and the behavioral states of arousal and sleep and of consciousness and coma are discussed in Chapter 11.

The role of afferent activity in maintaining the ongoing discharge of cortical neurons can be demonstrated by undercutting the cortex and chronically isolating a slab of cortex from afferent input. The cortical layers of an isolated cortical slab become atrophic and thinner than normal. The neurons in an isolated slab exhibit little or no so-called spontaneous electrical activity. However, isolated cortical slabs have a lower threshold than normal cortex for seizure activity evoked by direct electrical stimulation. Localized cooling of a specific thalamic relay nucleus, produced by inserting a chilled probe into the nucleus, will also produce a depression of rhythmic activity in the cortical sector to which the thalamic nucleus projects. In contrast, if the brainstem

is transected just behind the thalamus, leaving the thalamus and cortex interconnected but separated from ascending spinal and brainstem projections, the cortex exhibits high-voltage rhythmic synchronous ECoG activity at a frequency of about 8 to 12 Hz. If the brainstem of a cat or monkey is transected at a midcollicular level caudal to the third nerve nucleus (cerveau isolé preparation), the animal is immobile, has strongly constricted pupils, and appears to be in deep sleep. Visual and olfactory stimulation can still evoke a primary cortical response, but the stimuli will not arouse or awaken the animal. In contrast, if the brainstem is transected at the spinomedullary junction (encephale isolé), the electrical activity of the cortex will show synchronized rhythmic activity at times and desynchronized low-voltage fast activity characteristic of an aroused or awakened behavioral state at other times. The effects of successive transections of the brainstem on cortical electrical activity therefore suggest that the thalamus is in some way responsible for rhythmically synchronizing electrocortical activity and brainstem areas are responsible for desynchronizing electrocortical activity. These observations can be confirmed and extended by electrical stimulation of subcortical areas.

The effects of single-shock electrical stimulation of the specific and nonspecific thalamic nuclei and of the brainstem reticular formation on electrocortical activity have been described above in discussing the evoked potentials. Repetitive stimulation of specific and nonspecific thalamic nuclei with low-frequency (5 to 10 Hz) trains of shocks evokes synchronized incrementing of PSPs in cortical neurons. Trains of stimuli delivered at higher frequencies (20 to 300 Hz), both in the specific and nonspecific thalamus and in the brainstem reticular formation, generally produce a disruption of incrementing PSPs. The effects of repetitive low-frequency stimulation of each of these areas will now be considered in more detail.

The electrocortical effects of repetitive stimulation of specific nuclei have been largely studied in the ventral lateral and ventral posterior nuclei, and to a lesser extent in the medial and lateral geniculate nuclei of the cat. The effects appear to be similar in these nuclei in the cat, the monkey, and humans. However, there are differences in latencies and in some components of the cortical evoked responses when different specific nuclei are stimulated in different species. These differences require further investigation. Stimulation of the VL nucleus at frequencies of 5 to 10 Hz evokes a train of waxing and waning responses in the motor cortex (anterior sigmoid gyrus) of the cat. The intracellular and ECoG response to the first stimulus of the train is a primary response, as described above (Figs. 6-33 to 6-35) and in Figs. 6-40 and 6-41. However, the cortical response to the second and subsequent shocks of the train of stimuli is modified, and this modification is called the augmenting response. The augmenting response pattern of PSPs in pyramidal tract neurons, and in many nonpyramidal tract neurons as well, consists of an increased amplitude and latency of the EPSPs of the primary response and a marked reduc-

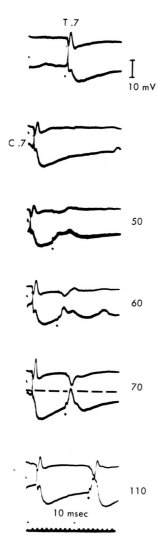

tion in the amplitude of the IPSP evoked by ventro-lateral stimulation. These changes in PSP pattern continue to augment in amplitude following the third to fifth shocks in the train. The responses to subsequent shocks in the train of stimuli remain augmented, but wax and wane in amplitude. Because the early (1.5- to 10-msec latency) EPSPs associated with the initial positive and negative waves of the primary evoked response increase in amplitude and in latency during the augmenting response, both the positive and negative waves of the ECoG primary response undergo similar increases in amplitude during augmenting.

The importance of the augmenting response lies in its indication of changes in the pattern of activity in thalamocortical pathways following repetitive usage of the pathways. In the VL nucleus such changes of activity probably occur in activation of the cerebellothalamic motor cortex pathway during voluntary movement. The changed pattern of activity of cortical cells during the augmenting response is probably caused by the initial shock of the train producing a reorganization of thalamic activity so that subsequent shocks evoke a different pattern of afferent thalamocortical discharge. Changes in reactivity of cortical circuits following the thalamocortical volley may also play a role in augmenting responses.

A model of thalamic activity in which neurons are interconnected by recurrent inhibitory pathways can explain many features of rhythmic, incrementing synchronization of thalamic and cortical activity produced

Fig. 6-40. The augmenting response. The PSP patterns of the primary and of the augmented responses evoked in a large pyramidal neuron of the motor cortex by conditioning *(C)* and testing *(T)* shocks, delivered at varying intervals to the ventral lateral nucleus. The time of delivery of the testing shock is marked with a dot. The ECoG response is shown on the upper line, and the intracellular response on the lower line of each pair of tracings. C-T intervals are given in milliseconds at the right of each pair of tracings (C and T, shock intensity of 0.7 mA). Note the marked increase in amplitude of the secondary EPSPs evoked by the testing shock at C-T intervals starting at about 60 msec and the smaller IPSP evoked by the testing shock.

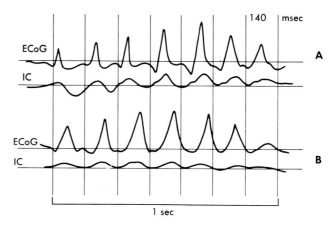

Fig. 6-41. Augmenting and recruiting patterns of response of cortical neurons to 7/sec repetitive thalamic stimulation. ECoG response is shown on the upper line, and the intracellular PSP responses of a large pyramidal neuron are shown on the lower line of each pair of tracings *(IC)*. Action potential responses are omitted. **A,** Augmenting response evoked by stimulation of a specific thalamic nucleus, recorded in the projection area of the nucleus. **B,** Recruiting response evoked by stimulation of a nonspecific nucleus. The thalamic stimuli are delivered at a rate of 7/sec at each vertical time marker.

by low-frequency thalamic stimulation. Whether such a neural network does underlie the rhythmic activity produced by stimulation of both specific and nonspecific systems is not known. However, synchronization of inhibition by each stimulus, producing inhibitory phasing of excitatory discharge, is undoubtedly important in developing rhythmic thalamocortical activity. The most general functional effect of repetitive low-frequency stimulation of a specific nucleus appears to be to increase the excitability of the cortical sector to which it projects. Low-frequency stimulation of the VL nucleus in patients with parkinsonian tremor will often augment the amplitude of the tremor, whereas electrocoagulation of the nucleus will often reduce the amplitude of the tremor.

Repetitive stimulation of the nonspecific thalamic nuclei also evokes incrementing EPSPs in cortical neurons. Unilateral stimulation within these nuclei evokes cortical responses bilaterally. In the cat the responses are largest over the frontal half of the hemispheres. The first shock of the train of stimuli evokes a large-amplitude, long-latency EPSP in cortical pyramidal tract neurons, which is associated with the negative wave of the ECoG response (Fig. 6-35). The response to the second and subsequent shocks of the train is modified, and these modifications are called the recruiting response (Fig. 6-41). The PSP pattern in cortical neurons during the recruiting response consists of an increased amplitude of the long-latency EPSP. The EPSP continues to increase in amplitude in response to the third to fifth shocks of the train and then waxes and wanes if the train of stimulation is prolonged. Because the late EPSP evoked by nonspecific thalamic stimulation corresponds to the negative waves of the ECoG response, this wave becomes larger during recruiting. The initial, positive wave does not increase in amplitude during recruiting, in contrast to the initial, positive wave of the primary evoked response.

The pathways to the cortex by which cortical activity is bilaterally synchronized by nonspecific thalamic stimulation are unknown. There is some evidence that the orbitofrontal cortex is most directly affected by nonspecific stimulation. The functional significance of the recruiting response is unknown. By stimulating the thalamus with chronically implanted electrodes, it is possible to evoke recruiting responses without producing any change in the behavior of freely moving unanesthetized animals. However, if the nonspecific nuclei are stimulated with intense currents at a frequency of 3 to 8 Hz, an arrest reaction can be produced both in animals and in humans. During the arrest reaction, ECoG activity at the frequency of the stimulus is evoked bilaterally in the cortex, and there is an abrupt cessation of ongoing locomotor movement without loss of the standing posture or muscle tone. The arrest reaction has electrocorticographic and behavior similarities to a petit mal seizure (p. 229). A major function of the nonspecific thalamic nuclei appears to be to modulate transmission through specific thalamic nuclei. The intranuclear interaction of the nonspecific nuclei with specific nuclei is largely inhibitory. Stimulation of nonspecific nuclei evokes moderate-latency IPSPs in VL neurons and blocks cerebellothalamocortical transmission. Stimulation of the VL nucleus evokes short-latency IPSPs in nonspecific thalamic nucleus neurons.

Stimulation of the reticular formation blocks or reverses the inhibition of VL nucleus neurons produced by stimulation of the nonspecific nuclei. High-frequency stimulation of the reticular formation also disrupts synchronized PSPs of cortical neurons evoked by low-frequency stimulation of specific and nonspecific thalamic nuclei. It is not known if the effects of reticular formation stimulation on cortical activity are mediated solely by reticular projections to the thalamus or whether direct reticulocortical projections are also involved. Nonrhythmic, continuous sensory stimulation will also desynchronize the ECoG. Many neurons of the reticular formation can be discharged by sensory stimulation, and many respond to more than one sensory modality.

Auditory and pain stimuli are particularly effective in discharging reticular neurons. The projections from sensory systems to reticular neurons appears to come from the spinal gray matter and from sensory relay nuclei of the brainstem. It is thought that sensory-evoked behavioral arousal is mediated by sensory projections to the reticular formation, which then influences thalamocortical activity.

The effects of low-frequency repetitive stimulation of the thalamus in evoking rhythmic cortical activity have been stressed here, but the tendency of thalamocortical systems to develop rhythmic activity can also be seen following single-shock stimulation of the thalamus. A single shock delivered to a specific thalamic nucleus in an animal lightly anesthetized with a barbiturate anesthetic will evoke the primary response PSP sequence in cortical neurons, followed by a waning sequence of alternating EPSPs and IPSPs lasting about a second (Fig. 6-42). This type of oscillatory corticoneuronal activity can also be observed after peripheral sensory stimulation, such as a flash of light, a click, or a shock to a peripheral nerve, and is known as the sensory after-discharge. The after-discharge is distributed bilaterally over wide areas of the cortex in contrast to the primary

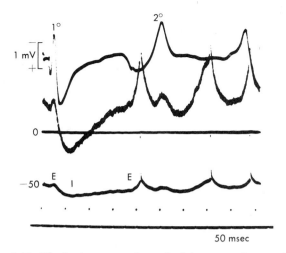

Fig. 6-42. Rhythmic potentials evoked by a single stimulus. The secondary response (2°) and rhythmic after-potentials following a primary response (1°) evoked by stimulation of a specific thalamic nucleus. ECoG shown on upper line, and intracellular potentials at high and low gain shown on second and fourth lines respectively.

response, which is localized to a specific sensory cortex. The initial ECoG response of the sensory after-discharge can be localized to the appropriate sensory cortex and has the appearance of the primary evoked response, and in such a case is called the secondary response. It is probable that the stimulus activity that evokes the primary response by activating a specific thalamic nucleus also activates the reticular formation and nonspecific thalamic nuclei. The after-discharge is probably mediated by nonspecific pathways.

Direct electrical stimulation of the somatic sensory or visual cortex in humans who are awake must be maintained for several hundred milliseconds to evoke sensory perception. It is probable that the intracortical events that occur during the time when secondary responses and sensory after-discharges occur are critical events for evoking perception. It is likely that nonspecific and reticular systems as well as the specific sensory pathways play a role in the intracortical elaboration of specific sensory activity that leads to perception.

To what extent are the synchronized rhythms of the human EEG caused by the activities of specific and nonspecific thalamic systems? This question is generally considered primarily for the alpha rhythm. The alpha rhythm (see the section on the electroencephalogram) or alphalike rhythm of nonhuman primates is generated in the parietotemporo-occipital cortex. In humans this is the eulaminate isocortex, which is the thalamic projection area of the lateral dorsal, lateral posterior, and pulvinar nuclei of the thalamus. Lesions of this cortex produce deficits of language, calculation, spatial relationship, and other so-called higher functions. Only a small number of studies of the electrophysiological relationships of this cortex to its thalamic projection nuclei have been made in higher primates and humans, in comparison with the large number of studies of the ventral lateral thalamic projection to the motor cortex in the cat. The similarity of wave form and duration of the alpha rhythm to potentials evoked by nonspecific thalamic stimulation has been stressed by many investigators. However, the spatial distribution of recruiting potentials over the cortex is not quite the same as that of alphalike rhythms. There is insufficient evidence at present to state that the alpha rhythm is like either an augmenting or a recruiting rhythm. The relative roles of different thalamocortical synchronizing mechanisms in generating the alpha rhythm and other natural cortical rhythmic activity are unknown at the present time.

What is the functional role of the thalamocortical activity that generates rhythmic PSP sequences in cortical neurons? Among the various hypotheses of the function of rhythmic activity are the following: it represents the activity of a scanning mechanism that sweeps the cortex and reads out patterns of afferent input; it represents the activity of an erasing mechanism that wipes out input; and it is a mechanism that maintains readiness or excitability of thalamocortical neurons. Evidence for the last hypothesis is that pyramidal tract neurons are more easily discharged during the EPSPs that occur during the negative peaks of alpha-rhythmlike waves. However, the functional significance of the alpha rhythm and other ongoing cortical rhythms is still unknown.

Malfunctioning of thalamocortical synchronized activity might be expected to occur, and there is evidence that the generalized epilepsies represent either a primary derangement or a secondary engagement of thalamocortical synchronizing mechanisms, as is discussed in the section on epilepsy.

Spreading depression of cortical activity

The cerebral cortex responds to intense localized electrical stimulation, to local application of KCl, or to local trauma with a local cellular depolarization. This depolarization, under certain conditions, can propagate slowly across the cortex at a rate of 2 to 5 mm/min. As the wave of depolarization advances, the neurons of the involved cortex discharge at high frequencies and then depolarize. The electrical activity of the depolarized areas remains depressed for several minutes and then recovers. This phenomenon is known as spreading depression (of Leão, after

A. A. P. Leão, the neurophysiologist who first described the phenomenon). During spreading depression the depolarization of apical dendrites and somata of cortical neurons occurs with respect to their axons in the subcortical white matter. Glial cells also depolarize. Na^+ and Cl^- enter cells from the extracellular space, and the electrical resistance of the cortex increases because of cell swelling and reduction in the size of the extracellular space. Cellular depolarizations make the gray matter of the cortex up to 25 mV negative with respect to the underlying white matter. The negative potential, which can be recorded with nonpolarizable electrodes and DC-coupled amplifiers (see Appendix I), is the characteristic electrical sign of spreading depression. The potential develops rapidly over a period of 15 to 30 seconds. The wave of depolarization spreads into a cortical area and remains strongly negative for 1 to 2 minutes and then declines in amplitude. There is a massive efflux of K^+ and amino acids, which are thought to be neurotransmitters (see below) from cells in the cortex that are undergoing spreading depression. It is likely that the release of depolarizing substances from cells is involved in propagating spreading depression.

Spreading depression can be evoked in the lissencephalic cortices of the rabbit and rat more easily than in the more complex cortices of carnivores or primates. In more complex cortices, localized depolarization will propagate into a spreading depression more easily if the cortex has been traumatized, as by repeated microelectrode punctures or by the removal of CSF and drying. Spreading depression can also be evoked in the retina and in subcortical nuclei. It is likely that some process like spreading depression can occur in the cortex of humans following intense seizure activity or when the cortex is injured by direct trauma or by ischemia. The paroxysmal depolarization of the cerebral cortex that can be recorded following cerebral ischemia has many similarities to spreading depression. Fig. 6-43 illustrates how depolarization of the intracortical portions of vertically oriented neural elements, such as presynaptic fibers, contributes to the anoxic or asphyxial negative cortical potential produced by cerebral anoxia or ischemia.

Neurotransmitters in the cerebral cortex

Because of the large number of afferent systems projecting to the cortex, as well as the variety of cortical cells, it is likely that many substances now being examined for possible roles as central nervous system transmitters will eventually be found to be transmitters in the cortex.

The substances for which most evidence has been accumulated for a role as cortical transmitters are acetylcholine (ACh) and the amino acids L-glutamic acid and gamma-aminobutyric acid (GABA). These substances are present in the neocortex, although not in as high concentrations as in some portions of the brain, such as parts of the basal ganglia.

Enzymatic systems appear to be present for synthesizing these substances in cortical neurons and in neurons that send axons to the cortex. These substances appear to be released from the cortex during cortical activity. They have been collected from the cortex by placing a cup perfused with artificial CSF on the cortical surface and activating the cortex. During EEG desynchronization (arousal), ACh and L-glutamic acid are released in larger amounts than when the EEG is synchronized. When the EEG is synchronized, larger amounts of GABA than of L-

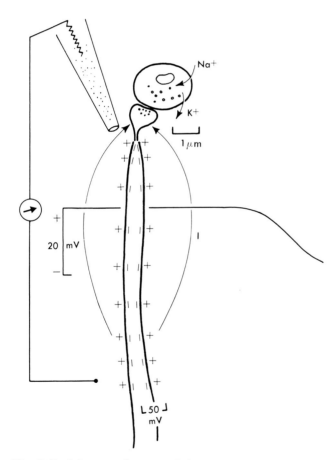

Fig. 6-43. Schematic diagram of the generation of a negative shift of transcortical potential recorded between a micropipette in layer 4 of the cortex and axons in the subcortical white matter, caused by differential depolarization of thalamocortical axon terminals produced by cerebral ischemia. Na^+ is shown entering a postsynaptic cellular process, and K^+ is shown leaking from the cell as a consequence of the failure of metabolic activity of the cell produced by ischemia.

glutamic acid are released. Iontophoretic application of ACh and L-glutamic acid has been shown to excite many cortical neurons. GABA generally has an inhibitory effect. However, localization of these substances to particular axon terminals and synaptic junctions, as can be done for the catecholamines in the basal ganglia, has not been accomplished. Therefore, it cannot yet be determined if these substances mimic the effect of stimulating particular presynaptic neurons.

True cholinesterase is present in cortical neurons, so an enzymatic system for removing ACh probably exists in the cortex. However, a well-defined system has not yet been described for removing putative amino acid transmitters from the postsynaptic membrane in the central nervous system.

It is likely that catecholamines do not play a large role as neocortical transmitters. Few dense-core vesicles of the type seen in axon terminals known to contain catecholamines are found on electron microscopy of the neocortex. Chemical studies reveal comparatively low concentrations of catecholamines in the neocortex. Putative neurotransmitters in the limbic cortex are discussed in Chapter 10. It can be said that much work will have to be done to establish the identity of cortical neurotransmitters.

ELECTROENCEPHALOGRAM

The electroencephalogram (EEG) and epilepsy, which is discussed in the next section, are very extensive subjects. However, an introduction to these subjects is justified here because of their medical significance and their importance in illustrating neurophysiological mechanisms and in stimulating research.

The existence of electrical potentials of the brain was first demonstrated by the English surgeon Caton in 1875. He implanted nonpolarizable electrodes (see Appendix I) over the cortex of monkeys and observed slow potentials. A number of investigators then described fluctuating cortical potentials. A very important contribution was made by Berger, the psychiatrist who in 1929 published the first description of human brain potentials and described the changes of rhythmic activity in changing states of alertness. However, it was not until the 1930s, when vacuum tube amplifiers and galvanometer recorders with penwriting outputs were developed, that electrocephalography became a practical method of clinical investigation.

The EEG is used clinically for two main purposes: to localize areas of brain dysfunction and to aid in the classification of the epilepsies. Clinical examination of the electrical activity of the cortex is obtained with silver–silver chloride electrodes ap-

plied to the scalp. It is not necessary to shave the head, because electrode paste, a concentrated salt solution in a jellylike form, is used to improve the contact with the scalp. Sixteen scalp electrodes are generally used and placed in a pattern that samples the activity of the convexity of the cerebrum. In the 10/20 electrode placement system, the head is divided into eight regions: frontal pole (FP), frontal (F), central (C), parietal (P), temporal (T), and occipital (O) (recordings are routinely taken from these areas), as well as basal and cerebellar areas. The distance from the nasion to the inion is divided into segments of 10% and 20% of the total distance, as shown in Fig. 6-44. Electrodes are placed on the regions of the head at the intersections of the dividing lines. The leads on the left side of the head are designated with odd numbers, those on the right side with even numbers. The numbering for the leads within an area, the frontal area for example, is not sequential; numbers are deliberately skipped so that if an additional lead is inserted, it can be designated with one of the intervening numbers. Reference electrodes are placed on the ears (A_1 and A_2) and on the vertex of the skull (Cz). For studying the ac-

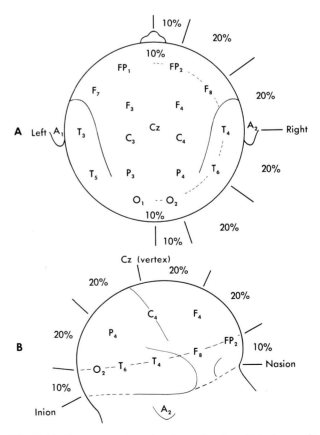

Fig. 6-44. Placement of scalp electrodes for clinical recording of the EEG in the 10/20 electrode placement system.

tivity of the orbitofrontal and mesial temporal lobes, special basal electrode insertions are made through the nasal and external auditory passages to the naso-pharyngeal and tympanic areas and through needles to the greater wing of the sphenoid bone (ala magna lead).

The patterns of interconnections of electrodes through which recordings are taken are called montages. The examination is started with monopolar recording, in which the electrodes on each side of the head are referred to the electrode on the ipsilateral ear. The ear electrode is considered indifferent, although it does pick up some temporal lobe activity. Recordings from homologous points on each side of the head are displayed on adjacent channels, with the left-sided trace above the right-sided trace, to facilitate comparison. Recordings are then made with bipolar derivations in which the electrodes are connected in parasagittal chains, or linkages, and in chains running from the left to the right sides of the head. If abnormal activity that is suspected to have a highly localized cortical origin is detected, the electrodes can be connected to each other in patterns that may localize the sinks and sources of the potential. This is done by finding points of phase reversal of potentials.

The clinical EEG examination includes periods of recording, with the patient in various states of arousal or alertness. The initial recording is made with the patient resting quietly with eyes closed. Recordings are then made in physiological states that activate the EEG, to attempt to evoke abnormal EEG activity. The commonly used technique to accomplish this is to have the patient hyperventilate and produce a respiratory alkalosis, which increases neuronal excitability. A recording during sleep will often be taken, as abnormal EEG activity frequently appears during sleep. Another type of activation procedure that is used in the study of some seizure disorders is metrazol activation. The patient is given carefully titrated doses intravenously of the convulsant metrazol while EEG and behavioral seizure activity is recorded. Photic stimulation with a flickering light at the alpha frequency (see below) is also used as an activation procedure.

EEG potentials are described in terms of their frequency, amplitude, and morphological characteristics. The frequency band has been divided into α, the alpha band, 8 to 13 Hz; β, the beta band, over 13 Hz; θ, the theta band, 4 to 7 Hz; and δ, the delta band, less than 4 Hz. These terms simply refer to the frequency of the waves. The presence of activity at the alpha frequency, for example, does not necessarily connote that a specific mechanism is generating the waves.

The potentials can then be characterized further as low-voltage or high-voltage potentials. In addition to ongoing or rhythmic potentials, the normal EEG exhibits transients, or special graphic elements, waves of unusual structure that occur singly or in groups, which will be described further below.

Because of the complexity of the potentials recorded in the EEG, there is considerably more information in an EEG recording than can be easily assimilated and extracted by visual inspection of the frequency, amplitude, and structure of the potentials. Computers and other electronic devices have been used to extract and display the percentages of potentials occurring in different frequency bands, the power spectrum of the potentials, and the phase relationships of the potentials over the hemispheres. At present such equipment is used more in research than in clinical practice.

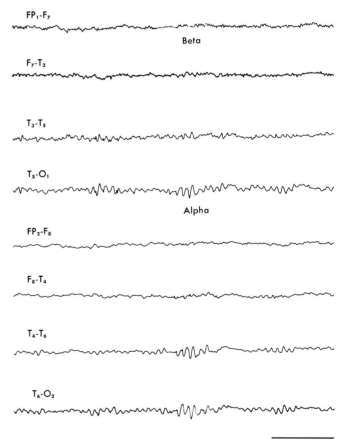

Fig. 6-45. Normal rhythmic EEG potentials and normal spatial distribution of potentials in a 13-year-old girl, with no medications. Montage of temporal chains, starting in the frontal region and proceeding to the occipital region, on each side of the head. See Fig. 6-44 for illustration of electrode positions. Note the frontal distribution of the beta rhythm and the posterior temporo-occipital distribution of the alpha rhythm, which tends to be symmetrical in left and right hemispheres. (Courtesy Dr. Robert J. Gumnit.)

EEGs recorded from individuals at increasing ages show changes that are referred to as maturation. The first evidence of spontaneous EEG activity is found in fetuses 6 to 7 months of age. At birth the EEG consists of very low voltage slow waves. During childhood the dominant frequencies are slow, and the EEG does not exhibit large amounts of activity at the alpha frequency until puberty. Some individuals do not exhibit what will be their adult patterns of EEG activity until their early twenties. In old age, slowing and loss of complexity of the EEG can be seen.

The mature EEG pattern varies with the state of arousal of the subject. When the patient is resting quietly with eyes closed, waxing and waning trains of potentials in the alpha (8 to 13 Hz) frequency band are recorded from the temporoparieto-occipital region. The activity in the central and frontal regions tends to be faster in the beta band (Fig. 6-45). The parieto-occipital distribution of the alpha rhythm and the frontal distribution of low-amplitude high-frequency beta rhythm, which are recorded through the skull and scalp, are a reflection of potential differences that can be recorded from different cortical areas. Jasper and Penfield have shown that distinctive differences exist between the temporoparieto-occipital region, where the dominant rhythm is at the alpha frequency, and the central sensorimotor region, where the dominant frequency is in the beta band at 20 to 25 Hz. The medial temporal limbic cortex exhibits a rhythm of 14 to 16 Hz, with some slower waves.

When the patient becomes alert or aroused, which may be brought about by sensory stimulation or by opening the eyes, the resting rhythms are replaced by lower voltage, higher frequency waves. Conversely, when the patient becomes drowsy, there is some slowing or disorganization of the alpha rhythm. When the patient is in light sleep, trains of spindles of 10- to 15-Hz waves are mixed with slower waves. The sleep spindles are slightly faster in frequency and are maximal in amplitude more parasagittally and anteriorly than the alpha rhythm potentials. In deep sleep, waves in the theta and delta band are found (see Chapter 11).

Transient potentials that are seen normally include lambda waves, which are positive potentials that occur in the occipital area and appear to be associated with opening the eyes and eye movements; vertex waves, sharp transients recorded from frontal and central areas in light sleep; and K complexes, consisting of one or more large slow waves, also recorded from frontal and central regions in sleep, which can also be evoked by auditory stimulation and may represent secondary responses.

In recent years the EEG has been used in conjunc-

tion with the neurological examination to establish the occurrence of irreversible damage to the brain. The criteria that are used to establish brain death include the total absence of somatic motor reflexes, the absence of spontaneous respiration, and two iso-electric EEG recordings taken, at high gain, 24 hours apart in the absence of central nervous system depressant drugs.

EPILEPSY

The epilepsies are characterized by abnormalities of behavior and electrical activity, which occur during seizures, and abnormal electrical activity, which can occur between seizures. The words used to describe seizures indicate the impression these conditions have made on people throughout history: seizure (*Latin,* to take possession of), ictus (*Latin,* to strike), convulsion (*Latin,* to tear up), fit (*Anglo-Saxon,* fight or strife), and epilepsy (*Greek,* to take or seize on). The modern classification of the epilepsies, in which electrical activity is correlated with behavioral manifestations of seizures, has been the work of many investigators. In the past 40 years notable contributions have been made by F. A. Gibbs, E. L. Gibbs, W. G. Lennox, H. Jasper, W. Penfield, A. Ajmone-Marsan, and H. Gastaut.

Clinical seizures can be divided into partial seizures, in which there is an abnormal electrical discharge of only part of the brain and the patient does not lose consciousness, and generalized seizures, in which abnormal electrical activity includes large areas of the brain and the patient loses consciousness. There are two major types of partial seizures. The first type is the focal seizure proper, in which there is high-frequency discharge of neurons in a local area of the cortex. These seizures are characterized by a focal EEG abnormality consisting of a train of spike discharges. The most common cortical regions involved are frontal or frontoparietal. The common behavioral manifestations of focal seizures of these cortical areas are focal motor activity or somatic sensory complaints. Focal epileptic activity of the motor cortex evokes twitching or cramplike contractions of muscles of the contralateral side of the body. The motor activity usually starts either in the face, the arm, or the leg. Typical evoked movements are rapid grimacelike contractions of half of the face; rapid jerking movements of the thumb or fingers, or pronating-supinating movements of the forearm; and repetitive jerking dorsiflexion movements of the foot. In epileptic activity of the sensory cortex, electric shocklike or paresthetic feelings are experienced, localized to the side of the body contralateral to the cortical discharge. Focal seizures are frequently both motor and sensory. If the cortical discharge is located in the frontal motor eye field, contraversive eye movements are produced. Frequently the muscular or sensory activity will start in one part of the body and then spread to involve adjacent areas of the body. This was vividly described by the English neurologist Jackson; therefore, a focal motor or sensory seizure is known as a jacksonian seizure, and the spread of activity is called a jacksonian march. Jackson inferred that the seizure activity must spread to contiguous cortical areas; and from the pattern of progression of sensory and motor symptoms during the march of the seizure he was able to construct maps of localization of function in the sensorimotor cortex, indicating that the arm area lay between the leg and the face areas. A similar attempt has been made to localize functions in the limbic lobe on the basis of the spread of symptoms of autonomic function in temporal lobe seizures. In some cases focal seizures will spread to involve progressively larger areas of the body and will become generalized seizures. In the period after a focal seizure it is not uncommon for there to be depression of either motor or sensory function in the affected limbs. This was described by Todd, and is now referred to as Todd's paresis. The occurrence of Todd's paresis is often associated with the presence of a structural abnormality of the brain at the site of the cortical epileptic activity. A structural abnormality of the brain is found more often in patients who have focal seizures than in patients who have seizures that are generalized from the outset.

A second type of partial epilepsy is psychomotor epilepsy, often called temporal lobe epilepsy because the locus of the abnormal electrical activity is generally in the limbic structures of the medial side of the temporal lobe. As is discussed in the section on the limbic lobe (see Chapter 10), it appears to be easier to induce epileptic activity in hippocampal pyramidal neurons than in neocortical pyramidal neurons. However, the epileptic activity evoked in limbic structures tends to remain localized within the limbic lobe and not to spread to neocortical neurons and their associated thalamic areas. This is probably why consciousness is not lost in psychomotor seizures. Psychomotor seizures are characterized by motor automatisms, in which the patient carries out fragments of coordinated motor activity, such as picking movements, running movements, posturing, and deviations of the head and eyes. In addition, repetitive motor activities that are associated with visceral functions, such as chewing movements and lip smacking, are often performed. Autonomic concomitants, such as changes of blood pressure and respiration, also occur. A psychomotor seizure is

characterized by a change in state of consciousness, but not a loss of consciousness. There is usually some depression or clouding of consciousness, and hallucinations, illusions, or both. Illusions refer to distortion of perception. Common examples are micropsia, in which the visual field is seen as if it were very far away (as if seen through the wrong end of a telescope); jamais vu (never seen), a sensation of unfamiliarity or strangeness; and déjà vu (already seen), a sensation of having been in or being familiar with the situation present. Hallucinations are the perception or experience of qualities that are not actually in the environment. These are commonly olfactory, in which the patient smells an unpleasant odor, such as that of burning rubber, or sees visual phenomena that are not there. In addition, there may be changes in speech, generally of the nature of speech arrest or garbled speech.

The EEG abnormalities in partial seizures are characteristically asymmetrical, in contrast to the generalized seizures, which are characterized by bilaterally synchronous electrical activity, termed primary bilateral synchrony. The finding of asymmetrical or symmetrical EEG abnormalities are of practical importance. The great majority of generalized seizures are idiopathic (primary disease not produced by another disease). They therefore are not caused by tumors or other structural abnormalities that would require further diagnosis and treatment, but can be managed with medication. Partial epilepsies are more often associated with some structural lesions that may be amenable to surgical or other treatment. Although partial epilepsies are typically characterized by asymmetrical EEG abnormalities, projected discharges from the focus of abnormal electrical activity may give rise to bilaterally synchronous EEG changes, so-called secondary bilateral synchrony. Therefore, it is of etiological and prognostic significance to determine if bilaterally synchronous discharges occur primarily or secondarily.

There are many modifications of the basic pattern of a generalized seizure. Ajmone-Marsan and his associates have made extensive studies of patterns of EEG and motor activity in generalized seizures. Many patients exhibit components of partial epilepsies, particularly of the psychomotor type, in combination with the generalized seizure.

The major generalized seizures are the grand mal and the petit mal seizures. Behaviorly, grand mal (tonic-clonic) seizures start abruptly or with an aura (breeze; a sensation as if a vapor were rising about the body). The aura is a sensory experience that tends to be stereotyped and can serve as a warning of the onset of a seizure. The aura usually is brief and may be sensed as an unpleasant feeling in the chest and abdomen, akin to an unpleasant emotional sensation, or the aura may be a more or less well-formed auditory, visual, or tactile experience. The grand mal seizure proper starts with an abrupt loss of consciousness and generalized contraction of the somatic musculature. This is the tonic (muscular tension) phase of the seizure. There frequently is an aversive pattern to the onset of the seizure, with a turning of the head, deviation of the eyes, and posturing of the limbs. This is followed in 30 to 60 seconds by the clonic (violent motion) phase of the seizure, in which there is relaxation of the initial tonic posture and repetitive contractions of the somatic musculature. This is followed by a period of relaxation, frequently with profound depression of respiration. Following this there frequently is a period in which the patient appears to be asleep, which may last from several minutes to half an hour. The patient generally awakens without any focal motor paresis. Electroencephalographically, the seizure is characterized by the abrupt appearance of high-voltage, bilaterally synchronous waves at a frequency of about 10 Hz, which last throughout the tonic period. These waves slow in frequency toward the end of the tonic period. They are then interrupted by slow waves, which correspond to the periods of muscular relaxation in the clonic phase. There is then a period of electrical silence corresponding to the period of postictal flaccidity, after which a normal pattern of electrical activity slowly returns.

The bilaterally synchronous appearance of spikes in both hemispheres in the classical grand mal seizure has suggested that there is a subcortical, probably thalamic, site of synchronization of the cortical epileptic discharge in generalized seizures. This concept has been elaborated by Jasper and Penfield, who termed seizures showing primary bilateral synchrony centrencephalic seizures. The fact that 3/sec stimulation of the nonspecific thalamic nuclei in animals and man can produce behavioral arrest and bilaterally synchronous 3/sec spike and wave discharges typical of a petit mal (absence) supports the concept of a role of the thalamus in the petit mal type of generalized seizure. However, one of the unanswered questions about the role of the thalamus as a centrencephalic system in generalized seizures is whether the seizure activity originates in the thalamus or whether the synchronizing role of the thalamus develops secondarily.

The second type of generalized seizure is the absence, or the petit mal, seizure. These may be simple absences, in which there is only impairment of consciousness, or complex absences, with changes of consciousness and changes of muscular activity, clonic contractions, motor automatisms, or autonomic phenomena. Simple absences may occur many times a day and involve a brief impairment of consciousness, which may last from several seconds up to perhaps a minute. These seizure disorders occur typically in children. At the present time no organic basis for these disorders has been found. Electroencephalographically, they can be associated with rhythmic 3/sec spike and wave discharges, which, when they occur, characterize the typical absence. However, similar behavior may occur with low-voltage fast activity, or rhythmic discharges at 10 Hz, or irregular sharp and slow waves. These are referred to as petit mal variants, or atypical absences.

In addition, such conditions as bilateral massive myoclonic seizures, infantile spasms, atonic seizures, and akinetic seizures can be distinguished as behavioral and EEG variants of generalized epilepsy. Gastaut, in his classification of the epilepsies, which has been followed here, also distinguishes a group of unilateral seizures that have behavioral manifestations of tonic or clonic seizures but without impairment of consciousness and with restriction of the motor activity to one side of the body. Because of the complexity of clinical seizures some investigators consider the present classifications of seizure disorders to be very inadequate. It should also be remembered that the descriptions presented here are of idealized types of seizures. Nevertheless, this classification is valuable in treating patients with epilepsy.

In practice the diagnosis and classification of a seizure disorder is generally made on the basis of the history of the behavioral manifestations of the seizure and on the basis of abnormalities of frequency or morphological characteristics of potentials in the EEG in the interictal period, because the opportunity to observe a naturally occurring seizure while recording an EEG does not occur often. These abnormalities in the interictal record generally consist of the appearance of single spikes, spikes and waves, or bursts of these abnormal transients. If only a single interictal EEG is taken, about one half of patients with epilepsy will have a normal EEG record. However, by obtaining serial tracings and using EEG activation techniques, one can find abnormalities in all but about 10% of patients with epilepsy. Conversely, about 10% of patients who never manifest a clinical seizure will have an EEG showing occasional changes similar to the interictal EEGs of patients who do have clinical seizures.

The aspects of seizure activity that have been studied most intensively with experimental neurophysiological techniques are the events that occur in single cortical cells in an epileptogenic focus and the spread of epileptic activity from a focus to another area of the brain. Experimental focal seizures can be produced by applying a number of drugs to the cortex, by strongly stimulating the cortex, and by damaging the cortex. The mechanisms of generation of seizure activity in these different models of focal seizure activity are probably somewhat different. However, the final electrocorticographic result is usually the same: the development of repetitive spike potentials recorded from the surface of the cortex. The discharging area is called an epileptogenic focus.

Intracellular recording in the cortical focus produced by the local application of penicillin to the cortex of the cat has provided the data for many of the current concepts of the cellular events occurring in focal epilepsy. Within a few minutes of applying penicillin to a small area of the cortex surface, negative potentials of high voltage, lasting 60 to 300 msec, appear. These spikes, which will hereafter be called paroxysmal waves, appear in the ECoG every few seconds. If the penicillin is applied over the sensorimotor cortex, each paroxysmal wave may evoke focal motor activity of the contralateral muscles. The paroxysmal waves may occur with increasing frequency and develop into a train of paroxysmal waves at a frequency of about 10 Hz. The repetitive parox-

ysmal wave activity is a model of the interictal spike activity of the EEG, and the transition from single paroxysmal waves to a continuous train of paroxysmal waves is a model of the onset of a focal cortical seizure (Fig. 6-46).

Three types of events have been described in neurons in the area generating the paroxysmal waves. Some neurons exhibit a paroxysmal depolarizing shift (PDS) of membrane potential, lasting about 60 to 300 msec. This has been shown to be a complex PSP, which is largely a giant EPSP. When the cell membrane potential reaches threshold, a burst of action potentials is generated, which may be followed by spike inactivation. The cell then repolarizes and may then hyperpolarize. In some cells the hyperpolarization has characteristics that suggest that it is caused by the same ionic mechanisms that generate IPSPs.

A second set of neurons, particularly around the circumference of the paroxysmal wave focus, exhibit only a prolonged IPSP during the paroxysmal wave. A third group of neurons does not exhibit any activity that can be correlated with the paroxysmal wave.

Pyramidal tract neurons exhibiting the PDS appear normal in other respects; in the intervals between the PDS, normal PSPs can be evoked in these neurons,

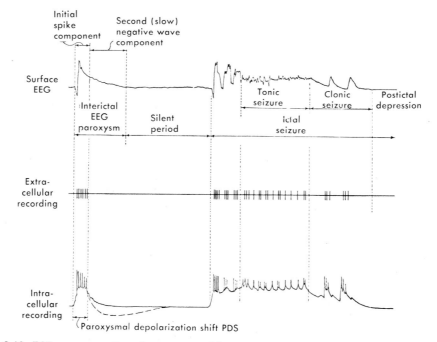

Fig. 6-46. PSP sequences in a large pyramidal neuron in an experimental cortical epileptic focus produced by applying penicillin to the motor cortex of the cat. The PDS associated with interictal spike potentials of the EEG is shown on the left. The pattern of intracellular depolarizations associated with the tonic and clonic phases of a generalized seizure are shown on the right. (From Ayala, G. F., Matsumoto, H., and Gumnit, R. J.: J. Neurophysiol. 33: 73-85, 1970.)

and their membrane properties appear to be unchanged. Therefore, the larger pyramidal neurons in the penicillin focus, in which intracellular recording can be carried out, do not appear to be intrinsically epileptic; rather, they appear to be responding to a massive, highly synchronous, excitatory barrage. It is thought that facilitation of the activity of recurrent excitatory pathways in the cortex plays an important role in producing the massive synchronous excitatory activity that generates the PDS. There is less evidence about the mechanisms generating the hyperpolarization following the PDS. The effect of the hyperpolarization appears to be a brake on the development of tonic seizure activity. In the transition from interictal to ictal activity, the PDS occurs progressively more frequently, and the subsequent hyperpolarization decreases until a prolonged depolarization of the neuron occurs, corresponding to the tonic phase of the seizure. Repetitive hyperpolarization of the membrane occurs in the clonic phase of the seizure. A marked hyperpolarization usually occurs during the period of postictal suppression of ECoG waves. Glial cells (astrocytes?) depolarize markedly during the tonic and clonic phases of the seizure. Some glial cells hyperpolarize during and after the period of postictal suppression of ECoG waves.

During tonic-clonic seizure activity there is a marked increase in metabolic activity and CO_2 production in the discharging area, and vasodilatation of cortical blood vessels occurs. If artificial ventilation is provided, metabolic substrates in the brain are not greatly depleted by a single seizure, possibly because of the increased blood flow to the discharging area. However, repetitive generalized seizures can produce hypoxic brain damage caused by hypoventilation during and after the seizure.

The cellular events occurring in a penicillin-induced acute cortical focus may not be completely the same as those that occur in a focus produced by trauma. Posttraumatic epilepsy in humans and in experimental animals usually develops subacutely. Some types of injury are more epileptogenic than others, for reasons that are not understood. A laceration of the cortex will produce epileptogenic activity in about 25% to 40% of cases. A freezing lesion of the cortex will produce marked epileptogenic activity in almost all cases.

The injection of cobalt powder or alumina cream into the cortex is another form of trauma that is highly epileptogenic. These substances produce epileptogenic activity over a period of months, during which a chronic granulomatous lesion develops in the cortex. The alumina cream lesion has been studied histologically in some detail. Penicillin-induced foci

are known to show histological changes, but these have not yet been well defined. Pyramidal cells in the alumina cream lesion show a loss of their dendritic spines and stunting of their dendrites. There is also a general loss of axon terminals ending on these cells, probably largely caused by damage to interneurons as well as to afferent fibers. The concept has been developed that the pyramidal neurons are partially denervated and are hyperexcitable. This might be because of changes in membrane properties and also because of the loss of inhibitory projections to them.

The spread of seizure activity from one part of the brain to another is also only partially understood. Seizure activity can be propagated by way of the major commissural fibers, the anterior commissure, and the corpus callosum, from one hemisphere to another. If a primary focus is set up in one hemisphere with one of the techniques for evoking epileptic discharge, a secondary focus can often be found at the homologous area of the contralateral cortex. An important finding made by Morrell was that after a period of time the secondary focus may become autonomous. The homologous cortical area may become epileptogenic as a result of the bombardment of impulses from the primary focus.

Attempts to find models of generalized seizure activity that resemble human idiopathic generalized epilepsy have led to the investigation of a number of species that exhibit generalized seizures precipitated by sensory stimulation. Generalized seizures can be induced in the baboon *Papio papio* by flickering light. Mutant strains of rabbits and mice that exhibit a tendency to have sensory-induced generalized seizures have also been identified. It is likely that the same mechanisms that generate large rhythmic EPSPs in thalamocortical neurons are driven into seizure activity by repetitive sensory stimuli.

Paroxysmal activity of the cortex and thalamus has been emphasized in this discussion. Fewer studies have been carried out on subcortical nuclei than on the cortex. Abnormal discharge in many subcortical nuclei can be produced by local freezing or application of various drugs. However, it is not clear if all central nervous system cell groups have the property of developing the type of rhythmic self-sustaining paroxysmal activity that can be evoked in the cortex. The tendency to epileptic activity of the cortex is probably caused by the structure of cortical neurons, their electrical properties, the intrinsic interconnections of the cortex, and the high level of synchronized synaptic activity impinging on cortical neurons.

It can be seen from the foregoing discussion that epilepsy is not a unitary process. It is likely that changes in a number of cellular processes and pathways can have the same final result of producing prolonged depolarization and high-frequency discharge of neurons that result in the electrical and behavioral signs of epilepsy.

The pharmacology of anticonvulsant drugs, such as phenobarbital and diphenylhydantoin (Dilantin), is outside the scope of this discussion. The mechanism of action of these drugs in preventing seizures is unknown, although many effects of these drugs on neural activity have been described. The anticonvulsant drugs in clinical use do not have a great effect on the appearance of interictal paroxysmal waves in the EEG. Their action appears to be one of preventing the transition from interictal to ictal activity. It is probable that such an effect is caused by actions on a number of processes and pathways.

REFERENCES
Thalamus

Angevine, J. B., Jr., Locke, S., and Yakovlev, P.: Limbic nuclei of thalamus and connections of limbic cortex; thalamocortical projections of the magnocellular medial dorsal mucleus in man, Arch. Neurol. **10**:165-180, 1964.

Bertrand, G., Jasper, H. H., and Wong, A.: Microelectrode study of the human thalamus, functional organization in the ventrobasal complex, Confin. Neurol. **29**:81-86, 1967.

Clark, W. E. L., and Powell, T. P. S.: On the thalamo-cortical connections of the general sensory cortex of Macaca, Proc. R. Soc. (Biol.) **141**:467-487, 1953.

Hassler, R.: Anatomy of the thalamus. In Schaltenbrand, G., and Bailey, P., editors: Introduction to stereotaxis with an atlas of the human brain, Stuttgart, 1959, Georg Thieme Verlag.

Mehler, W. H.: Further notes on the centre median nucleus of Luys. In Purpura, D. P., and Yahr, M. D., editors: The thalamus, New York, 1966, Columbia University Press.

Olivier, A., Parent, A., and Poirier, L. J.: Identification of the thalamic nuclei on the basis of their cholinesterase content in the monkey, J. Anat. **106**:37-50, 1970.

Olszewski, J.: The thalamus of the *Macaca mulatta;* an atlas for use with the stereotaxic instrument, Basel, 1952, S. Karger AG.

Papez, J. W.: Comparative neurology, New York, 1929, Thomas Y. Crowell Co.

Ralston, H. J. III, and Herman, M. M.: The fine structure of neurons and synapses in the ventrobasal thalamus of the cat, Brain Res. **14**:77-97, 1969.

Rinvik, E.: A re-evaluation of the cytoarchitecture of the ventral nuclear complex of the cat's thalamus on the basis of corticothalamic connections, Brain Res. **8**:237-254, 1968.

Rose, J. E., and Woolsey, C. N.: Organization of the mammalian thalamus and its relationships to the cerebral cortex, Electroencephalogr. Clin. Neurophysiol. **1**:391-404, 1949.

Scheibel, M. A., and Scheibel, A. B.: The organization of the nucleus reticularis thalami; a Golgi study, Brain Res. **1**:43-62, 1966.

Strick, P. L.: Cortical projections of the feline thalamic nucleus ventralis, lateralis, Barin Res. **20**: 130-134, 1970.

Walker, A. E.: The primate thalamus, Chicago, 1938, University of Chicago Press.

Cerebral cortex

Bailey, P., and von Bonin, G.: The isocortex of man, Urbana, Ill., 1951, University of Illinois Press.

Blackstad, T. W.: Cortical grey matter; a correlation of light and electron microscopic data. In Hydén, H., editor: The neuron, Amsterdam, 1967, Elsevier Publishing Co.

Bok, S. T.: Histonomy of the cerebral cortex, Amsterdam, 1959, Elsevier Publishing Co.

Chow, K. L., and Leiman, A. L.: The structural and functional organization of the neocortex, Neurosci. Res. Program Bull. **8**:153-220, 1970.

Colonnier, M.: Synaptic patterns on different cell types in the different laminae of the cat visual cortex; an electron microscope study, Brain Res. **9**:268-287, 1968.

Cragg, B. G.: The density of synapses and neurones in the motor and visual areas of the cerebral cortex, J. Anat. **101**:639-654, 1967.

Gray, E. G.: Axosomatic and axodendritic synapses of the cerebral cortex; an electron microscope study, J. Anat. **93**:420-433, 1959.

Jacobson, S., and Marcus, E. M.: The laminar distribution of fibers in the corpus callosum; a comparative study in the rat, cat, rhesus monkey and chimpanzee, Brain Res. **24**:517-520, 1970.

Jones, E. G., and Powell, T. P. S.: Connexions of the somatic sensory cortex of the rhesus monkey. II. Contralateral cortical connexions, Brain **92**:717-730, 1969.

Kaas, J., Hall, W. C., and Diamond, I. T.: Cortical visual areas I and II in the hedgehog—relation between evoked potential maps and architectonic subdivisions, J. Neurophysiol. **33**:595-615, 1970.

Lashley, K. S., and Clark, G.: The cytoarchitecture of the cerebral cortex of Ateles; a critical examination of cytoarchitectonic studies, J. Comp. Neurol. **85**:223-305, 1946.

Lorente de Nó, R.: Cerebral cortex. In Fulton, J. F., editor: Physiology of the nervous system, ed. 3, New York, 1949, Oxford University Press, Inc.

Marin-Padilla, M.: Prenatal and early postnatal ontogenesis of the human motor cortex; a Golgi study. II. The basket-pyramidal system, Brain Res. **23**:185-191, 1970.

Pandya, D. N., Gold, D., and Berger, T.: Interhemispheric connections of the precentral motor cortex in the rhesus monkey, Brain Res. **15**:594-596, 1969.

Penfield, W., and Rasmussen, T.: The cerebral cortex of man; a clinical study of the localization of function, New York, 1950, The Macmillan Co.

Peters, A.: Stellate cells of the rat parietal cortex, J. Comp. Neurol. **141**:345-374, 1971.

Ramon-Moliner, E.: The histology of the postcruciate gyrus in the cat. I. Quantitative studies, J. Comp. Neurol. **117**:43-62, 1961.

Rutledge, L. T., Duncan, J., and Beatty, N.: A study of pyramidal cell axon collaterals in intact and partially isolated adult cerebral cortex, Brain Res. **16**:15-22, 1969.

Sholl, D. A.: The organization of the cerebral cortex, New York, 1956, John Wiley & Sons, Inc.

Smit, G. J., and Colon, E. J.: Quantitative analysis of the cerebral cortex. I. A selectivity of the Golgi-Cox staining technique, Brain Res. **13**:485-510, 1969.

Valverde, F., and Ruiz-Narcos, A.: Dendritic spines in the visual cortex of the mouse; introduction to a mathematical model, Exp. Brain Res. **8**:269-283, 1969.

Woolsey, C. N.: Organization of somatic sensory and motor areas of the cerebral cortex. In Harlow, H. F., and Woolsey,

C. N., editors: Biological and biochemical bases of behavior, Madison, 1958, University of Wisconsin Press.

Woolsey, T. A., and Van der Loos, H.: The structural organization of layer IV in the somatosensory region (S I) of mouse cerebral cortex; the description of a cortical field composed of discrete cytoarchitectonic units, Brain Res. **17:**205-242, 1970.

Thalamocortical electrophysiology

Adrian, E. D., and Matthews, B. H. C.: The Berger rhythm; potential changes from the occipital lobes in man, Brain **57:**355-385, 1934.

Anderson, P., and Andersson, S. A.: Physiological basis of the alpha rhythm, New York, 1968, Appleton-Century-Crofts.

Bates, J. A.: The electrophysiology of the human thalamus, J. R. Coll. Physicians Lond. **1:**118-123, 1967.

Bergamini, L., and Bergamasco, B.: Cortical evoked potentials in man, Springfield, Ill., 1967, Charles C Thomas, Publisher.

Berger, H.: Uber das electrenkephalogramm des menschen, Arch. Psychiat. Nervenkr. **87:**527-570, 1929.

Brazier, M. A. B.: The electrical activity of the nervous system, ed. 3. Baltimore, 1968, The Williams & Wilkins Co.

Caton, R.: The electric currents of the brain, Br. Med. J. **2:**278, 1875.

Creutzfeldt, O. D., Watanabe, S., and Lux, H. D.: Relations between EEG phenomena and potentials of single cortical cells. I. Evoked responses after thalamic and epicortical stimulation, Electroencephalogr. Clin. Neurophysiol. **20:**1-18, 1966.

Dempsey, E. W., and Morison, R. S.: The electrical activity of a thalamocortical relay system, Am. J. Physiol. **138:**283-296, 1943.

Desiraju, T., and Purpura, D. P.: Organization of specific-nonspecific thalamic internuclear synaptic pathways, Brain Res. **21:**169-181, 1970.

Grossman, R. G., and Rosman, L. J.: Intracellular potentials of inexcitable cells in epileptogenic cortex undergoing fibrillary gliosis after a local injury, Brain Res. **28:**181-201, 1971.

Jasper, H. H.: Diffuse projection systems; the integrative activity of the thalamic reticular system, Electroencephalogr. Clin. Neurophysiol. **1:**405-420, 1949.

Jasper, H. H., and Koyama, I.: Rate of release of amino acids from the cerebral cortex in the cat as affected by brainstem and thalamic stimulation, Can. J. Physiol. Pharmacol. **47:**889-905, 1969.

Koike, H., Okada, Y., and Oshima, T.: Accommodative properties of fast and slow pyramidal tract cells and their modification by different levels of their membrane potential, Exp. Brain Res. **5:**189-201, 1968.

Krnjević, K., Reiffenstein, R. J., and Silver, A.: Inhibition and paroxysmal activity in long isolated cortical slabs, Electroencephalogr. Clin. Neurophysiol. **29:**283-294, 1970.

Li, C. L.: Cortical intracellular synaptic potentials, J. Cell. Comp. Physiol. **58:**153-167, 1961.

Lux, H. D., and Pollen, D. A.: Electrical constants of neurons in the motor cortex of the cat, J. Neurophysiol. **29:**207-220, 1966.

McLennan, H.: Inhibitions of long duration in the cerebral cortex; a quantitative difference between excitatory amino acids, Exp. Brain Res. **10:**417-426, 1970.

Moruzzi, G., and Magoun, H. W.: Brain stem reticular formation and activation of the EEG, Electroencephalogr. Clin. Neurophysiol. **1:**455-473, 1949.

Naito, H., Nakamura, K., Kurosake, T., and Tamura, Y.: Transcallosal excitatory postsynaptic potentials of fast and slow pyramidal tract cells in cat sensorimotor cortex, Brain Res. **19:**299-301, 1970.

O'Leary, J. L., and Goldring, S.: DC potentials in the brain, Physiol. Rev. **44:**91-125, 1964.

Phillips, C. G.: Intracellular records from Betz cells in the cat, Q. J. Exp. Physiol. **41:**58-69, 1956.

Phillis, J. W., and Ochs, S.: Occlusive behavior of negative-wave direct cortical response (DCR) and single cells in the cortex, J Neurophysiol. **34:**374-388, 1971.

Purpura, D. P., and Cohen, B.: Intracellular recording from thalamic neurons during recruiting responses, J. Neurophysiol. **25:**621-635, 1962.

Purpura, D. P., Shofer, R. J., and Musgrave, F. S.: Cortical intracellular potentials during augmenting and recruiting responses. II. Patterns of synaptic activities in pyramidal and nonpyramidal tract neurons, J. Neurophysiol. **27:**133-151, 1964.

Spencer, W. A., and Brookhart, J. M.: Electrical patterns of augmenting and recruiting waves in depth of sensorimotor cortex of cats, J. Neurophysiol. **24:**26-49, 1961.

Steriade, M., Apostol, V., and Oakson, G.: Control of unitary activities in cerebello-thalamic pathway during wakefulness and synchronized sleep, J. Neurophysiol. **34:**389-413, 1971.

Van Harreveld, A., and Khattab, F. I.: Changes in cortical extracellular space during spreading depression investigated with the electron microscope, J. Neurophysiol. **30:**911-929, 1967.

Waszak, M., Schlag, J. D., and Feeney, D. M.: Thalamic incremental responses to prefrontal cortical stimulation in the cat, Brain Res. **21:**105-113, 1970.

Whitehorn, D., and Towe, A. L.: Postsynaptic potential patterns evoked upon cells in sensorimotor cortex of cat by stimulation at the periphery, Exp. Neurol. **22:**222-242, 1968.

Electroencephalography

Fois, A., Low, N.: The electroencephalogram of the normal child, Springfield, Ill., 1961, Charles C Thomas, Publisher.

Gibbs, F. A., and Gibbs, E. L.: Medical electroencephalography, Reading, Mass., 1967, Addison-Wesley Publishing Co., Inc.

Hill, D., and Parr, G., editors: Electroencephalography; a symposium on its various aspects, ed. 2. London, 1963, MacDonald & Co. (Publishers) Ltd.

Kiloh, L. G., and Osselton, J. W.: Clinical electroencephalography, ed. 2, London, 1966, Butterworth & Co. (Publishers) Ltd.

Remond, A.: Integrated and topological analysis of the EEG. In Brazier, M. A. B., editor: Computer techniques in EEG analysis, Electroencephalogr. Clin. Neurophysiol., Suppl. 20, 1961.

Epilepsy

Ajmone-Marsan, C., and Abraham, K.: A seizure atlas, Electroencephalogr. Clin. Neurophysiol., Suppl. 15, 1960.

Ajmone-Marsan, C., and Zivin, L. S.: Factors related to the occurrence of typical paroxysmal abnormalities in the EEG records of epileptic patients, Epilepsia **11:**361-381, 1970.

Beresford, H. R., Posner, J. B., and Plum, F.: Changes in brain lactate during induced cerebral seizures, Arch. Neurol. **20:**243-248, 1969.

Dichter, M., and Spencer, W. A.: Penicillin-induced interictal discharges from the hippocampus. II. Mechanisms underlying origin and restriction, J. Neurophysiol. **32:**663-687, 1969.

Gastaut, H.: The epilepsies; electro-clinical correlations, Springfield, Ill., 1954, Charles C Thomas, Publisher.

Gastaut, H.: Clinical and electroencephalographic classification of epileptic seizures, Epilepsia 11:102-113, 1970.

Jackson, J. H.: Selected writings of John Hughlings Jackson; On epilepsy and epileptiform convulsions, vol. 1, edited by J. Taylor, London, 1931, Hoddler & Stoughton Ltd.

Jasper, H. H., and Droogleever-Fortuyn, J.: Experimental studies on the functional anatomy of petit mal epilepsy, Res. Publ. Assoc. Res. Nerv. Ment. Dis. 26:272-298, 1947.

Matsumoto, H., Ayala, G. F., and Gumnit, R. J.: Neuronal behavior and triggering mechanism in cortical epileptic focus, J. Neurophysiol. 32:688-703, 1969.

Penfield, W., and Jasper, H.: Epilepsy and the functional anatomy of the human brain, Boston, 1954, Little, Brown and Co.

Prince, D. A., and Futamachi, D. J.: Intracellular recordings from chronic epileptogenic foci in the monkey, Electroencephalogr. Clin. Neurophysiol. 29:496-510, 1970.

Schmidt, R. P., and Wilder, B. J.: Epilepsy, Philadelphia, 1968, F. A. Davis Co.

Sutherland, J. M., and Tait, H.: The epilepsies; modern diagnosis and treatment, Edinburgh, 1969, E. & S. Livingstone Ltd.

Ward, A. A., Jr.: The epileptic neuron; chronic foci in animals and man. In Jasper, H. H., Ward, A. A., and Pope, A., editors: Basic mechanisms of the epilepsies, Boston, 1969, Little, Brown and Co.

CHAPTER 7

Sensory systems

SENSORY ACTIVITIES AND THEIR NEURAL SUBSTRATES

Two aspects of the functional activity of the sensory systems should be distinguished. The first is the sensory input involved in reflex or unconscious activity. Such activity can be seen, for example, in impulses coming from muscle spindle and joint receptors that are involved in postural reactions that generally do not involve conscious sensation. The second and more obvious type of sensory activity is that which results in conscious sensation or perception. Afferent fiber activity involved in reflex behavior has been more extensively analyzed in terms of the information carried by the discharges than has afferent fiber ac-

tivity involved in perception. Reflex connections are emphasized in Chapter 4; the dominant theme of this chapter is the neural pathways involved in sensory perception.

If psychophysiologists are to describe the neural substrates and patterns of activity in neurons that are correlated with particular psychological or perceptual states, the first task of psychophysiologists must be to define those perceptual states or those features of sensation with which neural activity can be correlated. In general, the perception of sensation in all of the sensory spheres has at least three aspects: sensations have specific qualities and intensity, and they can be localized in space. For example, in auditory perception sounds can be described in terms of tone, loudness, and their source with respect to the observer. Visual perceptions have color and brightness, and they are localized in the visual field. The homologies between the psychophysiological aspects of different sensory systems are incomplete, however. The visual sphere is more complex than the other sensory spheres; and under the heading of quality, it is possible to include such modalities as form, size, direction, and speed of movement, as well as color.

ORGANIZATION OF SENSORY SYSTEMS
General anatomical plan

An idealized sensory system can be described, although the different systems cannot be homologized

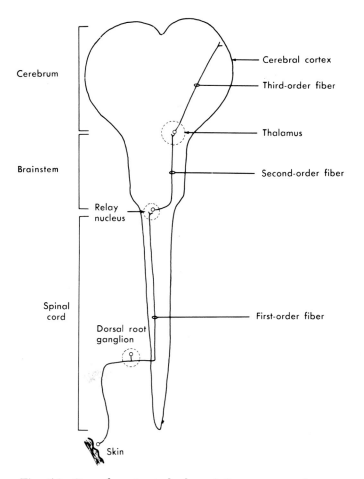

Fig. 7-1. General anatomical plan of the sensory pathways. The first-order neuron of a sensory pathway is shown innervating a sensory receptor in the skin. Its cell body is in a dorsal root ganglion, and the ascending fiber ascends in the spinal cord to end in the medulla. In this case, the second-order neuron has its cell body in the lower brainstem. The decussation of its axon is shown, and the second-order fiber ascends to the thalamus. Here it synapses with a third-order neuron, whose axon projects to a sensory area of the cerebral cortex.

in detail anatomically any more than they can be completely homologized psychophysically. The generalized plan of a sensory system would include a primary afferent fiber, or first-order neuron (Fig. 7-1). The cell body of a first-order fiber is characteristically located in a ganglion in the peripheral nervous system rather than in the central nervous system. A peripheral process, which, from the standpoint of the direction of information flow, is equivalent to a dendrite, connects with a sensory receptor organ (see Chapter 2), whereas a central process enters the spinal cord or brainstem to synapse on a second-order cell of the sensory pathway. The second-order neuron gives off an axon that decussates (crosses to the contralateral side) and ascends to a higher level of the central nervous system. Second-order neurons that decussate are referred to as lemniscal fibers. The lemniscal fiber then synapses with a third-order neuron. In general, the third-order neuron lies at the thalamic level, in a thalamic relay (specific) nucleus of the thalamus. The thalamic relay nucleus cell then gives rise to a projection fiber to a sensory region of the cerebral cortex, where fourth-order neurons receive the sensory information. The three neurons from the periphery to the sensory cortex comprise the central path of the sensory system. However, neurons in the pathway give off branches that synapse with other cells involved either in reflex activity or perceptual activity. Furthermore, some of the sensory pathways utilize more than three orders of neurons.

General physiological plan

Information about the physical properties of a stimulus, such as the pitch and loudness of a sound and its localization in space with respect to the listener, can be coded in the central nervous system by a number of different mechanisms. For purposes of illustration, it is best to consider a particular system, such as the auditory system. The representation of tone can be carried out by the firing of different sets of fibers by different tones. This is the method of coding postulated in the place theory of hearing. Alternatively, information about the frequency of a tone can be carried by fibers firing at the tone frequency or at a fraction of the frequency. This is the type of coding described by the pattern theory of hearing. Other and more complex neural activities can be postulated for coding of the stimulus. However, place and pattern codes appear to be the most common mechanisms that exist within the nervous system (Fig. 7-2). With respect to the other perceptual qualities, other coding mechanisms can be hypothesized. Loudness might be coded by means of an increasing number of fibers firing as the intensity of the stimulus increases, or loudness could be signified by an increased rate of discharge of a sensory neuron as the stimulus intensity increases. It is possible that the mechanisms that code qualities of stimulus are not mutually exclusive, but that the coding of the quality of the stimulus may be carried out in several ways to ensure accurate representation of the stimulus.

In general in sensory pathways, place coding of stimulus quality does occur; that is, there are specific receptors and ascending pathways for specific stimuli (place theory). In the auditory system, the structure of the basilar membrane is so arranged that low tones excite one group of nerve fibers in the cochlea, whereas high tones excite another group of nerve fibers. In the visual system, there are different receptors for different colors. In the somatosensory system, there are receptors that are activated preferentially by pressure and others that are activated by temperature. However, the specificity of peripheral receptors does not appear to be entirely clear-cut. In the auditory system, high tones may activate a portion of the basilar membrane preferentially, but they also activate other portions to some extent. In the somatosensory system, specificity of responses of skin receptors is not complete. For instance, some tactile receptors show an altered response when they

are cooled. The nervous system appears to have mechanisms for sharpening or heightening the specific quality of the information that is received from peripheral receptors. Among these mechanisms are centrifugal pathways to receptor organs and inhibitory synapses in the sensory relay nuclei. Nevertheless, the principle of topographic representation is an important one. Within the auditory system, the spatial separation of cells that respond most strongly to certain frequencies, referred to as their best frequency, is maintained throughout the levels of the auditory system from the peripheral receptors to the auditory cortex.

Another important aspect of the physiological plan of sensory systems is the frequency of discharge evoked by a stimulus. This has been most intensively studied for the coding of intensity of sensation. The human auditory system is able to respond to an immense dynamic range of stimuli. Between the faintest sound detectable and the most intense sound that can be heard without producing structural damage to the basilar membrane of the cochlea is a range of sound energy of 10^{10}. This dynamic range is so great that it is expressed on a logarithmic scale. The extremely large range of stimuli to which the organism can respond is of adaptive value. The transformation of stimulus energy into neural firing rates that represent that energy appears to follow a power-law relationship. This transformation appears to occur largely at the receptor level.

Another important concept about the functioning of sensory systems is the degree of preprocessing of information that occurs at the relay stations within the pathways to the cerebral cortex. This phenomenon has been best studied in the auditory and visual systems. Excitation of particular points within the auditory or the visual system produces excitation of secondary neurons that respond to the stimulus and inhibition of other neurons (surround inhibition). Complex interactions within the relay nuclei appear to occur and, within these nuclei, result in spatial patterns of activity that are thought to code the stimulus. The intrinsic organization of these excitatory and inhibitory lateral networks is thought to form mechanisms that serve as detectors. For example, certain ganglion cells within the retina that project axons by way of the optic nerve respond only to particular peripheral patterns of excitation, such as movement in one direction, or to particularly shaped surfaces in the peripheral field of vision of the cell. Interneurons in the retina are thought to be responsible for this capability of retinal ganglion cells.

A fourth principle of the organization of sensory systems is the control of the relay of information through nuclear centers by descending activity from

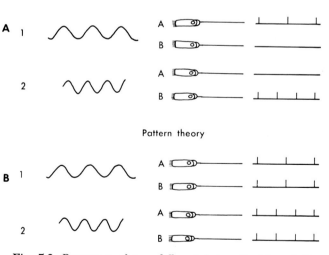

Place theory

Pattern theory

Fig. 7-2. Responses of two different hair cells (*A* and *B*) to auditory stimuli having two different frequencies (*1* and *2*). In **A**, one hair cell is shown to trigger a nerve impulse train in its cochlear nerve fiber in response to just one of the two stimuli, while the other hair cell selectively responds to the other stimulus. This is an example of place coding. In **B**, each of the hair cells responds to each stimulus. However, the frequency of discharge of the cochlear nerve fibers reflects the frequency of oscillation of the stimulus in each case. This is a case of pattern coding.

higher centers. For example, in the auditory system, stimulation of a bundle of fibers going from the superior olive to the cochlear nucleus (olivocochlear bundle) can modulate the amplitude of the response of the receptor cells themselves. Similar suppression (or, less commonly, facilitation) of transmission, frequently brought about by the mechanism of presynaptic inhibition, has been demonstrated in other sensory systems. For instance, a pathway from the cerebral cortex can presynaptically inhibit the synapse between the primary and secondary neurons of the somatosensory system in the dorsal column nuclei.

SOMATOSENSORY SYSTEM
Sensory modalities tested clinically

The choice of sensory modalities for clinical testing does not necessarily reflect psychophysical principles. The modalities are chosen partially for convenience and ease of testing and largely for the purpose of localization of the point of damage that has been done to pathways carrying sensory information within the spinal cord and brainstem in patients with nervous system disease.

For purposes of classification, the somatic sensations that are tested may be divided into the two categories of proprioception and exteroception (see Chapter 2); interoception is discussed later in the section on visceral afferent sensations. Proprioceptive information is concerned with the orientation of the body in space and is derived from sensory receptors that monitor, among other things, joint and head position. Exteroceptive information is concerned with the external environment. The sensory receptors for exteroception include the cutaneous receptors, as well as the auditory and visual systems, which are discussed in later sections of this chapter.

The most commonly tested somatosensory modalities can be grouped into two sets. One cluster of sensory modalities includes discriminative touch, vibratory sensibility, and joint position sense. The other includes crude (nondiscriminative) touch, pain, and temperature sensibility. Some aspects of the clinical testing of these sensory modalities are discussed in Chapter 12.

Complex sensations

Three complex sensations that are tested clinically are the abilities to discriminate between two stimuli applied at different points on the skin, to recognize that two stimuli are applied simultaneously on opposite sides of the body, and to determine the shapes and sizes of objects by manipulating them within the hand. The last is referred to as stereognosis (knowing the shape of objects). The ability to perform this type of discrimination is dependent on hand movement as well as on sensory input.

Two sensory modalities about which little is known are itch and tickle. It seems likely that these involve the activation of several types of sensory receptors and that the information is transmitted by a combination of pathways.

Abnormal sensations

Sensation may be decreased or increased as a result of disease. A loss of sensation, or numbness, is called hypesthesia if incomplete and anesthesia if complete. If particular sensory modalities are involved, special terms may be used (analgesia, loss of pain; athermia, loss of temperature sensation). Increased sensation is called hyperesthesia. Again, special names are used when individual sensory modalities are involved (for example, hyperpathia, increased sensitivity to touch, resulting in pain). In some pathological states there may be abnormal sensations called paresthesias. These commonly have a buzzing or tingling quality.

Somatosensory pathways

There are at least three important ascending pathways in the spinal cord that mediate somatic sensations arising in the extremities and trunk. These are the dorsal column pathway, the spinocervical tract, and the spinothalamic tract. The dorsal column pathway conveys discriminative touch, vibratory sensibility, and joint position sense. The spinothalamic tract mediates crude touch, pain, and temperature sensibility. The spinocervical tract appears to have functions that overlap those of the dorsal column pathway and the spinothalamic tract. It carries information concerning discriminative touch in addition to pain and temperature sensibility. In humans, the dorsal column pathway and the spinothalamic tract may be more important than the spinocervical tract. Although little is known as yet about the human spinocervical tract, in some mammals, including carnivores, the spinocervical tract seems to be as important as the dorsal column pathway and perhaps more important than the spinothalamic tract.

Somatosensory information from the face is conveyed largely by way of the trigeminal nerve, although a portion of the skin of the external ear is innervated by the facial, glossopharyngeal, and vagus nerves. The relay nuclei within the brainstem for somatosensory information from the face are the main sensory and spinal nuclei of the trigeminal nerve, and the ascending pathway is the trigeminothalamic tract. Some think that the part of the pathway that relays in the main sensory nucleus of the trigeminal nerve is comparable to the dorsal column pathway and the portion through the spinal nucleus of the trigeminal nerve resembles the spinothalamic tract in function.

All of the somatosensory pathways relay in the thalamus in the ventrobasal nuclei. The pathways from the spinal cord terminate in the ventral posterior lateral (VPL) nucleus; those from the face end in the ventral posterior medial (VPM) nucleus. The VPL and VPM nuclei project to the first and second somatosensory receiving areas (SI and SII) of the cerebral cortex.

In addition to joint position sense, the sensory equipment of the head includes a special proprioceptive system, the vestibular apparatus. For convenience, the vestibular apparatus is discussed along

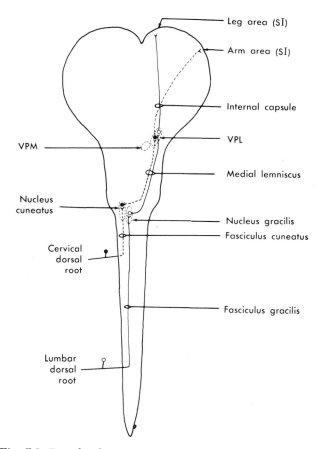

Fig. 7-3. Dorsal column pathway. Afferent fibers contributing to the dorsal column pathway are shown entering the spinal cord through dorsal roots at the lumbosacral and cervical levels. A collateral from the lumbosacral afferent ascends to the medulla through the fasciculus gracilis, ending in the nucleus gracilis. A collateral from the cervical afferent ascends in the fasciculus cuneatus to terminate in the nucleus cuneatus. Second-order fibers originate from neurons of the dorsal column nuclei, cross the midline in the decussation of the medial lemniscus, and ascend to the VPL nucleus of the thalamus. Third-order axons originate in the VPL nucleus and ascend through the posterior limb of the internal capsule to terminate in the appropriate part of the somatosensory cerebral cortex.

with the cochlea, but it should be kept in mind that its function in humans is proprioceptive rather than exteroceptive.

Dorsal column pathway. Information conveyed by the dorsal column pathway originates in sensory receptor organs, chiefly of the skin, but also of joints and muscle (Fig. 7-3). The sensory modalities thought to be represented in the dorsal column pathway include discriminative touch, pressure, vibratory sensibility, and joint position sense. The receptors known to have axons that project up the dorsal column include hair follicle endings, pacinian corpuscles, slowly adapting touch receptors, joint receptors (including paciniform endings), and muscle receptors. The vast majority of the dorsal column afferents are connected with rapidly adapting receptors. High-threshold receptors, which presumably mediate pain, do not have axon collaterals in the dorsal column pathway.

The afferent fibers arising from the sensory receptors travel in peripheral nerves and eventually enter the central nervous system through the dorsal roots. Each dorsal root contains the afferent fibers from a region of skin known as a dermatome (Fig. 7-4). The dermatomes of the embryo are the regions of skin associated with particular somites. Each segment of the neural tube innervates the adjacent myotome (precursor region for muscle) and dermatome (precursor region for skin). In the adult, the dermatome pattern of innervation is still quite clear for the trunk, where the segmental pattern of the rib cage and vertebral column persists, but is less clear for the extremities.

There is considerable overlap in the innervation of adjacent dermatomes. This is shown by the fact that sectioning of a single dorsal root results in practically no sensory loss in the distribution of its dermatome. To obtain complete anesthesia of an area of the skin, it is necessary to cut three successive dorsal roots.

Primary afferent fibers enter the spinal cord through the dorsal roots and divide into ascending and descending branches (Fig. 7-5). The larger fibers enter through the medial part of the dorsal roots, and their branches form a part of the ipsilateral dorsal column. Smaller afferent fibers enter the spinal cord through the lateral part of the dorsal roots and contribute to the dorsolateral fasciculus (of Lissauer). Although many types of afferent fibers course for some distance in the dorsal column, only 25% of afferent fibers project all the way to the medulla oblongata. In this text only these are considered to belong to the dorsal column pathway.

The fibers of the dorsal column pathway from lower spinal levels are displaced medially by those from more rostral levels. This kind of topographic organiza-

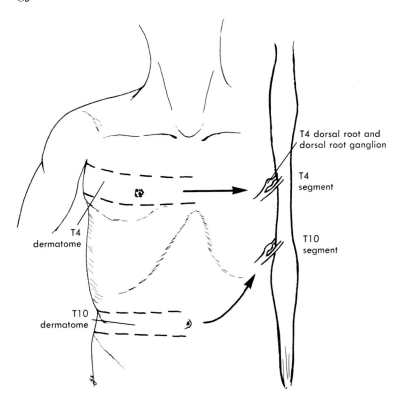

Fig. 7-4. Dermatomes and dorsal roots. The distribution of dermatomes T4 and T10 is shown on the left for the anterior chest wall. The dermatomes continue across the posterior chest wall to the midline of the back. Afferents from these two dermatomes enter the spinal cord through dorsal roots T4 and T10, and the cell bodies of the afferents are contained within the respective dorsal root ganglia.

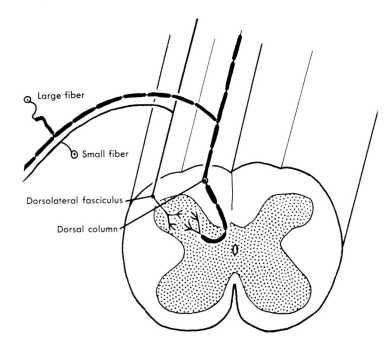

Fig. 7-5. Entry of primary afferent fibers into the spinal cord. The courses of a large myelinated afferent fiber and of an unmyelinated afferent fiber as they enter the dorsal aspect of the spinal cord are shown. The large myelinated fiber enters medially to the unmyelinated fiber and sends branches rostrally and caudally in the dorsal column. Collaterals from these branches descend into the dorsal horn. From cutaneous fibers, these collaterals curve back dorsally to terminate in the nucleus proprius and the substantia gelatinosa. The unmyelinated fiber sends branches rostrally and caudally in Lissauer's fasciculus. Collaterals from these descend into the substantia gelatinosa, where they synapse.

tion is quite common in the central nervous system. The fibers from the lumbosacral and lower thoracic dorsal roots form a compact bundle known as the fasciculus gracilis (Fig. 7-6). The fibers originating from upper thoracic and cervical levels form the fasciculus cuneatus. These two parts of the dorsal column can be distinguished only at the more rostral levels of the cord (above T6).

The fibers of the fasciculus gracilis synapse with cells of the nucleus gracilis in the caudal part of the medulla oblongata (Fig. 7-7). The fibers of the fasciculus cuneatus end on cells of the nucleus cuneatus. It should be noted that the lateral cuneate nucleus has no functional relationship to the dorsal column pathway. It serves as a relay nucleus for the cuneocerebellar tract, and it derives its afferent input from the upper extremities and the upper part of the trunk.

The neurons of the dorsal column nuclei are the second-order cells of the dorsal column pathway, and they project axons to the contralateral side of the brainstem. As the fibers cross, they form a part of a system of fibers known as internal arcuate fibers. Near the midline, these fibers merge to form a compact group of crossing axons known as the decussation of the medial lemniscus (Fig. 7-7). After crossing the midline, the fibers turn rostrally to ascend through the brainstem in a tract called the medial lemniscus (Fig. 7-8). The medial lemniscus terminates in the thalamus in a specific relay nucleus, the VPL nucleus (Fig. 7-9). The axons arising from third-order neurons of the VPL nucleus traverse the internal capsule to end in the appropriate part of SI of the cerebral cortex. Neurons of the VPL nucleus also project to SII, which in humans is found in the cortex forming the dorsal margin of the sylvian fissure.

The topographic arrangement that characterizes layering of axons in the dorsal column is preserved at the more rostral levels of the pathway. The medial lemniscus in the medulla is a vertical bundle of fibers positioned just dorsal to the pyramid and medial to

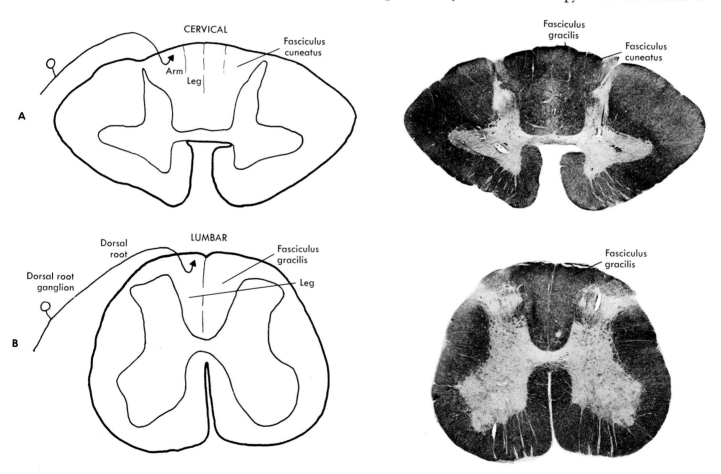

Fig. 7-6. Composition of fasciculus cuneatus and fasciculus gracilis. The dorsal column pathway consists of the ascending branches of afferent fibers. Fibers from receptors of the forelimb and upper trunk (**A**) ascend in the laterally placed fasciculus cuneatus, whereas fibers supplying receptors in the hindlimb and lower trunk (**B**) ascend in the medially placed fasciculus gracilis.

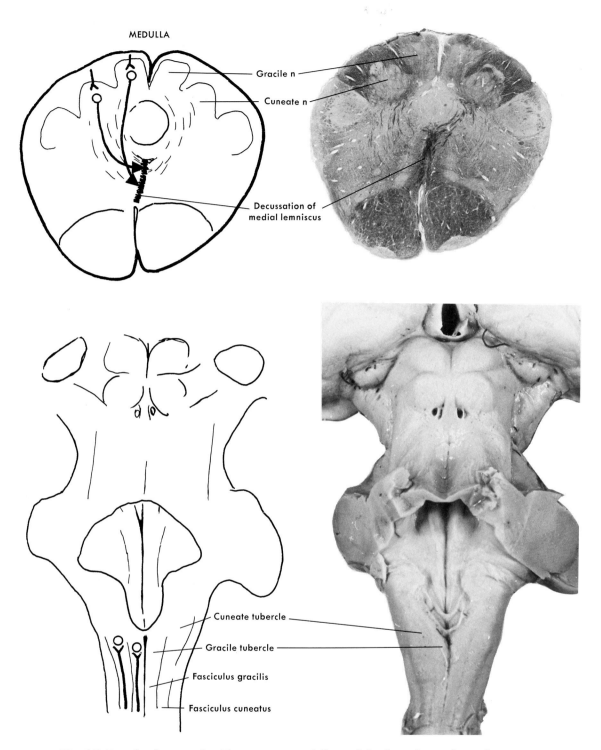

Fig. 7-7. Dorsal column nuclei. The termination of fibers of the fasciculi gracilus and cuneatus on cells of the nuclei gracilis and cuneatus is shown. Second-order axons leave the nuclei and cross the midline in the decussation of the medial lemniscus.

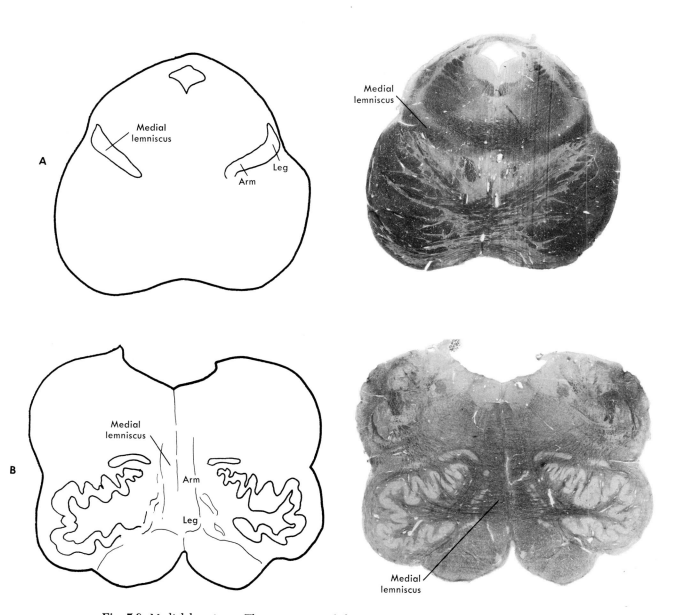

Fig. 7-8. Medial lemniscus. The orientation of the medial lemniscus is vertical in the medulla and oblique in the upper pons and midbrain. The medial lemniscus has a somatotopic organization, with the fibers carrying information from the forelimb and upper trunk coursing separately from those representing the hindlimb and lower trunk. The positions of arm and leg fibers are indicated for the medial lemniscus of the isthmus (**A**) and medulla (**B**).

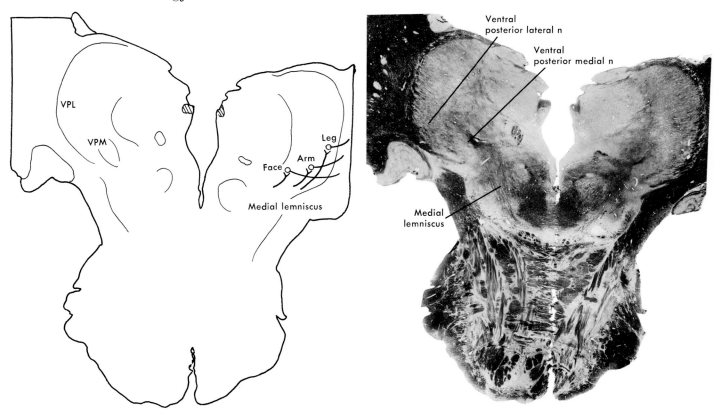

Fig. 7-9. Thalamic relay of dorsal column and trigeminothalamic pathways. The medial lemniscus terminates in a somatotopic fashion in the ventral posterior lateral *(VPL)* nucleus of the thalamus. The trigeminothalamic projection synapses in the ventral posterior medial *(VPM)* nucleus.

the inferior olivary nucleus. Fibers representing the lower body are in the ventral part of the medial lemniscus, whereas those from the upper body are in the dorsal part. As the medial lemniscus enters the pons, its fibers migrate relative to one another, so that the bundle assumes a nearly horizontal orientation. The fibers representing the lower body are now lateral to those for the upper body. In the midbrain and caudal diencephalon, the same general relationship holds, although the medial lemniscus is now angled, with the fibers representing the lower body dorsolateral to those for the upper body. The relay neurons in the VPL nucleus have an orientation that matches that of the medial lemniscus.

The third-order fibers project to the somatosensory cortex through the posterior limb of the internal capsule (Fig. 7-10). In this structure the fibers representing the lower body are located more posteriorly than those from the upper body. The thalamocortical terminals in the postcentral gyrus also have a somatotopic arrangement (Fig. 7-11). The lower body is represented on the vertex and on the medial aspect of the postcentral gyrus; the upper body is represented on the superior part of the lateral surface of the gyrus.

The topographic organization of tracts in the central nervous system and of the gray matter of the thalamus and cerebral cortex is often illustrated by a caricature of the human body called a homunculus. For the sensory system the representation is called a sensory homunculus (Fig. 7-12). The relative amount of nervous tissue devoted to processing information related to a given region of the body is symbolized by the size of that part of the sensory homunculus. For instance, a much larger part of the postcentral gyrus is devoted to the hand than to the thorax. For this reason, the sensory homunculus for the postcentral gyrus has a large hand and a small thorax.

Information conveyed by the dorsal column pathway is processed on its way to the cerebral cortex. This processing occurs at each of the relay stations in the pathway, the dorsal column nuclei and the VPL nucleus of the thalamus. Much more elaborate sensory processing occurs within the cerebral cortex. This pattern of sensory processing in the afferent pathway is characteristic of the various sensory systems of the vertebrate brain.

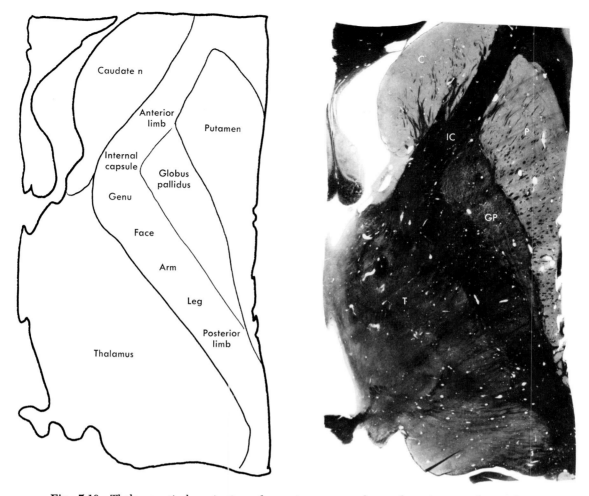

Fig. 7-10. Thalamocortical projection of somatosensory pathway through internal capsule. Third-order sensory fibers from the VPL and VPM nuclei project to the postcentral gyrus of the parietal lobe through the posterior limb of the internal capsule. The section shows the internal capsule cut in the horizontal plane, and the approximate locations of the fibers representing the face, arm, and leg are indicated. Abbreviations: *C,* caudate nucleus; *IC,* internal capsule; *GP,* globus pallidus; *P,* putamen; *T,* thalamus.

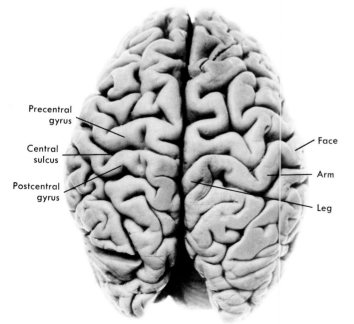

Fig. 7-11. Somatosensory cortex. The leg, arm, and face areas are indicated along the postcentral gyrus. The second somatosensory area (SII) is not shown.

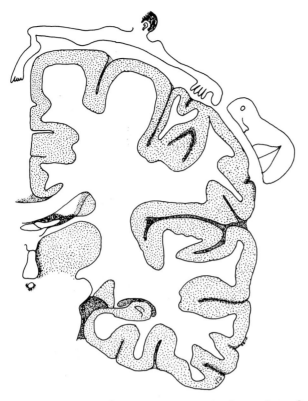

Fig. 7-12. The area of somatosensory cortex that is devoted to the representation of the various parts of the body surface is indicated by a distorted drawing of the human body, known as a sensory homunculus. More cortical tissue is devoted to the face and hand than to other parts of the body; thus these regions are proportionately larger in the homunculus.

Responses have been recorded from neurons of the dorsal column nuclei in an effort to provide an understanding of how these nuclei handle data that are then transmitted to higher levels of the central nervous system. The neurons have excitatory receptive fields, chiefly on the skin. The location of the neurons within the dorsal column nuclei and the position of the receptive fields on the body and limbs show the topographic relationship expected from the anatomy of the pathway. The majority of the cells fire in response either to movement of hairs or to touch or pressure applied to the skin. Some respond to movement of a joint or to stimulation of deep receptors. None appear to respond to noxious stimuli. The sizes of the receptive fields vary with the position of the fields on the skin. The smallest fields are those on the distal parts of the extremities, whereas large fields occur proximally on the extremities and on the body. The receptive fields of the neurons of the dorsal column nuclei are larger than those of the afferent fibers entering the nuclei from the dorsal funiculus. This is expected inasmuch as several afferent fibers converge on any given nuclear cell.

In addition to excitatory effects, stimulation of cutaneous receptors may produce inhibition of transmission to the relay neurons of the dorsal column nuclei. The inhibitory receptive fields are adjacent to the excitatory ones. At least a portion of the inhibitory action appears to be through the mechanism of presynaptic depolarization of the afferent fibers responsible for the excitatory drive. A morphological basis for this presynaptic inhibition is the presence of numerous axoaxonal synapses in the dorsal column nuclei. Fibers of the dorsal funiculus terminating within the nuclei have been shown to be the postsynaptic elements in these axoaxonal complexes. In addition, postsynaptic inhibition has been demonstrated by intracellular recordings of IPSPs from relay neurons of the dorsal column nuclei.

The dorsal column nuclei are subject to the control of the somatosensory region of the cerebral cortex. Stimulation of the sensory cortex results in an inhibition of transmission of information from peripheral nerves to cells within those dorsal column nuclei that project axons to the contralateral thalamus. The same volleys excite neurons within those dorsal column nuclei that do not project to the thalamus. Evidently, these are interneurons, and it has been suggested that the interneurons mediate the inhibitory action from the cortex onto the relay neurons. The inhibitory action of the cerebral cortex appears to depend largely on a presynaptic mechanism. The inhibition can be produced by stimulation of either the contralateral or the ipsilateral somatosensory cortex, although the contralateral action is the more powerful. The pathway descends in the medullary pyramids, so the cortical neurons involved are presumably corticobulbar projection cells with collaterals entering the medullary tegmentum from the pyramids.

The inhibitory action exerted by the cerebral cortex on the dorsal column nuclei illustrates the important principle of the centrifugal control of sensory input by the brain. The sensory cortex can select the information it will receive from that arriving at the level of the medulla in primary afferent fiber collaterals by allowing transmission of a part of the input and suppressing the rest.

The activity of neurons of the VPL nucleus of the thalamus and of the somatosensory region of the cerebral cortex are discussed after the following consideration of several other pathways that provide these higher centers with somatosensory information.

Spinocervical tract. Although the dorsal column pathway plays an important role in transmitting somatosensory information, the spinal cord has alternative routes for supplying this data to the brain. A major parallel pathway in the cat is the spinocervical tract.

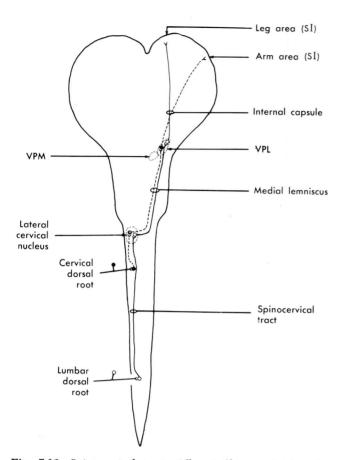

Leg area (SI)

Arm area (SI)

Internal capsule

VPL

Medial lemniscus

VPM

Lateral
cervical
nucleus

Cervical
dorsal
root

Spinocervical
tract

Lumbar
dorsal
root

Fig. 7-13. Spinocervical tract. Afferent fibers activating the spinocervical tract are shown entering the spinal cord through dorsal roots at the lumbosacral and cervical levels. The afferents terminate on second-order neurons located in the dorsal horn of the spinal cord near the level of entry of the afferents. The axons of these cells form a compact bundle of fibers, the spinocervical tract, in the dorsolateral white matter of the ipsilateral side of the spinal cord. The fibers end in the lateral cervical nucleus, which is located in the upper two cervical segments adjacent to the dorsal horn. Third-order axons arise here, decussate in the upper cervical spinal cord, then ascend with the medial lemniscus to the VPL nucleus of the thalamus. Fourth-order fibers connect the VPL nucleus with the somatosensory area of the cerebral cortex by way of the internal capsule.

A comparable tract has been found in a variety of other animals, including primates and humans; however, the path appears to be smaller in humans than in carnivores. The relative significance of the dorsal column pathway and the spinocervical tract in humans is as yet unclear.

The afferent fibers that activate the spinocervical tract enter the spinal cord through the dorsal roots (Fig. 7-13). They originate from both the lower and the upper extremities and from the trunk. The sensory modalities that are conveyed by the pathway appear to include touch, pressure, and (unlike the dorsal

column pathway) pain. The afferent fibers to the pathway originate from receptors giving rise to medium myelinated, small myelinated, and probably also unmyelinated afferents, but not from the largest cutaneous myelinated afferents. Some of the receptors include hair follicle endings of several types and pain receptors. Receptors that do not excite this pathway include pacinian corpuscles, the slowly adapting touch receptors, and joint receptors.

The first relay neurons of the spinocervical tract are located in the dorsal horn of the spinal cord at the segmental level corresponding to that of the afferent fibers. The cell bodies of the relay neurons have been found to lie within the region of the nucleus proprius (laminae IV and V) of the dorsal horn. The axons of these neurons leave the dorsal horn and join the spinocervical tract, which is a bundle of ascending fibers located in the dorsalmost part of the ipsilateral lateral funiculus, between the dorsal spinocerebellar tract and the dorsolateral fasciculus (of Lissauer). The spinocervical tract ends in the upper cervical spinal cord in a special nucleus called the lateral cervical nucleus. This nucleus consists of a column of neurons extending from the lower medulla to the second cervical segment. It is located just ventrolateral to the head and adjacent to the neck of the dorsal horn. The lateral cervical nucleus is the second relay nucleus of the pathway. Third-order axons from the structure cross the midline in the upper cervical cord to ascend in the ventral funiculus. In the medulla these fibers become associated with the medial lemniscus and ascend with it to the thalamus. The cervicothalamic fibers end in the VPL nucleus of the thalamus. Fourth-order fibers then transmit the information to SI and SII.

Recordings have been made of the activity of neurons giving rise to the spinocervical tract fibers and of neurons of the lateral cervical nucleus. Spinocervical tract neurons are excited by movement of hair, by touch or pressure applied to the skin, or by strong mechanical stimuli, including pinching. Firing may also be induced by changes of skin temperature. Few, if any, spinocervical neurons are discharged by proprioceptive input. There are inhibitory receptive fields, although these tend to be harder to demonstrate than those associated with the dorsal column pathway. The inhibitory fields include areas of skin adjacent to the excitatory fields and also distant regions of skin, including skin of limbs other than those having the excitatory receptive fields. IPSPs can be recorded from neurons of origin of the spinocervical tract in response to stimulation of the inhibitory receptive fields. In addition to postsynaptic inhibition, it is possible that presynaptic inhibition may play a role. The cells of origin of the spinocervical tract are subject to descending inhibitory control from the brain. This control is exerted both by the cerebral cortex and by pathways originating in the brainstem. An interesting and important feature of this supraspinal control is that the excitatory receptive fields of spinocervical tract neurons can be constricted by the brain. The sensitivity of the neurons to a given stimulus can be reduced, and the effectiveness of afferent fibers of particular types can be varied differentially.

Neurons of the lateral cervical nucleus display responses similar to those of the cells of origin of the spinocervical tract. However, the excitatory receptive fields of the cells in the lateral cervical nucleus tend to be larger than those of the tract cells. As is generally the case in the somatosensory system, the receptive fields vary in size with their position on the extremities, being smallest distally and enlarging proximally. The lateral cervical nucleus has a somatotopic organization, with representation from the hindlimb in the medial part of the nucleus and from the upper extremity in the lateral portion. Neurons of the lateral cervical nucleus may be inhibited by input from wide areas of the body. This inhibition is in addition to that exerted at the level of the cells of origin of the spinocervical tract, and it involves both presynaptic and postsynaptic mechanisms.

The effect of the spinocervical pathway at thalamic and cortical levels is considered later, along with the action of the other somatosensory pathways.

Spinothalamic tract. The third of the major somatosensory pathways of the spinal cord is the spinothalamic tract (Fig. 7-14). A distinction formerly was made between a lateral and a ventral spinothalamic tract, but there appears to be little anatomical or physiological basis for such a distinction.

The afferent fibers supplying information to this pathway enter through the dorsal roots at all levels of the cord. The sensory modalities that are thought to be represented by the pathway include a crude form of touch and, more important, pain and temperature sensibility. Some of the sensory receptors contributing to the tactile functions of the spinothalamic tract include hair follicle receptors and Meissner's corpuscles. Pacinian corpuscles do not appear to contribute, nor is there any evidence that the slowly adapting tactile receptors do. Insensitive mechanoreceptors, including mechanical nociceptors, provide pressure and pain input. Pain information is also provided by thermal nociceptors. Temperature sensibility depends on input to spinothalamic tract cells from thermoreceptors.

The afferent fibers from the sensory receptors enter the spinal cord through the roots appropriate to the dermatomes in which the receptors are located. The afferents sort themselves into a lateral bundle of small fibers and a medial bundle of large fibers. The small fibers appear to terminate in part on cells of the substantia gelatinosa, as do collaterals of the large fibers. A postulated role of the substantia gelatinosa will be discussed in the following section on the gate theory of pain. The afferents also synapse with the cells of origin of the spinothalamic tract (Fig. 7-15), which are located largely within the dorsal horn, although

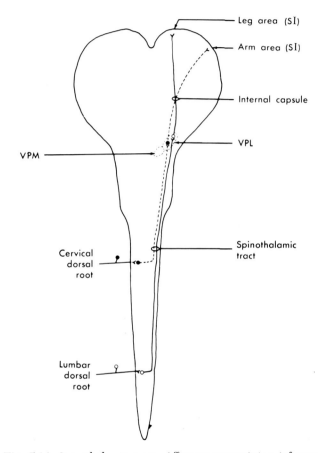

Fig. 7-14. Spinothalamic tract. Afferents transmitting information by way of the spinothalamic tract are shown entering the spinal cord through dorsal roots at the lumbosacral and cervical levels. The afferents synapse within the gray matter. The information may need to cross several synapses before it is relayed by a neuron of the spinothalamic tract to the brain. The axons of spinothalamic tract cells cross the midline at the segmental level in the anterior commissure of the spinal cord. The fibers then ascend in the ventral part of the spinal cord white matter on the side contralateral to the input (there may also be some ipsilateral projections). The somatotopic lamination of the spinothalamic tract as it ascends in the spinal cord is shown in Fig. 12-12. The spinothalamic tract terminates in the VPL nucleus of the thalamus and also in some adjacent nuclei of the posterior thalamus and in some of the intralaminar nuclei. The axons of neurons in the VPL nucleus project to the somatosensory region of the cerebral cortex.

some are also found in the intermediate region and the ventral horn. The spinothalamic tract cells that are responsible for pain and temperature sensibility are located in lamina I and in the nucleus proprius region, especially in lamina V. The tactile cells are in laminae IV and V.

The spinothalamic tract fibers arising from neurons of the spinal cord gray matter cross the midline in the anterior commissure. The axons then ascend in the contralateral white matter in the ventral funiculus and the ventral part of the lateral funiculus. They accompany other ascending tracts, including the ventral spinocerebellar tract, the spinotectal tract, the spino-reticular tract, and the ventral spino-olivary tract.

The spinothalamic tract has a somatotopic organization in the spinal cord. Fibers representing all levels of the body are found in the cervical cord (Fig. 7-15). Here the tract consists of layers, with the fibers from the lowest levels of the cord located at the periphery of the tract and those from the cervical region located medially in the tract. This arrangement is of considerable importance clinically because it determines the depth of incisions in the cord (cordotomy) made for the relief of chronic pain by sectioning of the spinothalamic tract. Pain arising from the lower part of the body can be relieved by a more superficial cordotomy than can pain arising from the chest or upper extremity.

In the medulla the spinothalamic tract is situated just dorsal to the inferior olivary nucleus in the lateral part of the tegmentum (Fig. 7-16). At this level the spinothalamic tract and the medial lemniscus are widely separated. However, in the pons the medial lemniscus shifts laterally; thus the medial lemniscus and the spinothalamic tract are adjacent at pontine levels and higher.

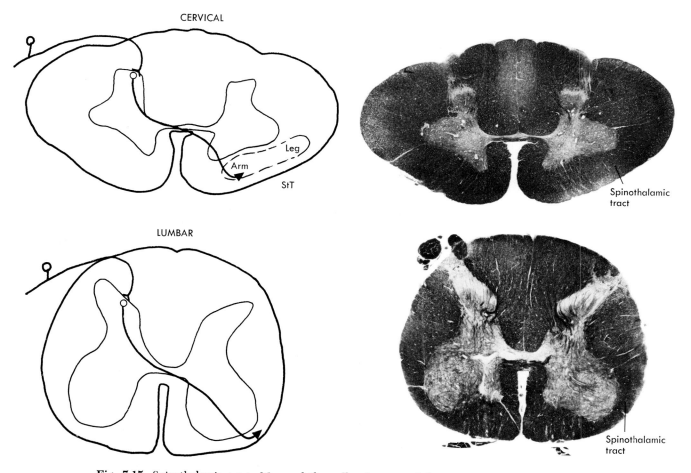

Fig. 7-15. Spinothalamic tract. Many of the cells of origin of the spinothalamic tract (*StT*) are in the dorsal horn, including lamina I. Afferents synapse on these cells after entering the spinal cord over the dorsal root. The spinothalamic tract cells project their axons across the midline in the ventral white commissure. The axons enter the ventrolateral white matter and ascend to the thalamus. The spinothalamic tract has a somatotopic organization, as shown. Fibers carrying information from the hindlimb and lower body ascend in a position lateral to the fibers representing the forelimb and upper body.

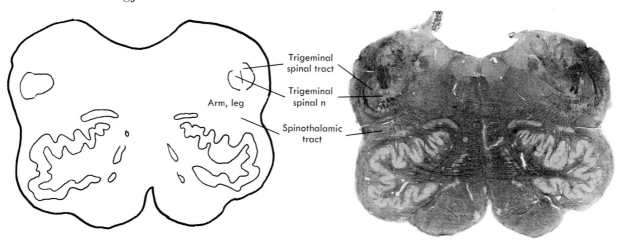

Fig. 7-16. Spinothalamic tract and trigeminal system in medulla. The position of the spino-thalamic tract in the medulla is just dorsal to the inferior olivary nucleus. There is probably a somatotopic arrangement, as indicated. The trigeminal spinal tract and nucleus are adjacent to the spinothalamic tract, but it should be remembered that the trigeminal structures represent the ipsilateral face, whereas the spinothalamic tract represents the contralateral body.

Much of the spinothalamic tract ends in the VPL nucleus of the thalamus, along with the medial lemniscus. However, a part of the spinothalamic tract ends in other thalamic nuclei, including a posterior region adjacent to the medial geniculate body and also in some of the intralaminar nuclei. The significance of the connections of the spinothalamic tract with these nuclei is not clear at present.

As for the dorsal column pathway and the spinocervical tract, the discussion of the actions mediated by the spinothalamic tract at the thalamic and cortical levels is deferred until all of the somatosensory pathways have been discussed.

Gate theory of pain. There is evidence that favors the view that pain is mediated by specific receptors, afferent fibers, and central pathways. This view is an example of the place theory of neural coding. However, an alternative proposal is that the perception of pain is signaled by an enhanced input over pathways whose activity is normally interpreted as touch or pressure. This approach can be considered an instance of the pattern theory. The most recent formulation of a pattern theory of pain is called the gate theory.

A number of observations led to the gate theory. It is well known that cutaneous pain can be antagonized or blocked by nonnoxious stimulation of the adjacent skin. This is the basis for the use of counterirritants for the treatment of painful areas and no doubt also for the tendency of people to rub or scratch such areas. The information interpreted as pain is carried to the central nervous system by small afferent fibers (A-delta myelinated fibers and C fibers),

whereas the counterirritant input is carried by large afferent fibers (A-beta). For some years, investigators interested in pain have believed that there is normally a balance between the inputs over large and small afferent fibers and that pain results when the input over small fibers becomes excessive relative to that over large fibers. For instance, certain kinds of peripheral nerve disease (for example, the neuralgia that sometimes follows an infection of peripheral nerve by herpes zoster, or shingles), result in the differential loss of large afferent fibers. The skin in such cases may have an increased threshold for detecting touch stimuli, yet it may become hyperpathic. A stimulus that is normally innocuous may produce severe pain. One interpretation of this finding is that the large fibers normally present produce central actions that suppress the input from small fibers. Without this suppression, the small fiber input from even mild stimuli may produce pain.

Two additional key observations led to the formulation of the gate theory. Neurons of the dorsal horn (laminae IV to VI) were found to respond to all gradations of mechanical stimulation of the skin; none responded just to noxious stimulation. If pain is relayed by these cells, the information would have to be signaled by a patterned input. The second observation was that small afferent fibers can evoke a positive dorsal root potential in large fibers. The most likely mechanism for such a positive dorsal root potential is the removal of a tonic depolarization. Inasmuch as presynaptic inhibition results from depolarization of afferent fibers, it may be supposed that removal of such a depolarization would result in a disinhibition,

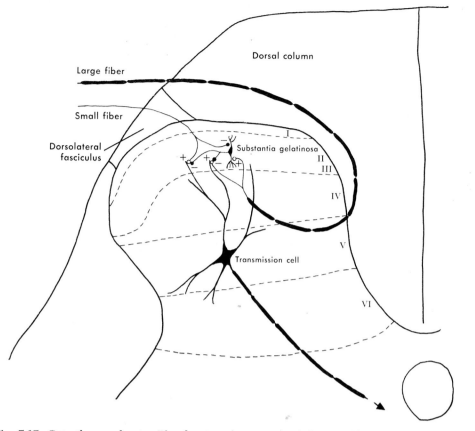

Fig. 7-17. Gate theory of pain. The drawing shows some of the possible neural substrates of the gating mechanism, which has been proposed for control of pain input. Large and small afferent fibers enter the dorsal horn through a dorsal root. The large fibers tend to course medially and loop back under the substantia gelatinosa, while small fibers tend to enter the substantia gelatinosa directly and laterally. In the recent version of the gate theory, large afferents would excite interneurons of the substantia gelatinosa (*SG*) and transmission cells (*T*) of the underlying nucleus proprius, as indicated by the plus signs. On the other hand, small afferents would inhibit the SG cells, as shown by the minus sign, while exciting the T cells. The SG cells would tonically inhibit the inputs over both large and small fibers by a presynaptic mechanism.

or facilitation, of transmission from the large afferent fibers.

A possible neural mechanism for the gate mechanism has been proposed (Fig. 7-17). Large fibers entering the dorsal horn would synapse on and excite two kinds of cells: large transmission (T) cells in the nucleus proprius and small substantia gelatinosa (SG) cells. The SG cells would cause presynaptic inhibition of both large and small afferent fibers. Thus, an input over large fibers would cause a modest response of the T cells but would interfere with further input. The small afferents also synapse on both kinds of cells; however, it is suggested that the synapse on the SG cells is inhibitory. Thus, an input over small fibers would activate the T cells but, in addition, would disinhibit the synapses made by the large fibers, making any ongoing input over these fibers much

more effective in firing the T cells. In this way, large fiber input results in damping of transmission by a negative feedback, whereas small fiber input opens the gate, a positive feedback mechanism. Pain would result when the T cell discharge exceeds some level monitored by higher centers.

There are a number of points of controversy about the gate theory. The first is that dorsal horn cells have now been found that respond selectively to intense stimulation of the skin. These are located in lamina I and the region of lamina V and were overlooked in the initial studies that led to the formulation of the gate theory. There may thus be a separate central pathway for pain transmission, just as there are separate nociceptive afferents in the peripheral nervous system. The other experimental basis for the gate theory was the observation of positive dorsal root potentials when fine afferent fibers were stimulated electrically. However, activation of pain afferents by natural stimulation, using a noxious level of radiant heat, has been shown to result in negative dorsal root potentials. Thus, the experimental evidence favoring the gate theory is no longer convincing. On the other hand, the evidence that large fibers inhibit pain transmission is firm. For instance, clinical studies have shown that pain can be reduced or eliminated by electrical stimulation of large afferents in peripheral nerves or in the dorsal columns.

Trigeminothalamic pathways. Somatosensory information from the face and from the oral and nasal cavities is carried primarily by afferent fibers of the trigeminal nerve (Fig. 7-18). The trigeminal nerve has three divisions—the ophthalmic, the maxillary, and the mandibular. These divisions supply dermatomelike areas of the skin and mucous membranes of the head (Fig. 7-19). The cell bodies of the afferent fibers are in the trigeminal (Gasserian, or semilunar) ganglion,

and the central processes of the ganglion cells enter the lateral aspect of the pons through the main root of the trigeminal nerve. A small area of skin of the external ear is innervated by somatic afferents of cranial nerves VII, IX, and X. The motor components of these nerves are discussed in Chapter 6.

Within the pons the trigeminal afferents generally bifurcate, sending a collateral branch rostrally to terminate in the principal sensory nucleus of the trigeminal nerve and another branch caudally in the spinal tract to terminate in the spinal nucleus of the trigeminal nerve (Fig. 7-20). Some afferents lack an ascending branch. The somatic afferents of nerves VII, IX, and X descend in the spinal tract of the trigeminal nerve and synapse in the spinal nucleus. The principal sensory nucleus of the trigeminal nerve is located at about the level of entry of the trigeminal nerve into the pons, whereas the spinal nucleus extends caudally from the level of the main sensory nucleus to the second cervical segment of the spinal cord. The spinal

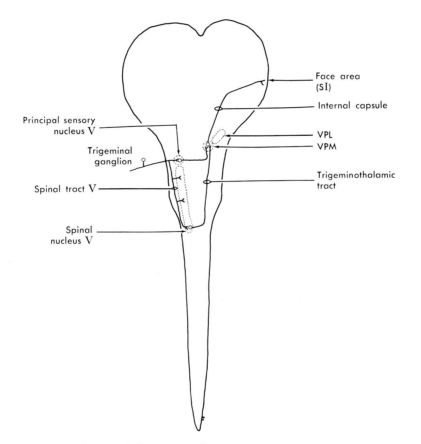

Fig. 7-18. Sensory pathways of the trigeminal nerve. Afferent fibers supplying the skin of the face and mucous membranes of the oral and nasal cavities enter the brainstem through the main portion of the trigeminal nerve, with their cell bodies located in the trigeminal ganglion. The afferents terminate in the principal sensory and spinal nuclei of the trigeminal. Second-order fibers decussate and ascend next to the medial lemniscus to the thalamus. The trigeminothalamic tract ends in the VPM nucleus of the thalamus. Third-order fibers ascend through the internal capsule to the face region of the somatosensory cortex.

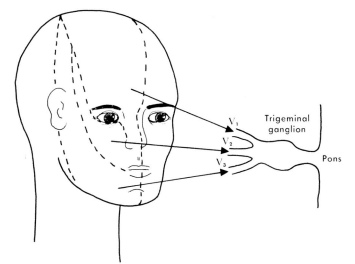

Fig. 7-19. The dermatomelike regions of distribution of the three divisions of the trigeminal nerve are shown for the face. The trigeminal nerve also supplies the mucous membranes of the nasal and oral cavities and parts of the dura mater. Note that the mandibular branch does not supply the skin over the angle of the jaw. V₁, V₂, V₃: ophthalmic, maxillary, and mandibular branches of trigeminal nerve.

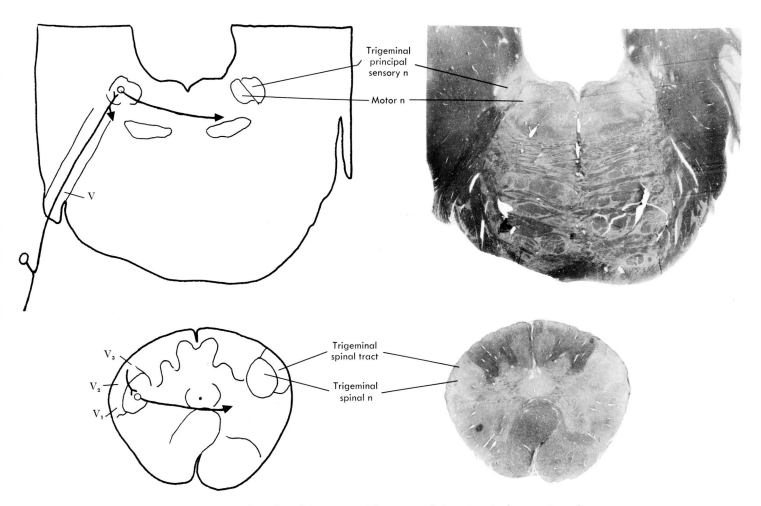

Fig. 7-20. Trigeminal nuclei of brainstem. The entry of the trigeminal nerve into the pons is shown. The trigeminal nuclei in the rostral pons include the principal sensory nucleus and the motor nucleus. The mesencephalic nucleus is shown in Fig. 7-21. Branches of trigeminal afferents also descend in the spinal tract and terminate in the spinal nucleus, as indicated. Second-order trigeminothalamic fibers arise from the principal and spinal nuclei, decussate, and ascend near the medial lemniscus to end in the VPM nucleus. V₁, V₂, V₃: ophthalmic, maxillary, and mandibular branches of trigeminal nerve.

nucleus has been subdivided on cytoarchitectural grounds into three parts—oral, interpolar, and caudal. Although the functional implications of such a subdivision are not as yet clear, the fact that some neurons in the rostral parts of the spinal nucleus project to the cerebellum and other neurons project to the thalamus indicates that the nucleus is by no means homogeneous.

Second-order neurons in the principal sensory and spinal nuclei that project to the contralateral thalamus send their axons across the midline in dispersed small bundles rather than in a well-defined decussation. The axons ascend in a position adjacent to the medial lemniscus. The crossed ascending pathway from the trigeminal sensory nuclei is called the trigeminothalamic tract (ventral trigeminothalamic tract, or trigeminal lemniscus). There is also an uncrossed component originating from the dorsal part of the main sensory nucleus (dorsal trigeminothalamic tract). The trigeminothalamic tract ends in the VPM nucleus of the thalamus (Fig. 7-9). Other fibers terminate in the posterior and intralaminar nuclei of the thalamus in a manner similar to that in the spinothalamic tract. Third-order neurons of the VPM nucleus project to the face region of SI and SII of the cerebral cortex. The face area in SI is on the lateral aspect of the postcentral gyrus (Fig. 7-11).

The trigeminal pathways have a somatotopic organization just as do the somatosensory pathways in the spinal cord. The afferent fibers in the spinal tract of the trigeminal nerve are arranged in layers (Fig. 7-20), with the most superficial fibers belonging to the mandibular division, the intermediate fibers to the maxillary division, and the deepest fibers to the ophthalmic division. Within the principal and spinal nuclei the neurons are ordered in a similar fashion. Neurons with receptive fields in the distribution of the mandibular branch are located most superficially; those with ophthalmic fields are deepest. The oral cavity is represented medially and the face laterally. There seems to be little rostrocaudal differential, although this point is disputed.

Clinical studies led to the view that the principal sensory nucleus of the trigeminal nerve is essentially a tactile relay nucleus and the spinal nucleus subserves pain and temperature. This hypothesis was based on the results of surgical interruption of the spinal tract of the trigeminal nerve. Such a procedure causes loss of pain and temperature sensibility of the face but not loss of touch. Thus, an analogy has been drawn between the principle sensory nucleus and the dorsal column nuclei and the spinal nucleus and the cells of origin of the spinothalamic tract. Until recently, the experimental evidence did not support such an analo-

gy. Neurons throughout the length of the trigeminal complex respond to tactile stimuli. Although only a few neurons that respond specifically to noxious or thermal stimuli have been found within the trigeminal nuclei, many of these are in the main sensory nucleus. Only recently have cells that might specifically relay noxious or thermal information been found in the caudal part of the spinal nucleus. These neurons are located in the marginal zone of the spinal nucleus and in the nucleus proprius and are thus in positions comparable to laminae I and V of the spinal cord. These neurons project to the contralateral VPM nucleus and appear to be similar to the spinothalamic tract cells that respond specifically to pain and thermal stimulation.

Like other somatosensory relay nuclei, the trigeminal sensory nuclei participate in the processing of sensory information. Neurons of these nuclei are sub-

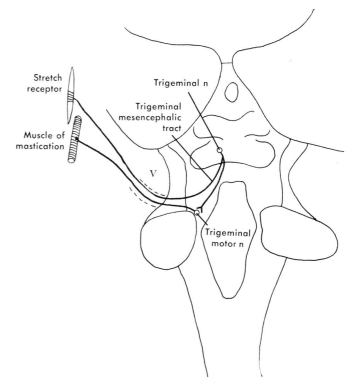

Fig. 7-21. Mesencephalic tract and nucleus of trigeminal nerve. The ending of a trigeminal proprioceptive afferent fiber is shown on a stretch receptor in one of the muscles of mastication. The afferent enters the pons through the portio minor of the trigeminal nerve and ascends in the mesencephalic tract to its cell body in the mesencephalic nucleus. The cell is a pseudounipolar neuron, similar to a dorsal root ganglion cell, but it is located within the central nervous system. The central process of the cell descends in the mesencephalic tract and synapses in the trigeminal motor nucleus, forming a monosynaptic reflex arc. The trigeminal motoneuron projects out through the portio minor to supply the muscle of mastication.

ject to inhibitory influences from peripheral receptors and are under the control of descending pathways from the sensorimotor cerebral cortex. Presynaptic inhibition seems to play a prominent role in these interactions.

Mesencephalic nucleus of the trigeminal nerve. The complex of trigeminal sensory nuclei includes the mesencephalic nucleus. This is actually the equivalent of a peripheral ganglion rather than a nucleus, because the neuron cell bodies in the mesencephalic nucleus are pseudounipolar ganglion cells and give rise to primary afferent fibers that connect with sensory receptors. These fibers reach the periphery by way of the mesencephalic root and portio minor of the trigeminal nerve and distribute to muscles of the head (Fig. 7-21). The receptors supplied include muscle stretch receptors, such as the muscle spindles of the masseter and other muscles of mastication. The central processes of the ganglion cells make reflex connections with motoneurons of cranial nerves, including those of the trigeminal motor nucleus. These connections underlie the stretch reflexes of the head musculature, including the jaw jerk reflex. It is likely that information from these neurons also reaches the cerebellum. However, as with other stretch receptors of the body, it is not certain that afferent information from stretch receptors of the head reaches the level of conscious perception.

Other ascending pathways that may contribute to somatic sensibility

In addition to the pathways just discussed, information that is important for somatic sensation may be transmitted by multisynaptic routes involving other pathways. For instance, it is likely that nondiscriminative touch, pain, and temperature sensations are mediated, at least in part, by propriospinal and spinoreticular tracts. The spinothalamic tract is more critical than these indirect pathways for this kind of sensory information, but the indirect pathways can supplement or even replace the spinothalamic tract function. A similar role of the reticular formation in transmitting sensory data related to the face is also likely.

Relay of somatosensory information in the thalamus

All of the somatosensory pathways transmitting information concerning the body, the face, and the nasal and oral cavities have a synaptic relay in the ventral posterior nuclei of the thalamus. These nuclei have a somatotopic organization, with the contralateral body represented in the VPL nucleus and the head in the VPM nucleus. The sensory homunculus would be in a recumbent position, with the feet placed dorso-

laterally and the shoulders placed ventrolaterally in the VPL nucleus and the head in the VPM nucleus. There is a small ipsilateral face area in the VPM nucleus in addition to the contralateral face representation. The VPL and VPM nuclei together are often referred to as the ventrobasal complex (VB).

The three main pathways bringing somatosensory information from the body appear to terminate, at least in part, on different cell groups in the thalamus. There may be some convergence of these pathways on particular neurons. The spinothalamic tract, in addition to its relay in the VPL nucleus, also has terminations in other thalamic loci. Some fibers terminate in the intralaminar nuclei and others in a posterior nuclear group adjacent to the medial geniculate body. The posterior terminations appear to be bilateral, whereas those in the VPL nucleus are contralateral to the cell bodies of origin of the spinothalamic tract. The dorsal column pathway and the spinocervical tract may also have small components terminating in thalamic nuclei other than the VB complex.

The response characteristics of neurons in the VB complex are well defined. They include excitation by a single stimulus modality, a small receptive field, and a short latency. The somatotopic organization of these thalamic nuclei is readily identified by comparison of the receptive fields of adjacent neurons. On the other hand, neurons in the posterior nuclear group often respond to several stimulus modalities; their cutaneous receptive fields are large, frequently bilateral, and sometimes discontinuous; the earliest discharges of the cells tend to have a longer latency than that of the VB neurons; and there is no obvious somatotopic organization of the posterior nuclei.

Most of the neurons of the VB complex respond to particular stimulus modalities, such as the bending of hairs or light pressure. A few neurons seem to respond best to a stimulus moving in a particular direction. Some respond primarily to intense mechanical stimuli, which in humans are associated with a sense of pain. However, the responsiveness of some of these neurons appears to depend in part on the state of consciousness of the animal. It is not clear at the present whether there are specific pain cells in the VB complex. Furthermore, the neurons that do respond to noxious stimuli seem not to have a somatotopic organization. It is possible that pain localization depends on a separate population of neurons than that responsible for pain recognition. Neurons that respond to thermal stimuli applied to the skin are uncommon in the VB complex. The neurons of the VB complex can often be inhibited by stimuli applied to areas of skin adjacent to their excitatory receptive fields. It is likely that part of this inhibition takes place at lower levels in the somatosensory pathways, but both postsynaptic and presynaptic inhibition have been demonstrated in recordings from the VB complex. It is significant that presynaptic inhibition is not limited to the first synapse of sensory pathways. Neurons in the posterior nuclei also show inhibitory responses from stimulation of the skin.

In addition to peripheral inhibition, neurons of the VB complex are subject to recurrent inhibition. Impulses in the axons of these cells produce IPSPs in the neurons, presumably by a pathway involving recurrent collaterals and inhibitory interneurons. The IPSPs last some 100 msec and are followed by a rebound excitation. It has been suggested that this excitation depends on intrinsic properties of the neuron membrane that cause the membrane potential to shift in a depolarizing direction following the termination of a prolonged hyperpolarization. Alternative explanations are a late EPSP mediated by a long recurrent pathway or a disinhibition. In any event, the rebound excitation may cause the discharge of a number of thalamic neurons, which would result in another period of recurrent inhibition. The entire sequence of discharge, recurrent inhibition, and rebound excitation may be repeated several times in response to a single initiating stimulus. This inherent rhythmicity of the thalamus may play an important role in the generation of the EEG, especially of the alpha rhythm, which has a frequency of about 10/sec. There are also corticothalamic projections to the VB complex. The forelimb and hindlimb areas of the somatosensory cortex project to the VPL nucleus, and the face area projects to the VPM nucleus. The sensory cortex also projects to the posterior nuclear group. The function of these corticothalamic connections is not known.

The axons of the neurons in the VB complex project through the posterior limb of the internal capsule to the cerebral cortex. The regions of termination of these axons include both SI and SII. A number of individual neurons of the VP nucleus have been shown to have a bifurcating axon that sends a branch to each of these regions of the cerebral cortex. Many of the neurons of the posterior nuclear group also project to the somatosensory receiving areas.

Somatosensory areas of the cerebral cortex

Information carried by the major somatosensory ascending pathways reaches the cerebral cortex first in the regions known as the somatosensory receiving areas. These are the areas of cerebral cortex that receive direct projections from the specific relay nuclei of the thalamus for somatosensory information, the VPL and VPM nuclei. The two best-known somato-

sensory areas are the first (SI) and the second (SII).* There may also be a third somatosensory area (SIII), although it has been less well investigated than SI and SII. Somatic sensory information is also transmitted to other regions of the cerebral cortex, although by a more indirect route. For instance, somatosensory data is utilized by the motor areas of the cerebral cortex and also by the parietal lobe association cortex.

In humans, SI is located in a vertically oriented strip along the postcentral gyrus of the parietal lobe. The region is coextensive with Brodmann's areas 1, 2, and 3. The cortex in these areas is of the granular variety (koniocortex), with prominent outer and inner granular layers (see Chapter 6). The specific thalamic afferents contribute to horizontal plexuses of axons in the fourth and adjacent parts of the third and fifth layers. The afferent projections are distributed in a somatotopic manner, with the contralateral surface of the head and body represented in a distorted fashion, as depicted by the sensory homunculus (Fig. 7-12).

SII is located along the upper margin of the sylvian fissure posterior to the central sulcus. The somatotopic organization of SII in humans has not been as well studied as SI because it is less accessible. However, in primates the face is represented medially and the lower extremity laterally. Other differences between SII and SI are that SII receives a bilateral input rather than just a contralateral projection, and the input to SII is only from superficial and not from deep receptors.

A prominent feature of the somatosensory cortex is its columnar organization. When a recording microelectrode is introduced into the cortex at right angles to its surface, all of the neurons encountered in a track through the width of the cortex tend to respond to stimulation of the same region of the body surface. If the microelectrode is shifted slightly along the cortical surface, all of the neurons from which recordings are made respond to stimulation of a distinctly different, although adjacent, part of the body. The proximity of the receptive fields is a function of the proximity of the microelectrode tracks. It seems likely that this columnar arrangement of the cortex depends on a discrete projection of somatotopically organized thalamocortical afferents from the VB nuclei. The thalamocortical afferents enter the cortex from the subjacent white matter and synapse on a series of

---

*In Chapter 8 the cerebral cortex is discussed from the point of view of motor effects elicited by electrical stimulation. The somatosensory area can produce movements, although these are less prominent than sensations. For this reason, it would perhaps be better to refer to the regions as sensorimotor regions, Sm1 and Sm2, rather than as SI and SII.

cortical neurons arranged in a vertical stack. A similar columnar organization is also characteristic of other regions of the cerebral cortex, including the other specific sensory receiving areas and the motor cortex.

In addition to an overall somatotopic arrangement of neuron columns, the somatosensory cortex shows a finer grain organization. Some columns contain neurons that have receptive fields on the body surface; other columns are concerned with receptive fields in deep structures. Furthermore, neurons of different cell columns respond to different sensory modalities. Some of the modalities in SI that have been investigated include touch (including hair bending), pressure, vibration, and joint position. A population of neurons has been found that responds specifically to temperature changes of the tongue. Neurons of SII respond chiefly to touch or pressure. Moving stimuli are especially effective. Some SII cells appear to fire only to noxious stimuli. Others are polymodal, and many have very wide receptive fields. In addition to excitatory responses, inhibition has been observed in both SI and SII. Surround inhibition is produced by stimulation of a region of skin adjacent to the excitatory receptive field. Inhibition may also be produced by stimulation of receptive fields at some distance from the excitatory receptive field. Another type of inhibition observed is cross-modality inhibition. Stimulation of one kind of sensory receptor produces excitation, and activation of another kind results in inhibition.

The receptive fields of cortical neurons tend to resemble those of cells at lower levels of the somatosensory pathways. The fields are often small when distal on an extremity and large when proximal on a limb or on the trunk. Discontinuous receptive fields are not uncommon at the cortical level. Furthermore, variable receptive fields have been described. For instance, receptive fields may increase in size during repeated stimulation, and sensory modalities that are initially ineffective may become effective. It seems possible that such lability depends on alterations in the excitability of the sensory pathways caused by modulation by descending pathways.

The afferent pathways responsible for the different forms of behavior of cortical neurons are still somewhat speculative. The input to SI neurons having discrete receptive fields is presumably conveyed over the dorsal column pathway or possibly over the spinocervical tract. Cortical neurons in SI with wide receptive fields presumably receive information over the spinothalamic tract. However, other indirect routes are also possible, including the spinoreticular tracts, with the linkage to the cortex through reticulothalamic projections and perhaps the nonspecific thalamocortical connections. Another possibility is an intracortical spread of activity. The input to SII is presumed to derive from all three major somatosensory pathways. The spinocervical tract may be more important for SII than for SI. The bilateral input to SII may reflect the projection to SII from the posterior group of thalamic nuclei in addition to the projection of the VB complex.

At the cellular level, cortical neurons have been found to generate excitatory and inhibitory postsynaptic potentials similar to those of neurons at other levels of the central nervous system. The IPSPs indicate that at least part of the inhibitory interactions involving cortical neurons occur at the level of the cerebral cortex, in addition to those that occur at levels of the subcortical relay nuclei, which have been discussed.

Perception of somatic sensation

The interpretation of sensory information at a conscious level requires the participation of the cerebral cortex. For the somatic sensations, the most important regions of the cerebral cortex are SI and SII. However, other regions of the brain, including the association areas of the cerebral cortex and subcortical structures, are undoubtedly also involved in the processing of sensory data.

Somatic sensations can be described in terms of several classes of responses to mechanical stimulation as well as pain and temperature sensibility. From a clinical standpoint, the most important sensory modalities associated with mechanical stimuli are discriminative touch, vibratory sensibility, and joint position sense. These modalities are perceived following the arrival of the appropriate information at the cortical level by way of the dorsal column pathway through the VB complex of the thalamus. The initial cortical data processing is in SI.

Pain and temperature sensations are thought to result from activity in the spinothalamic tract, although other pathways in the ventrolateral white matter of the spinal cord may contribute as well. The chief thalamic relay for these sensations may not be the VB complex. It is possible that the posterior nuclear group and the intralaminar nuclei are more important, at least for transmitting information related to noxious stimulation. Similarly, SII may play a more significant role than does SI in the perception of pain. Other regions of the cerebral cortex, including parts of the frontal lobes, are involved in the reaction to pain.

The role of the spinocervical tract in humans is not as yet clear. It may contribute both discriminative information and data relevant to pain, as it does in other mammals.

The coding of stimulus intensity in the somatosensory pathways seems to involve both the numbers of activated neurons and the discharge rates of individual neurons.

Localization of somatosensory stimuli in space is evidently related to the somatotopic organization of the somatosensory pathways. This is an instance of a place code. The sensory homunculus (Fig. 7-12) defines the relationship between stimulus location and specific regions of SI. A similar homunculus can be drawn for SII. However, it is not clear whether painful stimuli are localized on the basis of information transmitted by the spinothalamic tract or by the simultaneous activation of mechanoreceptors that project by way of the dorsal column pathway.

Clinical applications

The somatosensory pathways are important both for the diagnosis of nervous system disease and for therapy. Some specific examples are briefly mentioned here.

Central nervous system lesions frequently interrupt the long ascending somatosensory pathways. When the dorsal column system is interrupted, whether at the level of the spinal cord or in the brain, the patient is said to show dorsal column signs. These consist of a reduction in discriminative tactile sensibility and a loss of vibratory sensibility and joint position sense. The loss is referred to an area of the body caudal to the point of interruption of the pathway; it is ipsilateral if the lesion is in the spinal cord or dorsal column nuclei and contralateral if it is at higher levels. Although it is debatable that a lesion confined to a dorsal column would produce such sensory losses, there is a good clinical correlation between the occurrence of dorsal column signs and lesions of the dorsal column pathway.

Lesions that interrupt the spinothalamic tract cause a loss of pain and temperature sensibility at levels caudal to the lesion. Although tactile information is also carried by the spinothalamic tract, the patient experiences little reduction in ability to detect touch if the dorsal column pathway is intact. Because the spinothalamic tract is already crossed at the segmental level, the sensory loss will be contralateral to the lesion.

Brain lesions may produce sensory deficits both in the body and in the face. Destruction of the spinal tract or nucleus of the trigeminal nerve produces loss of pain and temperature on the ipsilateral side of the face. In the syndrome of the lateral medulla (Wallenberg syndrome, generally due to occlusion of the posterior inferior cerebellar artery), the spinothalamic tract is interrupted along with the spinal tract of the trigeminal nerve. The resultant sensory deficit is the loss of pain and temperature on the ipsilateral side

of the face and contralateral side of the body. Interruption of the trigeminothalamic tract or of higher levels of the somatosensory projection of the face causes a sensory loss on the side of the face contralateral to the lesion; the loss involves all sensory modalities. A common locus of damage to the somatosensory pathways is in the internal capsule, where cerebrovascular disease often causes hemianesthesia of the contralateral side of the face and body.

Cortical damage in SI is associated with a sensory deficit, generally of a limited area of the contralateral side of the body or face. All modalities may be lost at first, but there is often a partial recovery of some modalities, particularly of pain and temperature. The severest deficits are of the dorsal column modalities. It is not clear what deficits result from damage to SII.

The most important implications of the somatosensory pathways for therapy are in the management of pain. Acute pain, such as that following many surgical procedures, can usually be managed quite well with drugs. However, severe chronic pain caused by certain diseases, including cancer, may not be treated optimally with drugs, either because the drugs are insufficient or because of side effects. A number of options are available for surgical intervention. Peripheral nerves may be blocked with local anesthetics if the pain is restricted to the area of distribution of one or a few accessible nerves. For visceral pain, a sympathetic block may be helpful. Dorsal rhizotomy has been tried for more widespread pain, but this technique is often unsatisfactory. One problem is that there is so much overlap in the innervation of dermatomes that a large number of dorsal roots must be sectioned to render a region anesthetized. A defect of both peripheral nerve block and dorsal rhizotomy is that all forms of sensibility are lost, and the patient may complain of numbness. A more selective loss of pain and temperature sensation in the body without a loss of touch can be accomplished by cordotomy. In the past, this involved a laminectomy to expose the spinal cord, so that the spinothalamic tract could be sectioned under direct vision. Recently, techniques have been developed to allow the introduction of a needle electrode into the spinothalamic tract percutaneously under x-ray film control (Fig. 7-22). The fact that the needle is near the spinothalamic tract is confirmed by stimulation through the electrode, and then the tract is interrupted by electrocoagulation. Because the procedure is done with patients under local anesthetic, they can signify that there is a loss of pain and temperature sensation and indicate the level of the deficit. This information can be used for optimization of the lesion. Unfortunately, the pain may recur months or years after an initially successful cordotomy. The reason for this is unknown, although several possibilities have been suggested, including transmission of pain information over alternative pathways, sprouting of axons at the site of the cordotomy, and failure of the cordotomy to interrupt all of the spinothalamic tract. The first possibility seems the most likely, inasmuch as a second cordotomy often has no beneficial effect in such cases. Because of the problem of recurrence of pain, cordotomy is most successfully used in the treatment of pain in terminally ill patients.

Pain originating in the face is approached in a similar way. Generally, the painful input is interrupted at the level of the divisions of the trigeminal nerve, the trigeminal ganglion, or the portio major. It is possible to transect only the involved part of the portio major, because the afferent fibers retain their somatotopic orientation. A problem with pain in the ophthalmic distribution of the trigeminal nerve is the possibility that interruption of the afferent fibers of the ophthalmic division may lead to corneal insensitivity and hence damage. In an attempt to avoid

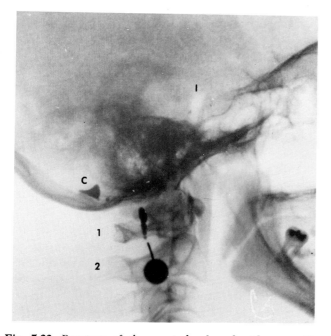

Fig. 7-22. Puncture of the cervical subarachnoid space. The tip of the spinal needle is seen entering the neural foramen between C_1 and C_2. The patient was in the supine position when the x-ray film was taken; a small amount of air and of radiopaque contrast material was injected. The contrast material is layered on the anterior surface of the dentate ligament, and a small amount has entered the cisterna magna (C). A small amount of air is visible above the clivus and in the interpeduncular cistern (I). The tip of the needle points to the location of the spinothalamic tract. The puncture was carried out to perform a percutaneous spinothalamic tractotomy for relief of intractable pain.

this, lesions were produced in the spinal tract of the trigeminal nerve at levels as low as the caudal medulla. Such lesions could produce a deficit in pain and temperature without a loss of touch. However, this approach has not been as widely used as trigeminal root section.

Lesions have also been made at higher levels of the brainstem. For example, the spinothalamic tract has been interrupted in the midbrain and at its relay in the thalamus. For the most effective pain relief with thalamic lesions, it has been found that it is important to intercept the connections into the intralaminar region, as well as those to the ventral posterior (and posterior?) nuclei. One danger with this approach is that inadequate lesions in the upper brainstem may result in the appearance of a central pain state much like that of the thalamic syndrome (caused by damage to the thalamus, usually by cerebrovascular disease). This central pain may be severe and in fact worse than the pain for which therapy was instituted. The explanation for central pain is in dispute, but presumably it reflects a change in the balance of excitatory and inhibitory inputs in the rostral parts of the somatosensory pathways.

Relief from the suffering produced by painful lesions can be produced by psychosurgical procedures, such as prefrontal leucotomy and cingulotomy. After such an operation, patients are not bothered by their pain, although they recognize that it is still present.

Another approach to the question of pain relief based on the gate theory involves stimulation of nervous system structures. The idea is that activation of large afferent fibers from receptors that signal other forms of sensation than pain will activate inhibitory mechanisms that interfere with pain transmission. The procedures used for this purpose include stimulation of peripheral nerve fibers, either transcutaneously or with electrodes implanted on a peripheral nerve trunk, and stimulation of the dorsal column. The dorsal column contains large afferents from a wide distribution, and implanted electrodes can be placed over the dorsal column so that these fibers can be stimulated by a system comparable to a cardiac pacemaker. These procedures have proved to be of value in selected patients, and they have the advantage that nervous tissue is not interrupted irreversibly by placement of a lesion. However, dorsal column stimulators often become ineffective over a period of months; thus their use is diminishing. Another approach that is now being tried is based on a different facet of the gate theory. Inasmuch as the pain circuit is under the control of pathways descending from the brain, it should be possible to inhibit pain transmission by stimulation within the brain. Some neurosurgeons are using electrodes implanted in certain regions of the brain, such as the periventricular region, which are known to interfere with the reactions of animals to painful stimuli. It is too early to predict how effective this kind of procedure will prove to be.

VISCERAL SENSORY SYSTEMS
Visceral afferent systems

Although the distinction between somatic and visceral portions of the nervous system is arbitrary, it is nevertheless useful. The somatosensory pathways provide the brain with information concerning the activity of receptors in the skin, in muscle, and in the joints, and visceral afferent pathways monitor sensory input from the receptors in the visceral organs, which include blood vessels as well as the heart, lungs, gastrointestinal tract, genitourinary system, and other structures of the body cavities.

The sensory receptors of the viscera proper are termed interoceptors, because they detect stimuli originating from within the body. The afferents from these interoceptors are classified as general visceral afferents. Certain exteroceptors, those mediating the sensations of olfaction and taste, are also considered visceral in function. The nerve fibers supplying these are known as special visceral afferents.

This classification emphasizes the more elaborate neural mechanisms involved in olfaction and in taste rather than those mechanisms involved in other sensory modalities. However, it should be noted that there are a number of highly specific and important linkages between particular visceral afferents and effector mechanisms. Many of these operate at a reflex level. An example is the stretch receptor afferents that supply the carotid sinuses. An increased blood pressure activates the afferents. Through their central connections, cardiovascular adjustments are made that tend to counteract the blood pressure elevation. Reflexes of this kind are of critical importance in medicine; however, a full consideration of them is beyond the scope of this book. The interested reader should refer to textbooks of general physiology or to monographs devoted to specific areas of research on visceral reflexes.

General visceral afferent pathways from the body

The best-studied general visceral afferents are those that supply receptors located in the body cavities. Afferents from blood vessels have been less well investigated. Much of the work on visceral afferent pathways is based on activation of afferent fibers in the greater splanchnic nerve, which supplies structures of the upper abdominal cavity.

The greater splanchnic nerve contains large (A beta) and small (A delta) myelinated afferent fibers and also unmyelinated afferent fibers. Many of the large myelinated fibers connect with pacinian corpuscles distributed in the mesentery and in the connective tissue about visceral organs. The small fibers supply other types of receptors, including those that respond to noxious stimuli, such as overdistension of hollow viscera.

Visceral afferents make reflex connections within the spinal cord (see Chapter 4). In addition, the information they convey is transmitted over ascending pathways to the brain. The large afferents give rise to collaterals that ascend in the dorsal column to the dorsal column nuclei. The remainder of the pathway to the cerebral cortex is comparable to that discussed in the previous section on somatic afferent information.

The small afferents may also contribute to the dorsal column pathway. More important, they activate fibers of the spinothalamic tract and related pathways of the anterolateral white matter of the spinal cord. The activity is evoked bilaterally in the anterolateral white matter, though the contralateral projection is greater than the ipsilateral. The information is relayed through the thalamus in a manner comparable to that described for the somatosensory system.

Ascending activity from visceral afferents of the splanchnic nerve activates neurons of the contralateral SI in the area devoted to the trunk. In addition, activity can be recorded from neurons of SII bilaterally. It is not clear how the information from the large visceral afferents is interpreted. Possibilities include body position as detected by shifts in the mesentery and the sense of visceral fullness, or satiation. Pacinian corpuscles would be poor candidates for relaying either of these kinds of sensations because they are rapidly adapting receptors. However, it is likely that other receptors in addition to pacinian corpuscles are connected with large afferents. It seems that the small afferents mediate, among other sensations, visceral pain. Perhaps the most prominent kind of visceral pain is that associated with overdistension of hollow viscera.

Many of the axons of the ventrolateral funiculus that are activated by splanchnic nerve input are also excited by somatic receptive fields. For instance, there may be convergence of excitatory input from distension of the bladder and from any of several stimulus modalities applied to the skin of the hindlimb. Inhibitory receptive fields from either visceral or somatic structures may also be demonstrated. There is also evidence of mutual presynaptic inhibition between visceral afferents and cutaneous afferents.

Referred pain

A phenomenon of major clinical significance is the referral of pain arising from viscera to somatic structures, especially the skin. A familiar example is the referral of pain arising in the heart caused by myocardial ischemia to the left arm. Several theories have been proposed to explain referred pain. There could be pain afferents that have peripheral connections both in the skin and in viscera; however, there is no evidence for this idea. More likely are theories that predict convergence of somatic and visceral input on central neurons, either at the spinal cord level or higher. The demonstration of such a convergence of input at the spinal cord level, mentioned in the preceding section, supports the hypothesis that referred pain depends at least in part on a spinal cord mechanism.

General visceral afferents in cranial nerves

Although visceral pain arising from structures within the body cavities reaches the central nervous system by afferent fibers carried in the components of the sympathetic nervous system (splanchnic nerves, sympathetic trunk), other kinds of afferent information from many of the same structures reach the central nervous system by way of cranial nerves. In large part, such information is used for reflex adjustments. In addition, general visceral afferents of the head also contribute to cranial nerve input.

The cranial nerves responsible for general visceral input are the facial (VII), the glossopharyngeal (IX), and the vagus (X) nerves. The areas of the head and neck that these nerves innervate include the pharynx and larynx. The glossopharyngeal nerve supplies the receptors of the carotid sinus and carotid body. The vagus nerve innervates receptors of the heart and great vessels, lungs, much of the gastrointestinal tract, and other structures of the thorax and abdomen. The motor components of these nerves are discussed in Chapter 6.

The cell bodies of the primary afferent fibers are located in ganglia of the respective cranial nerves (geniculate ganglion of nerve VII, petrosal ganglion of nerve IX, and nodose ganglion of nerve X). After the central processes enter the medulla, they turn caudally to join the solitary tract (Fig. 7-23). The solitary tract is laminated, with the fibers of nerve VII placed laterally and of nerve X placed medially, with nerve IX between. The afferents synapse in the nucleus of the solitary tract, which is just adjacent to the tract (Fig. 7-24). Second-order axons from the neurons of the nucleus of the solitary tract are believed to decussate and to ascend to the thalamus,

presumably to the VPM nucleus. It is likely that the information is then relayed to the face region of the sensory cerebral cortex.

Special visceral sensory pathway for taste

The receptors for taste are the taste buds. Within taste buds are two types of cells, both of which may function in taste. A pore at the apex of the taste bud allows entry of chemical agents into the bud. A gustatory process extends from each taste bud cell toward the pore. Peripheral processes of afferent fibers terminate in relation to the bases of the taste bud cells. Chemical substances that activate taste afferents presumably do so indirectly by altering receptors in the membranes of the gustatory processes of the taste

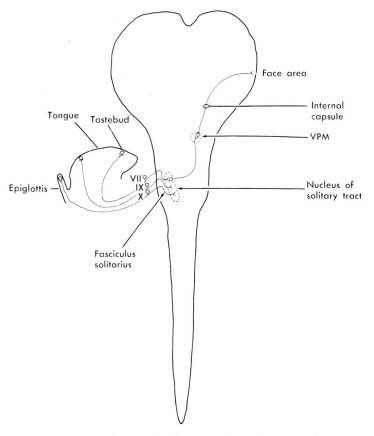

Fig. 7-23. Special visceral afferent pathway for taste. Shown diagrammatically are taste buds on the anterior two thirds of the tongue, on the posterior one third of the tongue, and in the region of the epiglottis. These are innervated respectively by the facial, glossopharyngeal, and vagus nerves. The central processes of the afferent neurons enter the brainstem and descend in the solitary tract, terminating in the nucleus of the solitary tract. Second-order gustatory fibers decussate and ascend to the VPM nucleus of the thalamus. Third-order fibers project from the VPM nucleus to the taste area of the cerebral cortex by way of the internal capsule.. The taste area is adjacent to the face area.

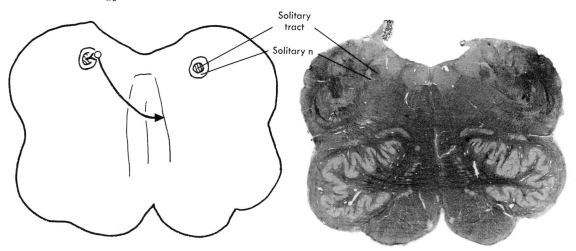

Fig. 7-24. Solitary tract and nucleus. Visceral afferents in cranial nerves VII, IX, and X enter the lower brainstem and descend in the solitary tract to synapse in the solitary nucleus. Second-order fibers from the solitary tract decussate and ascend to the VPM nucleus of the thalamus.

bud cells. A receptor potential would be generated that then activates the afferent nerve terminal.

The classes of stimuli that activate taste receptors are sweet, salt, bitter, and sour. The sensations commonly thought of as taste produced during food ingestion are actually complex mixtures of taste, olfactory, and somatic sensations. When specific chemical agents are used to map the locations of taste buds receptive to particular stimuli, it is found that the tip of the tongue responds to all four taste modalities, but it is most sensitive to sweet and salt. The lateral parts of the tongue are most sensitive to sour, but also respond to salt. The base of the tongue responds to bitter stimuli.

Taste buds on the anterior two thirds of the tongue are innervated by afferents belonging to the facial nerve (Fig. 7-23). The posterior third of the tongue has taste buds connected with the glossopharyngeal nerve. There may be a few taste buds in the pharynx and in the region of the larynx that are supplied by the vagus nerve (perhaps only in infancy). Usually, the taste fibers of nerve VII course in the chorda tympani nerve, although not invariably. The afferent cell bodies are in the same ganglia as the general visceral afferents of nerves VII, IX, and X (geniculate, petrosal, and nodose ganglia). The central pathways are also comparable to those of the general visceral afferents. The taste afferents enter the medulla, turn caudally in the solitary tract, and synapse in the nucleus of the solitary tract (Fig. 7-24). The second-order axons cross the midline and ascend to the VPM nucleus of the thalamus. The taste projection area in the cerebral cortex is adjacent to the face area.

Special visceral afferent pathway for olfaction

The sense of smell is much less developed in man, a microsmatic animal, in comparison with other mammals, such as rodents, which are macrosmatic. The relative importance of olfaction in mammals is reflected in the proportion of the brain devoted to the processing of olfactory information; only a small part of the human brain is employed in olfaction.

The olfactory receptors are hair cells that form a part of the olfactory epithelium in the nasal cavity. Other cell types in the olfactory epithelium include basal cells and sustentacular cells. The lower two thirds of the epithelium is composed of the sensory cells, whereas the nuclei of the sustentacular cells are located more superficially than those of the sensory cells. The sensory cells are actually neurons. They are quite different from the hair cells of other sensory epithelia, such as those of the ear. The olfactory hair cells have a sensory process that extends superficially through the olfactory epithelium between sustentacular cells toward the surface. Projecting from this process is a series of sensory hairs that are modified kinocilia. These kinocilia are presumed to bear on their surfaces the sensory receptive membrane for detecting olfactory stimuli. Beneath the olfactory epithelium are glands (Bowman's) that are believed to secrete a special fluid that bathes the epithelium. It is likely that the chemical agents that produce olfactory responses dissolve in this secretion and then diffuse to the receptive surface. Possibly this process is assisted by movement of the cilia.

The lower surface of the olfactory hair cell gives

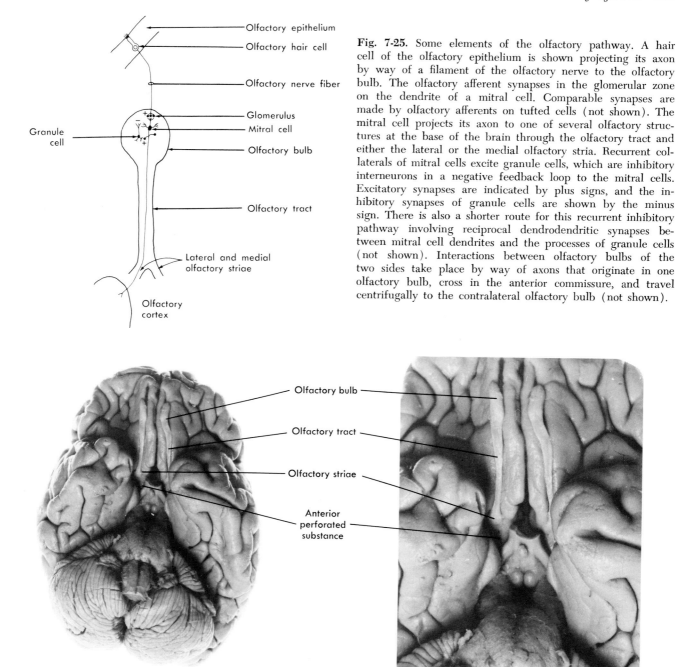

Fig. 7-25. Some elements of the olfactory pathway. A hair cell of the olfactory epithelium is shown projecting its axon by way of a filament of the olfactory nerve to the olfactory bulb. The olfactory afferent synapses in the glomerular zone on the dendrite of a mitral cell. Comparable synapses are made by olfactory afferents on tufted cells (not shown). The mitral cell projects its axon to one of several olfactory structures at the base of the brain through the olfactory tract and either the lateral or the medial olfactory stria. Recurrent collaterals of mitral cells excite granule cells, which are inhibitory interneurons in a negative feedback loop to the mitral cells. Excitatory synapses are indicated by plus signs, and the inhibitory synapses of granule cells are shown by the minus sign. There is also a shorter route for this recurrent inhibitory pathway involving reciprocal dendrodendritic synapses between mitral cell dendrites and the processes of granule cells (not shown). Interactions between olfactory bulbs of the two sides take place by way of axons that originate in one olfactory bulb, cross in the anterior commissure, and travel centrifugally to the contralateral olfactory bulb (not shown).

Fig. 7-26. Olfactory pathway. The base of the brain is shown to demonstrate parts of the olfactory pathway. The olfactory nerves (not seen) synapse in the olfactory bulb. Olfactory information is transmitted from the olfactory bulb to the base of the brain through the olfactory tract. The olfactory tract divides into lateral and medial olfactory striae. Caudal to these is the anterior perforated substance.

rise to an unmyelinated axon. Groups of hundreds of such axons form bundles that penetrate the cribriform plate of the ethmoid bone to enter the anterior fossa of the skull (Fig. 7-25). These bundles of olfactory axons form collectively the first cranial nerve. This arrangement of peripherally located neurons embedded in a sensory epithelium and projecting axons to distant portions of the nervous system is very primitive, resembling the very simple organization of the nervous systems of lower invertebrates.

The olfactory hair cells are very sensitive even in humans. For instance, mercaptan can be detected at a concentration of 0.00000004 mg per liter of air. The olfactory epithelium responds to a variety of odors, which may be divided into a number of major categories. Individual axons of olfactory hair cells have been recorded from, and it is possible to demonstrate some specificity of response to particular types of odorous substances.

The olfactory nerve fibers of one side of the body terminate in the ipsilateral olfactory bulb, which is located just above the cribriform plate. The olfactory bulb is actually a part of the central nervous system, although it is displaced for a considerable distance from the base of the brain. The connection between the olfactory bulb and the remainder of the brain is called the olfactory tract. The olfactory bulb serves to process olfactory information, which is then relayed to the base of the brain through the olfactory tract (Fig. 7-26). The olfactory tract in addition carries axons that connect with the contralateral olfactory bulb.

The olfactory bulb may be regarded as having a simple cortical structure, a primitive version of the cortical structure seen elsewhere in the cerebrum. The key cell type of the olfactory bulb is the mitral cell. These neurons resemble to a certain extent the pyramidal cells of the cerebral cortex. Both cell types have basal dendrites and an apical dendrite, and in both the axon arises from the base of the cell. The apical dendrite of the mitral cell is, however, quite different from that of a pyramidal cell. It terminates in a profusely branched tuft, which forms a part of a synaptic zone known as a glomerulus. Olfactory nerve fibers enter the glomeruli, arborize, and terminate in synaptic relationships with the branches of the apical dendrite. The axon of the mitral cell projects into the olfactory tract, thus serving as an output from the olfactory bulb. In its course, the axon gives off recurrent collaterals that ramify at right angles to the axon in a plexus below the layer of mitral cell bodies.

The olfactory bulb can be described as a layered structure by reference to the arrangement of the mitral cells and their processes. The superficial layer is composed of the incoming olfactory nerve fibers. Next is a layer of glomeruli. Beneath this is an external plexiform layer, which contains the basal dendrites of the mitral cells. Then there is the layer of mitral cell bodies, below which is an internal plexiform layer containing the collaterals of mitral cell axons. The deepest layer of the olfactory bulb contains another cell type, the granule cell, as well as white matter.

The granule cells are the most numerous cells of the olfactory bulb. They lack axons; instead, they have several short dendrites and a long one that extends superficially into the external plexiform layer.

The basis for classifying this long process as a dendrite includes the observation that its surface is covered with spines, which elsewhere in the nervous system are associated only with dendrites. The olfactory granule cells are thus an example of a cell type known as an amacrine (no long fiber) cell.

There are several other neuron types in the olfactory bulb. The tufted cells resemble small mitral cells. Their cell bodies are in the external plexiform layer. The tufted cells have apical dendrites that receive synaptic contacts from olfactory nerve axons in glomeruli, and they also have basal dendrites. Then axons leave the olfactory bulb, but they do not project centrally to the same regions as the mitral cells. Their exact projection is controversial. There are also Golgi type II neurons in the olfactory bulb, both in the glomerular layer and in the granular layer.

An interesting feature of the functional organization of the olfactory bulb is the demonstration of a recurrent inhibitory pathway from mitral cell axons (Fig. 7-25). Activation of these axons by antidromic volleys produces a long-lasting inhibitory effect in the mitral cells, rather like the recurrent inhibition of motoneurons by Renshaw cells (see Chapter 4). The pathway in the olfactory bulb appears to include the granule cells as the inhibitory interneuron. These cells are activated by a volley in mitral cell axons through synapses made by the axon collaterals on the granule cells, and they in turn inhibit the mitral cells by synapses on the basal dendrites. In addition to this pathway, there is another remarkable mechanism by which granule cells produce recurrent inhibition of mitral cells. A new type of synaptic region between mitral cell dendrites and the long dendrites of granule cells, a dendrodendritic synapse, has been described. Such synapses are polarized in both directions. Along a part of the synapse there is a cluster of synaptic vesicles in one process, and in an adjacent region another cluster of vesicles is found in the other process. There is electrophysiological evidence that the mitral cell dendrites excite the granule cell dendrites through one portion of these reciprocal synapses, and then the granule cell dendrites inhibit the mitral cells through the other portion.

The olfactory tract carries information centrally from the olfactory bulb (Fig. 7-26). In addition, it contains centrifugally directed fibers, some of which may arise in the contralateral olfactory bulb. The latter decussate in the anterior commissure. There is evidence that activity in these commissural fibers causes inhibition in the contralateral olfactory bulb.

As the olfactory tract approaches the base of the brain, its fibers separate into two bundles, the lateral and medial olfactory striae. Some fibers relay in the anterior olfactory nucleus, others in the anterior perforated substance, but most terminate in the medial part of the amygdaloid complex and in the prepiriform and periamygdaloid areas of the olfactory cortex. In humans, the olfactory cortex occupies only a small region in the anterior part of the temporal lobe. It should be noted that the olfactory pathway does not include a thalamic relay, in contrast to all of the other sensory modalities. The olfactory cortex has connections with other parts of the brain, including portions of the limbic system and the hypothalamus (see Chapter 10).

Clinical applications

As mentioned, the general visceral afferents are of major importance clinically, both because of their involvement in reflex adjustments through the autonomic and the somatic motor systems and because of sensory symptomatology in disease states. A consideration of some of the reflex mechanisms important in the control of autonomic actvity is given in Chapter 9. However, much of such information is beyond the scope of this text, as is a detailed consideration of the patterns of referred pain.

The special visceral sensations of taste and olfaction are of interest clinically. Loss of taste or olfaction can be helpful in the diagnosis of some lesions. For instance, the location of the point of interruption of the facial nerve in its peripheral course can be aided by examination of the integrity of the taste pathway, because taste afferents in most people leave the facial nerve with the chorda tympani. Damage to the olfactory pathway may occur in head injuries and as a result of subfrontal brain tumors, especially meningeal tumors (meningiomas) of the olfactory groove and cribriform plate. Olfactory hallucinations may occur during temporal lobe epileptic seizures (uncinate fits).

VESTIBULAR SYSTEM
Sensory apparatus of the ear

The evolutionary process of encephalization has resulted in the concentration of a number of important sense organs in the head. In addition to the somatic and visceral afferents of the head that have been discussed, there are the highly complex exteroceptors of the ear and eye. The sensory apparatus of the eye is discussed in the final section of this chapter.

The ear may be subdivided into external, middle, and internal portions. The external and middle ears form the pathway for the transduction of sound energy into mechanical energy in the process of audition. A part of the internal ear, the cochlea, acts as a sound analyzer and relays information concerning incoming sound to the brain. The auditory system is discussed later in this chapter.

The remainder of the internal ear is the vestibular apparatus. This is a sensory receptor that detects the position of the head and changes in the position of the head in space. The vestibular apparatus thus serves as a major organ of equilibrium.

Sense of head position

The dorsal column pathway, as described earlier, is thought to mediate the sense of joint position for the body. Presumably, a comparable sense of position of the jaw is conveyed through the trigeminal system. However, the most important detector of head position is the vestibular apparatus.

The ability to maintain orientation of the body and head in space depends in part on the proper functioning of the sensory systems for determining joint and head position. In addition, important cues are obtained from the visual system. Generally, loss of one set of information—body position sense, head position sense, or vision—will not produce a severe deficit in orientation.

The vestibular apparatus monitors both position and changes in position of the head. Information concerned with static position is transmitted from the otolith organs, and data signaling acceleration of the head originate in the semicircular canals. The afferent fibers carrying this information enter the brainstem through the eighth cranial nerve, accompanied by the afferents concerned with audition that arise from the cochlea. Most of the vestibular afferents synapse in the vestibular nuclei, a set of nuclei in the medulla and pons. Some vestibular afferents terminate in the cerebellum. Activity is generated in a number of pathways that interconnect the vestibular nuclei with a number of neural centers, most of which are concerned with motor function. These pathways are considered only briefly in this chapter but are considered in more detail in Chapter 8. In addition, there is a pathway from the vestibular nuclei to the cerebral cortex. Although the vestibular system operates largely at a subconscious level, modifying reflex activity, there is a component of vestibular activity that reaches the level of consciousness.

Vestibular apparatus

The vestibular apparatus is contained within the temporal bone in a complex cavity known as the bony labyrinth. The vestibular apparatus consists of a tubular structure, the membranous labyrinth, suspended within the bony labyrinth by fibrous strands (Fig. 7-27). The space between the bony and membranous labyrinths is filled with a fluid called peri-

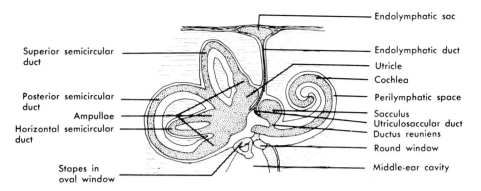

Fig. 7-27. Structure of the bony and membranous labyrinths. The temporal bone is indicated by the hatched area, while the bony and membranous labyrinths are white and stippled, respectively. Only a portion of the coil of the cochlea is shown. (After Sobotta, 1948.)

lymph, which closely resembles cerebrospinal fluid. The canal of the membranous labyrinth is filled with endolymph, which differs from perilymph in that it has a high potassium and low sodium content.

The vestibular apparatus is composed of two groups of sensory receptors, the otolith organs and the semicircular ducts.

Otolith organs. There are two otolith organs, the utricle and the saccule. Each consists of a sensory epithelium (a macula) contained within a dilatation of the membranous labyrinth. The utricular cavity is in continuity with the cavities of the semicircular canals. It is also connected with the cavity of the saccule through the utriculosaccular duct. The saccule is connected with the cochlea through the ductus reuniens. Thus, all of the spaces containing endolymph are in continuity. The endolymphatic duct penetrates the skull to end as the endolymphatic sac between layers of dura. It is thought that one of the functions of the endolymphatic sac is the reabsorption of endolymph.

Utricle. The utricle is an oval tube located medially in the vestibule. The sensory epithelium of the utricle is called the utricular macula (Fig. 7-28). When the head is upright, the utricular macula is essentially parallel to the ground. Covering the epithelium is a membrane in which are imbedded numerous calcareous granules called otoliths (or statoconia).

The sensory epithelium is composed of supporting cells and sensory hair cells. The supporting cells traverse the entire epithelium, whereas the hair cells are just in the superficial part, not extending to the basement membrane. Each hair cell has on its free surface a kinocilium and a group of stereocilia. The kinocilium is placed at one edge of the cluster of stereocilia, thus providing a polarized structure. There are two types of hair cells. Type I cells are pear-shaped and are nearly completely engulfed by a

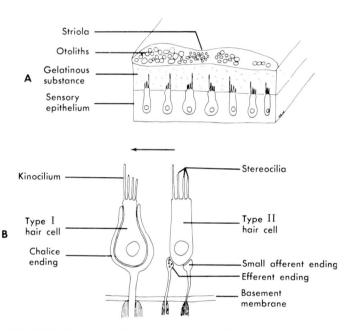

Fig. 7-28. Structure of the utricular macula. The sensory epithelium and its associated otolithic membrane are shown in **A.** The otoliths vary in size, the smallest tending to be in the region of the striola. The sensory hair cells also show a regional distribution. The free margins of the cells are largest, and the concentration of type I cells is highest at the striola. **B,** Expanded views of type I and type II hair cells. The type I cells are pear shaped, and they receive chalice endings from large afferent fibers. Type II cells are cylindrical, and they receive small terminals of afferent and efferent fibers. There are also efferents to the type I cells (not shown). The sensory hairs are cilia, including a kinocilium and several stereocilia. The cilia are the cause of functional polarization of the hair cells. When the cilia are bent in the direction of the kinocilium, the afferent fiber is caused to discharge. (After Lindeman, 1969.)

chalicelike sensory nerve ending. Type II cells are cylindrical, and they receive several small nerve endings at the base. The same cell types are characteristic of all the sensory epithelia of the vestibular apparatus.

Running in a curve through the central region of the utricular macula is a special area known as the striola. The hair cells in the striola have a broader free margin than elsewhere. The hair cells are polarized oppositely on the two sides of the striola, as shown by the pattern of their cilia. The kinocilia are on the striola side in each case. There are also regional differences in the concentrations of type I and type II cells: there are more type I cells in the striola, and at the periphery of the epithelium there are more type II cells.

The otolithic membrane (or statoconial membrane) overlies the sensory epithelium of the utricular macula. The otolithic membrane consists of a gelatinous substance in which are imbedded crystals of calcium carbonate (calcite) of various sizes (up to 30 μm in length). The thickness of the otolithic membrane varies regionally, being thinnest over the striola. The sensory hairs project into the gelatinous material.

The nerve fibers supplying the utricular macula include both afferents and efferents. The afferents end as chalices about the type I cells and as budlike endings on the type II cells. There are also efferent endings on these cells. These contain synaptic vesicles. The nerve fibers supplying the sensory epithelium are myelinated fibers of various sizes. The myelin is lost as the fibers penetrate the basement membrane. The large fibers each innervate a small group of type I cells that have the same polarity and are located close together. Small fibers innervate both cell types and may supply cells of different polarity. The large fibers end as chalices, and the small fibers end as boutons; the latter include both afferent and efferent terminals. The cell bodies of the afferent fibers are in the vestibular ganglion, which is located in the internal auditory meatus. The afferent neurons are bipolar cells that send one process into the vestibular apparatus and another process centrally through the vestibular portion of the acousticovestibular nerve (cranial nerve VIII) to the brainstem. The location of the cell bodies giving rise to the efferent fibers is thought to be the vestibular nuclei.

The afferent fibers of the utricular macula are affected whenever the otolithic membrane is shifted with respect to the sensory epithelium. Most of the afferents show a spontaneous discharge when the head is in an upright position. A given change in head position will cause some utricular afferents to increase and others to decrease their firing rates. The basis for the different responses of individual afferent fibers seems to be the direction in which the sensory hairs are shifted by the shear forces produced by a change in the position of the otolithic membrane. A given afferent fiber will discharge more frequently when the cilia of its hair cells are bent in the direction of the kinocilium and less frequently when they are bent in the opposite direction. As mentioned, there is a regional variation in the orientation of the hair cells of the utricular macula. For instance, the hair cells lateral to the striola are oriented in the direction opposite to that of the hair cells medial to the striola. Thus it would be expected that any tilt of the head would result in a patterned output from each utricle, with some afferents increasing and other afferents decreasing their discharges. The changes in afferent discharge are produced by a receptor potential originating in the hair cell. The receptor potential depolarizes the afferent terminal when the head is tilted in a direction that causes excitation and hyperpolarizes it when the tilt is in the opposite direction.

The response of the utricle is appropriate for a sensory receptor that acts to detect changes in head position. Because the afferent fibers are slowly adapting, the utricle will continue to signal a maintained change in position. The efferent fibers are thought to inhibit input through hair cells. This allows a degree of central control of the sensitivity of the utricle.

Saccule. The saccule is a flattened, irregular structure located in the medial part of the vestibule, just beneath the utricle. Its sensory epithelium is the saccular macula, and it is oriented approximately vertically in the upright human. The structure of the sensory epithelium and of the otolithic membrane of the saccular macula is essentially the same as that of the utricular macula. The saccule is innervated by two different branches of the vestibular nerve.

The function of the saccule in humans is not known. It could presumably aid the utricle in the detection of head position, although this is not established. In some lower forms, the saccule detects low-frequency vibrations and is therefore more akin to the cochlea in function.

Semicircular ducts. There are three semicircular ducts in each labyrinth. These are oriented in planes that are approximately at right angles to one another. One of the ducts is in a plane that is nearly horizontal; if the head is tilted forward 30°, it becomes horizontal. The other two ducts are upright, the second being superior and the third posterior. The semicircular ducts on the two sides of the head form pairs oriented in the same planes. The horizontal ducts of the two sides form one pair, and the superior and posterior ducts of opposite sides form the other pairs.

The lumina of the semicircular ducts connect with

the lumen of the utricle. Two of the semicircular ducts join before reaching the utricle, so that there are five openings in the utricle at points of junction with the semicircular ducts. Near the junction of one arm of each semicircular duct with the utricle there is a dilatation called an ampulla (Fig. 7-29). The sensory epithelia of the semicircular ducts, the cristae ampullares, are contained within the ampullae. The crista is oriented at right angles to the plane of the semicircular ducts. Each crista contains hair cells and supporting cells that are similar to those of the otolith organs. All of the hair cells of a given crista are polarized in the same direction. A separate branch of the vestibular nerve supplies nerve terminals to each crista. The innervation of the cristae is similar to that of the otolithic maculae.

The cilia of the hair cells of each crista project into a gelatinous structure known as a cupula. The cupula projects across the ampulla and divides it completely.

The function of the semicircular ducts is the detection of angular acceleration of the head. When the head rotates, the inertia of the endolymph within one or more pairs of semicircular ducts causes a relative movement of the endolymph in the direction opposite that of the head. The movement of the endolymph causes the cupula to bend in the direction of its flow. This causes a distortion of the sensory hairs, which either increases or decreases the rate of impulse discharge in the afferent fibers innervating the hair cells. If the rotation of the head continues, the friction between endolymph and the walls of the semicircular canal will eventually cause the endolymph to attain the same rate and direction of motion as the head. The cupula will no longer be bent, so the distortion

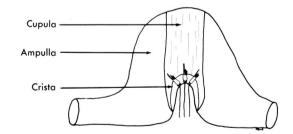

Fig. 7-29. Structure of the ampulla of a semicircular canal. The sensory epithelium covers a projection of the wall of the ampulla into its lumen. This projection is called the crista ampullaris. Sensory hair cells of both types I and II are present in the sensory epithelium. The cilia project into a gelatinous membrane called the cupula, which crosses the remainder of the lumen of the ampulla. Accelerative forces that deflect the cupula will bend the sensory hairs. This produces a receptor potential when the deflection is in one direction, with the result that the afferent nerve fibers discharge. A deflection of the cupula in the opposite direction tends to prevent the nerve fibers from firing.

of the cilia will subside and the rate of afferent discharge will revert to normal. When the head rotation stops, the reverse sequence of events will occur. The cupula will be bent in the reverse direction because of the continued flow of endolymph. After the inertial flow of endolymph stops, the cupula is restored to its original position, and the afferent discharge again reverts to normal. It is interesting that the cupula actually takes longer to return to its former position than is required for the endolymph flow to stop. The latter occurs within about 3 seconds, but the cupula returns to normal only after some 20 to 30 seconds.

The afferents from a given semicircular duct are most sensitive to movements in the plane of the duct. For instance, the most effective stimulus to the afferents of the horizontal canals in humans is a rotation of the individual in a plane parallel to the ground when the head is tilted 30° forward. The afferents of the other canals can best be stimulated by tilting the head in other directions. A convenient device for producing such rotations of human subjects is the Bárány chair. However, it should be emphasized that rotation of the entire body produces a stimulation of semicircular ducts on both sides of the body. When individual semicircular ducts are to be tested, caloric stimulation is used. This involves the introduction of warm or cool water into the external ear canal. Convection currents are apparently set up in the endolymph of semicircular ducts, especially of the lateral duct, which passes near the ear canal. The head is positioned so that the canal is being tested in a vertical plane. The effect of such stimulation is determined by the production of nystagmus, a type of eye movement produced by the central action of vestibular afferents (see Chapter 8).

Central connections of the vestibular nerve

As mentioned, the vestibular afferents have their cell bodies located in the vestibular ganglion, which is in the internal auditory meatus. The central processes of these bipolar cells travel in the statoacoustic nerve (cranial nerve VIII) to the brainstem. The vestibular portion of nerve VIII enters the pontomedullary junction between the restiform body and the spinal tract of the trigeminal nerve. It then branches, with fibers ascending and descending to terminate within the vestibular nuclei (Fig. 7-30).

The vestibular nuclei are located just beneath the floor of the fourth ventricle, chiefly in its lateral recess (Fig. 7-31). The nuclei include the descending, medial, lateral, and superior nuclei, as well as several minor cell groups that are not emphasized here. The vestibular afferents enter specific portions of the vestibular nuclei. In addition, some vestibular afferents bypass the vestibular nuclei and terminate in the cerebellum.

The afferents from the utricle appear to project to the lateral and to the descending vestibular nuclei, whereas the afferents from semicircular ducts project to the superior and medial nuclei.

The vestibular nuclei send second-order axons to each of these regions: the spinal cord, the cerebellum, the nuclei of the extrinsic eye muscles, the reticular formation, and the contralateral vestibular complex. In addition, there is a pathway to the cerebral cortex.

The bulk of the fibers to the spinal cord are in the vestibulospinal tract, which arises from the lateral vestibular nucleus (Fig. 7-30). However, some fibers reach the spinal cord through the MLF, originating from the medial vestibular nucleus. The vestibulospinal tract excites extensor motoneurons on the ipsilateral side of the body. This aids in tonic contractions of the antigravity muscles. The descending fibers of the MLF seem to end within the upper cervical spinal cord. It is probable that they activate motoneurons to muscles participating in movements of the neck, perhaps in synergy with eye movements.

The fibers going to the cerebellum come from the medial and the descending vestibular nuclei. These fibers end in the flocculonodular lobe. Besides the second-order fibers, there are also some primary vestibular fibers that go to the same cerebellar lobe.

The innervation of the nuclei of the extrinsic eye muscles by second-order vestibular fibers is through the MLF. This structure can easily be identified at levels between the medulla and mesencephalon. It continues into the spinal cord. The MLF contains fibers from all four vestibular nuclei. Some of these cross the midline, some ascend, some descend, and some branch and both ascend and descend. Fibers from the superior nucleus all appear to ascend. Many of these second-order vestibular fibers end in the somatic motor nuclei of nerves III, IV, and VI. Some continue rostrally and terminate in the interstitial nucleus of Cajal and in the nucleus of the posterior commissure.

Connections to the reticular formation are made by all of the vestibular nuclei. However, there is some specificity of connections between particular vestibular nuclei and particular regions of the reticular formation.

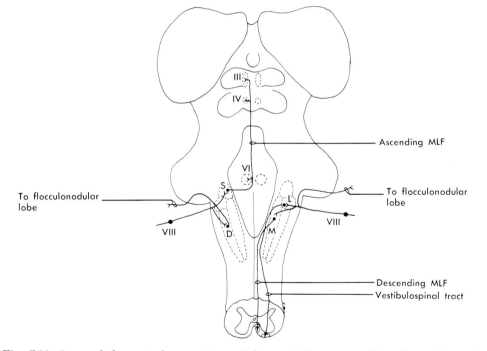

Fig. 7-30. Some of the central connections of the vestibular system. The afferent fibers of the two vestibular nerves are shown synapsing in the four vestibular nuclei. (*S,* superior; *L,* lateral; *D,* descending; *M,* medial). Direct afferents are also shown projecting to the flocculonodular lobe of the cerebellum through the inferior cerebellar peduncle. Second-order fibers are shown arising in the vestibular nuclei, including vestibulospinal fibers from the lateral nucleus, descending fibers of the medial longitudinal fasciculus (*MLF*) from the medial nucleus, ascending *MLF* fibers from the superior nucleus to the nuclei of the nerves to the extrinsic eye muscles, and second-order fibers to the cerebellum from the descending nucleus. Other connections, not illustrated, exist.

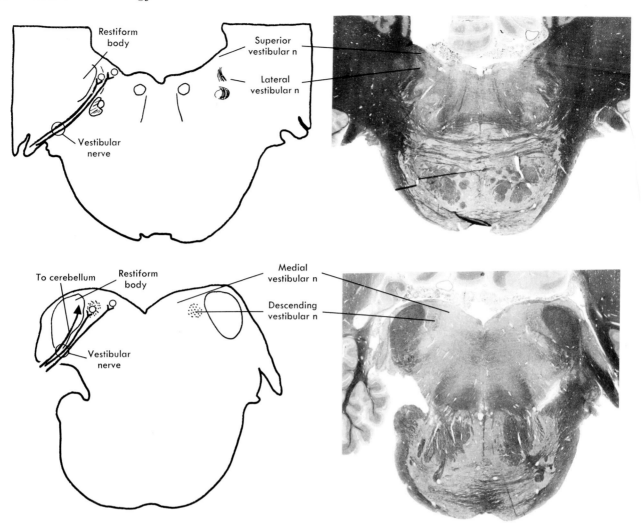

Fig. 7-31. Connections of the vestibular nerve. The vestibular nerve is shown to synapse in the superior and lateral vestibular nuclei in the caudal pons and in the medial and descending vestibular nuclei in the rostral medulla. Direct projections to the cerebellum are also indicated.

The spinal cord, cerebellum, upper brainstem, and reticular formation all give rise to fibers that project to the vestibular nuclei. The connections of the vestibular nuclei are clearly very rich and serve to make the nuclei a major coordinating center.

Pathway from vestibular nuclei to cerebral cortex

There is a pathway from the vestibular nuclei to the cerebral cortex. The sensory receiving areas probably include a portion of the superior temporal gyrus adjacent to the auditory cortex and a region near the face area of the SI somatic sensory cortex. Details about the route followed by vestibular input to the cerebral cortex are not known. It is believed that the pathway contributes to a sense of orientation of the head in space.

Reflex effects of the vestibular apparatus

Besides signaling to the cerebral cortex information concerning spatial orientation, the vestibular apparatus triggers reflex mechanisms that tend to stabilize the eyes, head, and body in space. The vestibular reflexes may be subdivided into three classes: acceleratory reflexes, positional reflexes, and righting reflexes. These reflexes are all organized in reference either to the direction of the gravitational field or to the horizontal plane.

The acceleratory reflexes oppose changes in position. The semicircular ducts are the receptors primarily responsible for these reflexes. If the head is subjected to an angular acceleration, the afferent discharges from the sensory epithelia of one or more pairs of semicircular ducts initiate reflex activity that affects eye, head, and body position in such a way as to counteract, at least partially, the imposed movement. The eyes are shifted conjugately in the direction opposite that of the imposed movement. This helps provide a stable visual target. A fine adjustment of the lines of vision is provided by the fixation reflex (for further discussion of fixation and accommodation see p. 292). If the movement exceeds the range of the eyes, a sudden shift of the eyes in the direction of the movement occurs and another visual target is sought. The alternation of slow eye movements in one direction with fast eye movements in the other is termed nystagmus. Nystagmus may be produced either through vestibular reflexes or through activity in the visual pathway. A detailed description of nystagmus is given in Chapter 8.

In addition to the production of nystagmus, the acceleratory reflexes evoked by semicircular duct activity produce changes in the state of contraction of the antigravity muscles. The muscles will act to counter the imposed movement. For example, if an individual is suddenly thrown to the right, the extensor muscles of the right lower extremity will contract to a greater degree and those of the left limb will relax somewhat. The result is that the body will tend to remain vertical. The neck muscles are also involved, and they will tend to keep the head in its normal position.

Positional reflexes tend to alter the placement of the eyes and body in keeping with the position of the head. The main receptors responsible for the positional reflexes are the otolith organs, especially the utricle. For instance, if the head is tilted, the eye muscles rotate the eyes in a direction opposite that of the head tilt. This tends to keep the visual fields horizontal. The acceleratory reflexes produce the initial change in eye movement, but the maintenance of the new eye position is caused by positional reflexes.

The antigravity muscles of the body are also subject to positional reflexes. The muscle contractions are adjusted in such a way as to keep the head oriented appropriately with respect to the gravitational field. The vestibular reflexes often act cooperatively with the tonic neck reflexes. The latter are triggered by afferent discharges from receptors located in the joints of the neck. It is possible to separate the actions of the labyrinthine and neck reflexes by altering the head position without bending the neck or by changing the angle of the neck while keeping the head in its normal orientation with respect to gravity. Another approach is to destroy the labyrinths or to denervate the neck receptors. The neck reflexes produce the following reflex alterations in the antigravity muscles of the limbs in the cat. If the neck is extended (dorsiflexed), the forelimbs extend and the hindlimbs flex. The op-

posite occurs when the neck is flexed. Turning of the head causes extension of the limbs on the side toward which the head moves. The changes in head position when the neck is extended or flexed are not in the direction of stabilization but are in the opposite direction. On the other hand, the labyrinthine reflexes tend to work in the direction of stabilization. If the body tilts forward, the neck is extended to keep the head horizontal. In addition, the forelimbs would extend and the hindlimbs flex. These actions continue after cessation of activity in the semicircular canals and are caused by the otolith organs.

The third group of reflexes involved in balance is the set of righting reflexes. These tend to cause the head and body to resume their normal position in space. They are initiated when the individual is displaced from the normal position. It is likely that both the semicircular ducts and the otolith organs are responsible for the labyrinthine component of the righting reflexes. In addition, the neck reflexes play a major role. The first compensatory adjustment during righting involves a movement of the head toward its normal position. This initiates neck reflexes that produce movements of the body musculature. The labyrinthine reflexes are minimized as the head assumes a horizontal position. The neck reflexes cease as the body position is normalized. In addition to signals from the vestibular apparatus and the neck receptors, righting can be triggered by the input from asymmetrically activated mechanoreceptors of the body wall. If an animal is lying on its side, the cues available from the force exerted on the flank bearing the animal's weight are sufficient to initiate righting even if the labyrinths are destroyed.

These various reflexes assist in the maintenance of equilibrium. In addition to the acceleratory, positional, and righting reflexes of the labyrinth, the neck reflexes, and the body mechanoreceptor reflexes, balance is maintained through the assistance of the stretch reflexes and other segmental reflexes (extensor thrust, placing responses, and others) and through vision.

Clinical applications

One of the most prominent results of malfunction of the vestibular apparatus is the occurrence of nystagmus and an associated complaint of dizziness. Nystagmus can be produced by an imbalance between the two labyrinths because of an irritative lesion or because of destruction of the labyrinth on one side. Care must be taken, however, to distinguish between nystagmus produced by vestibular system disease and that caused by lesions affecting other parts of the nervous system (for example, the cerebellum). Nystagmus is often horizontal, that is, occurring in a plane parallel to the ground, but in some cases it may be vertical or even rotatory. The direction assigned clinically to nystagmus is that of the quick phase, although the more important part of the activity from a physiological standpoint is the slow phase (the phase comparable to the slow deviation of the eyes that occurs as one turns). Accompanying the nystagmus, there may be a tendency for the patient with labyrinthine disease to fall. This is due to the postural adjustments of the neck and body, which are activated by vestibular stimulation and mediated by the descending lateral and medial vestibulospinal and reticulospinal pathways.

The occurrence of nystagmus and its direction can be usefully documented by electronystagmography. This technique takes advantage of the difference in potential across the eye. Electrodes are placed beside the orbits, and changes in electrical potential are recorded whenever the eyes move.

The integrity of the vestibular system can be tested by inducing nystagmus. This can be done in any of several ways. The entire system can be stimulated by rotation of a patient in a Bárány chair. The head is positioned in such a way as to orient the appropriate set of semicircular ducts parallel to the plane of rotation. Generally, the horizontal ducts are the ones tested. The chair (and with it the patient) is rotated rapidly for a long enough time to allow the endolymph to attain the momentum of the head, thus halting the vestibular input produced by the rotation; then the chair is stopped abruptly, and the effect of the tendency for the endolymph to continue its motion is examined. The nystagmus normally produced in this way is called postrotatory nystagmus. The individual labyrinths can also be tested separately by the caloric reaction. The external auditory canal on one side is irrigated by either warm or cold water. The semicircular duct to be tested is oriented vertically by prior positioning of the patient's head. The warmed or cooled endolymph sets up a convection current within the semicircular duct, and this current impinges on the cupula of the appropriate receptor.

In addition to nystagmus and dizziness, stimulation of the labyrinths may produce nausea and vomiting. These events are well known to individuals suffering from motion sickness. A similar reaction may occur in patients undergoing caloric testing.

The function of the otolith organs is more difficult to test. One reflex caused by otolith organ activity is the ocular torsion response to head tilt. When the head is tilted to one side, the eyes rotate in the opposite direction, thus maintaining a relatively horizontal position. However, this test is not commonly employed clinically.

AUDITORY SYSTEM
Acoustic apparatus

The sense of hearing depends on the acoustic apparatus, which consists of structures in the external, middle, and internal ear. The external ear includes the pinna and the external auditory canal. It is separated from the middle ear by the tympanic membrane.

Within the middle ear is an air-filled space that is kept at atmospheric pressure by means of the periodic opening of the auditory (eustachian) tube, which connects the middle ear with the pharynx. Also in the middle ear is a chain of three auditory ossicles: the malleus, incus, and stapes. The long process of the malleus is attached to the tympanic membrane. The incus bridges between the malleus and the stapes. The stapes is fastened into the oval window, which separates the middle and internal ears. Another membrane between these two cavities is the round window, which is covered by the secondary tympanic membrane. Two muscles, the tensor tympani and the stapedius, are found in the middle ear. The tensor tympani muscle is supplied by the trigeminal nerve, and the stapedius is innervated by the facial nerve. These middle ear muscles are attached to the long process of the malleus and the stapes respectively. Their contractions tend to rotate the ossicles into the middle ear cavity; this reduces the sensitivity of the ossicle chain to vibration. Another structure in the middle ear is the chorda tympani, a branch of the facial nerve.

The internal ear is contained within the bony labyrinth of the temporal bone (Fig. 7-27). It consists of the cochlea (Fig. 7-32). The portion of the cochlea adjoining the oval window is the vestibule. The membranous labyrinth of the vestibule connects with the saccule of the vestibular apparatus through the ductus reuniens. The cochlea is a spiral-shaped structure, having a coil of two and one-half turns in humans. The function of the cochlea depends both on the bony labyrinth and the membranous labyrinth, unlike the vestibular apparatus, which utilizes just the membranous portion. The membranous labyrinth of the cochlea forms a spiral tube that continues almost to the tip of the cochlea. This tube bridges across the bony labyrinth, dividing it into two compartments. The part of the bony labyrinth continuous with the vestibule is called the scala vestibuli. The other part is the scala tympani; this terminates at the round window. The membranous labyrinth stops short of the tip of the cochlea, and the scalae vestibuli and tympani meet at a point known as the helicotrema. The membranous labyrinth in the cochlea is often called the scala media. The coil of the cochlea is supported by a bony core,

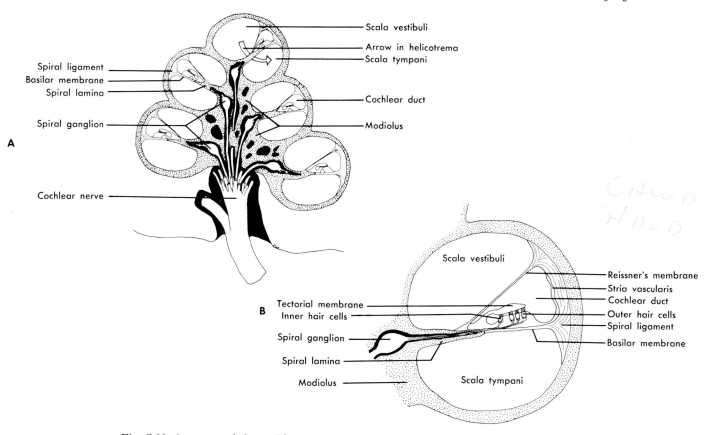

Fig. 7-32. Structure of the cochlea. **A,** cross section through the cochlea. The three ducts are each continuous through the 2½ turns of the cochlea. The scala vestibuli and the scala tympani join at the helicotrema, and the cochlear duct ends blindly adjacent to the helicotrema. Sounds of low frequency cause movements of the basilar membrane along much of its length; sounds of high frequency cause a vibration that is restricted to the proximal part of the basilar membrane. **B,** cross section of the cochlear duct showing the organ of Corti. Movements of the basilar membrane produce a shearing force between the tectorial membrane and the sensory hairs. This results in the development of a receptor potential called the cochlear microphonic, which in turn activates the cochlear nerve fibers terminating on the hair cells. (After Netter, 1962.)

called the modiolus. Along the edge of the modiolus is a spiral ridge of bone, called the spiral lamina. The scala media is attached to the spiral lamina along its internal border. The external border of the scala media is fastened to the wall of the bony labyrinth by a connective tissue structure known as the spiral ligament. The membranous labyrinth of the scala media has a triangular outline in cross section. The base of the triangle is formed by the basilar membrane, which is attached between the spiral lamina and spiral ligament. The upright portion of the triangle is formed by a vascularized membrane, called the stria vascularis, lining the external wall of the bony labyrinth. The stria vascularis may secrete endolymph. The hypotenuse of the triangle is formed by a structure called Reissner's membrane.

The sensory epithelium of the cochlea is in the organ of Corti, which lies on the basilar membrane. The receptor cells of the organ of Corti are hair cells closely resembling the type II cells of the vestibular apparatus. A striking difference, however, is that the cochlear hair cells have only stereocilia, whereas vestibular hair cells also have a kinocilium. Cochlear hair cells are cylindrical in shape, and both afferent and efferent nerve fibers terminate at the base. They are divided into a row of inner hair cells and three or four rows of outer hair cells distributed longitudinally along the basilar membrane. The hair cells are associated with several types of supporting cells. The margins of the hair cells bounding the scala media are joined into a firm platelike membrane called the cuticular membrane. The stereocilia of the hair cells pass through the cuticular plate and are imbedded in an overlying structure called the tectorial membrane.

The tectorial membrane is composed of a gelatinous material and is attached to tissue over the spiral lamina.

The hair cells are innervated by axons from the cochlear nerve. The sensory endings are formed by the peripheral processes of neurons whose cell bodies are contained in the spiral ganglion, which is found within the modiolus. These neurons are bipolar, and the central processes pass into the brainstem in the cochlear nerve. Efferent fibers also form synaptic endings on the hair cells. These fibers arise from cells located chiefly in the contralateral superior olivary nucleus; the axons of these cells cross the pons in the olivocochlear bundle (of Rasmussen). They travel for some distance in the vestibular nerve before they finally enter the cochlear nerve. There are also some uncrossed olivocochlear fibers. The function of the efferent fibers is to inhibit the hair cells, reducing their sensitivity to auditory input.

Functional operation of the acoustic apparatus

The acoustic apparatus serves to analyze sound waves of a range of frequencies between about 20 to 20,000 Hz. The various components of the ear aid in this process. The characteristics of the components in part determine the sensitivity of the ear to particular frequencies.

The external auditory canal has a resonant frequency of about 4,000 Hz, and the middle ear has one of around 1,700 Hz. The overall frequency response of the ear is maximal over a broad range from 800 to 6,000 Hz, with a sharp falloff above and a less sharp falloff below these frequencies. The frequency response of the ear can be altered somewhat by reflex contractions of the middle ear muscles.

The tympanic membrane acts rather like a loudspeaker, or microphone cone. It moves as a whole up to about 2,000 Hz. As it vibrates, it produces movements of the ossicular chain, resulting in movements of the membrane covering the oval window. The force applied at the oval window is about the same as that at the tympanic membrane, but it is concentrated on a smaller area. Almost all of the force is absorbed in driving the oval window.

As the oval window vibrates, a pressure wave is set up in the perilymph of the cochlea. This results in a shift in the fluid, because the secondary tympanic membrane over the round window is free to move. The fluid shift largely involves a displacement of the scala media, although some fluid can pass through the helicotrema. As the scala media is displaced, the basilar membrane becomes distorted and a shear force is developed between the stereocilia of the hair cells

and the tectorial membrane. This results in the production of a receptor potential that in turn causes a change in the discharge pattern of afferent nerve impulses.

The portion of the basilar membrane that moves as a result of a sound stimulus depends on the frequency of the sound waves. The basilar membrane is a continuous structure, so any displacement of it will occupy some length of the membrane. The lowest frequencies of sound are able to produce a displacement of membrane to a distal point along the cochlea. There is a rapid falloff in the amount of displacement beyond the point of maximum displacement. High-frequency sounds produce a displacement of the basilar membrane only near the base of the cochlea. Therefore, the basilar membrane is responsive throughout to low-frequency sounds, but it is sensitive to high-frequency sounds only at the base. These characteristics are responsible in part for the ability of the cochlea to act as a frequency analyzer. The patterns of nerve impulses that are produced by the various longitudinal distributions of the traveling waves set up in the basilar membrane are presumably interpreted in terms of pitch. Sound intensity may be signaled by the response of high-threshold units to sound or by overall input from the cochlea to the brain.

The receptor potentials that are developed in the cochlea are called the cochlear microphonic potentials. They can be recorded from individual hair cells, but more commonly they are recorded with a gross electrode placed in the scalae or on the round window. The cochlear microphonic potentials are oscillatory events that appear to be produced by the hair cells in response to auditory stimuli. They have a frequency that is the same as that of the sound. The distortional forces applied to the hair processes presumably result in a changed membrane potential between the hair cells and the endolymph. The endolymph is at a high positive potential (+80 mV) with respect to the perilymph and other body fluids. This potential is called the endocochlear potential. The hair cells have resting potentials of about –70 mV. The difference in potential across the hair cells with respect to the scala media is thus 150 mV. This may be an important factor in the production of the cochlear microphonic potentials. The endocochlear potential is thought to be maintained by the stria vascularis, but the exact ionic mechanism involved is not known.

Cochlear nerve and central auditory pathway

The primary auditory neurons, as mentioned above, have their cell bodies in the spiral ganglion. The peripheral processes of these cells supply the hair cells of the organ of Corti. Their central processes enter the

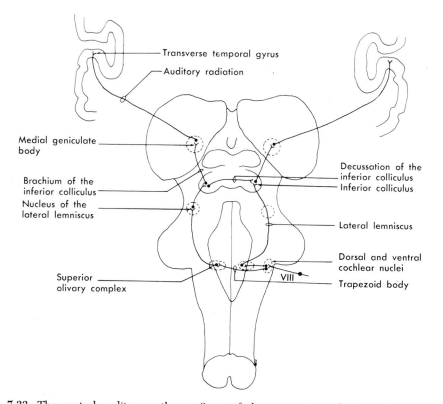

Fig. 7-33. The central auditory pathway. Some of the connections of the auditory pathway are shown for afferent fibers of one cochlear nerve. The first-order fibers synapse within the dorsal and ventral cochlear nuclei. Second-order fibers connect the cochlear nuclei with the superior olivary complex. Ascending fibers then project up each side of the brainstem in the lateral lemnisci. The ones that cross do so in the trapezoid body. There may be a synaptic relay on scattered cells in the trapezoid body (nucleus of the trapezoid body). Some fibers (not shown) of the cochlear nuclei, probably from the dorsal cochlear nucleus, cross in the trapezoid body to synapse either at the nucleus of the lateral lemniscus or at the inferior colliculus. There may be a synaptic relay in the nucleus of the lateral lemniscus, but most fibers of the lateral lemniscus terminate in the inferior colliculus. Information is transmitted from here to the medial geniculate body of the same side through the brachium of the inferior colliculus. Some recrossing of the pathway also occurs at the level of the inferior colliculus through its decussation. The medial geniculate body projects to the auditory cortex through the auditory radiation. The area of the cortex serving as the primary auditory receiving area is the transverse temporal gyrus.

medulla at the level of the restiform body. They terminate in the dorsal and ventral cochlear nuclei (Figs. 7-33 and 7-34). The dorsal nucleus produces the acoustic tubercle on the dorsal aspect of the restiform body; the ventral nucleus lies lateral to the restiform body. Primary cochlear fibers terminate in the two ipsilateral cochlear nuclei. The ventral cochlear nucleus can be subdivided into an anterior and a posterior part, each of which receives cochlear nerve afferents.

The central auditory pathway is complicated, so only the main features are emphasized here. The cochlear nuclei transmit information rostrally through the lateral lemnisci. However, the information is first processed in the superior olivary complex and in the nuclei of the lateral lemniscus. The dorsal cochlear nucleus projects entirely to the contralateral lateral lemniscus; the axons cross the midline in the dorsal part of the tegmentum. The ventral cochlear nucleus projects bilaterally in both lateral lemnisci. Most of the crossing fibers do so in the trapezoid body, although some decussate more dorsally. The fibers from the cochlear nuclei relay in the superior olivary complex or in the nuclei of the lateral lemniscus. Most of the axons of the lateral lemniscus terminate in the inferior colliculus, although a few may project directly to the medial geniculate body (Fig. 7-35). The inferior colliculus gives rise to fibers that ascend to the medial geniculate body in the brachium of the inferior colliculus and also to some fibers that decussate to the

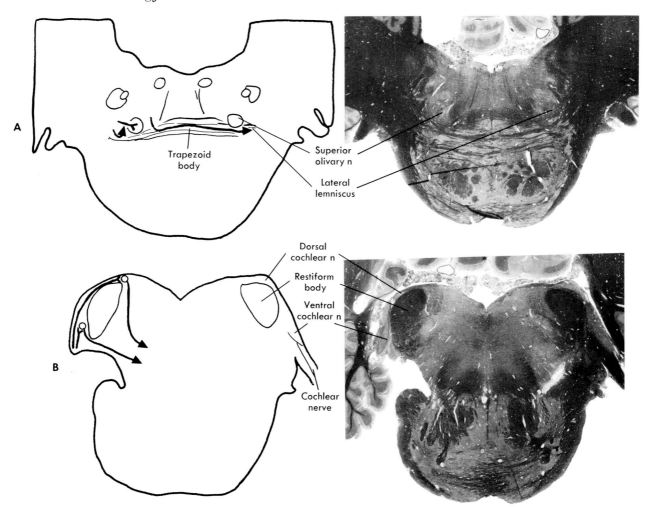

Fig. 7-34. The auditory pathway at the pons, **A,** and pontomedullary junction, **B.** The synapses of auditory nerve fibers in the dorsal and ventral cochlear nuclei are shown in **B.** The cells in the cochlear nuclei project to the superior olivary complex or into the lateral lemniscus. There are both crossed and uncrossed projections. The lateral lemniscus is the ascending auditory pathway.

opposite inferior colliculus. The medial geniculate body projects to the temporal lobe of the cerebral cortex through the auditory radiation. The auditory area of the cerebral cortex includes the transverse temporal gyrus, which is a portion of the superior temporal gyrus.

There are also descending fibers in the auditory pathway. These follow essentially the same course as the ascending fibers and provide a centrifugal control system. In addition, the auditory path has connections with the reticular formation and with the cerebellum.

Functional properties of afferent fibers of the cochlear nerve

The responses of neurons in the auditory pathway to sound are most often represented by tuning curves

(Fig. 7-36). The tuning curve is a graph showing the range of frequencies to which an auditory neuron responds at different intensities of sound. The sound intensity is expressed in terms of a unit of sound pressure level known as the decibel. The sound pressure level is a logarithmic function, and its calculation involves a comparison of the pressure on the acoustic apparatus produced by the stimulus with a reference level.

Tuning curves for single afferent fibers of the cochlear nerve are V-shaped. A fiber will respond to some minimum intensity of sound only when a very narrow range of frequencies is employed. This suggests that a given fiber is tuned to respond to some particular frequency, called its best frequency. If the sound intensity is increased, the fiber will respond to a wider

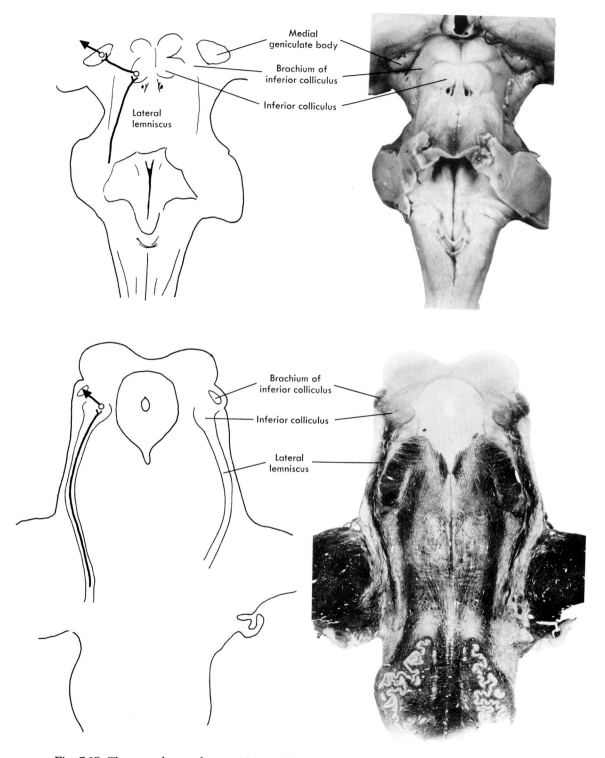

Fig. 7-35. The ascending auditory pathway. Fibers of the lateral lemniscus are shown to relay in the inferior colliculus. The next higher order projection is from the inferior colliculus to the medial geniculate body. From here, the auditory pathway is through the auditory radiation to the transverse temporal gyrus.

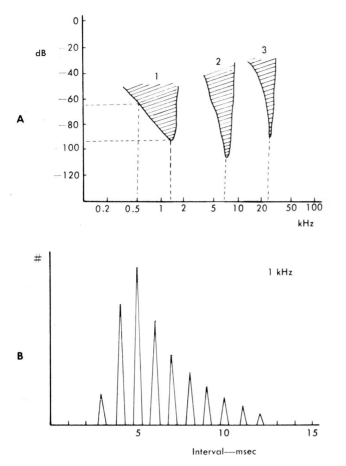

Fig. 7-36. Functional properties of auditory neurons. **A,** tuning curves for three neurons of the auditory pathway. The coordinates of the graph are decibels below a standard intensity level (ordinate) and frequency of a pure tone sound stimulus (abscissa). The neurons respond whenever the stimulus has the appropriate strength and frequency. The hatched areas within the V-shaped curves show the effective stimulus parameters for the three neurons. These are the tuning curves (or response areas) of the neurons. For instance, neuron 1 discharges when the stimulus frequency is 1.3 kHz at all stimulus intensities down to about 95 dB below the reference level. However, the same neuron would respond to a frequency of 0.5 kHz only if the stimulus intensity exceeded −65 dB. The best frequency of this cell is 1.3 kHz. The other two neurons have best frequencies of about 7 and 25 kHz. The graph in **B** is a poststimulus histogram showing the phase locking of an auditory neuron to the stimulus frequency. The stimulus has a frequency of 1 kHz. The abscissa shows the intervals between nerve impulses, and the ordinate the number of times a given interval occurs between impulses during a recording session. For this neuron, the intervals between successive discharges tend to be multiples of the basic stimulus interval, which is 1 msec (reciprocal of 1 kHz). Although there are no responses at 1- or 2-msec intervals, the cell often discharges at intervals of 3, 4, or 5 msec or at higher multiples of the basic frequency. The response is therefore phase locked to the stimulus frequency.

range of frequencies. This is undoubtedly related to the fact that a higher intensity sound stimulus will produce a wider excursion of the basilar membrane, so a given hair cell will be affected by a broader range of stimulus frequencies. A weak stimulus will produce a threshold movement of the basilar membrane for a restricted set for hair cells located at the point of greatest deflection of the membrane.

The complete tuning curve shows the ranges of frequencies that excite the afferent fiber at different levels of sound intensity. All combinations of effective stimuli fall within the margins of the tuning curve. The region of the effective stimulus combinations on the tuning curve is called the response area of the afferent.

Different afferent fibers of the cochlear nerve have different tuning curves. The range of best frequencies of the various afferents matches the spectral sensitivity of the ear to different frequencies of sound. However, the number of fibers having a given best frequency varies. There are more fibers responsive to intermediate frequencies than to either high or low frequencies. The ear therefore is best equipped for detecting and discriminating intermediate frequencies of sound.

A given cochlear afferent fiber will respond to a continuous sound by a discharge at a rate that depends in part on the frequency of the sound and in part on the intensity. If the frequency of the stimulus is kept constant, the discharge rate will vary with the intensity of the stimulus up to a point. Conversely, the discharge rate can be varied by changes in the frequency of a stimulus kept at a constant intensity.

The discharges of cochlear nerve fibers tend to have a constant phase relationship to the sound stimulus. An impulse may not occur with each cycle, but when an impulse does occur it is at a consistent point in time during the cycle. This observation is most easily understood if one considers that the sound wave produces a receptor potential, the cochlear microphonic, which oscillates at the same frequency as the sound. The cochlear microphonic potential produces an excitation of the afferent nerve fiber at this frequency. When threshold is exceeded, the nerve fiber will fire; this occurrence is most probable at the same point in each cycle. There is some variability in the timing of discharges, however. For this reason, the phase relationship becomes obscure for stimuli above 4,000 to 5,000 Hz.

Thus, frequencies of sound below about 5,000 Hz may well be coded by the discharges of a set of afferents that are phase-locked to the stimulus frequency. This would represent a case of a pattern coding of hearing. However, it is difficult to explain the coding of frequencies above 5,000 Hz based on this. The coding for the higher frequencies may be based strictly on the location of the hair cells on the basilar membrane, according to the place theory of hearing. A combination of the two coding mechanisms is proposed in the duplex theory of hearing.

Mechanisms for the centrifugal control of cochlear nerve discharges

There are two important mechanisms by which the central nervous system can regulate the sensitivity of the acoustic apparatus. One is the operation of the middle ear muscles, and the other is an efferent pathway to the cochlea, the olivocochlear bundle.

The middle ear muscles are the tensor tympani and the stapedius muscles. They are innervated by the trigeminal and facial nerves respectively. By reflex action, these muscles contract in response to loud noises, thus damping transmission through the ossicular chain of the middle ear. Loss of innervation of these muscles can produce hyperacusis (hypersensitivity to sound).

The olivocochlear bundle arises from neurons of the superior olivary complex. Most of the fibers cross the midline and reach the contralateral cochlea by way of the cochlear nerve. There is also a smaller uncrossed component. Stimulation of the olivocochlear bundle inhibits the discharges of cochlear afferents. This action is apparently mediated by the efferent endings on the cochlear hair cells. It is a typical postsynaptic inhibition in that it is blocked by strychnine. The function of the olivocochlear bundle seems to be the improvement of auditory frequency discrimination. Evidence for this has recently been obtained by interrupting the olivocochlear bundles as they cross the midline in monkeys trained to discriminate between stimuli of different frequencies. The ability of the monkeys to perform this task was impaired following the lesion.

Responses in the nuclei of the auditory pathway

The afferent fibers of the cochlear nerve terminate in the dorsal and ventral cochlear nuclei. Neurons in the cochlear nuclei respond to sound stimuli in a manner similar to that of the afferent fibers. A tuning curve can usually be constructed describing the response to different frequencies and intensities of sound. Although inhibitory actions can be demonstrated in cochlear nerve afferents, these are more prominent at the level of the cochlear nuclei and higher centers of the auditory pathway. Often, inhibition is produced by sounds having frequency and intensity parameters falling to either side of the tuning curve. It seems reasonable to suppose that such inhibitory actions explain, at least in part, the masking effect of ambient sounds that interfere with hearing in one's day-to-day activity.

The neurons of the cochlear nuclei are distributed spatially in such a way that their best frequencies vary systematically with the location of the cell. This organization resembles the somatotopic organization of the somatic sensory pathways, and so it is called tonotopic. There are actually several different tonotopic zones in cochlear nuclei (one in the dorsal and two in the ventral nuclei).

The dorsal cochlear nucleus projects to the contralateral nuclei of the lateral lemniscus. Little is known about the nuclei of the lateral lemniscus. The ventral cochlear nucleus projects to the superior olivary complex of each side of the brainstem.

Neurons in the superior olivary complex have many properties in common with those of neurons in the cochlear nuclei. In addition, olivary neurons are affected by sounds introduced into either ear. This is the result of their receiving a convergent input from both sets of cochlear nuclei. Some olivary neurons are excited by sound presented to either ear (EE cells); other neurons are excited by sound at one ear but inhibited by sound at the other ear (EI cells). The EE cells tend to be very sensitive to the general sound level (affecting both ears), but not to differences in the intensity of sound at the two ears. The EI cells are not sensitive to changes in the general sound level, but they are very good detectors of differences in the sound intensity at the two ears. Many olivary neurons are affected by differences in the phase of sound stimuli at the two ears. If the phase of the sound at one ear leads that at the other ear, a given neuron may discharge at a higher rate than it does when the sound reaches both ears in phase. Reversal of the phase difference causes the cell to fire at a lower rate than when there is no phase difference. It is believed that neurons having properties such as those described for the olivary neurons are involved in sound localization. Differences in the intensity of sound reaching the two ears are thought to provide the cue for localizing high-frequency sounds; differences in phase are implicated in the localization of low-frequency sounds. Animals in which the crossed input to the superior olivary complex through the trapezoid body is severed show a pronounced deficit in their ability to localize sound. Thus it appears that the initial integrative mechanism for sound localization is the superior olivary complex.

Most of the ascending fibers of the lateral lemniscus terminate in the inferior colliculus. There are several different nuclear regions within an inferior colliculus, and the pattern of connectivity is complex.

The inferior colliculus contains neurons with many of the response characteristics of the cells of the cochlear nuclei and superior olivary complex. For instance, there is a precise tonotopic organization of the inferior colliculus. In addition, there are neurons in the inferior colliculus that are sensitive to differences in the intensity or phase of sound stimuli presented at the two ears. However, the main nuclei of the inferior colliculi can be destroyed without impairment of an animal's ability to localize sound in a behavioral test. Therefore, the neurons showing a sensitivity to differences in binaural stimuli may be involved in the production of the appropriate reflex responses to sound, such as the appropriate movements of the head, pinna, and eyes, rather than in the perceptual aspect of sound localization. On the other hand, the inferior colliculi may participate in this function.

Animals can be trained to discriminate between sounds of two different frequencies even after removal of the input to centers of the auditory pathway higher than the inferior colliculi. It has therefore been suggested that the inferior colliculi are sufficient for a degree of frequency discrimination. However, the auditory cortex is required for the discrimination of sound patterns.

The medial geniculate body is the thalamic relay nucleus for the auditory pathway. It receives its chief afferent input from the ipsilateral inferior colliculus through the brachium of the inferior colliculus. (The magnocellular part of the medial geniculate body is not concerned primarily with audition; it is a part of the posterior nuclear group that receives terminals from the spinothalamic tract.)

Although it seems possible that the medial geniculate body has a tonotopic organization, this has not been clearly demonstrated. Otherwise, the responses of neurons in the medial geniculate body resemble those at lower levels of the auditory pathway.

Auditory cortex

The medial geniculate body projects through the auditory radiation to the temporal lobe. The auditory cortex lies in the transverse temporal gyrus, a part of the superior temporal gyrus situated deep in the sylvian fissure. The auditory cortex is thought to correspond to Brodmann's area 41. In animals, there are several auditory areas, just as there are several somatosensory areas. Presumably, the same is true of humans, although this is difficult to verify.

Whether there is a tonotopic organization of the auditory cortex is controversial. Some workers have found a tonotopic organization, but others have not. There may be a species difference. The cortex does appear to be organized in neuron columns, with cells having similar response characteristics arranged in a vertical array. However, the neurons in adjacent columns may have quite different response characteristics. In the cat, neurons with very high best frequencies are found in one region of the auditory cortex, but units of lower frequencies are scattered rather evenly across the cortex.

The auditory cortex does not seem to be necessary for frequency discrimination, although it is required for recognition of temporal patterns of sound stimuli. Single units may be more responsive to changing frequencies of sound than to a steady frequency. Furthermore, neurons of the auditory cortex may respond preferentially to sounds whose frequencies are changing in one direction but not to sounds whose frequencies are changing in the reverse direction. Some units discharge only when the frequency is increasing, others when it is decreasing, and still others respond to a change in frequency in one direction when the sound spectrum is at the high end and in the other direction when it is at the low end. Even more complex patterns of response have been described for some neurons of the auditory cortex. Furthermore, some aspects of a unit's response may change with time, suggesting that background input to the cells may alter their response characteristics.

Perception and the auditory pathway

The most important aspects of audition from the point of view of sound perception are the recognition of the frequency of a sound, its intensity, and its source in space. The frequency of sound is equatable with its pitch.

The frequency of sound appears to be coded in two ways. The frequency theory and the place theory can be combined in a duplex theory. For low frequencies of sound, below about 5,000 Hz, individual neurons may fire at the same frequency as the sound stimulus or at intervals that correspond to multiples of the period of the stimulus. A set of many auditory neurons would presumably represent the actual frequency, because some neurons would respond with each cycle. For frequencies above 5,000 Hz, this relationship breaks down because of the variability in the latency of impulses set up by the cochlear microphonic potentials. Furthermore, even lower frequencies are not represented in this manner at the higher levels of the auditory pathway.

On the other hand, the place theory seems best suited for explaining transmission of information about high frequencies of sound. The basilar membrane vibrates only to a limited extent in response to high frequencies, but it may vibrate throughout its length to low frequencies. Inasmuch as place coding would presumably be blurred as more hair cells are fired, the best discrimination based on place should be with high-frequency sounds. The discrimination of adjacent frequencies is improved by inhibitory interactions that tend to sharpen the response curves of units in the auditory pathway.

The ability to distinguish between two different frequencies appears to depend on subcortical structures and not on the auditory cortex. However, recognition of more complex sounds, such as those associated with speech, requires the integrity of the auditory cortex on at least one side of the brain.

It is thought that the perception of sound intensity depends in large part on the number of afferent fibers activated by a stimulus. Another factor is the discharge rate of individual fibers, which increases with stimulus strength in many neurons of the auditory path. Intensity discrimination appears to depend both on the auditory cortex and on subcortical centers, especially the inferior colliculi.

Sound localization depends on differences in the intensity and phase of sounds reaching the two ears. The masking effect of the head will reduce the intensity of sounds of high frequency reaching an ear directed away from the source of the sound. For low-frequency sounds, the wavelength is sufficient to prevent this. However, there will be a detectable phase difference for low-frequency sounds at the two ears if the source of the sound is not placed symmetrically with respect to the ears. Additional cues are available, however, because it is possible to localize sounds with just one ear. Localization is aided by movements of the head (and ears in animals) that provide a series of determinations.

The superior olivary complex appears to be the most significant structure in the auditory pathway for sound localization. Neurons of this structure have response properties that allow them to detect intensity or phase differences of sounds at the two ears. Presumably, higher structures of the auditory pathway make use of this information for discrimination.

Clinical applications

Damage to the auditory pathway may produce deafness. There are three categories of hearing impairment. Conduction deafness is caused by damage to the pathway that conducts sound, including structures of the external and middle ears. Perceptive, or nerve, deafness is caused by damage to the cochlea or to the cochlear nerve. The third type of deafness is that caused by lesions of the central nervous system. Because of the bilaterality of the auditory pathway at all levels above the cochlear nuclei, central deafness is generally of minimal degree and is not commonly recognized.

The differential diagnosis of conduction and nerve deafness can often be made on the basis of simple tuning fork tests. The normal ear can detect air-conducted sound more readily than bone-conducted sound. If a vibrating tuning fork is placed on a mastoid process until sound is no longer heard, movement of the fork to the vicinity of the external auditory meatus should restore hearing of the sound. If not, the most likely explanation is a conductive hearing loss. This is Rinne's test. If the tuning fork is placed on the vertex of the skull, the normal person will localize the sound to the midline. However, a patient with nerve deafness will localize it to the better ear, and a patient with a conductive deafness will hear the sound in the deaf ear. The reason for the latter finding is that ambient sound causes masking at the better ear, so bone conduction to the deaf ear is more effective. This is Weber's test.

In addition to decreased hearing, patients may experience a ringing sensation, known as tinnitus. This is often associated with damage to the cochlea or to the cochlear nerve.

VISUAL SYSTEM
The eye

The human eye is an elaborate sensory receptor organ designed for the detection of the portion of the electromagnetic spectrum, with a wavelength between 400 and 700 nm. This part of the spectrum is called visible light, although sensory receptors of other species may detect longer or shorter wavelengths than do human eyes.

The eyeball, which is nearly spherical, consists of three layers (Fig. 7-37). The outer layer is the fibrous tunic, which includes the transparent cornea and the opaque sclera. The junction of the cornea and sclera is known as the limbus. The middle layer is the vascular tunic. The anterior part of the vascular tunic includes the iris and the ciliary body. The lens is held in position behind the iris by suspensory ligaments. Light reaches the lens through an aperture in the iris called the pupil. Posteriorly located is the choroid. The inner layer is the nervous tunic, which consists of the retina.

The eye contains several spaces. The anterior chamber is the space between the cornea and the iris; the posterior chamber is between the iris and the lens. The anterior and posterior chambers contain a fluid called aqueous humor, which resembles cerebrospinal fluid. The large cavity behind the lens is filled with a viscous material called vitreous humor.

The aqueous humor is continually secreted into the posterior chamber by the epithelium covering the ciliary body. There is a circulation of the aqueous

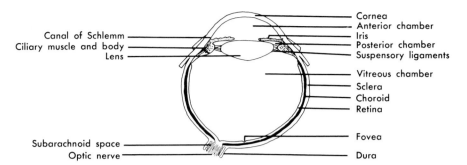

Fig. 7-37. Major components of the human eye. Note the three layers, including the fibrous, the vascular, and the nervous tunics. The anterior chamber, posterior chamber, and vitreous chamber are indicated. The light path through the cornea and lens to the retina is shown. The fovea and the optic nerve head mark special regions at the back of the eye.

humor out through the pupil into the anterior chamber, where the fluid enters a system of spaces (of Fontana) in the limbus. These spaces merge to form Schlemm's canal, which drains into the venous system of the eye. There is little turnover of vitreous humor.

Light entering the eye passes through the following sequence of structures called the refractive media. Light goes first through the cornea, which has a curved surface and a different refractive index than air. Therefore, light is refracted (bent) at the level of the cornea; in fact, the cornea is the main refractive surface of the eye. The light crosses the anterior chamber, passes through the pupil and posterior chamber, and then penetrates the lens. Although the lens does not refract light as much as the cornea does, it is crucial for proper focusing of the light because its refractile power can be changed. Proper focusing is accomplished by alterations in the shape of the lens produced by variations in the tension applied to the lens by the suspensory ligaments. Light that leaves the lens crosses the vitreous humor and strikes the retina.

The presence of pigment is a mechanism for preventing light scatter within the eye. There is pigment in several structures of the eye, including the iris, choroid, and the outermost layer of the retina.

Eye muscles. The operation of the eye is controlled by two sets of muscles, the intrinsic and the extrinsic ocular muscles. The intrinsic muscles of the eye are smooth muscles located in the iris and in the ciliary body. The sphincter of the iris causes pupillary constriction (miosis), and it is innervated by the parasympathetic nervous system (by way of cranial nerve III and the ciliary ganglion). The dilator of the iris enlarges the pupil (mydriasis), and it is innervated by the sympathetic nervous system (postganglionic neurons in the superior cervical sympathetic ganglion). The ciliary body contains several smooth-muscle layers that are attached in such a manner that

their contraction reduces the tension applied by the suspensory ligaments to the lens. Thus, contraction of the muscles of the ciliary body allows the lens to round up passively. This action results in accommodation of the lens for near vision, because the images of objects close to the eye are in focus on the retina. Relaxation of the ciliary muscle causes an increased tension on the suspensory ligaments, flattening of the lens, and focusing of the eye on the images of distant objects. The cilary muscle is innervated by parasympathetic fibers.

The extrinsic muscles of the eye determine the line of sight by positioning the axis of the eyeball. The extrinsic ocular muscles include the four rectus muscles (superior, inferior, lateral, and medial), the two oblique muscles (superior and inferior), and the levator of the eyelid (levator palpebra). There is also a smooth muscle of the upper eyelid (superior tarsal muscle), which is of clinical importance. The oculomotor nerve supplies all of the striated extrinsic muscles of the eye except the superior oblique and the lateral rectus muscles. The superior oblique muscle is innervated by the trochlear nerve, and the lateral rectus is supplied by the abducens nerve. The superior tarsal muscle is controlled by the sympathetic nervous system (superior cervical sympathetic ganglion). Another muscle involved in eye function is the orbicularis oculi, which serves to close the eyelids. It is supplied by the facial nerve.

The action of the extrinsic muscles of the eye is as follows. When the line of sight of the eye is horizontal, the lateral and medial rectus muscle produce temporal and nasal deviations of the eye respectively. If the line of sight of the eye is deviated temporally by 23°, the superior rectus muscle acts as a simple elevator and the inferior rectus muscle as a depressor of the eye. If the eye is deviated nasally by 51°, the superior oblique muscle is a depressor and the inferior oblique muscle an elevator of the eye. In other posi-

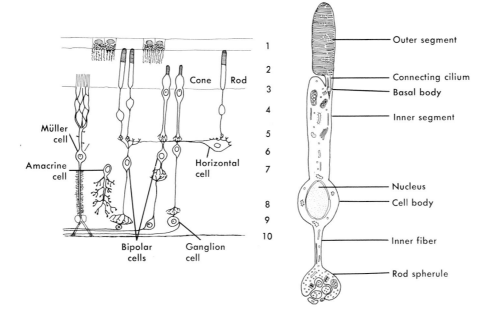

Fig. 7-38. The retina. **A,** Cellular components of the retina as they would be seen with the Golgi stain. The layers of the retina are: (1) pigment cell layer, (2) rods and cones, (3) outer limiting membrane, (4) cell bodies of rods and cones, (5) outer synaptic zone, (6) cell bodies of bipolar cells, (7) inner synaptic zone, (8) ganglion cells, (9) nerve fibers, and (10) inner limiting membrane. The ultrastructure of a rod is shown in **B.** (After Lentz, 1971.)

tions of the eye, rotatory components are added to these simple eye movements.

In general, movements of the two eyes are in concert, so that the images on the two retinas strike corresponding points. Such eye movements are called conjugate. However, when the lines of sight of the two eyes are brought to bear on near objects, the eyes converge instead of moving conjugately. A more detailed consideration is given to the control of eye movements in Chapter 8.

The retina. The nervous layer of the eye is the retina. The retina is derived embryologically from an outgrowth of the diencephalon. It is therefore a part of the central nervous system, a fact that is reflected by the complexity of this structure.

The retina can be described as having ten layers (Fig. 7-38). However, the basic organization of the retina centers around the first three neurons of the visual pathway. The receptor cells of the retina are located nearest to the choroid. These are the rod and cone cells. They synapse with the second-order cells of the visual pathway, the bipolar neurons, which are in the middle zone of the retina. The bipolar cells synapse with ganglion cells that are situated in the innermost part of the retina near the vitreous humor. Light must pass through the layers of ganglion cells and bipolar cells before it reaches the receptor cells.

In addition to the neuron types already mentioned, the retina contains numerous horizontal and amacrine cells that serve as interneurons within the retina. Furthermore, at least in lower vertebrates, there are efferent axons to the retina from the central nervous system. Finally, the supportive elements of the retina are the special glial cells known as Müller cells.

Photoreceptor cells of the retina. There are two distinct types of receptor cells in the retina, the rods and the cones. In the human retina, the rods outnumber the cones in a ratio of 100 million to 6 million. However, the proportions of rods and cones vary in retinas of different species, with limiting cases of retinas with only rods or cones.

The rod cell is thin and elongated, as its name implies. It can be subdivided into several regions: the outer segment, the connecting cilium, the inner segment, the cell body, the inner fiber, and the rod spherule. The outer segment is located at the apex of the cell and extends into the pigmented layer that forms the outer margin of the retina. The outer segment is actually a modified cilium and contains a stack of membrane lamellae that consist in part of the visual pigment characteristic of rods, rhodopsin. The outer segment is connected to the inner segment by a stalk called the connecting cilium. This structure contains nine pairs of filaments (but lacks the central pair of the typical cilium) that extend into the outer segment and terminate in a basal body in the inner segment. The cytoplasm of the inner segment contains numerous organelles distributed into two zones. The inner segment is connected to the cell body. A sheath of glial cytoplasm from Müller cells surrounds the photoreceptor cells and forms the outer limiting membrane of the retina. The cell body of a rod cell contains the nucleus. The cell body gives rise to one or more axons or inner fibers, which terminate in synaptic complexes. The terminal of a rod inner fiber is called a rod spherule. The rod spherules form synaptic relationships with the processes of bipolar cells and horizontal cells.

Cones have a structure that is basically similar to that of rods; however, there are a number of differences. The outer and inner segments and the cell body are generally broader, and the synaptic terminal of the inner fiber is larger than in the rod. The membrane lamellae of the cone outer segment are continuous with the surface membrane. The most important difference is the presence of pigments other than rhodopsin in the outer segments of cones. There are probably three different cone pigments, which would be involved in color discrimination. The pigments presumably occur in particular types of cone cells.

Photochemical reactions in rods and cones. Light energy must be absorbed to have a biological action. Substances that absorb light well are the pigments. The presence of rhodopsin in rod cells is well documented. When light strikes extracted rhodopsin, the reddish color of this substance disappears, indicating that photic energy has resulted in a changed molecular configuration of the pigment. The wavelengths of light that are absorbed by rhodopsin have been determined. The pigment is most sensitive to a wavelength of about 500 nm. Other adjacent wavelengths in the visible spectrum are absorbed to a lesser degree by the pigment. It has been shown that the sensitivity of the rods to light corresponds closely to the spectral sensitivity of rhodopsin extracted from the retina. It is thus plausible that the reaction between light and rhodopsin is responsible for the production of a receptor potential in rods. The receptor potential would initiate the neural activity signaling a visual stimulus.

A great deal is known about the biochemistry of the breakdown of rhodopsin and its resynthesis. Most of this information is beyond the scope of this book; however, the fact that vitamin A is involved in the rhodopsin cycle should be mentioned.

Less is known about the photochemistry of cones. At least three pigments appear to be associated with cones. The main difference between the cone pigments and rhodopsin is the structure of the protein component, which seems to be responsible for the fact that these pigments have different absorption spectra. One of the cone pigments is most sensitive to yellow, another to green, and the third to blue light.

The cones are probably not as sensitive to low levels of light as rods are. At night or in a dark room, most of the visual processing in the human retina depends on the action of rods. The dark-adapted eye is said to have scotopic vision (Gk. *skotos,* darkness), implying rod vision. With high light intensity, the rhodopsin of the rods becomes bleached, and the rods lose their capacity to respond. Daytime or photopic, vision depends largely on the cones. Color vision is an aspect of photopic vision.

Distribution of the rods and cones. The retinal photoreceptors are not uniformly distributed. When the eyes are fixed on an object of interest in the visual fields, light entering the eyes from that object is focused on a region of the retina known as the macula. At the center of the macula is a depression called the fovea. The center of the fovea contains only cones. Rods are found in the macula in increasing concentration toward its periphery. The density of the cone population decreases with distance from the fovea. The rod population reaches its maximum in a zone outside of the macula, then falls off toward the margin of the retina.

The resolution of images depends on the ability to discriminate between two closely adjacent points. Presumably, differences in the intensity of light striking three adjacent photoreceptors account for the resolution of the retina. However, this would not be the case if two or more photoreceptor cells utilized a common central pathway. There is a considerable convergence of input from adjacent rods on common bipolar cells. For this reason, the rod pathways are unsuited for fine resolution of images, but the cone pathways are well suited to this purpose. Because cones are broader than rods and so have a coarser grain, they might at first seem poorly designed for receiving images. However, the cones in the fovea are actually as narrow as rods. Furthermore, there is only a minor convergence of inputs from cones to bipolar cells and then to ganglion cells. The central pathways from cones are thus privileged-information channels. Another factor that enhances the resolving power of the retina is its neural interconnectivity.

Interconnections within the retina. The interneurons of the retina contribute much to the complexity of its organization. The horizontal cells, for instance, appear to establish synaptic contacts with the terminals of the rod and cone cells on bipolar cell dendrites.

The connections of the amacrine cells have also recently been described. These interneurons form vesicle-containing synapses with the synaptic terminals of the bipolar cells on ganglion cell dendrites or directly on the dendrites of ganglion cells. There are thus two different sets of axoaxonal synaptic complexes within the retina. To complicate the circuitry further, the bipolar cells also synapse with the amacrine cells. Thus, there is a reciprocal connection between the bipolar cells and amacrine cells that is reminiscent of the reciprocal synapses of the olfactory bulb (which also involve the amacrine cells of that structure, the granule cells). It seems reasonable to suppose that the horizontal and amacrine cells provide the basis for a major portion of the information processing that occurs at the level of the retina.

Early and late receptor potentials. With suitable techniques, it is possible to record the receptor potentials generated by photoreceptor cells of the retina in response to light. A very brief latency potential can be detected when intense stimuli are used. The onset of this early receptor potential occurs within less than 25 μsec. This is the briefest latency known for a bioelectric potential. It is believed that the early receptor potential is associated with the onset of the photochemical reaction of the visual pigment. Immediately following the early receptor potential is another electrical event, called the late receptor potential. This is thought to result from a changed membrane permeability of the photoreceptor cells, possibly resulting in a depolarization. The late receptor potentials of cones appear to have a briefer time course than those of rods.

Electroretinogram. When recordings are made by gross electrodes placed in such a way as to detect the electrical fields in front of and behind the retina, a characteristic sequence of potential changes occurs when the retina is illuminated. This response is called the electroretinogram because it has been shown to result from activity within the retina. Due to the complexity of the retina, it is not unexpected that the composition of the electroretinogram is also complex, inasmuch as it represents the sum of the activity of the individual elements of the retina. The sign of the electroretinogram is described by reference to an electrode on the corneal side of the retina. The sequential deflections of potential are an initial corneal negative wave (a wave) and a rapidly rising positive peak (b wave) followed by a slower rising positive wave (c wave). Sometimes a positive or negative wave (d wave) follows the cessation of the light stimulus.

The a wave of the electroretinogram appears to correspond to the late receptor potential and is thus caused by events within the photoreceptor cells. (The early receptor potential cannot be detected with gross electrodes.) The b wave may be a slow glial cell response to potassium liberated by the activity of neurons in the inner nuclear layer. The other components of the electroretinogram are thought to result from the activity of the bipolar cells and possibly the retinal interneurons. The ganglion cells do not appear to contribute.

The electroretinogram changes with the state of adaptation of the eye. In the light-adapted eye, the c wave is absent, the d wave is larger, and the time course of the potential sequence is briefer than in the dark-adapted eye. These changes can be attributed to a shift from rod to cone vision during light adaptation.

Single unit activity within the retina. It is very difficult to obtain intracellular recordings from most of the neuron types within the retina because of their small size; however, successful recordings have been made from horizontal, bipolar, and amacrine cells. The identity of these neurons was proved by marking the cells with a fluorescent dye contained in the recording microelectrode.

When records were made from horizontal cells in response to light, a membrane potential change occurred, called an S potential. In some horizontal cells, a hyperpolarizing S potential was evoked by all wavelengths of light, whereas in others the sign of the potential depended on the wavelength of the stimulating light.

Bipolar cells were of two types. Some were depolarized by light focused in the center of the receptive field and hyperpolarized by light striking the region surrounding the excitatory central region. In other bipolar cells the reverse pattern was seen. No action potentials were recorded.

Amacrine cells were depolarized both at the beginning and at the end of illumination. Spike potentials were generated in amacrine cells.

Much more information is available about the responses of retinal ganglion cells, because these neurons are relatively large and are thus easier to record from than are other retinal elements. Ganglion cells can be identified by antidromic activation of their axons in the optic nerve. Furthermore, the discharges of these cells can be recorded in the optic nerve or tract as well as in the retina.

Retinal ganglion cells of the mammalian eye conduct action potentials when the retina is exposed to no light at all. The response to light of a given cell may follow any of three patterns. Some ganglion cells respond to the onset of a light stimulus (on response), others to both the onset and cessation of the stimulus (on-off response), and still others just to the cessation of the period of illumination (off response).

The responses of ganglion cells in dark-adapted eyes have a spectral sensitivity pattern that matches the absorption spectrum of rhodopsin. However, more complicated response patterns are seen in the light-adapted state. Some ganglion cells respond to a broad range of wavelengths of light. These were called dominators by Ragnar Granit in his studies of retinal function. Other ganglion cells, termed modulators, responded only to a limited portion of the visible spectrum. Granit suggested that the dominators are responsible for signaling the intensity of light and the modulators are concerned with color detection.

The receptive fields of retinal ganglion cells (and of neurons at higher levels of the visual pathway) can be mapped by focusing a fine beam of light on the retina. By moving the beam across the retina, it is possible to determine the areas of the retina that excite or inhibit the neuron. The excitatory and inhibitory actions are chiefly caused by activity in the more proximal neural elements of the visual pathway (photoreceptors and horizontal, amacrine, and bipolar cells in the case of ganglion cells).

The receptive fields of ganglion cells are circular and vary in size but are typically up to a millimeter in diameter. The threshold for affecting the activity of the ganglion cell is much lower in the center of the field than at the periphery. Light falling on a zone around the receptive field often causes effects that are contrary to those produced by light striking the central region. For instance, if the effect of light in the center of the receptive field is an off response, then light striking the zone surrounding the center of the field may cause an on response. When the beam of light is spread across both the center zone and the surrounding zone, no action is observed. Some ganglion cells respond to a movement of a light stimulus across their receptive field; others do not.

Optic nerve and tract

The axons from the ganglion cells of the retina collect at a point medial to the anteroposterior axis of the eye and exit from the eye as the optic nerve. The term nerve is used in a general sense here, inasmuch as the fibers in the optic nerve are comparable to third-order fibers of central pathways and not to peripheral nerve fibers. The optic nerve in humans contains about 1 million axons.

The optic nerve enters the cranial cavity and meets its fellow of the opposite side at the optic chiasm (Fig. 7-39). Here the fibers from the nasal half of each retina cross into the contralateral optic tract and the fibers from the temporal half of each retina

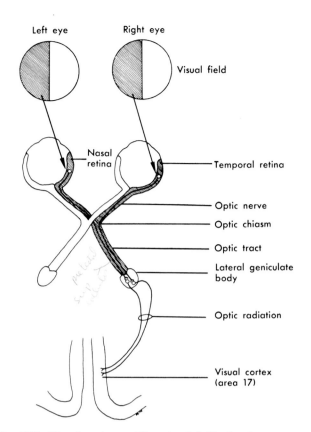

Fig. 7-39. Visual pathway. The visual fields for the two eyes are shown at the top. The left half of each visual field is shaded. Light from objects in the left visual field strikes the nasal retina of the left eye and the temporal retina of the right eye. Information about the visual stimulus is transmitted to the brain over the retinal ganglion cells. The axons of the ganglion cells are carried by the optic nerves. The axons of the ganglion cells of the nasal retina decussate in the optic chiasm, whereas those from the ganglion cells of the temporal retina continue ipsilaterally into the optic tract. The fibers of the right optic tract terminate in the right lateral geniculate body. Information is relayed from here through the optic radiation to the right occipital cortex, where it is first processed in the primary visual cortex. The left side of the visual field is thus "seen" by the right side of the brain.

continue into the ipsilateral optic tract. Note that the optic tracts are just continuations of the optic nerves, although the composition of axons has altered; the change in terminology from nerve to tract is not similar to the change in terminology from, for example, a peripheral nerve to the spinothalamic tract. In the latter case, at least one synapse lies between nerve and tract.

The optic nerve at its point of exit from the retina is called the optic nerve head. There are no photoreceptors in the optic nerve head; therefore the portion of the retina occupied by this structure is blind. Normally, the blind spot of the retina is not noticed, but it can be demonstrated by mapping the visual field of each eye.

Place coding of visual space

The portion of the external world detected as a visual stimulus by the eyes is called the field of vision. Each eye has a separate visual field, but in humans these overlap extensively because of the position of the eyes and because of the neural control mechanism that causes the eyes to move congruently. An object in visual space is thus usually detected by both eyes. The image is focused on corresponding points of each retina by the refractive system (cornea and lens) of each eye. An object situated to the left of the line of sight in visual space will have its image focused on the right half of each retina (Fig. 7-39). For the left eye, this is the nasal side of the retina; for the right eye, it is the temporal side. An object placed above the line of sight will have its image focused on the lower half of each retina. Therefore, at the level of the retina a given region in visual space is represented, or coded, by activity in neurons of specific regions of the two retinas.

The information conveyed by afferent fibers from these two retinal areas is transmitted through fibers of the optic nerves. A fiber within the optic nerve is located in a particular site that corresponds to its point of origin within the retina. Fibers from the upper retina are situated in the upper half of the optic nerve; those from the lower retina are in the lower half of the nerve. Fibers from the temporal side of the retina are in the temporal half of the optic nerve, and those from the nasal retina are in the nasal part of the nerve.

At the optic chiasm, the optic nerve fibers from the nasal halves of the two retinas decussate. Thus, the optic tracts contain fibers originating from the ipsilateral temporal retina and the contralateral nasal retina. Because these areas from the two retinas are the ones with corresponding visual fields, the visual representation has now been transformed from bilateral to unilateral; that is, the left side of visual space evokes activity in the right optic tract but not in the left optic tract. There is no comparable crossing of fibers in the dorsoventral direction.

Visual pathway behind the chiasm

Most of the axons in an optic tract terminate in the ipsilateral thalamus. The specific thalamic relay nucleus for the visual pathway is the lateral geniculate body (Figs. 7-39 and 7-40). It should be noted that some fibers of the optic tract terminate in the pretectal region and in the superior colliculus rather than in the thalamus. The function of these fibers is dis-

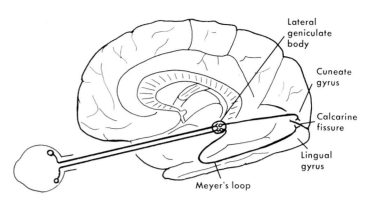

Fig. 7-40. Meyer's loop. The course of the visual pathway carrying information from the upper retina is shown to pass directly back to the cuneate gyrus in the occipital lobe. By contrast, the visual radiation fibers carrying information from the lower retina deviate into the temporal lobe in a band, called Meyer's loop, before continuing to their terminations in the lingual gyrus.

cussed separately from that of the ones belonging to the main part of the visual pathway.

The lateral geniculate body gives rise to the optic radiation (or geniculocalcarine tract), which projects to the primary visual cortex located in the occipital lobe. Visual information also reaches the visual association cortex, which surrounds the primary visual area.

Lateral geniculate body. The lateral geniculate body is a layered structure, containing six cellular laminae. Fibers from one retina end in three of the layers; those from the other retina terminate in the remaining layers (contralateral fibers end in layers 1, 4, and 6, and ipsilateral fibers end in layers 2, 3, and 5). The corresponding points of the two retinas are represented in adjacent regions of the layers receiving terminals from the two eyes. Because of this arrangement, a neuron in the lateral geniculate body will generally respond to a visual stimulus in just one eye, and the particular eye will depend on the layer in which the neuron is located.

There are about as many neurons in the lateral geniculate body as there are fibers in the optic nerve. However, some of the neurons of the nucleus are interneurons. Even so, the degree of divergence and convergence of optic tract afferents on lateral geniculate neurons is limited.

An evoked potential can be recorded from the lateral geniculate body in response to electrical stimulation of either optic nerve. The evoked potential consists of a compound action potential associated with activity in afferent fibers and a postsynaptic response. Following a single stimulus, there may be a series of oscillatory waves, rather like the rhythmic response previously described for the VPL nucleus following a single stimulus to the medial lemniscus (p. 256). Activity in one optic nerve can influence the response of the lateral geniculate body to stimulation of the other optic nerve. Much of this interaction is inhibitory and appears to involve both presynaptic and postsynaptic inhibition. Furthermore, transmission through the lateral geniculate body is affected by stimulation of corticofugal fibers originating in the visual cortex and by stimulation of the reticular formation. Both presynaptic and postsynaptic inhibition may be involved in these interactions.

The responses of single units of the lateral geniculate body to visual stimuli have been studied in some detail. There is activity of most of the neurons in the dark. The response of a given cell to a light flash may be an on, an on-off, or an off response, similar to the responses of retinal ganglion cells. The most common pattern is on-off. Although most geniculate neurons are activated by just one retina, a few are fired by stimulation of either retina. A simple stimulus can evoke a series of burst discharges occurring at about 100 msec intervals and lasting five or more cycles. As would be expected from the evoked potential studies, the single-unit response to stimulation of one eye can often be modified by stimulation of the other eye.

It is possible to distinguish between the responses of the lateral geniculate neurons, which project to the primary visual cortex, and the interneurons, both on the basis of their respective discharge patterns to stimulation of the optic nerve and on the basis that the projection neurons can often be fired antidromically following stimulation of the visual cortex, whereas the interneurons cannot. The interneurons are thought to be excited by recurrent collaterals of the projection cells, and in turn the interneurons may inhibit the projection cells postsynaptically. It seems likely that these interneurons produce a synchronization of the discharges of lateral geniculate projection neurons comparable to that mentioned earlier for the VPL nucleus.

The receptive fields of neurons of the lateral geniculate body have been mapped by discrete light stimuli focused on the retina. As in the case of retinal ganglion cells, the fields are circular, with a central and a surrounding field. The central region may be excitatory and the surround inhibitory, or vice versa.

The spectral sensitivity of lateral geniculate neurons corresponds to that of the retinal ganglion cells. There are two general categories of response, which are similar to the dominators and modulators. One type of geniculate neuron responds to or is inhibited by a broad range of wavelengths. These presumably signal light intensity, because they are much more sensitive to changes in intensity than in wavelength. The other category of neuron is excited by light within a narrow range of the spectrum; furthermore, it is inhibited when light falls into another range of the spectrum. There are several possible sets of wave bands having opposing actions (red excitatory–green inhibitory, yellow excitatory–blue inhibitory, green excitatory–red inhibitory, and blue excitatory–yellow inhibitory), each associated with a different population of geniculate neurons. These cells are presumed to signal color, because they are very insensitive to changes in intensity, yet very sensitive to wavelength.

Optic radiation. Neurons of the lateral geniculate body project to the primary visual cortex by way of the optic radiation. This tract passes adjacent to the posterior limb of the internal capsule (retrolenticular portion) and anterior to the lateral ventricle. Some of the fibers, those of the upper part of the radiation, course laterally and posteriorly to enter the occipital lobe by a fairly direct route (Fig. 7-40). These fibers end in the portion of the visual cortex that is superior to the calcarine fissure and carry information from the upper portions of the two hemiretinas. The lower fibers of the optic radiation follow a less direct route. These axons pass inferiorly and laterally over the temporal horn of the lateral ventricle before turning posteriorly to end in the portion of the visual cortex that is inferior to the calcarine fissure. The fibers thus loop into the temporal lobe (Meyer's loop), a fact of clinical importance. These fibers convey information from the lower portions of the appropriate hemiretinas.

Primary visual cortex. The part of the cerebral cortex that forms the primary visual receiving area is located on either side of the calcarine fissure on the medial aspect of the occipital lobe. The region is known as area 17 of Brodmann and also as the striate cortex. The term striate refers to a greatly thickened outer line of Baillarger (generally called the line of Gennari after the Italian medical student who first described it), which is visible on gross examination. The visual cortex has enlarged granular layers, as expected for a region devoted to sensory information processing.

The corresponding hemiretinas of the two eyes are represented topographically in the primary visual cortex. The largest region of the striate cortex corresponds to the macular projection. This region occupies much of the posterior part of the cortex above and below the calcarine fissure and extends back to the occipital pole. The remaining striate cortex in the anterior part of the occipital lobe is concerned with the nonmacular retina. The upper portions of the two hemiretinas are represented in the cortex superior to the calcarine fissure, whereas the lower portions of the hemiretinas are represented inferior to the fissure.

Electrical stimulation of the optic pathway produces a primary evoked response in the visual cortex. The initial part of the evoked response is more complex than that of evoked responses in other corticosensory areas. Light flashes also produce evoked potentials in the visual cortex. Both on and off effects are seen.

A number of studies have been done on single-unit responses of the primary visual cortex. Many cortical neurons do not seem to respond to diffuse light, whereas others have on, on-off, or off responses like those of cells at lower levels of the visual pathway. However, neurons that do not respond to diffuse light can be activated by light once the appropriate receptive field is found. Diffuse light no doubt causes a mixed excitatory and inhibitory input, with the result that some neurons may not appear to respond at all.

The receptive fields of cortical neurons of the primary visual area have been investigated in an elegant series of experiments by Hubel and Wiesel. In contrast to neurons at lower levels of the visual system, visual cortical neurons do not have circular receptive fields with concentric opposing surround fields. Instead, the cortical neurons respond to straight-line stimuli having a particular orientation. Their receptive fields can be classified in one of three categories, termed simple, complex, and hypercomplex by Hubel and Wiesel.

Simple receptive fields include excitatory and inhibitory areas located in a fixed region of the retina (Fig. 7-41). Light that occupies a larger area of the excitatory field produces a greater excitation through summation than does light focused on a more restricted region. Similarly, there is a summation effect in the inhibitory field dependent on the proportion of the field illuminated. Light spread across both the excitatory and the inhibitory fields causes antagonistic effects and may result in the cell not firing at all. It is possible to predict the responses to either stationary or moving light stimuli. Generally, the excitatory and inhibitory receptive fields of simple cortical neurons are arranged side by side, with a straight boundary. The boundary may be oriented vertically, horizontally, or obliquely on the retina.

Complex receptive fields are characteristic of many neurons of the primary visual cortex. These fields cannot be predicted from the responses to small spots of light. There are no separate excitatory and inhibitory fields. The stimulus required for a response is often restricted to a very specific pattern. For instance, a slit of light of a certain width and length

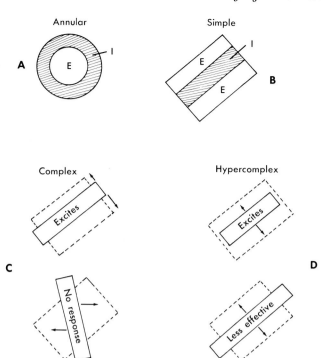

Fig. 7-41. Receptive fields of neurons in the visual pathway. **A** shows an annular receptive field characteristic of retinal ganglion cells and neurons of the lateral geniculate body. The center is excitatory and the periphery inhibitory in this case, although the converse could also be true. **B** shows a simple receptive field of a neuron of the primary visual cortex (area 17). There are parallel excitatory and inhibitory areas oriented linearly rather than in circular fashion as at lower levels of the visual pathway. **C** and **D** show examples of complex and hypercomplex receptive fields characteristic of cortical neurons both of the primary visual area and of the visual association cortex (areas 18 and 19). The neuron having the complex field (**C**) responds to a slit of light oriented in a particular direction. The length of the slit is not critical, but its precise orientation is. The neuron with the hypercomplex field (**D**) responds to a similar slit of light, but both the orientation of the stimulus and its length are critical. A longer slit, exceeding the length of the area marked by the broken-line box, is less effective than one of the same length as the box.

might give the optimum response as long as it falls anywhere over a region of the retina and as long as it is oriented properly, for example, horizontally. Some cells respond best not to slits but to edges. The position of the edge might not be important, although the orientation is. The neuron might fire when the light is to one side of the edge and be inhibited when the light is on the other side. Moving stimuli are particularly effective for activating neurons with either simple or complex fields. Many complex cells respond preferentially to movement in one direction.

Hypercomplex cells can also be found in the primary visual cortex. These can be excited by stimuli similar to those that activate complex cells, including slits, edges, or bars. However, extending the length of the stimulating form results in a decreased response.

Most of the neurons of the primary visual cortex are influenced by stimulation of both eyes. The receptive fields in these cases are in corresponding parts of the two retinas. The types of receptive fields are the same for both eyes, whether simple or complex. However, one eye may exert a more powerful effect than the other. Some units fire only when both eyes are stimulated simultaneously.

By mapping the receptive fields of cortical neurons encountered in sequence in each of a series of microelectrode tracks, Hubel and Wiesel were able to make some generalizations about the organization of the visual cortex. Neurons with receptive fields having a particular orientation tend to occur adjacent to one another in a track perpendicular to the cortex. Thus, the visual cortex has a columnar organization, like other regions of the sensory cortex.

Within a given column of visual cortical cells, neurons having simple, complex, or hypercomplex receptive fields could be found. Complex and hypercomplex cells were concentrated in layers 2, 3, 5, and 6; simple cells were most prominent in layer 4.

Thus there are a number of important differences in the responses of neurons of the primary visual cortex and of the lateral geniculate body that can be attributed to the more complicated organization of the cortex. These include a shift in the characteristics of the receptive fields from circular to linear, an emphasis on movement of the stimulus, a deemphasis in the ability of diffuse light to activate the cells, and binocular rather than monocular fields. Presumably, the receptive fields and other response properties of the cortical neurons can be accounted for by the convergence of input from different neurons of the lateral geniculate nucleus and by the effects of the input circuitry within the visual cortex itself. Simple fields can be explained on the basis of the direct connections from the lateral geniculate body, whereas the complex fields probably require higher order processing within the cortex, perhaps with a relay through neurons with simple fields. Hypercomplex cells may receive their input from complex ones.

Only a relatively small proportion of cortical units seem to display a differential sensitivity to the wavelength of the light used as a stimulus. However, such cells do occur, although their responses have not yet been sufficiently analyzed.

Visual association cortex. The region adjacent to the striate cortex is called the visual association cortex. It corresponds to Brodmann's areas 18 and 19. Experimental work has shown that this region receives projections from the primary visual cortex. Single-unit studies by Hubel and Wiesel reveal that neurons in this region have more complicated receptive fields than do neurons of the primary visual cortex. For instance, there are no cells belonging to the category called simple in the population studied in the striate cortex. The association area neurons are either complex or hypercomplex, and several orders of hypercomplex cells can be described. A higher order hypercomplex cell may show the responses of two different lower order hypercomplex cells. Area 18 contains mostly complex neurons, whereas area 19 has a higher proportion of hypercomplex neurons.

These findings are compatible with the notion that neurons of the visual cortex with different degrees of complexity of their receptive fields are interconnected in an orderly sequence that begins at the point of termination of the optic radiation in the striate cortex on neurons with simple receptive fields and progresses by connections of simple cells with complex cells of the striate and association cortices. Complex cells then project to hypercomplex cells of higher order. Both excitatory and inhibitory connections could be involved. The proportion of hypercomplex cells increases in the association cortex. It may be supposed that even greater degrees of complexity are introduced in adjacent regions of the cerebrum in which information from other sensory modalities is integrated in addition to the visual information.

Perception and the visual pathway

A large number of psychophysical observations have been made that relate to the visual pathway. These include such phenomena as the visualization of the retinal blood vessels, afterimages, the flicker-fusion frequency, and many others. Most of these are beyond the scope of this book; a few psychophysical questions are discussed briefly.

Visual acuity is of major concern in the testing of function in the visual pathway. Visual acuity depends on the smallest angle between two contours that can be distinguished by the subject. A test object, usually a standardized visual acuity chart, is placed at a known distance from the subject, who is asked to read characters that test for progressively smaller angles of resolution. The fovea can normally resolve objects having close to the minimum angle of resolution predicted from the grain of the cones and the optical imperfections of the eye, whereas the periphery of the retina has a much poorer resolving power, presumably because of the convergence and divergence in the rod pathway.

Besides acuity, two aspects of vision that are of special significance are the discrimination of color and intensity. Color vision depends on the presence in the retina of three different cone pigments. The trichromacy theory of color vision (Young-Helmholtz theory) is based in part on the observation that a normal person can match the color of a light by mixing the light emitted from three other colored lights. Similarly, the absorption of three wavelengths of light in the proper proportions should provide the cue for the recognition of any color. The activation of pathways in the retina by three different types of cones, each with its own pigment, would initiate the neural events responsible for color discrimination. Retinal elements that generate electrical activity that is dependent on stimulation by specific narrow ranges of the visible spectrum include horizontal cells whose membrane potentials may either hyperpolarize or depolarize according to the wavelength of the light and ganglion cells of the modulator type. Neurons of the lateral geniculate body that are excited by light in one spectral region and inhibited by light in another would presumably also be concerned with color vision, as would the color-sensitive neurons of the cerebral cortex.

Intensity, on the other hand, is signaled by rods or cones, depending on the state of light adaptation of the retina. In photopic vision, it is not clear whether cones of each type contribute to the signaling of light intensity or to what degree rods add to the information. The horizontal cells and ganglion cells (dominators) that respond to a broad range of the spectrum are presumably involved in the discrimination of light intensity, as are the neurons of the lateral geniculate body having similar response characteristics.

Other visual qualities of interest include the detection of the form, size, and direction of movement of objects. Fragments of the necessary information can be observed in single-unit recordings at various levels of the visual pathway. However, at the cortical level, the cells that were classified by Hubel and Wiesel as simple, complex, and hypercomplex appear to receive information of progressively higher degrees of organization. A given cell may respond selectively to a particular contour or to a movement of a contour in one direction across the retina. These kinds of neurons are therefore likely to be a part of the neural mechanism responsible for the recognition of the sensory qualities listed above.

Lower centers receiving visual input

Visual information is received not only by neurons of the lateral geniculate body and the visual cortices but also by neurons of lower centers (Fig. 7-42). The

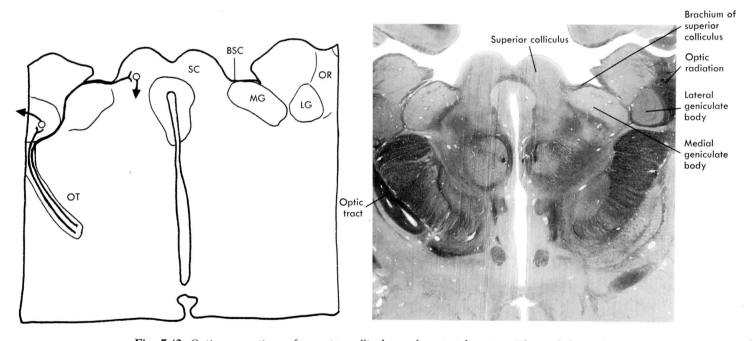

Fig. 7-42. Optic connections of superior colliculus and pretectal region. Fibers of the optic tract may end either in the lateral geniculate body or pass through the brachium of the superior colliculus to terminate in the superior colliculus or pretectal area. The latter establish reflex connections. The pretectal areas serve as a coordinating center for the pupillary response to light through connections to the Edinger-Westphal nuclei. Abbreviations: *BSC*, brachium of the superior colliculus; *LG, MG*, lateral and medial geniculate bodies; *OR*, optic radiation; *OT*, optic tract.

main lower centers involved include the pretectal region and the superior colliculus. The connections to these structures in humans do not permit vision in the absence of function in the structures of the main visual pathway. Instead, these lower centers appear to be involved in reflex activity.

The pretectal region is concerned with the coordination of the response of the pupils to light. This is a mechanism for protecting the retina against excessive light. When a light strikes the retina of one eye, the pupils of both eyes constrict. The pathway involves the neurons of the retina, including ganglion cells whose axons project to the pretectal region. From here, information is distributed bilaterally to Westphal's nuclei. The crossing fibers decussate in the posterior commissure.

The function of the superior colliculi in humans is not clear. Animal experiments suggest that they may be involved in the control of eye movements. There is a point-to-point projection of the retina on the superior colliculus, suggesting that a highly organized topographic relationship is required. Lower vertebrates can evidently utilize the superior colliculi as a major visual center.

Accommodation and fixation reflexes

Although the light reflex is strictly subcortical, pupillary constriction may also occur from cortical activity as part of the accommodation reflex. This reflex is involved when the eye becomes adapted to looking at near objects. The afferent pathway is the optic path from the optic nerves through the lateral geniculate bodies to the primary visual cortex. The efferent pathway begins with a corticofugal path to the superior colliculus, and then there is a connection with the parasympathetic outflow to the eye.

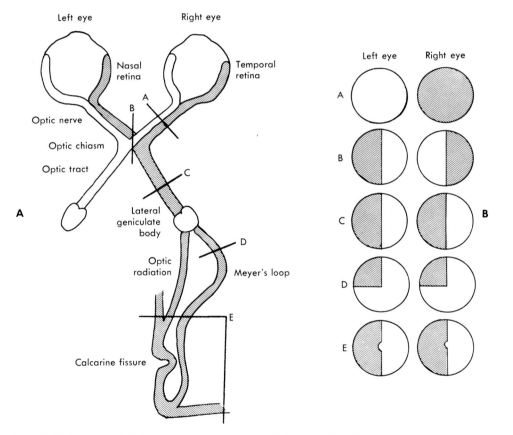

Fig. 7-43. Effects of lesions interrupting parts of the visual pathway. Parts of the visual pathway concerned with detection of objects in the left visual field are shown by the hatched areas (**A**). Lesions at various levels of the visual pathway are indicated by lines *A* to *D* and by the blocked off area in *E*. The results of the lesions are shown by the hatched areas in the representations of the visual fields (**B**). *A,* Transection of the right optic nerve produces blindness of the right eye. *B,* Sectioning the optic chiasm results in a bitemporal hemianopsia. *C,* Interruption of the right optic tract produces a left homonymous hemianopsia. *D,* Lesion in Meyer's loop on the right causes a left upper homonymous quadrantanopsia. *E,* Vascular lesion of the right occipital pole results in a left homonymous hemianopsia with macular sparing.

The accommodation reflex is generally accompanied by the fixation reflex. As the eyes adapt to near vision, they become oriented properly for viewing a particular object. The center involved in the fixation reflex appears likewise to be the occipital cortex.

Lesions of the visual pathways

A large number of disease processes cause changes in visual function. Generally it is possible to detect these changes through a neurological examination, although special diagnostic techniques, such as visual-field examination by means of a perimeter, may be necessary.

Lesions of the retina or optic nerve produce partial or complete blindness of one eye (Fig. 7-43). A discrete region of blindness in one eye is called a scotoma. However, damage to the optic tract, optic radiation, or optic cortex may result in visual-field defects in both eyes; this is caused by the decussation of part of each optic nerve in the optic chiasm. A complete interruption of the optic pathway at any of these sites produces a homonymous hemianopsia. If the left visual field is affected, as by interruption of the right optic tract, the condition is called left homonymous hemianopsia. Quadrantanopsia sometimes results from a partial lesion of the optic radiation, such as an interruption of Meyer's loop. Vascular damage to the occipital pole may result in a homonymous hemianopsia with macular sparing. The sparing of macular vision may be produced by an incomplete loss of macular representation, which is substantial at the cortical level.

Lesions of the sella turcica region may damage the optic chiasm and result in a visual-field defect in both temporal fields. This is called bitemporal hemianopsia.

If the optic axes do not allow objects to be focused on corresponding points of the two retinas, double vision (diplopia) results. If of long standing, the perception of one of the images will be suppressed; the visual acuity of the eye having the suppressed image may decrease even to the point of blindness. This condition is known as amblyopia. Common causes of diplopia are congenital defects in the external eye muscles and lesions involving pathways affecting the motor nuclei of the eye muscles. When the oculomotor nerve is interrupted, the eyelid cannot be raised; the condition is known as ptosis. Another cause of ptosis, in this case a partial ptosis, is loss of the sympathetic innervation of the superior tarsal muscle as part of Horner's syndrome.

In central nervous system syphilis it may be possible to demonstrate an Argyll Robertson pupil. This consists of a curious dissociation of disturbance to the visual pathways. The pupillary response to light is lost, but the response of accommodation is retained. Apparently the lesion affects the fibers entering the pretectal region from the optic tracts.

BIBLIOGRAPHY

Andersen, P., and Andersson, S. A.: Physiological basis of the alpha rhythm, New York, 1968, Appleton-Century-Crofts.

Andersen, P., Andersson, S. A., and Landgren, S.: Some properties of the thalamic relay cells in the spino-cervico-lemniscal path, Acta Physiol. Scand. 68:72-83, 1966.

Andersen, P., Eccles, J. C., Schmidt, R. F., and Yokota, T.: Depolarization of presynaptic fibers in the cuneate nucleus, J. Neurophysiol. 27:92-106, 1964.

Babel, J., Bischoff, A., and Spoendlin, H.: Ultrastructure of the peripheral nervous system and sense organs, St. Louis, 1970, The C. V. Mosby Co.

Bishop, P. O., and Davis, R.: Synaptic potentials, after-potentials and slow rhythms of lateral geniculate neurones, J. Physiol. (Lond.) 154:514-546, 1960.

Bowsher, D.: The anatomophysiological basis of somatosensory discrimination, Int. Rev. Neurobiol. 8:35-75, 1965.

Brindley, G. S.: Physiology of the retina and the visual pathway, London, 1960, Edward Arnold (Publishers) Ltd.

Brodal, A.: Neurological anatomy, New York, 1969, Oxford University Press, Inc.

Brodal, A., Pompeiano, O., and Walberg, F.: The vestibular nuclei and their connections, anatomy and functional correlations, Edinburgh, 1962, Oliver & Boyd, Ltd.

Brooks, V. B., Rudomin, P., and Slayman, C. L.: Peripheral receptive fields of neurons in the cat's cerebral cortex, J. Neurophysiol. 24:302-325, 1961.

Brown, A. G.: Cutaneous afferent fibre collaterals in the dorsal columns of the cat, Exp. Brain Res. 5:293-305, 1968.

Brown, A. G., and Franz, D. N.: Responses of spinocervical tract neurones to natural stimulation of identified cutaneous receptors, Exp. Brain Res. 7:231-249, 1969.

Burke, R. E., Rudomin, P., Vyklicky, L., and Zajac, F. E.: Primary afferent depolarization and flexion reflexes produced by radiant heat stimulation of the skin, J. Physiol. 213:185-214, 1971.

Burke, W., and Sefton, A. J.: Discharge patterns of principal cells and interneurons in lateral geniculate nucleus of rat, J. Physiol. (Lond.) 187:201-212, 1966.

Capps, M. J., and Ades, H. W.: Auditory frequency discrimination after transection of the olivocochlear bundle in squirrel monkeys, Exp. Neurol. 21:147-158, 1968.

Carreras, M., and Andersson, S. A.: Functional properties of neurones of the anterior ectosylvian gyrus of the cat, J. Neurophysiol. 26:100-126, 1963.

Casey, K.: Unit analysis of nociceptive mechanisms in the thalamus of the awake squirrel monkey, J. Neurophysiol. 29:725-750, 1966.

Christensen, B. N., and Perl, E. R.: Spinal neurons specifically excited by noxious or thermal stimuli; marginal zone of the dorsal horn, J. Neurophysiol. 33:293-307, 1970.

Cohen, M. J., Landgren, S., Strom, L., and Zotterman, Y.: Coritcal reception of touch and taste in the cat; a study of single cortical cells, Acta Physiol. Scand. 40(Suppl. 135):1-50, 1957.

Darian-Smith, I.: Neural mechanisms of facial sensation, Int. Rev. Neurobiol. 9:301-395, 1966.

Darian-Smith, I., Isbister, J., Mok, H., and Yokota, T.: Somatic sensory cortical projection areas excited by tactile stimulation of the cat; a triple representation, J. Physiol. (Lond.) 182:671-689, 1966.

DeValois, R. L., Abramov, I., and Mead, W. R.: Single cell analysis of wavelength discrimination at the lateral geniculate nucleus in the macaque, J. Neurophysiol. 30:415-433, 1967.

Dilly, P. N., Wall, P. D., and Webster, K. E.: Cells of origin of the spinothalamic tract in the cat and rat, Exp. Neurol. 21:550-562, 1968.

Dowling, J. E., and Boycott, B. B.: Neural connections of the retina; fine structure of the inner plexiform layer. In Cold Spring Harbor Symposium on Quantitative Biology, vol. 30, Sensory receptors, 1965, pp. 393-402.

Eisenman, J., Landgren, S., and Novin, D.: Functional organization in the main sensory trigeminal nucleus and in the rostral subdivision of the nucleus of the spinal trigeminal tract in the cat, Acta Physiol. Scand. 59(Suppl. 214):1-44, 1963.

Erulkar, S. D., and Fillenz, M.: Single-unit activity in the lateral geniculate body of the cat, J. Physiol. (Lond.) 154: 206-218, 1960.

Glees, P., and Soler, J.: Fibre content of the posterior column and synaptic connections of nucleus gracilis, Z. Zellforsch. 36:381-400, 1951.

Gordon, G., Landgren S., and Seed, W. A.: The functional characteristics of single cells in the caudal part of the spinal nucleus of the trigeminal nerve of the cat, J. Physiol. (Lond.) 158:544-559, 1961.

Granit, R.: Receptors and sensory perception, New Haven, 1955, Yale University Press.

Grillner, S., Hongo, T., and Lund, S.: The vestibulospinal tract; effects on alpha-motoneurones in the lumbosacral spinal cord in the cat, Exp. Brain Res. 10:94-120, 1970.

Hongo, T., Jankowska, E., and Lundberg, A.: Post-synaptic excitation and inhibition from primary afferents in neurones of the spinocervical tract, J. Physiol. (Lond.) 199:569-592, 1968.

Horrobin, D. F.: The lateral cervical nucleus of the cat; an electrophysiological study, Q. J. Exp. Physiol. 51:351-371, 1966.

Hubel, D. H., and Wiesel, T. N.: Integrative action in the cat's lateral geniculate body, J. Physiol. (Lond.) 155:385-398, 1961.

Hubel, D. H., and Wiesel, T. N.: Receptive fields, binocular interaction and functional architecture in the cat's visual cortex, J. Physiol. (Lond.) 160:106-154, 1962.

Hubel, D. H., and Wiesel, T. N.: Receptive fields and functional architecture in two non-striate visual areas (18 and 19) of the cat, J. Neurophysiol. 28:229-289, 1965.

Jones, E. G., and Powell, T. P. S.: Electron microscopy of the somatic sensory cortex of the cat, Philos. Trans. R. Soc. Lond. [Biol. Sci.] 257:1-62, 1970.

Kaneko, A.: Physiological and morphological identification of horizontal, bipolar and amacrine cells in goldfish retina, J. Physiol. (Lond.) 207:623-633, 1970.

Kerr, F. W. L.: Facial, vagal and glossopharyngeal nerves in the cat, Arch. Neurol. 6:264-281, 1962.

Kerr, F. W. L., Kruger, L., Schwassmann, H. O., and Stern, R.: Somatotopic organization of mechanoreceptor units in the trigeminal nuclear complex of the macaque, J. Comp. Neurol. 134:127-144, 1968.

Kiang, N. Y. S., Watanabe, T., Thomas, E. C., and Clark, L. F.: Stimulus coding in the cat's auditory nerve, Ann. Otol. Rhinol. Laryngol. 71:1009-1026, 1963.

Kruger, L., Siminoff, R., and Witkovsky, P.: Single neuron analysis of dorsal column nuclei and spinal nucleus of trigeminal in cat, J. Neurophysiol. 24:333-349, 1961.

Landgren, S.: Thalamic neurones responding to cooling of the cat's tongue, Acta Physiol. Scand. 48:255-267, 1960.

Lindeman, H. H.: Studies on the morphology of the sensory regions of the vestibular apparatus, Ergeb. Anat. Entwicklungsgesch. 42:1-113, 1969.

Lund, R. D., and Webster, K. E.: Thalamic afferents from the spinal cord and trigeminal nuclei, J. Comp. Neurol. 130: 313-327, 1967.

Masterton, R. B., Jane, J. A., and Diamond, I. T.: The role of brain-stem auditory structures in sound localization. I. Trapezoid body, superior olive, and lateral lemniscus, J. Neurophysiol. 30:341-359, 1967.

Mehler, W. R., Feferman, M. E., and Nauta, W. J. H.: Ascending axon degeneration following anterolateral chordotomy; an experimental study in the monkey, Brain 83:718-750, 1960.

Melzack, R., and Wall, P. D.: Pain mechanisms; a new theory, Science 150:971-979, 1965.

Mendell, L. M., and Wall, P. D.: Presynaptic hyperpolarization; a role for fine afferent fibers, J. Physiol. (Lond.) 172: 274-294, 1964.

Mosso, J. A., and Kruger, L.: Receptor categories represented in spinal trigeminal nucleus caudalis, J. Neurophysiol. 36: 472-488, 1973.

Mountcastle, V. B.: Modality and topographic properties of single neurons of cat's somatic sensory cortex, J. Neurophysiol. 20:408-434, 1957.

Mountcastle, V. B., Henneman, E.: The representation of tactile sensibility in the thalamus of the monkey, J. Comp. Neurol. 97:409-439, 1952.

Mountcastle, V. B., and Powell, T. P. S.: Neural mechanisms subserving cutaneous sensibility, with special reference to the role of afferent inhibition in sensory perception and discrimination, Bull. Johns Hopkins Hosp. 105:201-232, 1959.

Moushegian, G., and Rupert, A. L.: Response diversity of neurons in ventral cochleal nucleus of kangaroo rat to low-frequency tones. J. Neurophysiol. 33:351-364, 1970.

Nelson, P. G., Erulkar, S. D., and Bryan, J. S.: Responses of units of the inferior colliculus to time-varying acoustic stimuli, J. Neurophysiol. 29:834-860, 1966.

Noordenbos, W.: Pain; problems pertaining to the transmission of nerve impulses which give raise to pain, Amsterdam, 1959, Elsevier Publishing Co. Ltd.

Nyberg-Hansen, R.: Origin and termination of fibers from the vestibular nuclei descending in the medial longitudinal fasciculus, J. Comp. Neurol. 122:355-367, 1964.

Nyberg-Hansen, R., and Mascitti, T. A.: Sites and mode of termination of fibers of the vestibulospinal tract in the cat, J. Comp. Neurol. 122:369-387, 1964.

Penfield, W. G., and Boldrey, E.: Somatic motor and sensory representation in the cerebral cortex of man as studied by electrical stimulation, Brain 60:389-443, 1937.

Petit, D., and Burgess, P. R.: Dorsal column projection of receptors in cat hairy skin supplied by myelinated fibers, J. Neurophysiol. 31:849-855, 1968.

Poggio, G. F., and Mountcastle, V. B.: A study of the functional contributions of the lemniscal and spinothalamic systems to somatic sensibility, Bull. Johns Hopkins Hosp. 106: 266-316, 1960.

Powell, T. P. S., and Mountcastle, V. B.: Some aspects of the functional organization of the cortex of the postcentral gyrus of the monkey; a correlation of findings obtained in a single unit analysis with cytoarchitecture, Bull. Johns Hopkins Hosp. **105**:133-162, 1959.

Rall, W., Shepherd, G. M., Reese, T. S., and Brightman, M. W.: Dendrodendritic synaptic pathway for inhibition in the olfactory bulb, Exp. Neurol. **14**:44-56, 1966.

Ramon y Cajal, S.: Studies on the cerebral cortex (limbic structures). Translated by L. M. Kraft, London, 1955, Lloyd-Luke.

Rinvik, E.: A re-evaluation of the cytoarchitecture of the ventral nuclear complex of the cat's thalamus on the basis of corticothalamic connections, Brain Res. **8**:237-254, 1968.

Roberts, T. D. M.: Neurophysiology of postural mechanisms, New York, 1967, Plenum Publishing Corporation.

Rose, J. E., Brugge, J. F., Anderson, D. J., and Hind, J. E.: Phase-locked response to low-frequency tones in single auditory nerve fibers of the squirrel monkey, J. Neurophysiol. **30**:769-793, 1967.

Rose, J. E., and Galambos, R.: Microelectrode studies on medial geniculate body of cat. I. Thalamic region activated by click stimuli, J. Neurophysiol. **15**:343-358, 1952.

Rose, J. E., Greenwood, D. D., Goldberg, J. M., and Hind, J. E.: Some discharge characteristics of single neurons in the inferior colliculus of the cat. I. Tonotopical organization, relation of spike counts to tone intensity, and firing patterns of single elements, J. Neurophysiol. **26**:294-320, 1963.

Selzer, M., and Spencer, W. A.: Convergence of visceral and cutaneous afferent pathways in the lumbar spinal cord, Brain Res. **14**:331-348, 1969.

Taub, A., and Bishop, P. O.: The spinocervical tract, dorsal column linkage, conduction velocity, primary afferent spectrum, Exp. Neurol **13**:1-21, 1965.

Trevino, D. L., Coulter, J. D., and Willis, W. D.: Location of cells of origin of the spinothalamic tract in the lumbar enlargement of the monkey, J. Neurophysiol. **36**:750-761, 1973.

Truex, R. C., Taylor, M. J., Smythe, M. Q., and Gildenberg, P. L.: The lateral cervical nucleus of cat, dog and man, J. Comp. Neurol. **139**:93-104, 1969.

Walberg, F.: Axoaxonic contacts in the cuneate nucleus, probable basis for presynaptic depolarization, Exp. Neurol. **13**:218-321, 1965.

Wall, P. D., and Taub, A.: Four aspects of trigeminal nucleus and a paradox, J. Neurophysiol. **25**:110-126, 1962.

White, J. C., and Sweet, W. H.: Pain, its mechanisms and neurosurgical control, Springfield, Ill., Charles C Thomas, Publisher, 1955.

Whitfield, I. C.: The auditory pathway, London, 1967, Edward Arnold (Publishers) Ltd.

Whitlock, D. G., and Perl, E. R.: Afferent projections through ventrolateral funiculi to thalamus of cat, J. Neurophysiol. **22**:133-148, 1959.

Willis, W. D., Trevino, D. L., Coulter, J. D., and Maunz, R. A.: Responses of primate spinothalamic tract neurons to natural stimulation of hindlimb, J. Neurophysiol. **37**:358-372, 1974.

Wilson, V. J., Kato, M., Peterson, B. W., and Wylie, R. M.: A single-unit analysis of the organization of Deiters' nucleus, J. Neurophysiol. **30**:603-619, 1967.

Wilson, V. J., Wylie, R. M., and Marco, L. A.: Synaptic inputs to cells in the medial vestibular nucleus, J. Neurophysiol. **31**:176-185, 1968.

Winter, D. L.: N. gracilis of cat; functional organization and corticofugal effects, J. Neurophysiol. **28**:48-70, 1965.

CHAPTER 8

Motor systems

MUSCULAR ACTIVITIES AND THEIR NEURAL ORIGINS

Animals exhibit a number of different types of muscular activity: their muscles have tone; they maintain postures; they make reflex movements in response to sensory stimuli; and they make spontaneous rhythmic movements and voluntary movements that can occur independent of external stimuli. Motor activities can be intimately associated with the most complex mental processes, as in speech. Some characteristics of normal movement and the types of neural activity that generate them are discussed on the following pages.

Background muscular activity (tonus)

Many muscles are maintained in a state of mild contraction achieved by the firing of a portion of the motor units of the muscle. The tension of muscles varies with the role of the muscle in maintaining posture and resisting gravity, the state of alertness of the individual, and the degree of stretch placed on the muscle. A way of describing the tonus of a muscle is to describe its resistance to stretching. This provides a measure of the degree of excitatory and inhibitory influences playing on the motoneurons innervating the muscle. Muscle tonus can be regarded as the background on which more active phasic muscular contraction, which produces movement, occurs. The maintenance of muscular tonus is closely related to maintenance of posture, and it is likely that vestibulospinal and reticulospinal systems playing on the alpha and gamma motoneuron systems are important in maintaining tonus.

Coordination of muscular activity (synergy)

Almost any useful muscular activity requires the coordinated activity of groups of muscles. Muscles that act together are called synergists, usually a group of flexors or extensors. The term synergy is used here in a broader sense, derived from clinical observations of disturbances of synergy, to mean the cooperative activity of all of the muscles used in performing a motor act. For example, in the act of making a fist, several groups of muscles contract nearly simultaneously. The hand is dorsiflexed at the wrist and stabilized, and the finger flexors contract. Most motor acts require similar coordination between flexion, extension, and stabilizing activity.

The spinal cord (and the brainstem in the case of cranial nerve motor nuclei) contains some of the mechanisms necessary for synergy. Sensory input to the spinal cord is arranged so that when certain inputs are activated, synergistic muscular activity occurs. These reflex activities of the spinal cord, the myotatic and flexion reflexes, and the reciprocal inhibition of contraction of antagonistic muscles are organized within the spinal cord (see Chapter 4). Spinal mechanisms are probably utilized to provide reciprocal inhibition when descending impulses evoke motor activity, but it is not known how or to what extent spinal reflex mechanisms are engaged or integrated into synergistic voluntary movements. It is not known, for example, if stimulation of a point on the motor cortex that evokes dorsiflexion of the foot engages the same interneurons as when a painful stimulus is applied to the sole of the foot, which also produces dorsiflexion.

Reflexes

A distinction can be made between motor activities that are under the control of afferent input (reflex activity) and those that are generated within the organism (spontaneous and voluntary activity).

In neurophysiological laboratories great emphasis has been placed on the study of reflex activity. One objective of these studies has been to see if complex or patterned movements such as walking are built on a series of simple reflex activities in which each response generates a new sensory state that in turn evokes the next response of the sequence.

This concept can be illustrated as follows:

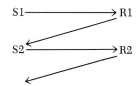

It can be seen how this type of activity could lead to rhythmic movement if R2 produces sensory state 1 (S1).

At present it appears that most repetitive or patterned movements are not generated in this manner but are controlled by a central program. The new sensory state set up by each response can modulate, but does not determine, the next response.

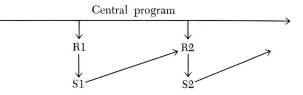

Reflex activity therefore appears to be integrated into the majority of mammalian motor activities rather than to dominate motor activity. However, reflex activity appears to be very important for the accurate performance of complex patterned movements. This is suggested by the observation that animals can use deafferentated limbs, but movements of such animals are clumsy and not normal.

Postural reflexes are an important group of reactions in mammals, who generally maintain a posture that keeps the horizontal meridian of the visual field at right angles to the gravitational field. Any perturbation of this position results in movements to restore the posture. The stimuli for postural adjustments come from muscle, joint, and skin receptors and from the vestibular and visual systems.

The postural effects of the proprioceptive impulses from neck muscles and joints are difficult to detect in intact animals. However, in decerebrate animals rotation of the head and neck to one side of the body will produce a pattern of limb movement, including ipsilateral forelimb extension and contralateral forelimb flexion (and, in the monkey, grasping of the contralateral hand). Such reactions are known as tonic neck reflexes and were studied in detail by

Magnus and his co-workers. Similar reactions can be seen in decerebrate humans.

The functional significance of most of the reactions is more apparent for animals than humans. Extension of the neck, for instance, produces extension of the forelimbs and flexion of the hindlimbs, the position assumed by an animal when it is looking upward and is going to jump upward.

Centrally programmed movement (rhythmic-automatic movements)

Certain movements of the somatic musculature are repeated rhythmically without voluntary effort, although the rate and amplitude of the movements can be modulated by sensory input and by voluntary effort. Such movements are largely produced by alternating contractions of antagonistic muscles. The movements of respiration are the prime example of rhythmic-automatic movements. (The central organization of the respiratory system is described in Chapter 9.) Rhythmic-automatic movements are not dependent on sensory input for their execution, although sensory input may trigger them. Such movements appear to be controlled by a central program. Locomotor movements should probably be classified as rhythmic-automatic movements, because coordinated locomotor movements of the limbs can occur in primates whose spinal cords are deafferentated. Licking and chewing movements are also probably controlled by a central program.

Little is known about the neural organization of centrally programmed movement in mammals. Recent studies of invertebrate nervous systems, however, have provided a number of interesting models of central control of movement. In invertebrates such as the crayfish, command neurons have been found that have connections with larger numbers of interneurons and effector neurons. The command neurons can be under the control of a particular sensory input, and, when activated by the sensory input, they produce coordinated activity of a group of muscles leading to a response, such as the tail movement used in escape activity by the crayfish.

No definite information is available about how the rhythmicity of centrally programmed movements is generated. Two types of central mechanisms are thought to produce repetitive activity, independent of a constant sensory input. (A constant sensory input, such as vestibular input, can be transformed into repetitive motor activity, such as nystagmus, described in the section on the oculomotor system.) One type of generator of so-called spontaneous rhythmic activity is pacemaker neurons. These are neurons that undergo rhythmic depolarization, firing, and hyper-

polarization that are independent of neuronal circuitry. The pacemaker activity is related to the metabolic activity and membrane properties of the cell. Such neurons have been shown to exist in some invertebrates. However, there is no strong evidence for the existence of pacemaker neurons in the mammalian nervous system.

The second mechanism for the generation of rhythmic activity is a loop of neurons that are excitatory to each other. The actual demonstration of such loops, with recording from all of the types of neurons in the circuit, has not been achieved in the mammalian nervous system. The respiratory system is an example of a system that exhibits so-called spontaneous rhythmic activity. Recordings have been made from the inspiratory neurons of the medulla that drive the spinal motoneurons that innervate the muscles used in inspiration. The inspiratory neurons of the medulla fire autonomously even when the medulla is isolated from afferent input, although their discharge is much more regular when the pons and spinal afferent input are intact. However, physiological and anatomical identification of a local excitatory circuit has not been accomplished for the respiratory neurons.

Some idea of the possible neuronal makeup of such circuits can be obtained from the study of models of recurrent excitation and inhibition described in Chapter 4 and elaborated with respect to repetitive epileptic discharge in Chapters 6 and 10.

Voluntary movement

From a psychological viewpoint volition is part of our conscious experience, and further introspective analysis does not seem to be possible. What appears to characterize willed movement is the act of initiating movement. Once the movement is started it is possible that it may be carried on by centrally programmed or reflex mechanisms. Another characteristic of willed movements is that they are usually willed with the purpose of reaching some goal. This may be a goal in the individual's sensory field or one that is represented in the individual's memory. The motivational aspect of voluntary movement suggests that the descending motor systems are being driven from sources that, from a psychological viewpoint, are related to consciousness, emotion, and memory. This "core" of the person is closely bound up with what we feel is our basic identity.

It has been suggested that structures with projections to large portions of the cortex are important in the initiation of movement, and therefore the nonspecific thalamic system (see Chapter 6) might function in voluntary movement. Limbic structures and their thalamic and frontal lobe projections appear to function in emotion, motivation, and memory, and these areas may also be important in the generation of voluntary movement. At the present time studies of the neural correlates of willed movement are being performed by simultaneously recording from a number of central structures in primates performing motor tasks. These studies show that there is a large amount of variability of the time of onset of firing of different central neurons with respect to the onset of movement. Changes in the firing patterns of cerebellar neurons appear to occur prior to the changes in firing of motor cortex neurons.

Associated movements

Associated movements are movements that normally occur as part of the total pattern of motor activity but that are not necessary to the performance of the basic motor activity. For example, during walking, people will normally swing their arms, although the arm swing can be voluntarily suppressed. Associated movements are clinically important because disruption of the normal linkage between voluntary and associated movements can be produced by lesions of central motor pathways. With lesions of descending motor pathways there is a tendency for the arm swing on the weak side of the body to be greatly diminished.

In addition, certain movements, particularly of the facial muscles, are associated with emotional activity without being specifically willed. Learning undoubtedly plays an important role in developing these responses, but there appear to be innate responses on which the learned responses are based. These movements are clinically interesting because patients with lesions of central motor pathways and with facial paralysis, who may be unable to smile volitionally, may smile in response to pleasure or to hearing a joke.

The term associated movements can also be used to describe movements that occur in pathological states, such as the extensor and flexor synergies that occur in hemiparetic patients. In such cases the attempt to flex a limb at one point will lead to flexion at all of the joints.

ABNORMAL MUSCULAR ACTIVITY

Clinically observed abnormalities of muscular activities are described in this section and are related, when possible, to the mechanisms producing abnormality.

Because the parts of the motor system are heavily interdependent, disturbance of almost any part of the system produces abnormalities in several types of muscular activity. Clinically observed syndromes of motor abnormalities produced by various central nervous system lesions are as follows:

I. Motoneuron lesions
   A. Abnormal tonus: hypotonia
   B. Decreased movement: paresis or paralysis
   C. Changes in muscle: fasciculation, fibrillation, atrophy
II. Descending motor tract lesions
   A. Abnormal tonus: hypotonia progressing to spasticity, decerebrate rigidity in midbrain injury
   B. Decreased movement: paresis or paralysis
   C. Improperly controlled voluntary movement: decreased rapidity and delicacy of movement
III. Cerebellar lesions
   A. Neocerebellar lesions
      1. Abnormal tonus: hypotonia
      2. Disturbances of synergy: ataxia
      3. Tremor: intention tremor
      4. Improperly controlled voluntary movement: decreased rapidity of movement, ataxia
   B. Flocculonodular lesions
      1. Disturbances of posture and equilibrium
IV. Dorsal root and dorsal column (sensory) lesions
   A. Disturbances of posture and equilibrium
   B. Improperly controlled voluntary movements
V. Parkinsonism
   A. Abnormal tonus: rigidity
   B. Decreased movement: akinesia
   C. Tremor: tremor at rest

Common clinical syndromes, including sensory changes, produced by lesions of various levels of the nervous system are discussed in more detail in Chapter 12.

Abnormal tonus

Hypotonia. Hypotonia means laxness or flaccidity of muscles. It is usually caused by motoneuron damage, but it may appear as an early result of damage to descending motor pathways and after cerebellar injury.

Hypertonia. Hypertonia can be classified as either spasticity or rigidity. In both of these states the muscle resists passive stretching at a time when there is no voluntary contraction of the muscle.

Spastic muscle is characterized by development of increasing tension as the muscle is stretched. There may then be an abrupt collapse of tension, the so-called clasp knife phenomenon, which is caused by inhibition of the monosynaptic reflex by Golgi tendon organ afferents (see Chapter 4).

Spasticity is a late result of injury to descending motor tracts. Following complete spinal cord transection, flaccid paralysis occurs. Over a period of weeks myotatic and superficially evoked reflexes return and become hyperactive (as described in more detail for clinical cases in Chapter 12). The limb muscles are usually spastic at this point. In humans the flexors of the arm and the extensors of the leg, the antigravity muscles, exhibit the greatest spasticity. Similar findings occur after brain lesions that injure tracts descending to the spinal cord. Inasmuch as spasticity is the end result of many brain and spinal injuries, it is of great clinical importance. The mechanism of production of spasticity is not clear. It is possible that lesions of the various descending tracts are synergistic in producing spasticity. Lesions of the motor cortex or of the lateral corticospinal tract do not produce marked spasticity. It is likely that removal of reticulospinal inhibitory influences is important in producing spasticity.

Dorsal rhizotomy is effective in reducing the severity of spasticity, probably because it represents, in part, hyperactivity of the monosynaptic reflex. A horizontal section of the spinal cord, Bischof's myelotomy, which separates the motoneurons from dorsal root input, will also relieve spasticity. Certain drugs can reduce spasticity, although their mechanism of action is not completely understood. However, the treatment of spasticity remains rather unsatisfactory at the present time.

Rigidity of muscles is typically seen in Parkinson's disease and is often associated with akinesia and tremor. The tension of the muscles during stretching is greater than in a normal muscle, but a marked increase in tension and clasp knife reactions during stretching are absent. There may be a series of little increases and relaxations of tension during stretching, named the cogwheel phenomenon. Turning a watch stem and feeling the catching of the ratchet gives this type of sensation. The cogwheel phenomenon may be related not to rigidity but to tremor in the muscle.

The rigidity of a muscle can be reduced by blocking the gamma motoneuron discharge to the muscle. This can be accomplished by injecting a weak solution of procaine around the nerve to the muscle, which depresses activity in small fibers, with much less effect on the large alpha motoneuron fibers. This is not a practical method of relieving rigidity in parkinsonism, which affects many muscles. The rigidity of parkinsonism, as well as the akinesia, can be improved by administration of L-dopa.

Decerebrate rigidity. This is an acute and marked increase in extensor tonus following transection of descending motor tracts at the level of the midbrain. The mechanism of this effect is probably different from that of rigidity, and it is unfortunate that the names of these states are somewhat similar. The clinical picture of decerebrate rigidity is rather similar in animals and humans. The limbs become rigidly extended, and the tonus of the extensor muscles of the neck and back (antigravity muscles) increases. If the cerebellum is also removed, extreme extensor rigidity ensues, with the head thrown back and the spine arched (opistho-

tonos: Gk. *opisthen,* behind, *tonos,* tension). The decerebrate preparation, in which the midbrain is often sectioned just between or just rostral to the colliculi of the midbrain, was employed by Sherrington for many of his experiments because changes in posture are readily detected in decerebrate animals. Inhibitory actions were particularly apparent, being seen as reductions in the extensor tonus. The appearance of decerebrate rigidity in humans is a grave sign. The midbrain damage is commonly caused by hemorrhage in the midbrain, by compression of the midbrain by tumor, by herniation of the temporal lobe through the tentorial notch (see Chapter 12), or by ischemia. Bilateral carotid artery and high basilar artery ligations will produce an anemic decerebration.

The cause of decerebrate rigidity has not been fully determined, although a number of contributing factors may be mentioned. In general, it is apparent that the balance between descending excitatory action and inhibitory action on extensor motoneurons has been disturbed, with the balance shifted in favor of excitation. The loss of the corticospinal tracts, which are predominantly excitatory to flexor motoneurons, may contribute somewhat to the rigidity, but this could not be a major cause inasmuch as removal of the motor cortex does not produce decerebrate rigidity. The interruption of the rubrospinal tracts, which also are largely devoted to facilitation of flexor motoneurons, should certainly add to the extensor bias. The vestibulospinal tract is probably overactive, with a concomitant increase in excitatory drive to motoneurons. However, destruction of the lateral vestibular nuclei will not eliminate decerebrate rigidity, although it will reduce it. Another major factor may be the change in the activity of the descending control system that inhibits flexion reflex interneurons. This inhibitory pathway is probably reticulospinal, and it is more active in the decerebrate state than in the intact animal; that is, decerebration removes an inhibitory control of the descending inhibitory pathway.

In short, decerebrate rigidity is a complex phenomenon that can probably be fully explained only when the activity of the entire motor system is explained.

Disturbances of synergy (ataxia)

There are various types of disturbances of synergy seen in motor disease. These are often subsumed under the heading of ataxia (without order). The incoordination may be an inability to perform rapidly alternating movements, such as pronation and supination of the forearm and hand. Such movements require rapid reciprocal contraction and relaxation of antagonists. The inability to perform such movements smoothly and rapidly is called dysdiadochokinesia.

There may be decomposition of movement, in which a limb movement that is normally composed of simultaneous movements at several joints will be performed as a series of movements. The most striking form of ataxia is intention tremor (described below and in Chapter 12). Disturbances of synergy are most strikingly seen in lesions of the neocerebellum (see the section on the cerebellum).

Disturbances of reflexes

In disease states, reflexes that are normally present may be increased or decreased, and reflexes that are not normally present may appear. Reflexes that are clinically tested include the phasic stretch reflex (myotatic reflex, deep-tendon reflex) of various muscles and certain superficial reflexes.

Phasic stretch reflex is the response to a quick stretch of a muscle, activation of the group Ia afferents from muscle spindles (see Chapter 2), and excitation of the motoneurons to the muscle stretched and to its synergists (see Chapter 4). A concomitant inhibition of motoneurons to the antagonistic muscles also occurs. Typical reflexes of this sort commonly elicited clinically include the biceps, triceps, and brachioradialis jerks and the finger flexion reflex (Hoffmann's sign) in the upper extremity and the knee and ankle jerks in the lower extremity. The reflex occurs in both extensor and flexor muscles. Weak reflexes can often be enhanced by reinforcement, as in Jendrassik's maneuver, which consists of having the patient clasp his hands together and pull against himself while the reflex is tested. Phasic stretch reflex is typically increased in cases of spasticity. Enhanced phasic stretch reflex may lead to the appearance of clonus, a rhythmic alternation of contractions of a set of muscles followed by contraction of the antagonistic muscles. Apparently, the contraction of one set of muscles produces a sufficient stretch of the antagonists to serve as an effective stimulus of their phasic stretch reflex. This does not happen normally because there is sufficient damping in the system to prevent such oscillations from occurring. Phasic stretch reflex is often not increased in rigidity. A decrease in the phasic stretch reflex occurs when the reflex arc is interrupted, as in peripheral nerve disease, dorsal or ventral root damage, or in diseases affecting the motoneurons, such as poliomyelitis. The reflex may also be diminished in cerebellar disease and following acute injury to the descending motor pathways, prior to the development of spasticity.

Superficial reflexes that are often tested include the abdominal reflex and the plantar reflex. Abdominal reflexes are elicited by stroking the skin adjacent to the umbilicus. The abdominal muscles normally con-

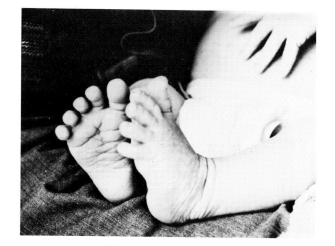

Fig. 8-1. Sign of Babinski. The dorsiflexion of the great toe and fanning of the other toes are shown on the left in this normal infant. The right foot also showed the response, but the great toe is no longer in dorsiflexion.

tract and move the umbilicus toward the side stimulated. Generally, the testing is done by stroking the skin in each of the four quadrants of the abdomen. The reflex may be absent in some normal individuals. However, its absence on one side may indicate an interruption of the corticospinal tract, because the descending effects of this pathway include support of this reflex.

A more important indicator of corticospinal tract damage is Babinski's sign. The normal response in adults to stroking the lateral margin of the sole of the foot, beginning near the heel and continuing to and across the ball of the foot, is a flexion of the toes. Some individuals will show little response; others may have a flexion withdrawal of the foot and leg. With interruption of the corticospinal tract, a positive sign of Babinski consists of a dorsiflexion of the great toe and fanning of the other toes. A similar response may be produced by stimulation of other areas of the foot and leg. Children below 2 years of age normally show Babinski's sign, presumably because the corticospinal tracts are not yet fully operational (Fig. 8-1).

Disturbances of posture and equilibrium

The neurology of postural disturbances, sometimes called disturbances of station, is a complex subject. Disturbances of posture and of equilibrium are most clearly produced by lesions of the peripheral and central vestibular system, by lesions of the flocculonodular lobe of the cerebellum, which receives vestibular projections, by lesions of large sensory fibers from muscle spindles and joints, and by dorsal column lesions. Impaired equilibrium and mispositioning of the limbs caused by dorsal column lesions is sometimes referred to as dorsal column ataxia. There are also postural disturbances in parkinsonism, and it is likely that many central structures contribute to postural regulation.

Decreased movement (paresis, paralysis, akinesia)

The term paresis (to relax, let go) can be used to mean impaired movement, as in referring to a paretic limb or a hemiparesis in which the face, arm, and leg of one side of the body are weak. Impaired voluntary movement is implied. Paresis may also be used to mean weakness of contraction of a muscle.

Paralysis (to loosen, dissolve, weaken) or palsy refers to a total lack of movement or contraction. The combining form plegia means stroke; unilateral paralysis is termed hemiplegia. Paraplegia (besides, stroke), which refers to paralysis of the legs, is most commonly caused by spinal cord injury. The motor states are affected by damage to motoneurons or to descending motor tracts.

Akinesia refers to difficulty in initiating movement, with a resulting decrease in the frequency of movements. Akinesia is a prominent feature of parkinsonism.

Increased movement (hyperkinesia)

Increased frequency of normal movements is called hyperkinesia. Hyperkinesia not produced by increased emotional activity but by lesions of motor areas is uncommon. Hyperkinesia has been reported to occur in some patients with surgical lesions of the caudate nucleus.

Tremor (physiological tremor, intention tremor, tremor at rest)

Tremor, or shaking of a part of the body, is caused by rhythmic involuntary contraction of muscles.

Tremors can be classified on the basis of their relationship to voluntary movement. Physiological tremor is present in all persons. The tremor appears when a person maintains a fixed posture, such as holding the hand outstretched. Therefore, the tremor is sometimes called sustention tremor. The tremor is normally of small amplitude and is rapid, about 10 Hz. In some persons this type of tremor may become clinically noticeable.

Intention tremor refers to a tremor that develops during the course of voluntary movement. The tremor is particularly marked during goal-directed movements as the limb reaches its goal. Shoulder-girdle muscles participate in intention tremor of the arm. Intention tremor is produced by neocerebellar damage.

Tremor that occurs in the absence of voluntary movement is called resting tremor. This type of tremor is suppressed or reduced during movement and is the tremor characteristic of Parkinson's disease. There is alternate flexion and contraction of antagonistic muscles, particularly of the forearm muscles, with the finger flexor movements appearing more marked than the extensor movements. This is called pill-rolling tremor, because the movements are similar to those which are made when rolling a pill between thumb and forefinger. Resting tremor involves distal limb muscles more than proximal limb-girdle muscles.

Involuntary movement

This term is used here to describe involuntary movements more elaborate than tremor and ataxia. Three major types of involuntary movements occur clinically: ballistic movement, in which a limb is thrown (associated rather specifically with partial destruction of the subthalamic nucleus); choreiform (dancelike) movements of the trunk and limbs, in which the limbs are thrown out as in ballistic movements but with less violence and with a more writhing quality (seen in Huntington's chorea, in which there is degeneration of the caudate nucleus and in the cortex); and athetoid (without a fixed position) and dystonic movements, which are slow, writhing movements of the trunk and limbs. Such movements may in some cases be associated with lesions of the neostriatum and paleostriatum. Torticollis, or spasmodic twisting of the head and neck, may be part of a generalized athetosis or may appear alone.

Improperly controlled voluntary movement

Several types of improper control of voluntary movement can be seen clinically. *Ataxia* has been described above. Dysdiadochokinesia may occur as part of a syndrome of cerebellar ataxia. However, *decreased speed of movement,* where movement is otherwise well controlled, may also occur after lesions of descending motor tracts. Rapid alternating movement of distal muscles, such as pronation-supination of the hand or tapping with the fingers or toes, are most affected.

A further level of complexity of impaired motor control is seen in *apraxia* (Gk. *a-*, without, *praxis,* doing), in which skilled motor acts are performed as if for the first time. Apraxia is seen in lesions of the parietal lobes. It appears that the learned central program of the motor act has been damaged. For example, the patient may be unable to use a fork, comb his hair, or dress.

Pyramidal and extrapyramidal systems and syndromes

The term pyramidal system is often used to designate the corticospinal projections and is generally used in a restricted sense to mean those fibers that pass through the pyramid. The term pyramidal syndrome is used to describe the type of paresis and reflex changes seen after injuries of descending motor pathways, in which corticospinal projections as well as other descending motor pathways are usually injured.

An important clinical distinction is made between lesions that affect descending pathways making connections to motoneurons and those that injure motoneurons directly. The former are called upper motoneuron lesions, and the latter lower motoneuron lesions (see Chapter 12). When motoneurons are damaged (either the cell body or the motor axon), certain results ensue (see Chapter 3). The muscles supplied by the motoneurons become weak or paralyzed. Muscle tone is reduced and voluntary movements and reflex responses are diminished, the severity of effects depending on the proportion of motoneurons injured. If motoneurons are irreversibly damaged, the muscle they supply atrophies unless reinnervated. As motoneurons die, they discharge repetitively; this produces fasciculations of the muscles innervated. When a muscle has been denervated and begins to atrophy, it shows spontaneous electrical activity called fibrillation. Fasciculation may be observed readily through the skin because entire motor units are discharged simultaneously; fibrillation cannot be seen because single muscle fibers are contracting asynchronously. The diagnosis of fibrillation requires electromyography. Other changes in the muscle, such as hypersensitivity to acetylcholine, a decrease in electrical excitability, and various biochemical and histologic changes, result from denervation.

Upper motoneuron diseases produce changes that depend on the site or sites of damage. A typical upper motoneuron lesion is that caused by cerebrovascular disease affecting the internal capsule. A number of descending systems are involved in this kind of lesion. The motor effects include paresis or paralysis, but there are an eventual late increase in muscle tone (spasticity), increased myotatic reflexes, and the presence of pathological reflexes, including Babinski's sign. There is no muscle atrophy (except secondarily to disuse) and no fasciculation, fibrillation, or other changes in muscle. Many of the effects are quite similar to those observed in the decerebrate animal. Although the typical upper motoneuron lesion is often referred to as producing a pyramidal syndrome, it has been pointed out above (and in Chapter 12) that the complete pyramidal syndrome is probably caused by concurrent damage to a number of descending tracts in addition to the corticospinal tract.

The term extrapyramidal system is often used in two ways. It may designate the basal ganglia, particularly when extrapyramidal motor diseases, which are largely but not entirely diseases of the basal ganglia, are being discussed. The term extrapyramidal may also be used to designate descending motor projections other than the fibers in the pyramids or corticospinal tracts. At one time it was thought that the basal ganglia had significant descending projections, but this does not now appear to be the case. Therefore, extrapyramidal descending projections arise from cortical areas other than the precentral gyrus, from the precentral gyrus, which does not send all its fibers into the pyramids, and from brainstem nuclei.

Because of the lack of precision of these terms and the somewhat incorrect description they give of the anatomical bases for disease states, they probably should now be discarded. However, they have served useful purposes for many years, and extrapyramidal motor disorder and pyramidal syndrome are conveniently short ways of referring to neurological syndromes. Therefore, it is unlikely that these terms will soon be dropped from the neurological lexicon.

TECHNIQUES USED IN STUDYING MOTOR ACTIVITY

The starting point in the study of movement is to describe accurately the sequence of muscle activities that occur during different movements. With the development of mechanical and photographic recording equipment in the second half of the last century, notable studies of human and animal locomotion were made by Duchenne, Muybridge, Maray, and others.

Description of muscular activities can be obtained by electromyography, by the use of sensors that measure muscle tension and joint angles, and by photography. However, it is generally felt that these techniques still require refinement and that complete descriptions of the sequences of muscle activity that occurs in most of the common movements of humans have not been achieved. Computers are now being used for collecting and correlating the large amounts of data that are obtained in this type of study.

To obtain precisely controlled and reproducible movements for study, animals are trained to perform motor tasks in which a particular aspect of motor control is emphasized, for example, to exert a constant force or to make a movement of constant amplitude.

We would understand a motor activity if we could give a complete description of the neural events that occur during the activity. Because of the complexity of the central pathways for control of movement, it is unlikely that this goal can be soon achieved except for simple reflexes.

Another approach to the understanding of motor activity that is applicable to reflex activity is to plot motor output against sensory input and, from these data, to investigate the gain of the system and to see whether there are positive or negative feedback loops in the system. The muscle stretch, postural, and pupillary reflexes have been treated as control systems, or servomechanisms, in recent years with such techniques. These are powerful techniques because identifying the functional characteristics of the central portion of the control system can provide hypotheses for electrophysiologically and anatomically identifying the neurons that make up the system.

Recording of the electrical activity of single neurons in primates making controlled movements is a relatively new and highly promising technique, developed extensively by Evarts and his co-workers.

Electrical stimulation has been used to determine which brain areas evoke movement and modulate reflex activity. However, it has been difficult to interpret what the evoked movements signify about the organization of the areas stimulated. For example, stimulation of the motor cortex can evoke contraction of individual limb muscles but also can produce simple synergistic movements of the limbs. Some of the variability of the effects of electrical stimulation is probably a function of electrode size and stimulus parameters, as well as the fact that electrical stimulation is a very abnormal way of activating systems that are normally synaptically activated.

Ablation was the first method of studying the motor function of the brain. Interpretation of ablation studies has often been difficult. A major technical problem of ablation studies is that lesions damage not only the cell bodies of the area under study but also the fiber systems passing through the area.

In interpreting ablation studies it is important to remember that the motor abnormalities produced by lesions reflect the activity of the remaining neural structures. The effect of a lesion of an area on an area to which it projects is generally not just to subtract the effect of the lesioned area but also to add the disturbed function of other areas. For example, a lesion of the motor cortex not only has a direct effect on motoneurons but will change the activity of other pathways projecting to motoneurons.

A further complicating factor in lesion studies is that after lesions are made, poorly understood processes of compensation and relearning usually produce progressive changes in the character of motor deficits. It has been suggested that new synaptic contacts produced by collateral sprouting of intact axons take the place of degenerating axon terminals after injuries and that such changes may produce changing patterns of motor activity after lesions.

The motor effects of ablating the same structure in different species are often different. There is a much greater encephalization of motor control in primates than in lower species. For example, the cat is able to walk quite well immediately after the entire brain rostral to the subthalamus is removed, but the primate cannot.

Finally, it should be mentioned that surgical attempts to reproduce the clinical effects of disease-induced lesions have often been unsuccessful, particularly for the diseases of the basal ganglia. This is probably because disease processes will often selectively damage only some cells, whereas surgical ablations damage all of the cells of an area as well as axons of passage.

ORGANIZATION OF MOTOR SYSTEMS
Organization of the motoneurons and projections to them

The motoneurons of the brainstem cranial nerves and of the spinal cord are the final common pathway for effecting movement. The motoneurons are under the control of local sensory fibers, local interneurons, and descending and ascending tracts. The different projections to the motoneurons and to local interneurons probably control different aspects of motor activity. For example, the corticospinal tract appears to control fine movements of distal musculature; the vestibulospinal tracts mediate postural reflexes. Activity in all of the tracts probably occurs in a complex act such as walking, in which voluntary and reflex postural mechanisms interact.

Each of the descending motor tracts has a particular distribution to motoneurons and to interneurons. There are differences in the density of synaptic terminals of descending fibers on motoneurons of flexor and extensor muscles and on motoneurons to distal and proximal limb muscles. The lateral corticospinal tract is most heavily distributed to motoneurons of flexor muscles of the hand and forearm. The corticospinal tract also has a topographic, or point-to-point, projection from its sites of origin to its sites of termination, as does the rubrospinal tract. In contrast, there does not appear to be any somatotopic organization of reticulospinal tracts, although such an organization may yet be found. The fine details of the terminal distributions of descending motor tracts are currently under intensive study.

Descending tracts appear to modulate spinal motor activity in two ways: by direct commands or programs of impulses, and by facilitation or inhibition of spinal reflex arcs. Direct commands generally excite both alpha and gamma motoneurons to a given muscle. The activation of gamma motoneurons prevents the unloading of muscle spindles and thus loss of the excitatory support provided the alpha motoneurons by the stretch reflex. Excitation of gamma motoneurons by descending pathways may in addition assist in the production of alpha motoneuron discharge by way of the gamma loop (see Chapter 4). Descending effects on spinal reflexes are produced by EPSPs and IPSPs evoked in spinal neurons that raise or lower their excitability. Presynaptic inhibition of transmission in spinal reflex arcs can also be produced by activity in some descending pathways.

Organization of suprasegmental areas projecting to motoneurons

The organization of brain areas that give rise to descending motor tracts will be discussed in this and the next sections. Fig. 8-2 shows the major projections of brain areas that are most directly related to movement, the major descending motor tracts, and their major effects on spinal motoneurons. It is important to remember that many of these central structures have functions other than modulating motor activity. In particular the neostriatum (caudate nucleus and putamen) receives input from wide areas of the cortex and appears to participate in many different types of activity.

There are two closely related questions that can be asked about the motor organization shown in Fig. 8-2. What is the motor function of each of the areas, and what areas mediate the different types of motor activity, such as tonus, postural reflexes, rhythmic automatic movements, and voluntary movement, which were described in the first section of this chapter? Precise answers cannot be given to these questions; however, some general answers can be given.

These structures can be divided into four main groups:

1. The first group consists of the *thalamus* and the *corticobulbospinal system.* The cortex is modulated by the thalamus, which in turn receives input from the sensory systems, the cerebellum, and the basal ganglia. The cortex in turn modulates these structures and sends descending tracts to brainstem motor nuclei and to motoneurons.

There has been a strong tendency to equate voluntary control of motoneurons with the corticospinal system, discussed in more detail below. For the present it can be said that the corticospinal system in its *restricted* sense, meaning the fibers from the motor

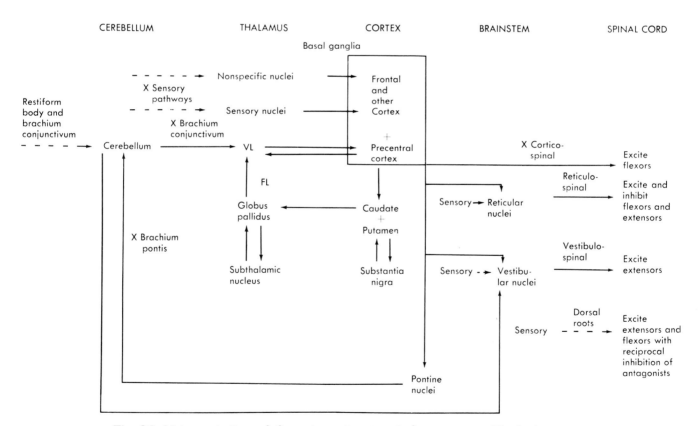

Fig. 8-2. Major projections of the motor system to spinal motoneurons. The broken arrows in the diagram indicate major points of sensory input. The predominant effects of electrical excitation of descending pathways on spinal motoneurons are also indicated. x predominantly decussating pathways. Abbreviations: *FL,* fasciculus lenticularis; *VL,* ventrolateral nucleus of thalamus.

cortex to the pyramids and the lateral corticospinal tract, is only one system mediating voluntary movement, and it largely mediates fine movement of the hand. However, it can also be said that in adults, descending tracts from the cortex, including cortical tracts to brainstem nuclei, in a *broad* sense either mediate or facilitate any useful voluntary movement to a very great extent.

2. The *brainstem nuclei* are modulated by sensory input, the cerebral cortex, and the cerebellum. The brainstem nuclei send descending tracts to motoneurons. They mediate postural reflexes and are important in providing impulses that set the tone of muscles. There is reason to believe that voluntary movement, particularly of the musculature of the trunk and proximal extremities, can be mediated via brainstem nuclei. In addition, the brainstem contains interneurons that mediate chewing, licking, and the rhythmic-automatic activity of respiration.

3. The *cerebellum* is modulated by sensory input and by the cerebral cortex. It largely modulates the activity of the cerebral cortex and the brainstem vestibular and reticular nuclei. The cerebellum appears to coordinate motor activity, producing synergistic action of muscles. It appears to function as an error-correcting device for goal-directed movement. It receives information about the position of the body and then provides an output that is used by descending motor systems to correct the position in terms of reaching the goal.

4. The *basal ganglia* receive input largely from the cerebral cortex. They modulate thalamic activity. The type of control they exert over thalamocortical activity is unknown.

Hierarchical order of motor systems

The motoneurons are accessible to a number of systems that play on them continuously and simultaneously. However, certain systems dominate the motoneuron's activity at different times. For example, a cervical spinal cord motoneuron innervating the diaphragm muscle will fire regularly with each inspiration. The same neuron will change its firing pattern during a body movement requiring postural and voluntary control. It will also change its activity during swallowing, coughing, and speaking. Little is known of how the switching of neurons from one activity to another occurs. In some cases the switching appears to be done simply by overriding, that is, by providing a massive input, as when painful stimulation produces flexion of a limb. Although voluntary inhibition of respiration requires as little effort as any voluntary act, voluntary inhibition of inspiration cannot be maintained no matter how much effort is expended, proba-

bly because of massive stimulation of the inspiratory neurons by CO_2.

The general dominance of descending activity of the cortex over brainstem and spinal activity in adults is seen when transections of the neuraxis are made. Exaggerated motor activities that appear when descending tracts are interrupted at certain levels of the brain, such as decerebrate rigidity, are often called release phenomena, implying that the activity that appears is normally suppressed or dominated by higher or more complex systems. However, the details of the hierarchical control of the motor systems are very poorly known.

Motor-sensory integration

There is reason to believe that the motor systems send information about body movements into the sensory systems and that this information is used by sensory systems in interpreting the sensations received during the movement. For example, if an eye is moved by pressing on it with a fingertip, objects in the visual field appear to move; however, if the same movement is made voluntarily, the same sensation of movement of objects does not occur. The presumed motor-to-sensory discharge is called corollary discharge and is thought to provide information used by perceptual mechanisms that provide constancy of our perceptions of the world (see Chapter 11).

SUPRASEGMENTAL MOTOR SYSTEMS
Corticobulbospinal system

Anatomy. The corticospinal tracts arise in part from cells of the principal motor area (Ms1) of the cerebral cortex. The motor cortex was first demonstrated by Fritsch and Hitzig (1870), who stimulated the brain of a dog electrically and observed movements of the animal when certain areas of the cerebral cortex were excited. Most of the motor cortical cells are located in the precentral gyrus in primates, although some are located in front of the precentral gyrus and in the parietal cortex. However, the largest pyramidal cells of the precentral gyrus, the Betz cells, give rise to only about one thirtieth of the axons participating in the corticospinal tracts. The electrically excitable primary motor area therefore does not correspond exactly with either a gyrus or with a cytoarchitectural area, although a large part of it does correspond to Brodmann's area 4.

The primary motor area is somatotopically organized. The region controlling the face is situated laterally on the cortex; dorsal to it is the arm area; and the hindlimb area is on the vertex and medial surface of the hemisphere (Fig. 8-3). The relationship between the various parts of the motor cortex and the

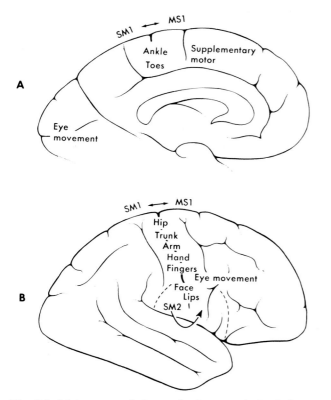

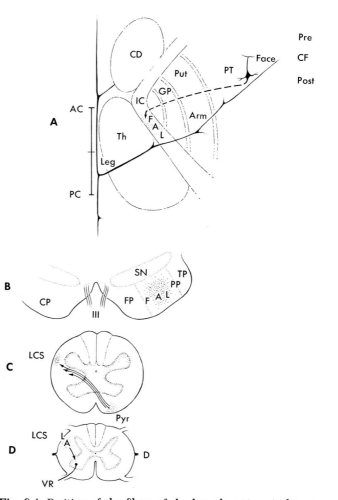

Fig. 8-3. Motor areas of the cerebral cortex. **A,** Medial aspect of hemisphere. **B,** Lateral aspect. *Sm1, Ms1,* primary sensorimotor and motor sensory areas. *Sm2,* secondary sensory and motor area. The parts of the body in which movement is evoked by stimulation of different parts of the primary motor cortex are shown. The labeling of body parts extends across the primary sensory and motor cortices to emphasize two points: that in man, as in lower animals, these cortices are best regarded as sensorimotor cortices and that the sensory sequence and the representation of the body follows a similar sequence in adjoining parts of the postcentral and precentral gyri. *Sm2* lies at the foot of the precentral and postcentral gyri and extends in the parietal operculum, as indicated by the arrow.

Fig. 8-4. Position of the fibers of the lateral corticospinal tract at different levels of the neuraxis. **A,** Horizontal section of the right cerebrum showing the internal capsule *(IC),* caudate nucleus *(CD),* globus pallidus *(GP),* putamen *(Put),* thalamus *(Th),* and the location of the anterior *(AC)* and posterior *(PC)* commissures. The position of the central fissure *(CF)* and of the precentral *(Pre)* and postcentral *(Post)* cortices of the right cerebrum are shown as in a view of the superior aspect of the cerebrum. The contribution of an axon of a pyramidal tract cell of the precentral cortex *(PT)* to the fibers of the corticospinal tract is shown. **B,** Transverse section through the right midbrain shown in a posterior-anterior view (that is, seen from behind). *CP,* cerebral peduncle; *SN,* substantia nigra; *III,* exiting fibers of the oculomotor nerve; *TP, PP, FP,* temporal, parietal, and frontal pontine tracts; *F, A, L,* fibers projecting to motoneurons for face, arm, and leg musculature respectively. **C,** Decussation of axons from the pyramid *(Pyr)* into the lateral corticospinal tract *(LCS);* view as in **B. D,** Spinal cord, showing the lateral corticospinal tract in the lateral column above the level of the dentate ligament *(D).* The arrow indicates projections to ventral horn neurons. *VR,* ventral root.

parts of the body they innervate can be shown figuratively by a homunculus drawn over a representation of the precentral gyrus. The motor homunculus is a distorted version of the body, with the various parts having a size roughly in proportion to the area of cortex devoted to their control. The motor homunculus looks rather like the corresponding sensory homunculus of the postcentral cortex (Fig. 7-12).

Knowledge of the position of the corticobulbar and corticospinal tracts is of clinical importance. The fibers of the lateral corticospinal tract are shown at various levels of the neuraxis in Figs. 8-4 to 8-9.

Corticospinal axons pass through the internal capsule, the cerebral peduncles, the pons, and the pyramids of the medulla to reach the spinal cord. Corticobulbar fibers project along with the corticospinal

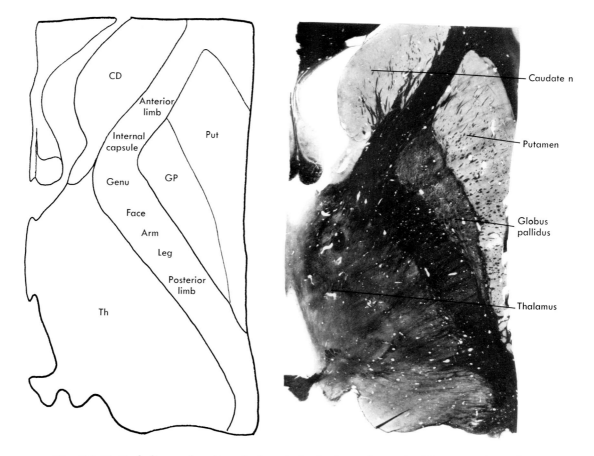

Fig. 8-5. Corticobulbar and corticospinal tracts in the internal capsule. The section is in the horizontal plane and shows the anterior limb, genu, and posterior limb of the internal capsule. The approximate positions of the corticobulbar and corticospinal fibers are indicated.

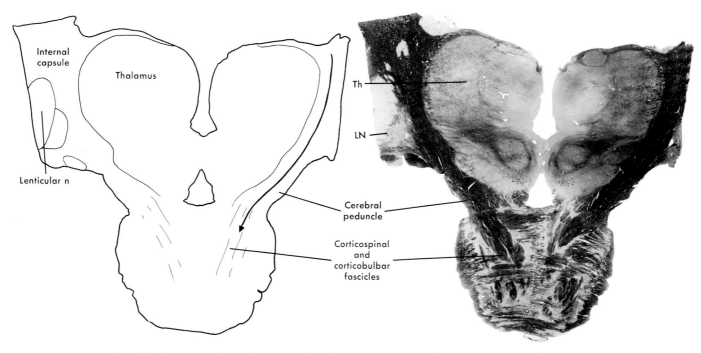

Fig. 8-6. The internal capsule, cerebral peduncle, and corticobulbar and corticospinal fascicles in the pons. The posterior limb of the internal capsule is shown descending between the thalamus and the lentiform nucleus to enter the cerebral peduncle; the fibers continue as corticobulbar and corticospinal fibers through the base of the pons.

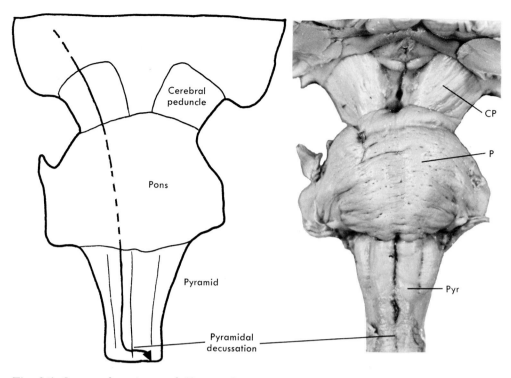

Fig. 8-7. Course of corticospinal fibers in brainstem. A corticospinal fiber is shown diagrammatically at the left emerging from the internal capsule to enter the cerebral peduncle, descending through the pons to form a part of the pyramid, and finally crossing in the pyramidal decussation. The fiber is shown in buried structures by dashed lines and in superficial structures by solid lines.

fibers into the brainstem but terminate before reaching the spinal cord. In the caudal medulla, most of the corticospinal fibers decussate to form the lateral corticospinal tract, which descends in the lateral funiculus. Some fibers also enter the lateral corticospinal tract of the ipsilateral cord, and a few enter the ventral corticospinal tracts bilaterally. The ventral corticospinal tracts traverse the ventral funiculi. All four tracts supply all segmental levels of the cord, although the thoracic cord is less richly endowed with terminations than are the cervical and lumbosacral parts of the cord. The main pathway in humans appears to be the crossed lateral corticospinal tract. This path is organized in lamellar fashion, like several of the ascending tracts already described (Figs. 7-6, 7-15, and 8-9). The fibers of the lateral corticospinal tract leading to the cervical cord are situated medially in the tract, and fibers traveling further down the cord are placed more laterally because their course is longer. The great majority of axons in the lateral corticospinal tract are very fine. Only 60% are myelinated, and almost all of these are less than 4 μm in diameter. Only about 2% of the myelinated fibers are large (10 to 20 μm).

The mode of termination of corticospinal axons depends on the species and age of the animal. In the cat, corticospinal axons end on interneurons in Rexed's laminae IV to VIII and not directly on motoneurons. The heaviest projections are to the lateral parts of laminae V and VI. The more dorsal projections appear to arise from the region of the cerebral cortex just caudal to the main motor area. This is a sensory region of the cerebral cortex, although closely related to the motor area. The connections through the corticospinal tract to the dorsal horn might suggest a role for these fibers in the control of sensory input. The corticospinal fibers from the area of cerebral cortex generally regarded as chiefly motor in function end in laminae V to VIII and form the predominant projection to the spinal cord. The terminations presumably excite interneurons that relay the actions of the corticospinal tract to motoneurons.

In the primate the corticospinal tract has endings on interneurons of the same pattern as in the cat. The pattern of termination in the very young primate is very similar to that in the cat; however, in the adult primate there are also many endings of the corticospinal tract on motoneurons within lamina IX. The density of such terminations is greatest on motoneurons supplying the distal musculature, such as the muscles of the hand. Furthermore, the density of direct projections to motoneurons appears to be

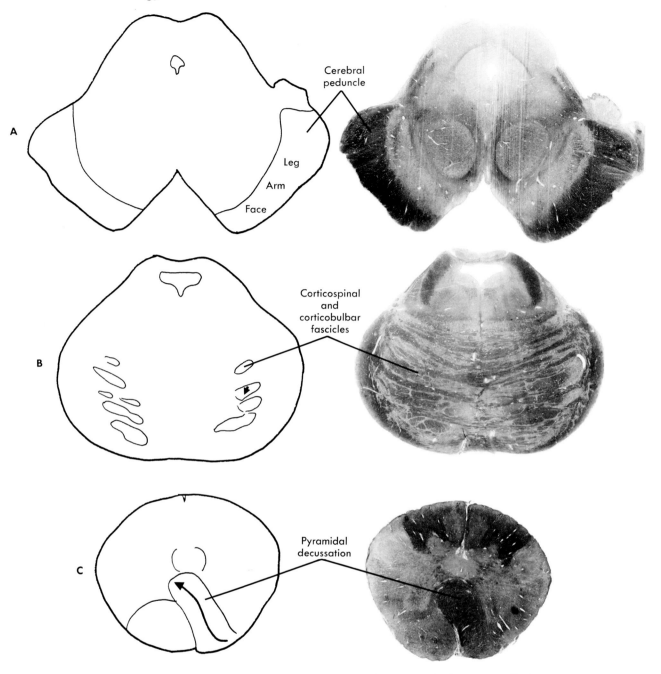

Fig. 8-8. Course of the corticobulbar and corticospinal fibers in the brainstem. The position of the corticobulbar and corticospinal tracts is shown for the midbrain and pons in **A** and **B**. The pyramidal decussation (corticospinal tract) is shown in **C**.

greater in anthropoid apes than in monkeys. These observations suggest a relationship between the degree of development of fine motor control and the density of projection from motor cortex directly to the motoneurons responsible. Support for this idea comes from the findings that there are some direct corticospinal-motoneuronal connections in the raccoon that seem to relate to its manual dexterity, and there are heavy projections of this kind to the motoneurons supplying the tail muscles in New World monkeys with prehensile tails.

The corticobulbar tract arises from the face area in the motor cortex and adjacent sensory cortex. The fibers course through the genu of the internal capsule and enter the brainstem as a bundle just medial to the corticospinal fibers in the basis pedunculi. Some of

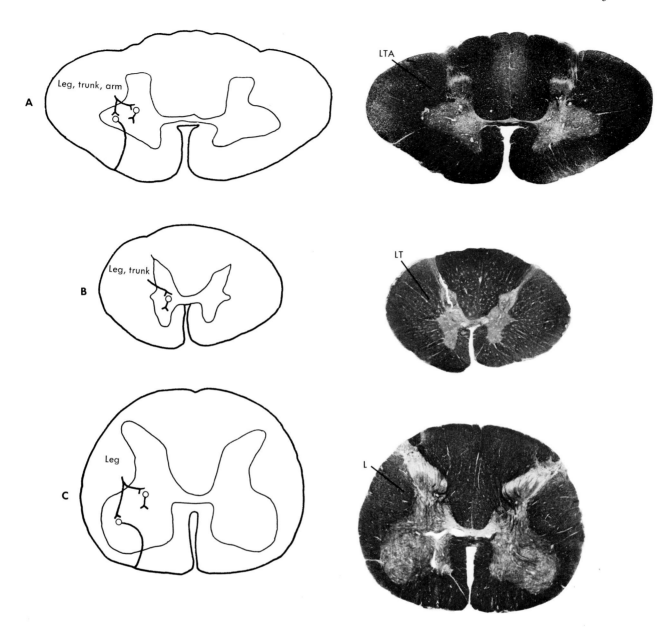

Fig. 8-9. Corticospinal tract in the spinal cord. **A,** Most of the corticospinal fibers occupy the lateral corticospinal tract and are contralateral to their cells of origin in the motor cortex. **B,** The lateral corticospinal tract has a somatotopic organization, as indicated. **C,** In the cervical cord, the fibers distributing to the cervical enlargement are medial to those distributing to the thoracic cord and to the lumbosacral enlargement. The ventral corticospinal tract is not shown, but includes uncrossed fibers; it distributes to motoneurons supplying axial muscles.

the corticobulbar fibers continue caudally along with the corticospinal projection through the base of the pons and into the pyramid. However, throughout the brainstem parts of the corticobulbar tract separate from the main descending system to terminate in the tegmentum in association with cranial nerve nuclei or other brainstem structures, including the reticular formation. For the purpose of the present discussion,

emphasis will be placed on the projections to cranial nerve nuclei. From the standpoint of clinical application, the most important consideration is which cranial motor nuclei receive bilateral connections from the corticobulbar tract and which ones receive a crossed projection. Bilateral connections are found for all of the cranial motor nuclei except that part of the facial nucleus that supplies muscles below the orbit and the part of the hypoglossal nucleus that supplies the genioglossus muscle. These nuclei are exceptions and receive only a crossed innervation from the corticobulbar tract (Fig. 8-10). This arrangement is reminiscent of the corticospinal tract, which is essentially a crossed projection for control of distal muscles, especially those of the hand, but includes a bilateral projection for the supply of axial and proximal muscles. The crossed corticobulbar supply of the muscles of the lower face and tongue has the important clinical consequence that interruption of the corticobulbar tract on one side in disease produces weakness of the contralateral muscles of the lower face but not of the frontalis muscle or the orbicularis oculi. A facial nerve palsy results in weakness of all of the facial musculature on the same side. Weakness of the tongue on one side can result from either a contralateral interruption of the corticobulbar tract or ipsilateral damage to the hypoglossal nucleus or nerve. These can be distinguished on the basis of atrophy in the case of damage to the motoneurons.

Responses evoked in the corticospinal tract by cortical stimulation. Recordings of field potentials and of single-axon discharges in the corticospinal tract have generally been obtained in the pyramids, with

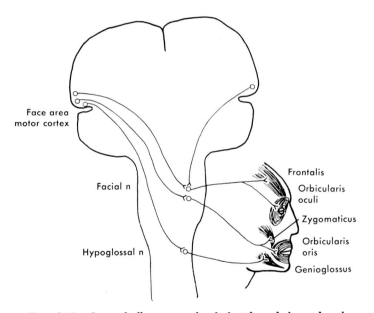

Fig. 8-10. Corticobulbar control of facial and hypoglossal motoneurons. The corticobulbar tract provides a bilateral innervation of most cranial nerve motor nuclei. For example, the illustration shows a bilateral corticobulbar projection to the facial motoneurons that innervate the frontalis and orbicularis oculi muscles. However, there is only a crossed corticobulbar supply to motoneurons innervating the muscles of facial expression below the orbit, such as the zygomaticus and the orbicularis oris, and to motoneurons supplying the genioglossus muscle.

microelectrodes inserted through an opening in the base of the skull. The responses of the large corticospinal fibers dominate the activity recorded from the pyramids. Single-shock cortical stimulation in the monkey evokes a single positive wave in the pyramid, with a latency of about 1 msec followed by a series of positive waves lasting several milliseconds. The response looks something like that evoked by stimulating the pyramid and recording in the cortex. The initial wave (direct, d wave) is produced by direct excitation of the Betz cells giving rise to the largest axons in the pyramids; the later waves (indirect, i waves) are caused by interneuronal excitation of pyramidal neurons; directly excited, more slowly conducting axons of smaller pyramidal cells may also contribute to the i waves.

Recording of single-axon discharges in the pyramidal tract has also been used as a way of monitoring the output of the motor cortex when inputs to it, such as ventrolateral nuclei, are stimulated.

Effects of stimulation of the motor cortex. The effect of electrical stimulation of the motor cortex in carnivores such as the cat is somewhat different from that in primates. In the cat, descending volleys in the pyramidal tract generally facilitate the activity of flexor motoneurons and inhibit extensor motoneurons through polysynaptic pathways involving one or more spinal cord interneurons. As a rule, the effects on alpha and gamma motoneurons are comparable. In the primate, the action of the corticospinal tract is more complex. Electrically evoked volleys produce an early facilitation through a monosynaptic pathway. This is followed by a mixture of inhibitory and facilitatory actions through a polysynaptic pathway, but, as in the cat, the degree of inhibition is greater than facilitation in extensor motoneurons and vice versa in flexor motoneurons.

The type of movement evoked in the primate by motor cortex stimulation varies with the stimulus parameters. The responses are easily depressed by general anesthesia. Single-shock stimulation at low strength of the face, hand, and leg areas produces very quick flicklike contralateral movements of the angle of the mouth, the thumb, and the great toe respectively. With minimal stimulation, contractions of some individual muscles can occur. With repetitive stimulation and with stimulation with increasing current intensities, large portions of the limb respond, with a greater variety of responses. The responses in the anthropoid apes and in humans are rather similar. The responses include flexion of a limb or grimacelike contractions of the face. Complex patterned movements involving rhythmic or repetitive activity are not typically evoked from the motor cortex.

Bilateral movements can be evoked in the face area. These include jaw, lip, and swallowing movements. Vocalization can be produced by stimulation near the lateral fissure. This response consists of expiration and a vowel sound.

Several features of the organization of the projection from motor cortex to alpha motoneurons in the primate are of particular interest. The strength of the linkage depends on the location in the extremity of the muscle innervated. Motoneurons supplying the muscles of the hand, for instance, are more powerfully excited by the monosynaptic corticospinal pathway than are motoneurons to proximally placed muscles. This presumably reflects the richer innervation of the motoneurons to distal muscles by corticospinal fibers. The density of innervation no doubt accounts for the size of the part of the motor homunculus devoted to control of the hand. The dependence of humans on the integrity of the corticospinal tract for the control of fine movements of the hand is presumably caused by an organization of the linkage between motor cortex and the motoneurons to distal muscles similar to that in the primate.

In the awake human, about 20% of stimulations of the primary motor cortex evoke sensations as well as movement. Similarly, about the same percentage of motor responses are evoked by stimulating the primary sensory cortex of the postcentral gyrus. Therefore, these areas are best considered as sensorimotor structures, and designated as Ms1 and Sm1 respectively.

Effects of ablations of the corticobulbospinal system. The effects of ablations of the primary motor cortex and of the corticobulbospinal tracts in the adult human cannot yet be stated with complete certainty. That this should be so after 100 years of investigation of the motor cortex may seem surprising, but it is very difficult to obtain satisfactory clinicopathological correlations of the effects of human brain lesions.

In adults extensive damage to the primary motor cortex produces a paralysis of the contralateral somatic musculature. At first, muscle tone and the stretch reflexes are diminished, but after a few weeks these return and may increase somewhat. Voluntary movement improves over a longer period. Mass movements,

largely caused by proximal limb muscles, are better performed than fine movements of distal limb muscles. Recovery of function after lesions of the primary motor cortex depends on a number of factors. The size of the ablated area, the age of the individual, and the species all affect the extent of recovery. Prognosis is worse with large lesions, in older individuals, and in humans than with small lesions, in children, and in monkeys or lower mammals.

The effects of lesions of the corticobulbospinal tracts at different levels of the neuraxis also are not known with certainty. It must be remembered that the descending tracts have wide cortical origins and distributions that can be indicated as in the diagram below.

This diagram indicates that an internal capsule lesion will produce a greater deficit than a lateral corticospinal tract lesion, because a lesion in the internal capsule interrupts the lateral corticospinal fibers plus all the other cortical influences that are relayed to motoneurons through descending pathways originating in the brainstem nuclei.

The corticospinal tract in humans appears to be only one of several tracts mediating voluntary movement. Most important, it mediates fine hand movement. For a spinal cord or brainstem injury to produce the severe and lasting changes observed following internal capsule lesions, other descending tracts, which run in the anterolateral white columns of the cord, must also be damaged. These tracts are probably largely reticulospinal in origin.

Secondary and supplementary motor areas. Stimulation of areas of the cortex other than the primary motor area can also evoke simple movements. The delineation of the secondary and supplementary motor areas in humans has largely been carried out by Penfield and his co-workers.

The second motor area lies at the base of the precentral and postcentral gyri, just above the lateral fissure, and it extends into the parietal operculum (Fig. 8-3). This area is coextensive with the second sensory cortex, and sensory phenomena are more prominent than motor phenomena when this area is stimulated. The area should probably be designated Sm2. Contralateral, ipsilateral, and bilateral

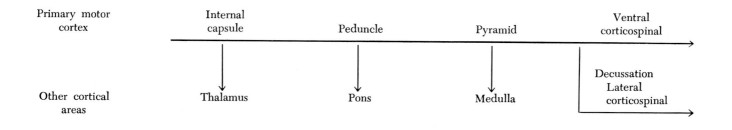

responses can be evoked from Sm2. Contralateral responses predominate. Movements of the contralateral body (generally of the hand), inhibition of movement, or a sensation of a desire to move the contralateral arm or hand are evoked by stimulation of Sm2. This area has been studied much less extensively than the primary sensorimotor areas. The face appears to be represented in Sm2 just above the lateral fissure; the arm and then the leg are represented proceeding into the lateral fissure, with the representation extending on to the parietal operculum. Ablations of the area have not been extensively studied, but no obvious motor or sensory deficits appear to result from injury to this area.

The supplementary motor area lies on the medial surface of the frontal lobe in front of the primary motor cortex representation of the lower leg (Fig. 8-3). Stronger currents must be used to evoke responses from the supplementary motor cortex than from the primary motor cortex. There appears to be a crude topographic representation of the body in the supplementary cortex in the monkey, although this has not been found in humans. Stimulation of the supplementary motor area in people evokes largely contralateral movements, but some ipsilateral responses occur as well. Stimulation evokes posturing, often a turning of the head to the contralateral side of the body and raising the contralateral arm. Posturing of the ipsilateral arm may also occur. There may be rhythmic movements. Fine movements of the hand, like those produced by stimulation of the primary motor area, are not evoked. Vocalization can be produced. Supplementary motor stimulation may also slow or arrest voluntary movement. Autonomic effects, such as changes in pulse and visceral sensations, can also be evoked.

Ablation of the supplementary motor area produces lasting slowness of movement of the contralateral limbs and transient forced grasping. The grasp reflex is evoked by stroking the palm of the hand. Forced grasping is a clinical sign of frontal lobe damage.

Eye movements can be evoked from the motor and frontal cortex and from the occipital visual cortex, as well as from many subcortical structures. Eye movements are discussed further in the last section of this chapter.

Reticular formation

Anatomy. The core of the brainstem contains neurons that form nuclear groups with indistinct boundaries and many fibers that are not organized into well-circumscribed tracts. This area is named the reticular formation because the cell bodies, dendrites, and axons in it give it a reticulated appearance that

is different from the more tightly organized appearance of the periphery of the brainstem, where most of the nuclear groups and tracts have sharp boundaries. However, distinct cytoarchitectual areas of the reticular formation and specific projections of these areas to other parts of the brain have been established in recent years. It is possible that the term reticular formation, which suggests an unmapped portion of the brain, will eventually not be used when all the reticular nuclei are assigned to functional systems. At present the area that is considered the reticular formation is a core of the brainstem extending from the caudal medulla to the mesencephalon, which can be divided into medullary, pontine, and mesencephalic clusters of neurons (Fig. 8-11). Each of these three areas can be subdivided into a medial and a lateral portion. This distinction is clearest in the medulla and becomes progressively less clear in the pons and mesencephalon. The medial reticular formation comprises about two thirds of the reticular area. It contains the gigantocellular portion of the reticular formation. Medium-sized and small neurons are intermingled with the giant cells. The lateral reticular formation, the parvicellular portion, contains mostly medium-sized and small neurons.

Long ascending and descending projections arise from the medial reticular formation. The lateral reticular formation appears to function as a local system of interneurons, with shorter ascending and descending projections that project to the medial reticular neurons. The lateral reticular formation probably also projects to brainstem sensory relay and cranial nerve nuclei.

The neurons of the medial reticular formation that have long projections transmit reticular influences largely to the thalamus and spinal cord. These reticular cells have comparatively long, sparse dendrites. This has been called an isodendritic pattern and is typified by the motoneuron. In contrast, sensory relay nucleus neurons typically have shorter, more highly branched dendrites.

Many of the neurons of the medial reticular formation have axons that bifurcate, with one axonal branch ascending and the other descending. In addition, many collateral branches are given off that appear to synapse on other reticular neurons as well as on neurons in the terminal distributions of the reticular projections. Cells with predominantly ascending axons are located a little caudally to cells with predominantly descending axons in both the medial medullary and pontine reticular areas (Fig. 8-12). Most of the mesencephalic reticular neurons with long axons appear to project rostrally. Collateral branches and interneurons probably interconnect neurons that have pre-

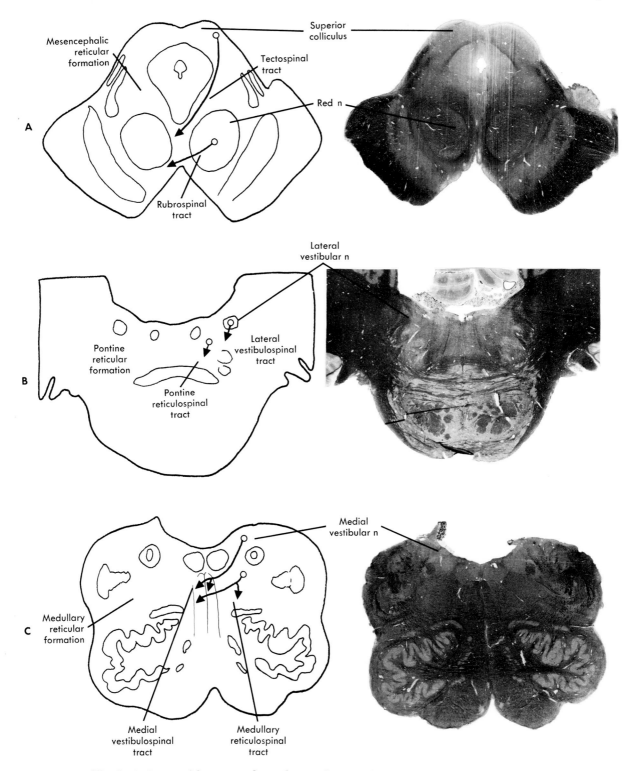

Fig. 8-11. Origin of brainstem descending pathways. The structures that give rise to descending pathways are shown at midbrain, pontine, and medullary levels. **A,** The tectospinal and rubrospinal tracts arise from the superior colliculus and red nucleus respectively; both tracts cross before descending to the spinal cord. **B,** The lateral vestibulospinal and pontine reticulospinal tracts originate in the lateral vestibular nucleus and the pontine reticular formation respectively; these tracts descend uncrossed to the spinal cord. **C,** The medial vestibulospinal and medullary reticulospinal tracts come from the medial vestibular nucleus and the medullary reticular formation respectively; these tracts descend bilaterally into the spinal cord.

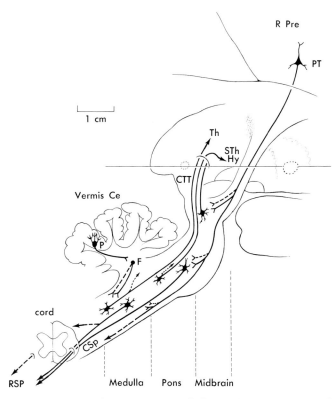

Fig. 8-12. Interrelationships of medial medullary, pontine, and mesencephalic reticular formation neurons with cerebellar, thalamocortical, and spinal areas. Schematic diagram of sagittal section of the brain. Note both ascending and descending projections of the medial medullary and pontine reticular neurons, and the ascending projections of the mesencephalic reticular neurons. Abbreviations: *Ce*, cerebellum; *CSp*, corticospinal tract; *CTT*, central tegmental tract; *F*, fastigial nucleus; *Hy*, hypothalamus; *P*, Purkinje neuron; *PT*, pyramidal tract neuron; *R Pre*, right precentral gyrus; *RSP*, reticulospinal projections; *STh*, subthalamus; *Th*, thalamus. Bilateral projections shown by broken lines.

dominantly ascending axons with those that have predominantly descending axons. It is not known to what extent the caudal and rostral projections of the reticular formation represent collaterals of the same cell.

Afferent and efferent connections of the reticular formation

A major relationship of the reticular formation is with the spinal cord. The medial medullary reticular formation sends axons to the ipsilateral and contralateral medullary reticulospinal tracts (Figs. 8-11 and 8-13). The pontine reticular formation projects only ipsilaterally. The reticulospinal tracts lie in the ventrolateral quadrant of the spinal cord. The medullary reticulospinal tract terminates more dorsolaterally in the ventral horn than the pontine reticulospinal tract,

which terminates ventromedially in the ventral horn. Reticulospinal axons appear to terminate largely on interneurons of the ventral horn; however, there are direct connections with motoneurons.

The medullary and pontine reticular formations receive a heavy projection of spinoreticular fibers that ascend in the ventrolateral quadrant of the spinal cord. They are distributed bilaterally, largely to the areas of the medial reticular formation that project to the thalamus.

The projections of the reticular nuclei to the thalamus are probably the most important ascending reticular projections. They have a profound effect on thalamocortical activity (see Chapter 16). The details of the reticular projections to the thalamus are of great physiological importance but have not been completely clarified. The medullary, pontine, and mesencephalic reticular nuclei send axons that ascend ipsilaterally and contralaterally in the area of the central tegmental tract, which is a complex fiber bundle. The mesencephalic reticular formation makes a heavy contribution to this tract. Most of these fibers project to the nonspecific thalamic nuclei. A smaller group diverges at the level of the posterior thalamus and appears to project to the hypothalamus and subthalamus.

The reticular formation, again largely the medial portion, receives bilateral projections from the cortex, particularly from the sensorimotor cortex.

The reciprocal connections made between the reticular formation and the cerebellum are discussed later.

Functions of the descending reticular pathways

The functions of the reticulospinal tracts are manifold, including both somatic and autonomic activity. In the somatic sphere, they are involved in excitatory and inhibitory control of spinal motoneurons. Stimulation of a large area in the caudal reticular formation, the inhibitory center of Magoun and Rhines, results in the inhibition of all types of spinal cord motoneuronal activity. Stimulation in a more rostral area (the facilitatory center) causes an excitation of motoneurons. An exact correlation of the brainstem sites that produce inhibition or excitation and of the structures actually stimulated is still in progress. Reticular formation inhibition has been found to be caused by both presynaptic and postsynaptic inhibition of spinal motoneurons. Reticular formation neurons may also inhibit spinal interneurons. A monosynaptic excitatory pathway from some reticular neurons to motoneurons has recently been described. The same reticular neurons also excite interneurons directly, and the latter in turn excite motoneurons.

The autonomic functions of reticulospinal neurons

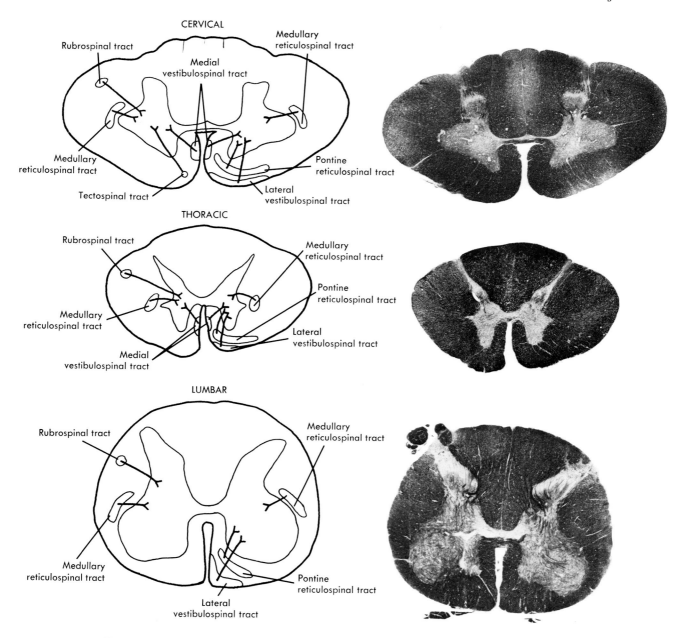

Fig. 8-13. Locations of descending pathways from the brainstem in the spinal cord white matter. Tracts originating from the right side of the brainstem are shown. The crossed tracts are the rubrospinal and tectospinal tracts; the uncrossed tracts are the lateral vestibulospinal and pontine reticulospinal tracts; the bilateral tracts are the medial vestibulospinal and medullary reticulospinal tracts. The region of the spinal cord gray matter in which each of the tracts terminates is shown.

include the control of vasomotor and respiratory activity. Although respiratory activity logically should be discussed as a somatic motor activity, the medullary location of the inspiratory center makes it convenient to include respiration with autonomic activities that are organized in the medulla (see Chapter 9 for further discussion of these topics).

Brainstem nuclei and tracts

Rubrospinal tract. The red nucleus gives rise to the rubrospinal tract (Figs. 8-11 and 8-13). This pathway is a powerful one in animals such as the cat, but its function has probably been largely superseded in humans by other pathways, including the corticospinal tract. The rubrospinal tract decussates shortly after leaving the red nucleus. The fibers descend through the lateral part of the brainstem, and in the spinal cord they occupy a position adjacent to the lateral corticospinal tract in the dorsal part of the lateral funiculus. The red nucleus is somatotopically organized, one part of the nucleus projecting to the cervical spinal cord and another part projecting to lumbosacral levels. In the cat the rubrospinal tract terminates in much the same areas as the terminations of the corticospinal tract in this animal. The predominant action of the rubrospinal tract in the cat, like the corticospinal tract, is to excite flexor motoneurons and to inhibit extensor motoneurons. In humans, direct rubrospinal connections may have little significance.

Neurons of the red nucleus are activated by inputs from several major sources. One of these is from the motor areas of the cerebral cortex. Others are from the deep nuclei of the cerebellum and possibly from the basal ganglia, although probably not by direct projections.

Lateral vestibulospinal tract. The lateral vestibulospinal tract is composed of fibers originating in the lateral vestibular nucleus (Deiters' nucleus). The tract is located in the ventral funiculus of the cord and contains only uncrossed axons (Fig. 8-11 and 8-13). The tract extends throughout the length of the cord. Its activity is influenced by the vestibular nerve, probably by way of interneurons located in other portions of the vestibular nuclear complex, because the primary afferent fibers of the vestibular nerve do not seem to end on the cells of origin of the vestibulospinal tract. The cerebellum also exerts control over the activity of the vestibulospinal tract. It has been found that some Purkinje cell axons from the cerebellum end directly on the cells that give rise to the vestibulospinal tract and inhibit them postsynaptically. Another source of afferent input to the lateral vestibular nucleus is the spinovestibular tract. The axons of the vestibulospinal neurons end directly on extensor motoneurons in the spinal cord, exciting them monosynaptically. The excitatory effect on the extensor motoneurons of the neck (antigravity muscles) are particularly strong. Lateral vestibulospinal axons also end on interneurons of the ventral horn.

Medial vestibulospinal tract. Fibers reach the spinal cord through the descending component of the medial longitudinal fasciculus. This pathway is sometimes called the medial vestibulospinal tract (Figs. 8-11 and 8-13). The nucleus of origin of the vestibulospinal fibers in the MLF is the medial vestibular nucleus. The tract is located adjacent to the ventral medial fissure in the ventral funiculus. Each medial vestibular nucleus projects bilaterally, although there are more

fibers on the ipsilateral side. The axons terminate in the medial part of the ventral horn.

Tectospinal tract. One of the deep layers of the superior colliculus gives rise to the tectospinal tract. The fibers cross to descend in the contralateral ventral funiculus near the ventral median fissure (Figs. 8-11 and 8-13). Most of the fibers terminate in the ventral horn of the upper four cervical segments.

Interstitiospinal tract. There is a small bundle of fibers descending bilaterally in the ventral funiculus from the interstitial nucleus of Cajal. These end in the ventral horn.

REGULATION OF MOTOR OUTPUT

The activity of the descending pathways that have just been described is regulated by two major brain systems, the cerebellum and the basal ganglia. This regulation is required for normal motor behavior, and abnormalities of motor control are of major clinical importance. The gross morphology of the cerebellum is described in Chapter 5, and the internal organization of the cerebellum and the arrangement of the basal ganglia are introduced in Chapter 6. It is recommended that the reader review these sections before continuing with the discussion of the connectivity and functions of the cerebellum and basal ganglia.

CEREBELLUM
Microscopic structure of the cerebellum

The cerebellum consists of a cortex of gray matter, the underlying white matter, and several deep nuclei:

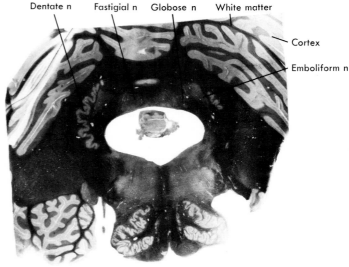

Fig. 8-14. Deep cerebellar nuclei. The section is through the cerebellum and medulla and shows the deep cerebellar nuclei: fastigial, globose, emboliform, and dentate. The cortex and white matter of the cerebellum are also indicated.

dentate, emboliform, globose, and fastigial (Fig. 8-14). There are numerous infoldings of the cortex, called folia. Because of this arrangement, only a fraction of the cortical area is visible from the surface. White matter extends into each folium.

The cerebellar cortex is organized in three distinct layers: molecular, Purkinje cell, and granular. The molecular layer is the most superficial, the granular layer is adjacent to the cerebellar white matter, and the Purkinje cell layer is between the other two layers (Fig. 8-15).

Cerebellar neurons (Fig. 8-16)

The five major kinds of neurons found in the cerebellar cortex are the Purkinje cells, granule cells, Golgi cells, basket cells, and stellate cells.

The key structure for understanding the organization of the cerebellar cortex is the *Purkinje cell*. This is a large neuron that has parts within all three layers of the cerebellar cortex, although its soma is located within and defines the Purkinje cell layer. The most striking feature of the Purkinje cell is its huge dendritic system, which extends across the molecular layer. The dendrites are arranged in a plane oriented at right angles to the long axis of the folium (Fig. 8-17). The dendrites of the various Purkinje cells in a given folium are thus in parallel planes. The primary dendrite arises from the soma at the junction between the Purkinje cell layer and the molecular layer. The primary dendrite branches into secondary dendrites, and these in turn branch into tertiary and higher

order dendrites. The surface of the primary and secondary dendrites is smooth, whereas the tertiary and smaller branches have numerous spines, which are postsynaptic membrane specializations. There are also synapses on the soma and dendritic membrane. The axon of the Purkinje cell arises from the pole of the soma opposite to the origin of the primary dendrite. After a short distance, the Purkinje cell axon acquires a myelin sheath. It gives off recurrent collaterals before crossing the granular layer and entering the white matter of the cerebellum. Purkinje cell axons terminate either on cells of the deep nuclei or, in the case of a fraction of them, on neurons of the lateral vestibular nucleus. The Purkinje cell axons are the sole efferents of the cerebellar cortex.

Granule cells form the major neuronal component of the granular layer. They are small, their somata having a diameter of about 10 μm. Each has about four or five clawlike dendrites. There are apparently no synapses on the somata of the granule cells. The axon arises either from the soma or from a dendrite. Granule cell axons ascend from the granular layer through the Purkinje cell layer to the molecular layer (Fig. 8-17). Within the molecular layer, they bifurcate. Each branch runs parallel to the long axis of the folium, a distance of about 1 to 1.5 mm. The axons of the granule cells of the lower part of the granular layer run within the deeper strata of the molecular layer, whereas those of the more superficial granule cells course near the surface of the molecular layer. The granule cell axons within the molecular layer are called paral-

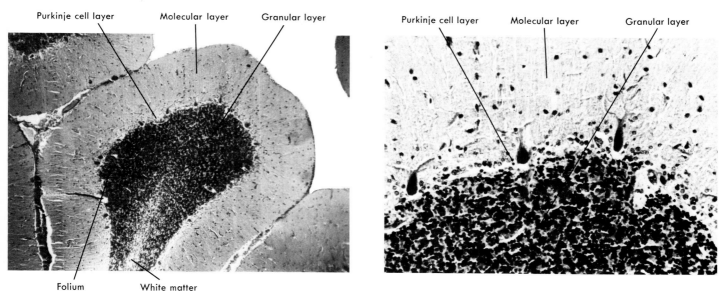

Fig. 8-15. Cerebellar cortex and underlying white matter. The light micrographs show sections through the cerebellar cortex at low and high magnifications. The molecular, Purkinje cell, and granular layers are indicated, as well as the white matter, which underlies the cortex.

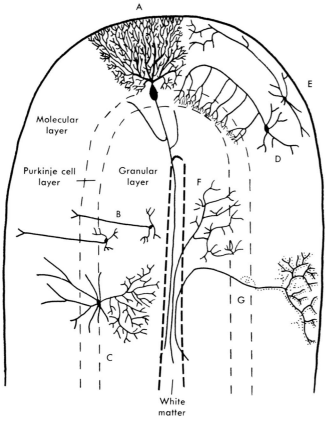

Fig. 8-16. Neural elements of the cerebellar cortex. The neuron labeled *A* is a Purkinje cell. This type of neuron has its cell body in the Purkinje cell layer; its dendrites extend across the molecular layer, and its axon crosses the granular layer to enter the white matter. The Purkinje cell is the output cell of the cerebellar cortex. The small neurons at *B* are granule cells. Their cell bodies and dendrites are in the granular layer, and their axons ascend into the molecular layer to form parallel fibers. The other neuron whose cell body is in the granular layer is the Golgi cell, *C*. Its dendrites protrude into the molecular layer, and its axon ramifies extensively in the granular layer. Neurons of the molecular layer include the basket cell, *D*, and the stellate cell, *E*. The axons of these cells are transverse fibers, and the basket cell axons terminate with basketlike endings on the cell bodies of Purkinje cells. The afferents to the cerebellum include mossy fibers, *F*, and climbing fibers, *G*.

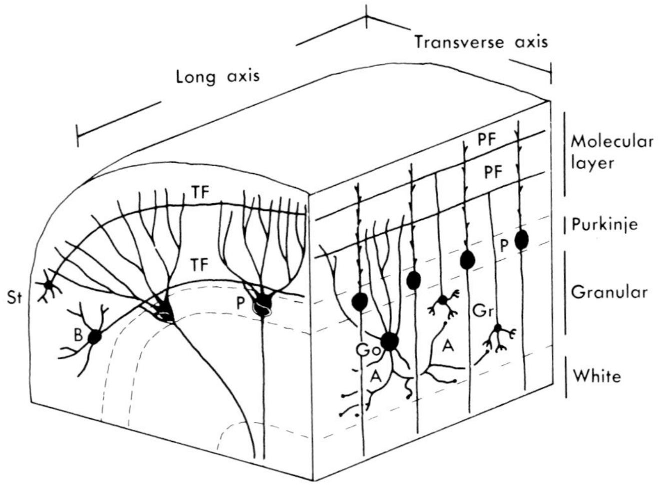

Fig. 8-17. Cellular organization of the cerebellar cortex. The cutaway drawing shows the neuronal elements that are intrinsic to a folium of the cerebellar cortex. Cell types: *P*, Purkinje cell; *St*, stellate cell; *B*, basket cell; *Gr*, granule cell; *Go*, Golgi cell. The axons of several of the neuron types are specially indicated: *A*, Golgi cell axon; *PF*, parallel fiber, granule cell axon; *TF*, transverse fibers, basket and stellate cell axons. The Purkinje cell axons are shown leaving the cortex to enter the underlying white matter.

lel fibers. They synapse with the spines on dendrites of Purkinje, basket, stellate, and Golgi cells. Each parallel fiber may synapse with numerous dendrites, because the synapses occur in passing rather than as terminal boutons.

Golgi cells are also found in the granular layer but are much less numerous than the granule cells. These are large neurons, and their somata are generally found just below the Purkinje cell layer. The dendrites emerge from the soma in all directions, but most turn upward to enter the molecular layer. The dendrites

branch several times, and the smaller branches have spines. The axon branches profusely within the granular layer, making these cells a prime example of Golgi type II cells. The axon endings are on granule cell dendrites.

Basket cells are medium-sized cells primarily found in the lower half of the molecular layer near the Purkinje cell layer. Their dendrites form a planar arborization similar to that of the Purkinje cells, although much less profuse. The plane of the dendrites is at right angles to the long axis of the folium. The dendrites have spines that are postsynaptic to parallel fiber synapses. The somata also receive synapses. The axon of a basket cell leaves the soma and runs transversely to the folium; thus the name transverse fibers. The neurons are called basket synapses because there are side branches from the axon that end on the somata of a series of Purkinje cells. About ten Purkinje cells aligned in the same transverse plane receive contacts from a single basket cell axon.

The *stellate cells* are very similar to the basket cells except for their position within the molecular layer and the course of their axons. These small cells are located in the outer half of the molecular layer. Their axons may branch diffusely near the cell body or they may form transverse fibers that synapse on the dendrites of the Purkinje cells.

Types of afferent terminals in the cerebellar cortex

Afferent fibers that enter the cerebellar cortex end either as mossy or as climbing fibers. These have quite distinct structural and functional characteristics.

The mossy fibers enter the white matter of the cerebellum as coarsely myelinated axons. Within the white matter they may branch, so a given fiber may terminate within two adjacent folia. Some branches end in the deep nuclei. As a mossy fiber courses within the white matter of a given folium, it gives off collaterals that enter the granular layer on either side of the folium. Within the granular layer more branching occurs, and finally there are numerous synaptic expansions in relation to the dendrites of granule cells. The areas of synapse between mossy fibers and granule cells are called glomeruli. Golgi cell axon endings also take part in the complex synaptic arrangement of the glomerulus. The sources of mossy fibers are numerous and include the spinocerebellar tracts, the pontocerebellar tract, vestibulocerebellar fibers, and reticulocerebellar fibers.

The other type of afferent fiber to the cerebellar cortex is the climbing fiber. This fiber forms a much more discrete projection. A given climbing fiber enters the cortex without branching and ends on the dendritic tree of a single Purkinje cell. The termination consists of a series of branches paralleling those of the Purkinje cell dendrites. The climbing fiber appears to make numerous synaptic contacts with the dendritic surface. Some of the branches may continue past the Purkinje cell to end on basket or stellate cells. The only known origin of the climbing fibers is the contralateral inferior olivary nucleus (and accessory olivary nuclei). Climbing fiber branches in the cerebellar white matter terminate in the deep cerebellar nuclei.

Information processing within the cerebellar cortex

Both types of afferent fibers to the cerebellar cortex have been shown in physiological experiments to be excitatory (Fig. 8-18). The mossy fibers end on and activate granule cells. The excitatory effect tends to be diffuse because each mossy fiber has a wide distribution. The climbing fibers produce a powerful excitation of Purkinje cells, firing them repetitively. However, a given climbing fiber probably excites just one, or at most a few, Purkinje cells.

Granule cells are excitatory interneurons. Their axons, the parallel fibers, excite the dendrites of Purkinje, stellate, basket, and Golgi cells. If a group of granule cells is activated by a mossy-fiber pathway, the parallel fibers from these granule cells may form a group of discharging axons arranged as a beam

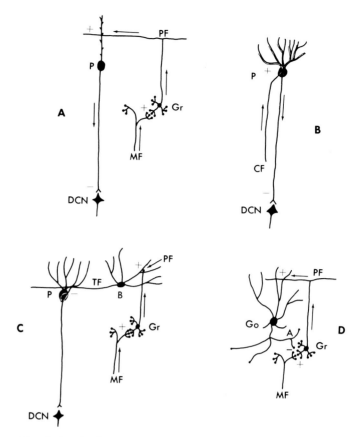

Fig. 8-18. The basic cerebellar circuits. The input to the cerebellum is carried by two types of afferent fibers, known as mossy and climbing fibers. The output is by the axons of the Purkinje cells. Two circuits by which cerebellar afferents excite Purkinje cells are shown in **A** and **B**, and two pathways that result in a reduced output are diagrammed in **C** and **D**. In **A**, granule cells are excited by mossy fibers. The granule cells in turn excite Purkinje cells. The action of the Purkinje cells on neurons of the deep cerebellar nuclei is inhibitory, as indicated. In **B**, a climbing fiber is shown ending directly on a Purkinje cell and exciting it. **C** shows a circuit in which a mossy fiber excites a granule cell, which in turn excites a basket cell; the basket cell then inhibits a Purkinje cell. The inhibition of the Purkinje cell would result in disinhibition of the deep cerebellar nuclear cell. The basket cell circuit is a mechanism for feed-forward inhibition of Purkinje cells. **D** shows a mechanism for feedback inhibition. A mossy fiber excites a granule cell, which excites a Golgi cell. The Golgi cell then inhibits the granule cell. Abbreviations as in Fig. 8-17. *DCN*, deep cerebellar nuclear cell; *MF*, mossy fiber; *CF*, climbing fiber.

within the cerebellar cortex. Thus a series of Purkinje cells and other elements may be excited in sequence longitudinally along a folium for the length of the parallel fiber beam.

The basket cells produce a powerful inhibition of Purkinje cells. The basket synapses are strategically located on the cell body, an ideal situation for inhibition inasmuch as the IPSP would prevent all but the most powerful synaptic excitation from causing the axon hillock to reach threshold for producing an action potential. The inhibition would be equally effective in counteracting excitation of any dendritic branch. Even the climbing-fiber response of a Purkinje cell is largely blocked by the inhibition produced by basket cells, although in this case one or two spikes may be set up.

The stellate cells are also inhibitory to Purkinje cells. However, their axons end on Purkinje cell dendrites, and so the inhibition is much less effective than that

of the basket cells for generalized background excitation, although the stellate cells could no doubt be quite effective in counteracting synaptic excitation of the same dendrites on which their axons terminate.

The Golgi cells inhibit granule cells by way of their axon endings within the glomerulus. The circuit from mossy fiber to granule cell to Golgi cell and back to granule cell is thus a negative feedback. It is speculated that the Golgi cells serve as a focusing device, eliminating all but the strongest input to the granule cells from the mossy-fiber pathways.

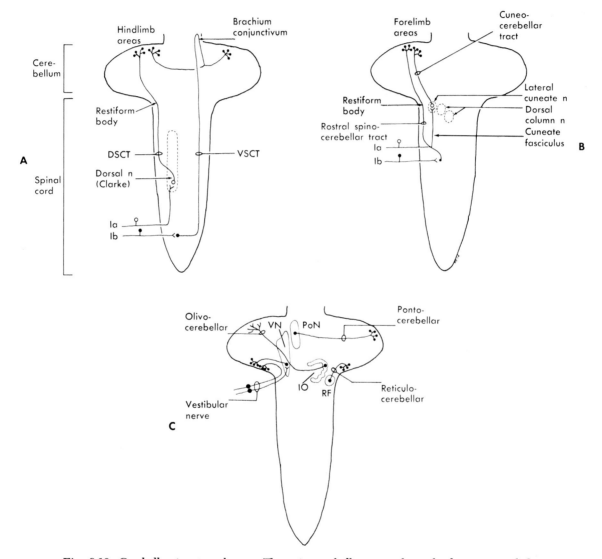

Fig. 8-19. Cerebellar input pathways. The spinocerebellar tracts from the lower part of the body are diagrammed in **A**. These are the dorsal and ventral spinocerebellar tracts. The spinocerebellar tracts from the upper body, the cuneocerebellar tract, and the rostral spinocerebellar tract are shown in **B**. Other cerebellar inputs are outlined in **C**. These include vestibulocerebellar, reticulocerebellar, olivocerebellar, and pontocerebellar tracts. All of the pathways terminate as mossy fibers except the olivocerebellar tract, which ends as climbing fibers. Abbreviations: *IO*, inferior olive; *VN*, vestibular nerve; *RF*, reticular formation; *PoN*, pontine nucleus.

The Purkinje cells thus a receive a variety of information from afferent fibers to the cerebellum. They are excited by mossy fibers by means of the granule cells and directly by the climbing fibers. They are inhibited by mossy fibers through a longer circuit involving granule cells and then basket or stellate cells. If these events are considered in terms of the Purkinje cells in line with a beam of active parallel fibers and those just off this beam, the on-beam Purkinje cells are excited by the mossy fibers and then later inhibited by the basket and stellate cells; the off-beam Purkinje cells are just inhibited. The excitability of the Purkinje cells can be monitored continuously by the climbing fiber input. When the Purkinje cells are excited by the mossy-fiber volley, the climbing-fiber response will be a train of impulses. When the Purkinje cell is inhibited, the climbing-fiber response will be just one or two spikes. This type of activity resembles to some extent the behavior of a computer, in which the memory consists of a set of magnetic devices that operate in two states, magnetized or nonmagnetized. The state of each memory site can be tested and the information used for some purpose. The purpose of the cerebellum as a computer is to smooth and coordinate movements.

Afferent pathways to the cerebellum

There are a number of pathways that are afferent to the cerebellum (Fig. 8-19). The major ones transmit information from the spinal cord, the vestibular nerve, several structures of the brainstem, and the cerebral cortex. The afferent pathways may terminate in the cerebellar cortex and in the deep cerebellar nuclei.

Spinocerebellar tracts. There are at least two separate spinocerebellar tracts serving the lower portion of the body and another two serving the upper part. Comparable information reaches the cerebellum from the head through cranial nerves and their nuclei.

The pathways from the lower part of the body (below about T6) to the cerebellum are the dorsal and ventral spinocerebellar tracts (Fig. 8-19, A). The dorsal spinocerebellar tract originates from the nucleus dorsalis (Clarke's column), which is a column of neurons located in Rexed's lamina VII just lateral to the central canal at segmental levels from about T1 to the upper lumbar region (Fig. 8-20). Afferents of a number of different categories reach the cells of the nucleus dorsalis through the dorsal column. Monosynaptic excitatory connections are made by afferents that come from muscle spindles (groups Ia and II) and Golgi tendon organs (group Ib). Excitation also occurs from stimulation of cutaneous receptors. The receptive field of the cells of origin of the dorsal spinocerebellar tract is ipsilateral, and the projection of the

tract is almost entirely ipsilateral. The axons pass laterally from the nucleus dorsalis into the lateral column, assuming a position at its dorsolateral border. The tract ascends in this position to the lower medulla, where it enters the cerebellum through the inferior cerebellar peduncle. The axons terminate in the cortex as mossy fibers. The region of termination is in the hindlimb area of the cerebellum, which includes parts of the anterior lobe and also a portion of the posterior lobe (Fig. 8-21).

The ventral spinocerebellar tract originates from cells located within the base of the dorsal horn and the intermediate region at the lumbosacral enlargement (Fig. 8-22). The neurons giving rise to the tract are excited monosynaptically by afferent fibers from muscle spindles and Golgi tendon organs of the ipsilateral muscles (groups Ia and Ib). They also receive polysynaptic excitatory and inhibitory actions from a variety of afferent types. The axons from these neurons cross to the opposite side of the cord, ascending in a position at the ventrolateral border of the lateral column. The tract continues through the medulla and pons until it reaches the level of the isthmus, where it moves dorsally to enter the cerebellum along the lateral aspect of the superior cerebellar peduncle. Part of the ventral spinocerebellar tract crosses within the white matter of the cerebellum. Some terminals occur within the cerebellar cortex on the side of the tract, but most occur on the side ipsilateral to the side in which the cells of origin of the tract lie. The endings are mossy fibers. The area of termination is similar to that of the dorsal spinocerebellar tract.

The cuneocerebellar tract relays information from the upper extremities and trunk. Its input resembles closely that of the dorsal spinocerebellar tract for the lower part of the body. Afferent collaterals ascend through the cuneate fasciculus to the lower medulla, where they terminate in the lateral cuneate nucleus (Fig. 8-23). The neurons of this nucleus give rise to axons that enter the cerebellum through the ipsilateral inferior cerebellar peduncle. The cuneocerebellar tract fibers terminate as mossy fibers in the forelimb areas of the anterior and posterior lobes.

The rostral spinocerebellar tract is the equivalent of the ventral spinocerebellar tract, except that the former relays information from the upper part of the body. Another major difference is that the rostral spinocerebellar tract stays on the ipsilateral side of the spinal cord and brainstem. The information it conveys, however, is like that carried by the ventral spinocerebellar tract. The cells of origin of the rostral spinocerebellar tract are in the gray matter of the cervical spinal cord. The axons enter the cerebellum through either the superior or the inferior cerebellar

Text continued on p. 328.

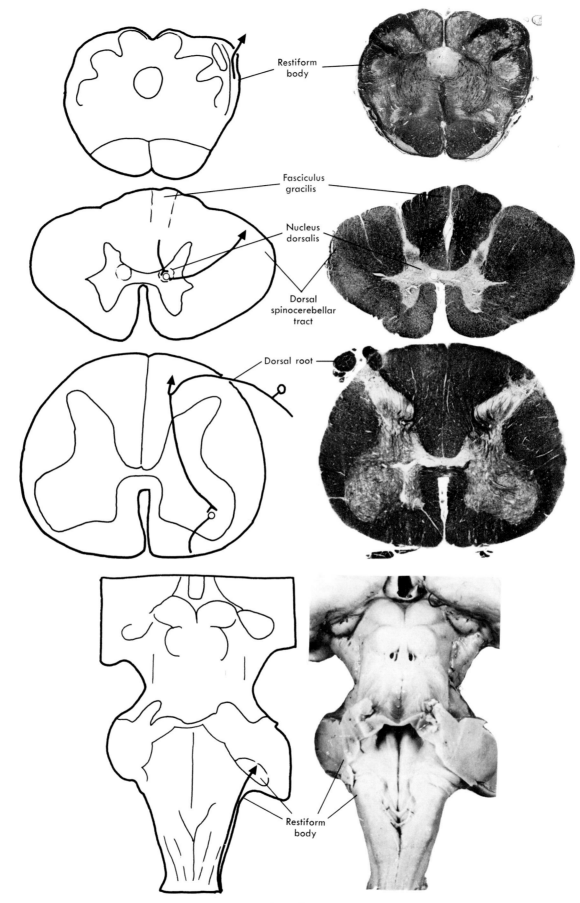

Restiform body

Fasciculus gracilis

Nucleus dorsalis

Dorsal spinocerebellar tract

Dorsal root

Restiform body

Fig. 8-20. For legend see opposite page.

Fig. 8-20. Dorsal spinocerebellar tract. The afferents to the nucleus dorsalis (Clarke's column) enter through dorsal root supplying the hindlimb and lower body, ascend in the fasciculus gracilis, and synapse. The axons of the cells of the nucleus dorsalis project laterally into the dorsal part of the lateral funiculus and then ascend in that position to the level of the caudal medulla, where they shift dorsally to enter the cerebellum through the restiform body.

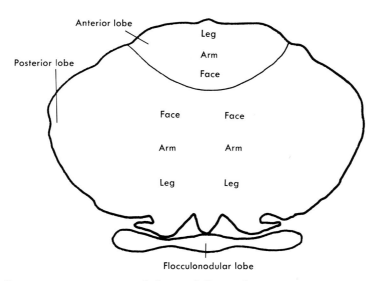

Fig. 8-21. Somatotopic organization of the cerebellum. There are separate somatotopic maps in the anterior and posterior lobes. The hindlimb is represented rostrally in the anterior lobe, and there is a bilateral representation caudally in the intermediate region of the posterior lobe. The forelimb and face representations are in sequence from the hindlimb area toward the primary fissure in each lobe.

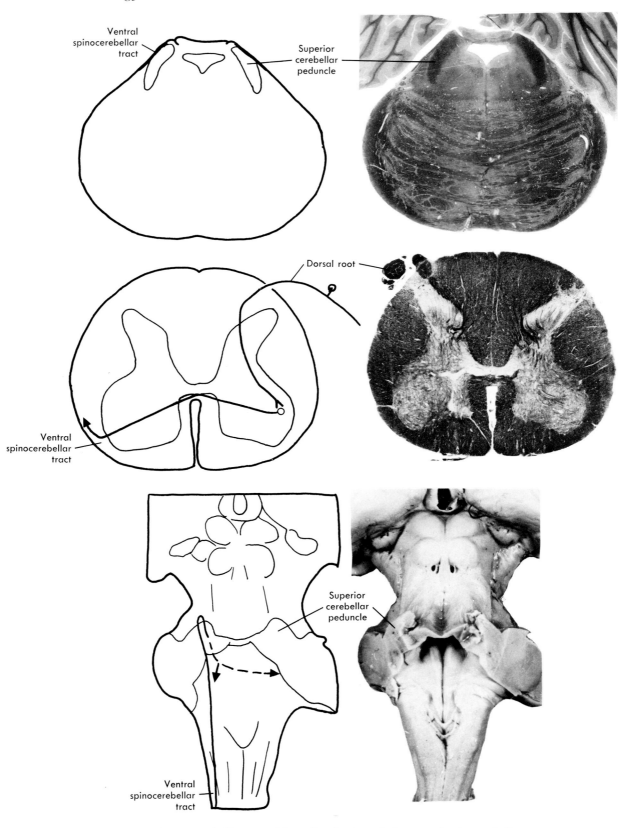

Fig. 8-22. Ventral spinocerebellar tract. The cells of origin of the ventral spinocerebellar tract are in the gray matter of the lumbar enlargement. Some of the cells are actually in the motor nucleus. The axons decussate and ascend in the ventral part of the lateral funiculus. They pass rostrally through the medulla and pons and then turn dorsally at the isthmus to enter the cerebellum through the superior cerebellar peduncle. The terminals are bilateral.

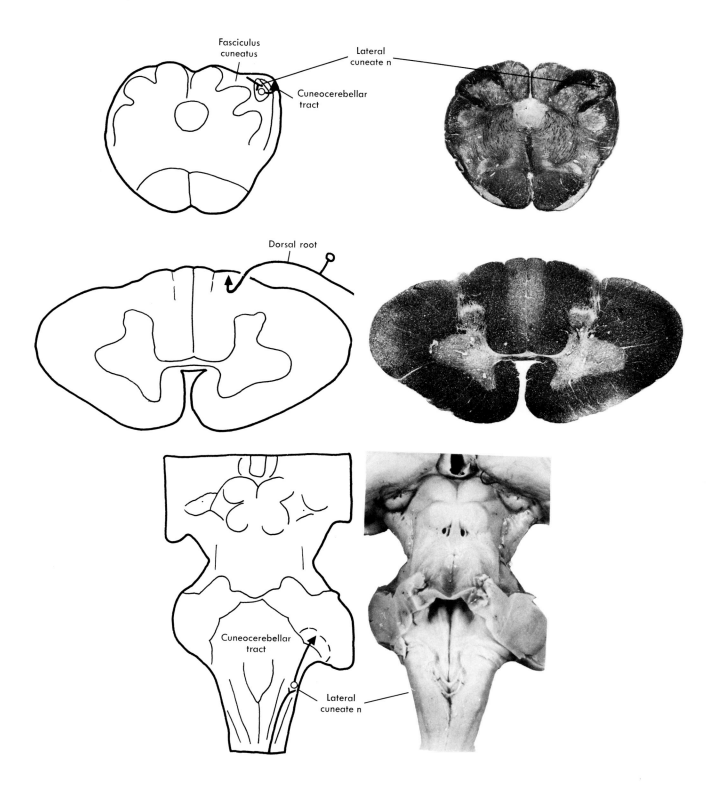

Fig. 8-23. Cuneocerebellar tract. Afferents to the cuneocerebellar tract supply the forelimb and upper trunk. They enter through the dorsal roots and ascend in the fasciculus cuneatus to the medulla, where they synapse in the lateral cuneate nucleus. Second-order axons from the lateral cuneate nucleus enter the cerebellum through the restiform body.

peduncle, and they end in the forelimb areas of the anterior and posterior lobes as mossy fibers.

Vestibular afferents. A substantial number of primary afferents enter the cerebellum directly from the vestibular nerve. These pass through the inferior cerebellar peduncle and end within the cortex of the flocculonodular lobe. Second-order connections are also made from the vestibular nerve by way of the vestibular nuclei (Fig. 8-24). The terminals are of the mossy-fiber type.

Reticulocerebellar connections. Several of the nuclei of the reticular formation project to the cerebellum (Fig. 8-24).

Corticopontocerebellar tract. There is a very strong projection to the cerebellum from several regions of the cerebral cortex. Projection fibers originate from pyramidal cells of areas of the frontal, parietal, and temporal lobes and pass through the internal capsule and the cerebral peduncle to end within the pontine nuclei of the same side (Fig. 8-4, *B*). These are col-

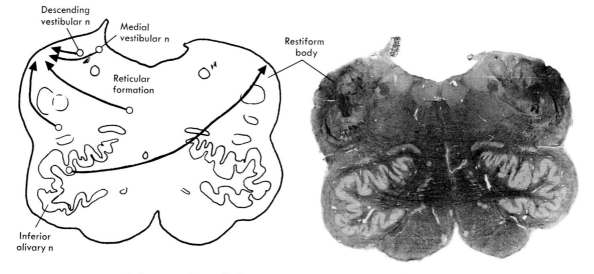

Fig. 8-24. Vestibular, reticular, and olivary projections to the cerebellum. Vestibular afferents to the cerebellum are shown to arise from the medial and descending vestibular nuclei and to enter the cerebellum through the ipsilateral restiform body. Reticulocerebellar afferents also project largely ipsilaterally through the restiform body. However, the olivocerebellar pathway is crossed.

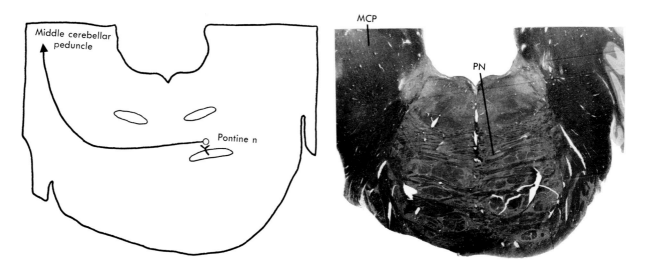

Fig. 8-25. Pontocerebellar tract. The cells of the pontine nuclei receive descending connections from the cerebral cortex over the frontopontine, parietopontine, and temporopontine tracts. The neurons of the pontine nuclei project into the contralateral side of the cerebellum through the middle cerebellar peduncle (brachium pontis).

lectively called corticopontine fibers, and the sub-component paths are the frontopontine, parietopontine, and temporopontine tracts. Neurons of the pontine nuclei send their axons contralaterally to enter the cerebellum through the middle cerebellar peduncle (Fig. 8-25). These fibers are responsible for the bridgelike appearance of the ventral surface of the pons, thus giving it its name. The pontocerebellar fibers end within the cortex of the hemisphere as mossy fibers.

Olivocerebellar tract. Fibers from the inferior olivary nucleus and its associated accessory olivary nuclei cross the medulla to enter the contralateral inferior cerebellar peduncle, forming the olivocerebellar tract (Fig. 8-24). The axons terminate as climbing fibers throughout the cerebral cortex of the side opposite the nucleus of the origin of the tract. The inferior olivary and accessory olivary nuclei appear to relay information from the spinal cord (from the spino-olivary tracts) and from higher levels of the brain (from the central tegmental tract).

Efferent pathways from the cerebellum

All of the output from the cerebellar cortex is by way of the axons of Purkinje cells. The main portion of the axon of a typical Purkinje cell passes through the white matter of the cerebellum to end in one of the deep cerebellar nuclei (Fig. 8-26). The Purkinje cells of the cerebellar hemispheres project to the dentate nuclei, those of the intermediate cortex project to the globose and emboliform nuclei, and those of the vermis project to the fastigial nuclei. Most of the Purkinje axons end in the appropriate deep nucleus of the ipsilateral side. A few Purkinje cell axons pass directly out of the cerebellum to end in the brainstem.

Physiological studies have shown that the Purkinje cells inhibit the neurons with which their axons connect. This is a startling finding because it implies that the entire output of the cerebellum is inhibitory. However, it should be noted that the neurons in the deep nuclei fire continuously because they are excited continuously through mossy-fiber and climbing-fiber collaterals. The inhibition produced in these cells by the cerebellar cortex modulates their activity. A reduction in inhibition results in an increased discharge of a deep cerebellar nuclear cell, and an increase in inhibition causes it to fire less frequently. The significant point is that the cerebellum exerts a full range of control over the neurons in the deep nuclei; the effects of the cerebellar cortex are thus passed on to the next neurons in the pathway by means of the deep nuclear cells. The transmitter utilized by Purkinje cells in producing the inhibitory action is gamma-aminobutyric acid (GABA).

There are a number of pathways through which the cerebral outflow acts. These include connections with the red nucleus, thalamus, vestibular complex, and reticular formation.

Dentatothalamic pathway. Axons from the dentate nucleus (Fig. 8-14) of one side of the cerebellum project through the superior cerebellar peduncle, cross in the decussation of the brachium conjunctivum, pass around or through the contralateral red nucleus, and terminate in the contralateral ventrolateral nucleus of the thalamus (Figs. 8-26 and 8-27). The effect of these axons is to excite the thalamic cells. They in turn project through the internal capsule to the motor areas

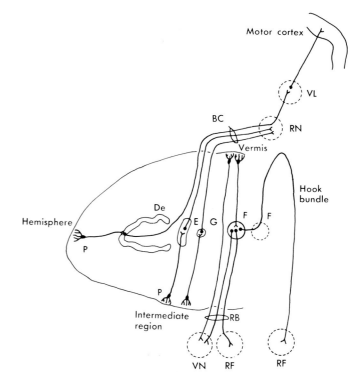

Fig. 8-26. Cerebellar output pathways. The Purkinje cell axons form the output system of the cerebellar cortex. The Purkinje cells *(P)* of the cerebellar hemisphere project to the dentate nucleus *(De)*, which is the lateralmost of the deep cerebellar nuclei. The dentate nucleus then projects axons through the brachium conjunctivum *(BC)* to the contralateral ventral lateral nucleus *(VL)* of the thalamus, which is connected to the motor cortex. The intermediate cerebellar cortex sends its output to the emboliform *(E)* and globose *(G)* nuclei, which in turn project to the contralateral red nucleus *(RN)* through the brachium conjunctivum. The Purkinje cells of the vermis may either project directly to the vestibular nuclei *(VN)* or terminate in the fastigial nucleus *(F)*. The fastigial nucleus projects in part ipsilaterally to the vestibular nuclei and reticular formation *(RF)* by way of the restiform body *(RB)* and in part contralaterally to the reticular formation by way of the opposite brachium conjunctivum. The latter path is known as the hook bundle, which passes through the contralateral fastigial nucleus *(broken circle)*.

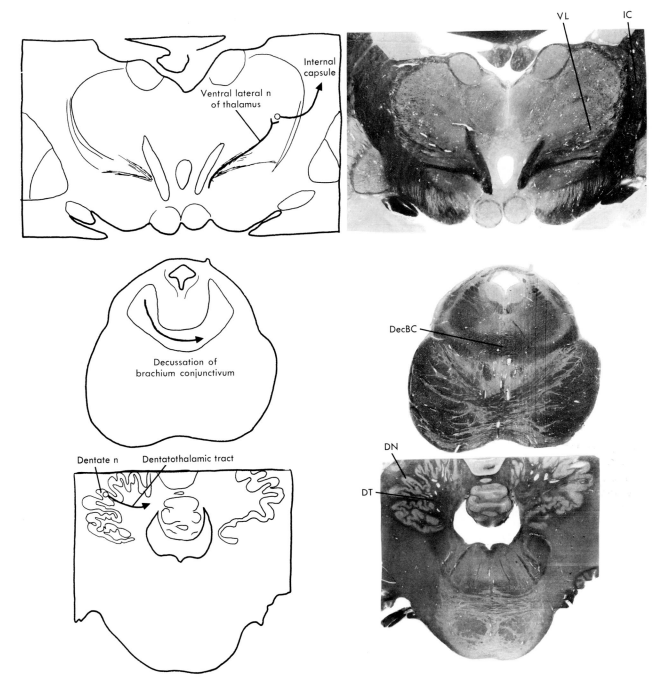

Fig. 8-27. Dentatothalamic pathway. The output of the cerebellum from the dentate nucleus is through the brachium conjunctivum. The dentate axons decussate and then ascend past the red nucleus to enter fields H and then H₁ of Forel. The axons terminate in the ventral lateral nucleus of the thalamus. The ventral lateral nucleus in turn projects to the motor areas of the cerebral cortex.

of the cerebral cortex. The information transmitted from the cerebellum is probably used to correct the output of corticospinal neurons. In addition, the corticopontocerebellar tract provides a feedback loop to the cerebellum.

Globose-emboliform-rubral pathway. Neurons of the globose and emboliform nuclei (Fig. 8-14) project through the superior cerebellar peduncles, cross in the decussation of the brachium conjunctivum, and end on neurons of the contralateral red nucleus (Figs. 8-26 and 8-28). The action on these cells is excitatory. The red nucleus projects through the rubrospinal tract

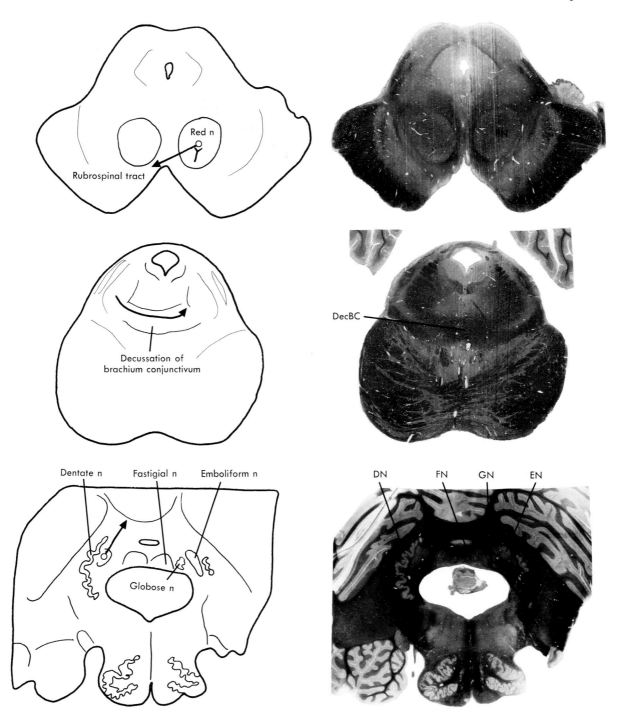

Fig. 8-28. Globose-emboliform-rubral pathway. The efferent pathway from the globose and emboliform nuclei is through the decussation of the brachium conjunctivum to the contralateral red nucleus. The rubrospinal tract crosses and descends into the spinal cord.

to the spinal cord. Because the rubrospinal tract crosses in the midbrain tegmentum, the action of the intermediate nuclei of one side of the cerebellum is eventually on neurons of the ipsilateral spinal cord.

Projections of the fastigial nucleus. The vermis projects to the fastigial nucleus (Fig. 8-14), which in turn projects to the lateral vestibular nucleus and the reticular formation (Figs. 8-26 and 8-29). Some Purkinje cells project directly to the lateral vestibular nucleus, which acts on the spinal cord through the vestibulospinal tract. Part of the output to the reticular formation is through the inferior cerebellar peduncle

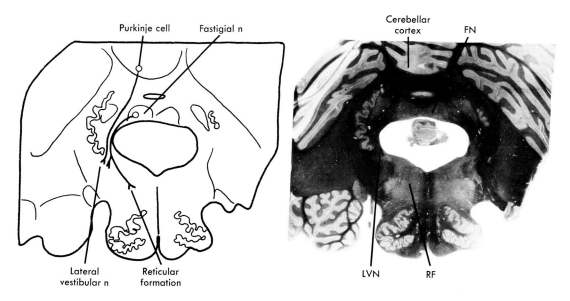

Fig. 8-29. Fastigial projection. Efferents from the fastigial nucleus pass through the juxta-restiform body into the brainstem, where they terminate in the vestibular nuclei and the reticular formation. There are also some direct projections from Purkinje cells through the juxtarestiform body to the lateral vestibular nucleus. Not shown are crossed projections from the fastigial nucleus rostrally around the superior cerebellar peduncle in the hook bundle. These also terminate in the vestibular nuclei and reticular formation.

Table 8-1. Cerebellar divisions and syndromes

Cerebellar division	Component	Connections	Syndrome
Archicerebellum (vestibulocerebellum)	Flocculonodular lobe	Input from vestibular nerve and vestibular nuclei Output to vestibular nuclei via fastigial nuclei and directly	Gait disturbance, head rotation, nystagmus, disturbance in station (eyes open or closed)
Paleocerebellum (spinocerebellum)	Vermis, inter-mediate region	Input from spinocerebellar tracts and brain-stem nuclei receiving spinal input (reticular formation, inferior olive) Output to brainstem nuclei giving rise to bulbospinal paths (reticular formation, lateral vestibular nucleus, red nucleus) via fastigial nuclei and interposed nuclei (globose and emboliform)	Gait disturbance, rigidity in animal models
Neocerebellum (pontocerebellum)	Hemispheres	Input from corticopontocerebellar pathway; indirect connections from cerebral cortex through inferior olivary nucleus and reticular formation Output to ventrolateral nucleus of thalamus via dentate nucleus; thalamic projections to motor cortex	Hypotonia, pendular knee jerk, disturbance in station, weakness, delay in starting and stopping muscular contractions, disturbances in rate of voluntary movements, dysmetria, decomposition of movement, dysdiadochokinesia, speech disturbance, gait disturbance, intention tremor

and part is through the superior cerebellar peduncle by way of the hook bundle.

Functional regions of the cerebellum and clinical applications

In the literature concerned with experimental studies of the cerebellum, a functional distinction is often made between the anterior and the posterior lobes. However, the phylogenetic development, anatomical connections, and the patterns of deficits that result from cerebellar damage suggest another approach to a functional subdivision of the cerebellum. This involves dividing the cerebellum into three regions known as the archicerebellum, the paleocerebellum, and the neocerebellum (Table 8-1). Synonyms for these, based on the dominant connections with other regions of the central nervous system, are vestibulocerebellum, spinocerebellum, and pontocerebellum.

Archicerebellum (vestibulocerebellum). The cerebellum appears to have evolved in relationship to the vestibular system and the lateral line in primitive vertebrates. For this reason, the portion of the mammalian cerebellum that is most closely interconnected with the vestibular system is called the archicerebellum or vestibulocerebellum. This is essentially coextensive with the flocculonodular lobe, although part of the uvula is also involved.

The input to the flocculonodular lobe consists of both primary vestibular afferents and second-order afferents arising in the vestibular nuclei. The afferents in mammals enter the cerebellum through the restiform body and end as mossy fibers. It is not yet clear which vestibular sensory epithelia convey information to the cerebellum, although it seems likely that both the otolith organs and the semicircular ducts do so. The output from the flocculonodular lobe consists of direct projections from Purkinje cells to the vestibular nuclei and indirect projections from Purkinje cells to the fastigial nucleus and from there to the vestibular nuclei. The direct projection and part of the fastigial projection pass through the ipsilateral restiform body, and the rest of the fastigial projection is in the hook bundle, which crosses and passes out through the contralateral superior cerebellar peduncle.

Damage to the archicerebellum in lower mammals results in alterations in otolithic reflexes of the eye, circling movements, nystagmus, and abnormal positions of the head or trunk. Tremor of the head and neck and an ataxic gait occur in primates. There is no tremor in the extremities, nor is there hypotonia or alteration in reflexes. In humans, there is a comparable picture, the archicerebellar syndrome, in cases which presumably affect chiefly the flocculonodular lobe. The most common pathological state in which this happens is medulloblastoma, a tumor of the cerebellum that occurs in children and damages the midline cerebellum. The archicerebellar syndrome consists of one or more of the following: gait disturbance, rotation of the head, and nystagmus. The gait disturbance is characterized by difficulty in maintaining balance during walking, but without ataxia of the extremities. The head rotation is a maintained postural abnormality resulting from an asymmetrical lesion of the flocculonodular lobe or of the output fibers in the restiform body. Nystagmus is sometimes present in quickly developing lesions, but not in slowly progressive ones; it is generally horizontal.

Paleocerebellum (spinocerebellum). The dominant region of the cerebellum in many mammals, such as the carnivores, is the paleocerebellum. Much of the experimental work on the cerebellum has been done with the cat as an animal model; thus this part of the cerebellum is the best understood. However, generalizations about the human cerebellum based on the animal work must be made with caution, because the dominant part of the human cerebellum is the neocerebellum.

The paleocerebellum consists of most of the vermis and part of the intermediate region. The input lines to the paleocerebellum are the various spinocerebellar tracts. These include the dorsal and ventral spinocerebellar tracts (carrying information from the lower body and hindlimbs), the cuneocerebellar and rostral spinocerebellar tracts (carrying information from the upper body and forelimbs), and the spino-olivary and spinoreticulocerebellar tracts. Most of these pathways enter the cerebellum through the restiform body and terminate as mossy fibers. However, the ventral spinocerebellar tract, which is crossed in the spinal cord, enters the cerebellum through the superior cerebellar peduncle and largely recrosses within the cerebellar white matter. The rostral spinocerebellar tract stays uncrossed, although it is equivalent in other respects to the ventral spinocerebellar tract, and enters the cerebellum partly through the restiform body and partly through the superior cerebellar peduncle. The olivocerebellar projections, which form the input to the cerebellum in the spino-olivary pathways, end in the cerebellar cortex as climbing fibers. Information from the head presumably reaches the cerebellum by way of projections from the spinal nucleus of the trigeminal. However, this pathway has not been well studied.

The cerebellar cortex has a somatotopic organization similar to that of the cerebral cortex. A dual representation of the body surface has been mapped on the cerebellar surface. One side of the body is represented ipsilaterally in the anterior lobe and bilaterally in the posterior lobe. The homunculus is arranged so that the head areas are near the primary fissure and the forelimb and hindlimb areas are progressively rostral in the anterior lobe and caudal in the posterior lobe (Fig. 8-21). The spinocerebellar tracts end in the appropriate regions. For example, the dorsal spinocerebellar tract, carrying information from the lower body and hindlimb, terminates in the hindlimb areas of the anterior and posterior lobes.

The information carried by the various spinocerebellar pathways is rather heterogeneous. There is information from muscle receptors, including muscle spindle and Golgi tendon organ afferents, from joint receptors, and from cutaneous receptors. Several of the pathways appear to signal the current state of activity in spinal reflex pathways, particularly the flexion reflex pathway.

There are a number of output paths from the paleocerebellum. In general, these are arranged like the input paths; thus motor effects are evoked chiefly on the side of the body ipsilateral to the side of the cerebellum under consideration. The vermis projects to the fastigial nucleus. Activity in the fastigial nucleus is relayed either through the ipsilateral restiform body or through the contralateral superior cerebellar peduncle by way of the hook bundle. The brainstem connections of the fastigial efferents are with cells of the vestibular nuclei or with neurons in the reticular formation. Motor activity at the spinal cord level is then influenced by way of the vestibulospinal and reticulospinal tracts.

The intermediate region of the cerebellar cortex projects to the interposed nuclei (globose and emboliform nuclei in humans). The neurons of the interposed nuclei send their axons to the contralateral red nucleus by way of the decussation of the brachium conjunctivum. The red nucleus gives rise to the rubrospinal tract, which crosses in the ventral tegmental decussation and descends into the spinal cord.

Damage to the paleocerebellum in lower mammals produces a marked extensor hypertonus. This is characteristic, for example, of the decerebellate cat. The arching of the head and back is termed opisthotonos. In addition to this postural change, the gait becomes ataxic and there is a tremor of the head and trunk. The effect of paleocerebellar damage is not nearly as dramatic in primates. In humans, a paleocerebellar syndrome has been described but is rarely seen. The main difficulty appears to be in gait, without hypotonia or reflex changes. The upper extremities tend not to be greatly involved.

Neocerebellum (pontocerebellum). The neocerebellum is the dominant part of the cerebellum in primates, including humans. The neocerebellum consists of the hemispheres and part of the intermediate region, as well as some of the middle zone of the vermis. The name pontocerebellum is derived from the large projection to this region from the pontine nuclei. However, the most significant relationship is with the cerebral cortex, particularly with the motor cortex.

The main input to the neocerebellum is by way of the corticopontocerebellar pathway. The corticopontine fibers originate widely in the cerebral cortex and descend through the internal capsule and cerebral peduncle with the corticospinal tract. Within the cerebral peduncle, the frontopontine projection is just medial to the corticospinal tract, and the projection from other lobes is lateral to the corticospinal tract

(Fig. 8-4). The corticopontine fibers terminate within the pontine nuclei. Axons from neurons of the pontine nuclei decussate and enter the cerebellum through the contralateral brachium pontis. They end in the cortex of the neocerebellum as mossy fibers. The corticopontocerebellar pathway from the motor cortex is organized somatotopically. For example, the axons of pontocerebellar neurons influenced by the arm area of the motor cortex terminate in the arm areas of the cerebellar cortex. There are also other inputs to the neocerebellum. These include a corticoreticulocerebellar pathway and a cortico-olivocerebellar pathway. The former terminates as mossy fibers, whereas the latter ends as climbing fibers.

The main output line from the neocerebellum is from the cortex of the cerebellar hemisphere to the dentate nucleus. From here, the dentatothalamic tract projects to the contralateral thalamus through the decussation of the brachium conjunctivum. The dentatothalamic tract fibers ascend past the red nucleus and through the fields of Forel to end in the ventrolateral nucleus of the thalamus. Relay cells of the ventrolateral nucleus project to the motor regions of the frontal lobe. There is a somatotopic arrangement, with the arm representation of the cerebellar cortex being connected with the arm representation of the motor cortex.

The function of the neocerebellum appears to include the modulation of the activity of the motor outflow from the cerebral cortex. Experimental studies show that activity in cells of the deep cerebellar nuclei may precede voluntary movements, suggesting that the influence of the cerebellum on the motor cortex serves not only to correct movement but is also involved in its initiation. In addition, the neocerebellum may play an important role in determining postural tone.

Isolated damage to the neocerebellum in lower mammals is difficult to produce because the paleocerebellum is the dominant part in these animals. However, when successful, the most striking effect is postural hypotonia. This may be accompanied by tremor of the head and the limbs ipsilateral to the side of the damage. Neocerebellar damage in primates produces hypotonia and disturbances of skilled movements. There may also be an intention tremor. Experiments have been done in which a cooling probe inactivated the neurons of the dentate nucleus in awake, behaving monkeys. The monkeys had been trained to make alternating movements of an arm. When the dentate nucleus was cooled, the movements became uncoordinated, with overshooting and undershooting.

In humans, cerebellar damage most commonly produces one or more elements of the neocerebellar syndrome. The signs of neocerebellar damage can be sub-divided into changes in posture and reflexes and disturbances in voluntary movement. The postural change typical of neocerebellar damage is hypotonia, which may cause the knee jerk reflex to become pendulous. Another finding is a disturbance of station. When asked to stand with the feet together, the patient tends to fall. This tendency is unchanged when the eyes are closed (unlike the ataxia of dorsal column disease, in which the tendency to fall is minimal with the eyes open but appears when the eyes are closed). In most instances, falling is toward the side of the lesion.

The changes in voluntary movement due to neocerebellar damage may include the following. The patient may complain of weakness. Muscular contractions on the affected side may be weak and irregular. Movements are often delayed in onset and in cessation. The rate of movement is disturbed, being too fast or too slow at different times. Movements involving several joints may under- or overshoot a target (dysmetria). It is difficult for the patient to perform rapidly alternating movements (dysdiadochokinesia). There may be a speech disturbance (scanning or ataxic speech), as well as difficulty in writing. There is often an intention tremor, an oscillation of the limb during and at the end of voluntary movement. The gait may be disturbed.

Other functions of the cerebellum. It seems clear that the cerebellum is not involved in conscious sensation; however, it undoubtedly has a wider role in the regulation of body function than is generally recognized. There are known visual and auditory inputs to the cerebellum. These presumably could be related to reflex adjustments of the head and neck to visual or auditory cues. Participation of the cerebellum in the learning of motor behavior seems likely, and a specific theory of how the climbing-fiber pathways may be involved has been proposed. There is also some evidence for an input to the cerebellum from visceral structures and for cerebellar influences on autonomic function. An intriguing series of experiments has shown that neurons of the fastigial nucleus can evoke large changes in cardiovascular function that can be interpreted to be a part of the adjustments involved in postural changes. Other visceral functions, including respiration and micturition, are also known to be influenced by the cerebellum.

BASAL GANGLIA

The basal ganglia (Fig. 8-30) include the caudate nucleus and putamen (neostriatum) and the globus pallidus (paleostriatum). Important connections are made between the basal ganglia and certain nuclei of the brainstem, including the subthalamic nucleus and the substantia nigra.

The phylogenetic development of the basal ganglia provides information about their function. The paleostriatum appears first as a well-developed part of the vertebrate brain in fish. The paleostriatum augmentatum, which is present in reptiles and is better developed in birds, appears to be homologous with the mammalian neostriatum.

Microscopic structure of the basal ganglia and associated nuclei

The neostriatum is the major receptive nucleus of the basal ganglia. The cells in the caudate and putamen resemble sensory neurons. The caudate nucleus contains four types of neurons. The commonest neurons are medium sized, with branching dendrites that exhibit spines. The second type is similar, but with dendrites devoid of spines. There are also small numbers of very large fusiform cells and very small neuroglioform neurons. The putamen has been less well studied than the caudate nucleus, but its structure seems to be similar.

The globus pallidus (paleostriatum) is the major output structure of the basal ganglia. Its neurons have an isodendritic pattern, like reticular neurons and motoneurons. The cells in the medial segment of the globus pallidus are larger than those in the lateral segment, and most of the output is from the medial segment.

The subthalamic nucleus (of Luys) consists of moderate- to small-sized cells with highly branched dendrites. The medial part of the nucleus has smaller, rounder, and more densely packed neurons than does the lateral part.

The substantia nigra contains moderately large, plump cells and some smaller cells in a dorsally placed compact zone. Some of the cells form clusters. The ventral region of the substantia nigra, or reticular zone, contains fewer neurons. The substantia nigra derives its name from the melanin pigment found in its cells. (Melanin is also found in cells of the nucleus locus ceruleus, the dorsal motor nucleus of the vagus, and other brainstem nuclei.) The accumulation of this pigment is undoubtedly related to the metabolism of tyrosine and the formation of catecholamines by these cells.

Afferent pathways to the basal ganglia

The major input to the basal ganglia comes from the cerebral cortex and enters the caudate nucleus and the putamen (Fig. 8-31). There are also projections from the substantia nigra (discussed below) and from the intralaminar nuclei of the thalamus to the caudate

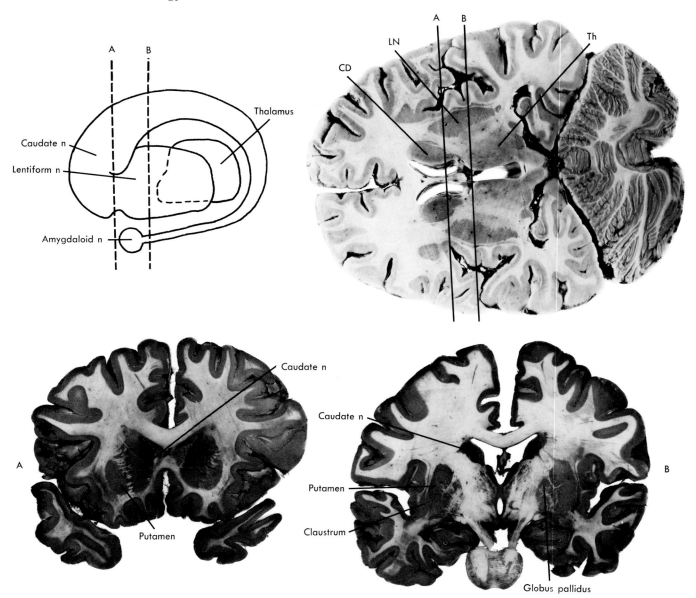

Fig. 8-30. Basal ganglia. Relationships between some of the basal ganglia and the thalamus. The caudate nucleus has two parts, a rostrally located head and a tail. The tail curves ventrally into the temporal lobe, runs along the roof of the inferior horn of the lateral ventricle, and ends rostrally at the level of the amygdaloid nucleus. The caudate nucleus is separated from the lentiform nucleus (putamen and globus pallidus) by the internal capsule. The lentiform nucleus is also separated from the thalamus by the posterior limb of the internal capsule. These relationships are shown on the coronal and horizontal sections of the brain. The coronal sections are at levels *A* and *B*.

nucleus and the putamen. The afferent projections from the cerebral cortex are extensive and are topographically organized. The anterior regions of the cerebral cortex, such as the frontal lobe, project on the head of the caudate and rostral part of the putamen; more posterior regions of the cortex connect with the body and tail of the caudate and with the caudal part of the putamen. There is also a mediolateral topographic arrangement. The cerebral cortex of the dorsal and medial surface of the hemisphere projects to the caudate, and the cortex of the lateral surface of the hemisphere connects with the putamen. Most of the cortical projections are ipsilateral, although there are some crossed projections through the corpus callosum.

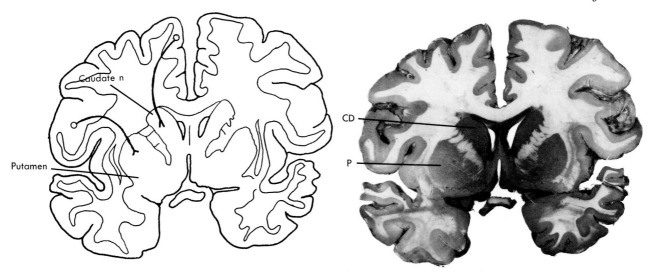

Fig. 8-31. Connections of cerebral cortex with neostriatum. Projections are shown from the cerebral cortex to the caudate nucleus and the putamen. These projections have a topographic organization.

Connections between the basal ganglia and related nuclei

The flow of information through the basal ganglia is primarily from the neostriatum to the globus pallidus (Fig. 8-32). However, there are reciprocal connections between the neostriatum and the substantia nigra and between the globus pallidus and the subthalamic nucleus.

The caudate nucleus and the putamen project to the globus pallidus. This projection is topographically organized, suggesting that the entire system, from cortex to globus pallidus, has a highly specific arrangement.

The neostriatum also projects to the substantia nigra, with synaptic endings chiefly in the reticular zone (Fig. 8-33). The main efferent projection from the substantia nigra is from the compact zone back to the neostriatum. These fibers include a dopaminergic component, although there may also be axons that use some other transmitter. There is also a non-dopaminergic projection from the substantia nigra to the ventral lateral (VL) and ventral anterior (VA) nuclei of the thalamus. The activity of the substantia nigra can thus modulate the basal ganglia circuit either at the level of the neostriatum or in the thalamus.

The lateral segment of the globus pallidus sends fibers to the subthalamic nucleus (Fig. 8-33) through the dorsal comb bundle, a system of fibers that crosses through the internal capsule, forming a structure resembling a comb. The subthalamic nucleus projects back to the globus pallidus, but to the medial segment. The interconnections of the globus pallidus and sub-

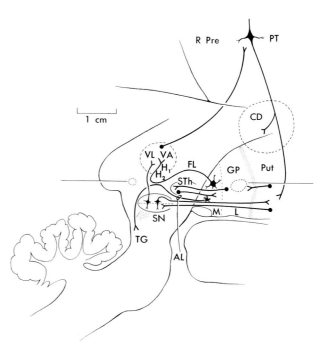

Fig. 8-32. Interrelationships of the basal ganglia, lateral thalamus, and motor cortex. Schematic sagittal section. Abbreviations: *AL*, ansa lenticularis; *CD*, caudate nucleus; *FL*, fasciculus lenticularis; *GP*, globus pallidus, medial *(M)* and lateral *(L)* segments; H_1 (thalamic fasciculus), H_2, fields of Forel; *Put*, putamen; *SN*, substantia nigra; *R Pre*, right precentral gyrus; *STh*, subthalamic nucleus; *TG*, tegmental neurons; *VA*, ventral anterior nucleus; *VL*, ventral lateral nucleus. For simplicity the efferent projections of the neostriatum (caudate-putamen) and the nigrostriatal afferents are shown only for the putamenal portion of the neostriatum.

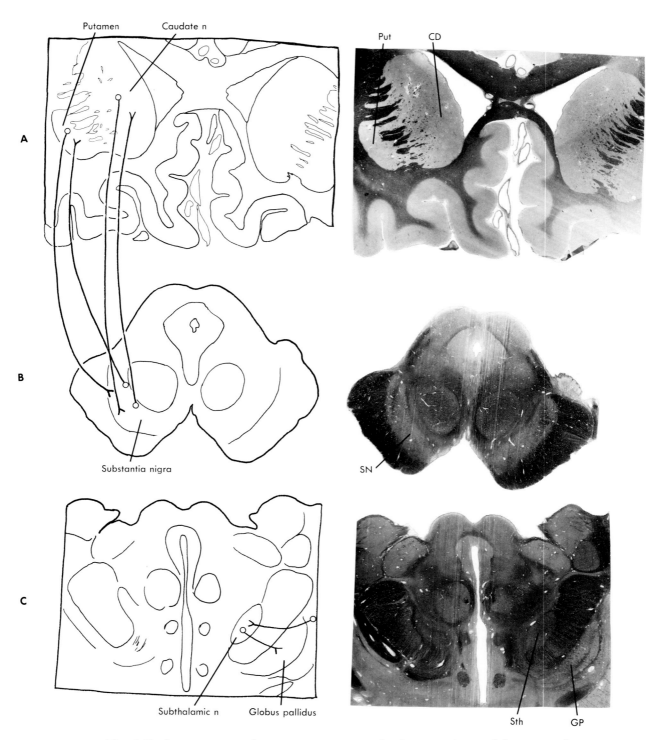

Fig. 8-33. Interconnections between neostriatum and substantia nigra and between paleostriatum and subthalamic nucleus. **A** and **B,** Interconnections between the caudate nucleus and putamen and the substantia nigra. **C,** Interconnections between the globus pallidus and the subthalamic nucleus.

thalamic nucleus are called the subthalamic fasciculus. The subthalamic nucleus can thus modulate activity in the basal ganglia circuit at the level of the paleostriatum.

Efferent connections of the basal ganglia

The main output of the basal ganglia is from the globus pallidus (Fig. 8-34). The output is to the thalamus and from there to the motor areas of the cerebral cortex. The major efferent pathway is from the medial segment of the globus pallidus. The ventral part of this structure projects rostrally and ventromedially; the axons swing around the edge of the posterior limb of the internal capsule as the ansa lenticularis and turn caudally to enter field H of Forel (Fig. 8-35). The H fields (G. *Haubefeld*, cap field or tegmentum field) were so named by the Swiss neuroanatomist Forel. These fields are parts of the subthalamus. The pallidal efferents pass through field H and then along the dorsal surface of the zona incerta in field H_1. Here they are part of the thalamic fasciculus. Finally, they terminate in the VA and VL nuclei of the thalamus.

Efferents from the dorsal part of the medial segment of the globus pallidus penetrate the posterior limb of the internal capsule and turn medially just ventral to the zona incerta. The fiber bundle is called the fasciculus lenticularis, which forms Forel's field H_2 (Fig. 8-32). These fibers course medially and caudally to enter field H, where they join the fibers of the ansa lenticularis. They then project laterally with the thalamic fasciculus to the VA and VL nuclei of the thalamus.

Some of the fibers of the thalamic fasciculus turn dorsally to terminate in the intralaminar nuclei of the thalamus (Fig. 8-34). The thalamic fasciculus also contains fibers that do not originate from the basal ganglia but from the dentate nucleus of the contralateral cerebellum; these are destined to end in the VL thalamus.

There appears to be a minor descending projection from the medial segment of the globus pallidus to the midbrain tegmentum; otherwise, the basal ganglia appear to have access to the motor outflow of the brain primarily by actions on the thalamus and motor cortex.

Neurochemistry of the basal ganglia

More is known about the identity, content, and distribution of substances that probably function as neurotransmitters in the neostriatum than in most other regions of the brain. For many years it was known that certain cell groups in the substantia nigra degenerated in Parkinson's disease. In the early 1960s, Hornykiewicz found that the normally high dopamine content of the neostriatum was also greatly reduced in Parkinson's disease. He and Cotzias found that some of the motor symptoms of Parkinson's disease could be alleviated by the administration of 3,4-dihydroxyphenylalanine (DOPA), the precursor of dopamine. An important technical advance made at this time was the application of the fluorescence histochemistry method for visualizing the monoamine-containing neurons of the nervous system (see Appendix I). The chemical and anatomical methods combined showed that dopamine is stored in nerve terminals of the nigrostriatal pathway. In addition to a high dopamine

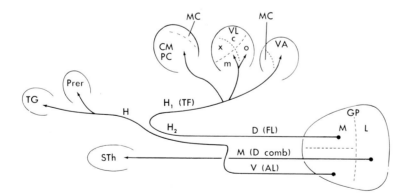

Fig. 8-34. Efferent projections of the globus pallidus. Abbreviations: *GP*, globus pallidus, medial *(M)* and lateral *(L)* segments. Projections: *D*, dorsal stratum of fibers, or *FL*, fasciculus lenticularis; *M*, middle stratum of fibers, or *D comb*, dorsal comb bundle; *V*, ventral stratum of fibers, or *AL*, ansa lenticularis; *H*, H_1(*TF*, thalamic fasciculus), and H_2, fields of Forel. Thalamic nuclei receiving projections: *CM*, centromedian (*PC*, parvicellular portion of *CM*); *VL*, ventral lateral (*c, o, m, x*, subdivisions of *VL* in the rhesus monkey); *VA*, ventral anterior (*MC*, magnocellular portion of *VA*). Subthalamic and mesencephalic nuclei receiving projections: *Prer*, nucleus of prerubral field (H field of Forel); *STh*, subthalamic nucleus; *TG*, tegmental neurons. (After Nauta and Mehler, 1966.)

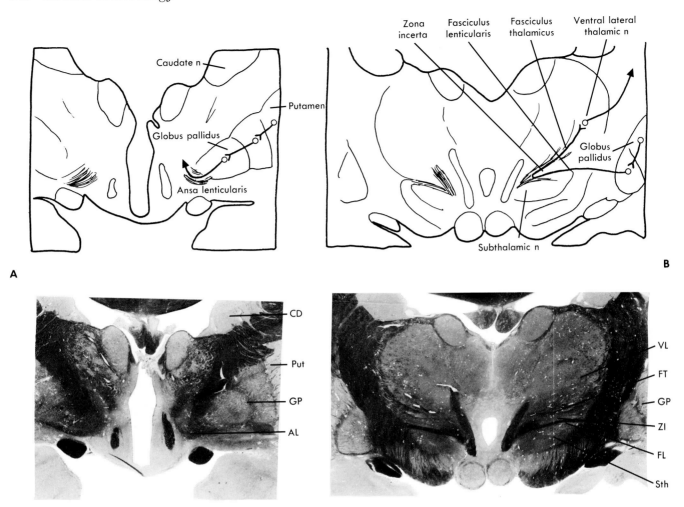

Fig. 8-35. Output pathways of the globus pallidus. **A,** The internal segment of the globus pallidus projects around the edge of the internal capsule into the ansa lenticularis. These axons pass caudally and join the thalamic fasciculus (field H₁). **B,** Other pallidal efferents cross the internal capsule, run medially just ventral to the zona incerta in the lenticular fasciculus (field H₂), and then bend back laterally just dorsal to the zona incerta in the thalamic fasciculus (H₁). The pallidal efferents terminate in the ventral anterior and ventral lateral nuclei of the thalamus and also in the centrum medianum nucleus.

content, the neostriatum has the highest concentration of acetylcholine of any part of the brain and also contains large amounts of 5-hydroxytryptamine (5-HT) and gamma-aminobutyric acid (GABA). Which neuronal elements in the neostriatum contain these substances is not yet clear. However, striatonigral axons stain for cholinesterase, and so these may be cholinergic.

Information processing in the basal ganglia

The excitatory and inhibitory circuits within the basal ganglia are under study. In general, it can be said that the cerebral cortex largely excites neurons of the neostriatum. The neostriatum generally inhibits pallidal neurons. The pallidum excites neurons of the

VA and VL thalami. The VL thalamus excites and inhibits neurons in the motor cortex. However, the details about the operation of this complex pathway and the interactions with the substantia nigra and subthalamus are only just beginning to be understood. It can be assumed at the present time that the substantia nigra and the subthalamic nucleus inhibit activity in the basal ganglion circuit. Thus, destruction of either of these regions results in a release of activity in the corticospinal tract, although the patterns of this released activity differ.

Stimulation and ablation studies

The effects of stimulation and ablation of the basal ganglia have been difficult to determine because of the intermingling of cell bodies and fibers of passage. In the cat, stimulation of the caudate nucleus produces turning of the head and eyes and circling locomotion away from the side stimulated. Arrest of motor activity has also been produced by caudate stimulation, but it is not clear if this effect is caused by spread of stimulus current to adjacent fiber systems. Lesions of the caudate nucleus in the monkey have been reported to produce slight hyperkinesia in some studies, but no effects in others.

Stimulation of the globus pallidus in the cat produces contraversive running movements. Similar movements can be produced by stimulation in the area of the zona incerta, which is adjacent to the pallidal outflow path. Lesions of the pallidum in cats and monkeys produce a mild hypokinesia.

Lesions of the subthalamic nucleus in animals are more dramatic than other basal ganglion lesions. If more than 20% of the subthalamic nucleus is destroyed, a monkey will develop hyperkinesia, choreiform movements, and some ballistic movements of the contralateral limb. These involuntary movements are abolished by lesions of the ipsilateral pallidum or ventrolateral thalamic nucleus without producing weakness. Motor cortex lesions also abolish the involuntary movements but produce weakness as well. Evidently, removal of the modulating effect of the subthalamic nucleus on the pallidum results in a disturbed transmission through the basal ganglion circuit.

Stimulation of the substantia nigra in the cat produces chewing movements. Bilateral lesions of the substantia nigra in the monkey cause hypokinesia and impaired chewing movements. The tremor of parkinsonism has not been produced by nigral lesions in the monkey. However, a tremor is produced by lesions in the ventral tegmentum, just above the substantia nigra, which interrupt nigral, cerebellar, and red nucleus projections. This tremor is ameliorated by lesions of the VL thalamus and by DOPA, as is the tremor of parkinsonism in humans.

Clinical applications

Diseases that involve the basal ganglia produce abnormal movements and disturbances of muscle tone. The abnormal movements may include tremor at rest (as in parkinsonism), chorea, athetosis, and ballism. The disturbed muscle tone of parkinsonism is termed rigidity.

Parkinson's disease

Although the detailed description of neurological diseases is beyond the scope of this book, the medical importance and physiological significance of Parkinson's disease (paralysis agitans, or shaking palsy) as an example of the extrapyramidal motor disorders requires that an introductory description of the disease be given here. The following motor signs are seen in patients with Parkinson's disease:

1. Rigidity of muscles
2. Tremor of the resting type, with a frequency of about 4 to 7 Hz; some patients also exhibit a type of sustention tremor that appears when the arm is held in an outstretched posture
3. A posture in which flexion of the limbs and trunk predominates
4. Difficulty in making motor choices
5. Loss of associated movements
6. Poverty of movement; signs four, five, and six can be subsumed under the terms bradykinesia or akinesia
7. Autonomic disturbances

Although tremor at rest is the most dramatic symptom of parkinsonism, the majority of patients are most functionally disabled by akinesia and rigidity. These three major motor signs of parkinsonism occur in varying degrees in individuals, some having only a little tremor but considerable rigidity or akinesia or both.

Parkinsonism is associated with the degeneration of certain neurons of the substantia nigra (probably the medial cell groups of the compact zone, in particular) that project to the neostriatum (caudate nucleus and putamen). Degeneration is also often found in other nuclei of the brainstem, such as the locus ceruleus, that, like nigral neurons, contain catecholamines and melanin pigment. The melanin appears to be related to the biosynthesis and degradation of the catecholamines in some as yet unknown way. The motor signs of parkinsonism often first appear on one side of the body but usually become bilateral over a period of years. In unilateral parkinsonism the nigrostriatal pathway contralateral to the side of the muscular abnormalities is found to be degenerated. The catecholamine contained in the largest amount in the neurons of the nigrostriatal pathway is dopamine. Dopamine is almost certainly a neurotransmitter substance in this pathway. The activation of the nigrostriatal projection, or the iontophoresis of dopamine onto caudate and putamen neurons, depresses the firing of most but not all neostriatal nuerons. Some caudate-putamen neurons are unaffected, but others increase their firing.

The biosynthesis and degradation of catecholamines in central nervous system neurons is represented in the diagram at the top of p. 342, in a simplified manner.

When administered into the bloodstream, dopamine does not penetrate the blood-brain barrier very well. However, L-dopa, the precursor of dopamine, will

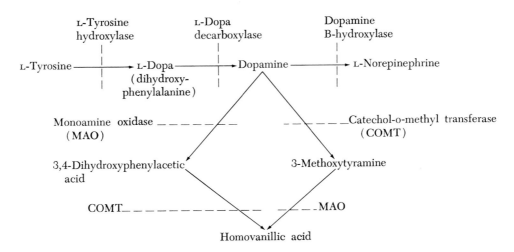

enter the brain from the blood, although still in rather small amounts. The intravenous or oral administration of large doses of L-dopa has been found to ameliorate rigidity and akinesia in a considerable percentage of patients with parkinsonism. The tremor improves more slowly, usually over a course of weeks or months, during L-dopa administration, and tremor is less improved than akinesia and rigidity in most patients. The most obvious explanation of these effects is that residual neurons of the nigrostriatal pathway are utilizing the L-dopa to make new dopamine and that this tends to restore normal transmission in the nigrostriatal pathway. However, there is no direct evidence that this is the mechanism of action of L-dopa. It is interesting that overdosage of L-dopa will produce involuntary movements, including rhythmic beating of the limbs, forced protrusion of the tongue, forced closure of the eyes, and tonic postures.

It has also been found that the administration of atropinelike anticholinergic drugs will have a mildly ameliorating effect on the symptoms of parkinsonism. The corticoneostriatal and neostriatal-nigral projections may be in part cholinergic projections. Many investigators have taken as a working hypothesis that there normally is a certain ratio of activity, or balance, between basal ganglia pathways utilizing biogenic amines (including 5-hydroxytryptamine) and pathways utilizing acetylcholine as transmitter substances. Their hypothesis is that this balance is disturbed in parkinsonism because of depression of dopaminergic transmission. The balance between transmission in these systems can be thought of as being corrected to some degree by administration of L-dopa and anticholinergic drugs.

Rigidity in parkinsonism can also be reduced by reducing afferent input to the spinal cord by cutting the dorsal roots or by blocking their function with local anesthetics. Blocking the gamma motoneuron axons in the ventral roots will also reduce rigidity.

Neither of these procedures has much effect on tremor. These findings suggest that in rigidity there are disturbances in the central control of the gamma loop. However, it is not definitely established that there is overactivity of the gamma loop in parkinsonism.

The origins of tremor appear to be related to rhythmic thalamocortical activity. Recording in the thalamus at the time of stereotaxic surgery for relief of parkinsonism has revealed that neurons lying at the border of the caudal pole of the ventral lateral nucleus and the rostral pole of the ventral posterior nucleus fire synchronously with the tremor. Sensory neurons in the thalamus and cortex also fire synchronously with the tremor but in response to sensory stimuli set up by the tremor. However, the site of origin of the abnormal discharge in parkinsonism has not yet been localized. Nor is the origin of the suppression of the tremor during voluntary movement understood. The tremor depends on an intact primary motor cortex and on the corticospinal system for its expression. The tremor can be abolished by ablation of these structures, but such procedures also produce paresis. Destruction of the ventral lateral nucleus of the thalamus ameliorates tremor and to a lesser degree rigidity in carefully selected cases of parkinsonism. Thalamotomy has been found to be more effective than interrupting the cortical-basal ganglia-thalamic-cortical circuit at the level of the globus pallidus (pallidotomy). The mechanism of action of thalamotomy in relieving tremor and other signs of parkinsonism is not understood. Thalamotomy has little effect on normal movement, producing only slight, transitory cerebellar-lesion-like disturbances of movement of the contralateral limbs.

The other movement disorder that is directly correlated with a specific lesion of the basal ganglion circuitry is ballism. Damage to a subthalamic nucleus on one side results in hemiballism of the contralateral limb. The movements are so violent that they can result in serious damage. As with the tremor of parkinsonism, the movements disappear during sleep.

Basal ganglion lesions are found, often along with lesions of various other parts of the central nervous system, in a variety of other conditions that are generally referred to as extrapyramidal system disease. Chorea is a dramatic sign of Sydenham's chorea, a movement disorder that may be a sequel to a streptococcal infection. Choreiform and athetoid movements and mental deterioration are characteristic of Huntington's chorea, a debilitating genetic disorder (dominant gene) affecting young adults. Athetosis is a prominent sign in a number of diseases damaging basal ganglia, including cerebral palsy (congenital brain damage). Wilson's disease (hepatolenticular degeneration), a genetic disorder of copper metabolism (recessive gene), is associated with a tremor and with rigidity. Another form of motor disorder produced by basal ganglion disease is dystonia musculorum deformans.

OCULOMOTOR SYSTEM

The oculomotor system is considered separately from other motor systems because of the necessity of introducing additional material about the anatomy of oculomotor structures and about eye movements. The organization of the oculomotor system does not appear to be different in principle from that of other motor systems that are under voluntary control mediated by descending pathways and under reflex control mediated largely by vestibular and other sensory pathways. Recent research on the electrophysiology of oculomotor motoneurons suggests that the oculomotor system may be an ideal system for investigating the mechanisms of motor control.

Peripheral oculomotor structures

The oculomotor system of each eye consists of six extraocular striated muscles, which move the eye, and three intraocular smooth muscles, one of which focuses the lens, whereas the other two constrict and dilate the pupil respectively.

Closely related to the activity of the muscles of the eye are the activities of two muscles that elevate the upper eyelid, and the sphincter muscle, which closes the lids.

The six extraocular muscles that move each eye are as follows:

1. Superior rectus, innervated by nerve III (oculomotor)
2. Inferior rectus, innervated by nerve III
3. Medial rectus, innervated by nerve III
4. Inferior oblique, innervated by nerve III
5. Superior oblique, innervated by nerve IV (trochlear)
6. Lateral rectus, innervated by nerve VI (abducens); the eye movements produced by these muscles are described later

These muscles are innervated by large motoneurons located in the cranial nerve nuclei of nerves III, IV, and VI. (See Chapter 6 for a description of the somatic efferent nuclei of the brainstem.) Characteristic of the innervation of the extraocular muscle fibers is the small size of their motor units, which often contain five to ten muscle fibers. This is a mechanism for producing fine control of movement.

The upper eyelid is strongly elevated by the levator palpebrae muscle, a striated muscle supplied by nerve III, and less strongly elevated by the tarsalis muscle (Müller's muscle), a smooth muscle applied to the underside of the levator palpebrae. The tarsalis muscle is innervated by postganglionic sympathetic neurons. The eyelids are closed by the orbicularis oculi muscle, which is innervated by nerve VII (facial). There are associated eyelid and eye movements; for example, when the eyelids are closed, the eyeballs roll upward.

Cranial nerves III, IV, and VI contain sensory afferent fibers from muscle spindles, as well as motor efferent fibers. The course of the afferent fibers is not completely clear. They probably leave the eye-muscle nerves and enter the first (ophthalmic) division of nerve V (trigeminal). Their cell bodies are probably in the mesencephalic nucleus of nerve V, which also contains the cell bodies of the spindle afferents from the jaw muscles.

The intraocular muscles are the ciliary muscle, the pupillary sphincter, and the pupillary dilator. The ciliary muscle focuses the lens in the following manner. When the ciliary muscle contracts, it relaxes the tension of the suspensory ligament of the lens, allowing the lens to assume its natural spherical shape, thereby focusing the image of nearby objects on the retina (accommodation for near vision). The pupillary sphincter muscle of the iris constricts the iris (miosis). The ciliary and sphincter muscles contract in concert in accommodation for near vision (the near reflex, p. 348). They are innervated by postganglionic parasympathetic neurons that have their cell bodies in the ciliary ganglia. The axons of these cells enter the eye by way of the short ciliary nerves. The cell bodies of the preganglionic neurons lie in the Edinger-Westphal nuclei of the oculomotor complex in the brainstem (see next section). Nerve III, therefore, unlike nerves IV and VI, whose motor component is purely somatic motor, contains both somatic motor and preganglionic parasympathetic neurons. These preganglionic parasympathetic neurons appear to lie on the dorsal surface of nerve III. Their separation from the motoneurons of the nerve appears to explain how compression of nerve III, if it is not too severe, can produce an internal ophthalmoplegia, which is paralysis of accommodation, and, more striking, a fixed, dilated (mydriatic) pupil, without producing a significant external ophthalmoplegia, which is paralysis of eye movement and ptosis (drooping of the upper eyelid and weakness of upper eyelid elevation).

The pupillodilator muscle and the tarsalis muscle of the upper eyelid are innervated by postganglionic sympathetic neurons that enter the eye as a plexus around the ophthalmic artery. The postganglionic neurons have their cell bodies in the superior cervical ganglion, and their axons form a plexus around the internal carotid artery. The plexus passes from the carotid to the ophthalmic artery. The preganglionic sympathetic neurons lie in the intermediolateral column of the thoracic spinal cord at T1 to 2. Stimulation of the sympathetic fibers to the eye produces dilatation of the pupil (mydriasis) and slightly elevates the upper eyelid. Damage to the sympathetic innervation to the eye produces Horner's syndrome: miosis, caused by unopposed action of the parasympathetically innervated pupilloconstrictor; ptosis, caused by paralysis of the tarsalis muscle; and enophthalmos, a retracted appearance of the eyeball, which usually is not very apparent. The ptosis, which is usually only moderate and does not produce a complete closure of the upper lid, disappears on voluntary upward gaze because of automatic contraction of the levator palpebrae (nerve III), an action that is associated with upward gaze.

Central oculomotor structures

The nuclei of nerves III, IV, and VI lie in a short segment of the brainstem, extending from the midbrain to the pons. Nerve III nuclei lie on either side of the midline of the midbrain, below the superior colliculi. The oculomotor nucleus of each side can be divided into several groups of motoneurons innervating extraocular muscles and the Edinger-Westphal nucleus, a dorsomedial column of parasympathetic neurons. The motoneurons innervating the four extrinsic muscles of the eye supplied by nerve III, and the levator palpebrae, are probably somatotopically arranged. Their axons innervate ipsilateral muscles, except for those to the superior rectus, which may project contralaterally. Westphal's nuclei and Perlia's nuclei innervate the ciliary and pupilloconstrictor muscles.

The nucleus of nerve IV lies below the inferior colliculus. The neurons of nerve IV decussate in the rostral part of the anterior medullary velum and innervate the superior oblique muscle of the contralateral eye. The functional reason for this decussation and for that of the crossing axons of nerve III is not clear.

The nucleus of nerve VI lies in the pons. Its axons innervate the ipsilateral lateral rectus.

Associated with the nuclei are other neurons that appear to act as interneurons for the motor system of the eye. The interstitial nucleus of Cajal and Darkshevich's nucleus are two such groups near the nucleus of nerve III. The functions of these interneuronal groups are not definitely known. Other interneuronal systems for the motor system of the eye are not well defined, either anatomically or functionally; however, the presence of such groups in the pretectal area, in the superior colliculus, and near the nucleus of nerve VI has been inferred from the effects of clinical and experimental lesions.

The medial longitudinal fasciculus (MLF) is the major projection system interrelating nuclei III, IV, and VI and associated interneurons. The vestibular projections to nuclei III, IV, and VI make up a large part of the MLF. These projections come largely but not exclusively from the superior vestibular nucleus (uncrossed) and from the medial vestibular nucleus (crossed and uncrossed projections).

Afferents to nuclei III, IV, and VI and to associated interneurons come from the retina, the cortex (especially from the frontal and occipital lobes) and the superior colliculus, as well as from the vestibular nuclei. There are probably reticular projections as well. The exact sites of termination of many of these projections are not yet known; many probably terminate on interneurons.

Eye movements

The eyes normally move so as to keep the image of the point of fixation on the equivalent part of the retina of each eye. This point is usually the macula lutea (yellow spot), where the resolving power (visual acuity) of the eye is greatest. If all objects were infinitely far away and light from them reached the eye by means of parallel rays, the visual axes of the eyes, the line from the center of the lens to the fovea (pit) of the macula, could remain parallel in the primary position (Fig. 8-36). The eyes could then be brought to fixate on objects either by moving the head with the eyes kept in the primary position or by purely conjugate movements of the eyes. To bring the images of nearby objects onto the maculas of each eye, the eyes must converge. Most eye movements are a combination of conjugate and convergence movements. Eye movements must also be coordinated with head and neck movements.

To accomplish its movements each eye has six extrinsic muscles. The superior rectus, inferior rectus, medial rectus, and inferior oblique are supplied by nerve III (oculomotor); the superior oblique is sup-

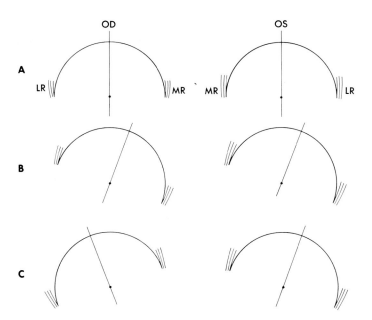

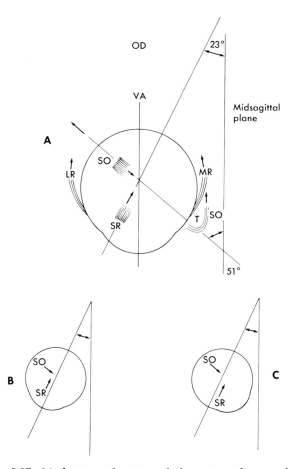

Fig. 8-36. Eye movements. **A**, Primary position. **B.** Conjugate deviation. **C**, Convergence. Abbreviations: *OD*, oculus dexter, or right eye; *OS*, oculus sinister, or left eye; *LR, MR*, lateral and medial recti.

Fig. 8-37. Mechanism of action of the extraocular muscles. **A**, Sites of attachment and direction of pull of the extraocular muscles. Superior aspect of the right eye *(OD)*. The eye is shown in the primary position. *VA*, visual axis of the eye; *SO*, superior oblique muscle. The inferior oblique muscle is attached in a similar position on the inferior aspect of the globe. *T*, trochlea; *SR*, superior rectus muscle. The inferior rectus muscle is attached in a similar position on the inferior aspect of the globe. *LR*, lateral rectus muscle; *MR*, medial rectus muscle. **B**, Actions of superior oblique and superior rectus muscles with the eye in abduction. **C**, Actions of the muscles with the eye in adduction.

plied by nerve IV (trochlear); the lateral rectus is supplied by nerve VI (abducens).

The muscles are arranged about the eye as shown in Fig. 8-37. All of the muscles except the inferior oblique originate from a common tendinous ring around the apex of the orbit. The inferior oblique originates in the area of the lacrimal (tear) sac. The superior oblique takes a different course than the other muscles originating at the apex of the orbit. It runs through a tendinous ring on the medial wall of the orbit, the trochlea (pulley), and then attaches to the globe so that its direction of pull is as shown in Fig. 8-37, *A*.

The medial and lateral recti are attached to the globe in a plane that is parallel to the floor of the orbit. They move the eye nasally (medially) and temporally (laterally) respectively. Movement of an eye nasally is adduction; movement temporally is abduction.

The superior and inferior recti are attached to the globe at an angle of 23° to the midsagittal plane, or to the medial wall of the orbit. When the eye is in abduction, with the optic axis of the eye parallel to the long axis of the superior and inferior recti, these muscles elevate and depress the eye respectively (Fig. 8-37, *B*). As various eye muscles move the eye, the direction of movement produced by the contraction of individual muscles changes. The situation can be simplified by considering the effects of contraction

of muscles with the eye in either adduction or abduction. When the medial rectus moves the right eye into adduction, the right superior rectus then acts to rotate the top of the right globe toward the medial wall of the orbit. This movement of the right eye is called intorsion. The right inferior rectus muscle extorts the eye with the eye adducted.

The superior and inferior oblique muscles are attached to the globe so that their direction of contraction is at 51° to the midsagittal plane. With the eye in adduction, the superior oblique depresses the eye and the inferior oblique elevates the eye. With the eye in abduction, the superior oblique intorts the eye and the inferior oblique extorts the eye. There appears to be the same type of reciprocal innervation of eye muscles as in the rest of the body. In making conjugate movements contraction of a muscle is accompanied by relaxation of its antagonist.

The motor effects of contraction of the individual muscles with the eyes starting near the primary (straight-ahead) position is shown in Fig. 8-38, *A*. To simplify recognition of the muscles used in making conjugate eye movements, movements in six directions (the cardinal directions of gaze, Fig. 8-38, *B*) can be considered. A very important eye movement is medial downward convergence, which is used in reading. This is produced by the superior oblique (IV, depression), the medial rectus (III, adduction), and the superior rectus (III, intorsion). The near point of convergence in young persons is about 30 mm from the nose.

If the images of the fixation point do not fall on equivalent points of each retina, double vision (diplopia) results. The central input of visual information from both retinas is important in maintaining proper alignment of the eyes. In psychological terms the stimulus for maintaining alignment is maintaining fusion of the images from each eye and suppressing

divergence or blurring of the images. If one eye is covered or becomes blind, there is a tendency for the eye to abduct.

Deviation of an eye is called a squint. Although in common usage squint now means to stare through half-closed lids, an older meaning was a glance out of the corner of the eye. Another term for a deviation of the eye is strabismus (twisting). Abnormalities of eye movement are a complex subject beyond the scope of this book, and neuro-ophthalmology is a discipline in itself. Briefly, eye deviations may be divided into comitant deviations, in which the deviation of the abnormal eye is the same in all directions of gaze, and noncomitant deviations, in which the deviation becomes greater in certain directions of gaze. The origin of most of the cases of comitant deviation, such as childhood strabismus, is not understood. The noncomitant type of deviation is generally the type produced by neurological lesions.

In some cases of noncomitant deviation of the eye, the deviation may not be apparent to an observer, although the patient has diplopia. To determine which eye muscle is weak, a qualitative test, the red-glass test, can be performed. As an example, consider weakness of the right lateral rectus muscle (Fig. 8-39). When fixating on an object in right lateral gaze, there is diplopia: the patient sees two objects that are side

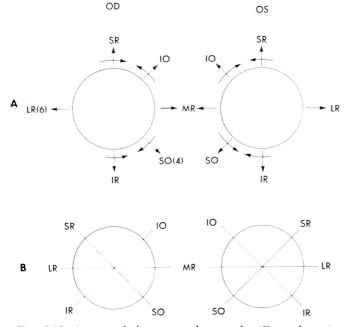

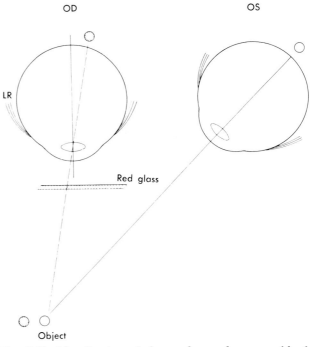

Fig. 8-38. Actions of the extraocular muscles. From the primary position, the *SO* and the *IO* each abduct the eye; however, their major functional use is as shown. **A,** Deviations (*centrifugal arrows*) and torsions (*circumferential arrows*) produced by individual muscles. **B,** Major muscles used for moving each eye in the six cardinal directions of gaze. Abbreviations: *SR*, superior rectus; *IR*, inferior rectus; *MR*, medial rectus; *IO*, inferior oblique; *SO*, superior oblique; *LR*, lateral rectus; *OD*, right eye; *OS*, left eye.

Fig. 8-39. Identification of the weak muscle responsible for diplopia, by means of the red glass test. Diplopia in right lateral gaze, caused by weakness of the right lateral rectus muscle is illustrated.

by side. This, however, could also be produced by weakness of the medial rectus muscle of the left eye. To determine which is the weak muscle, a piece of colored glass is placed before one eye, or one eye is covered. One of the two images then becomes colored or disappears. This identifies the image that is referable to the eye with the weak muscle in the following way. Because of the failure of the right eye to abduct, the image of the object falls on the nasal side of the right retina. The brain interprets this image as being in the right temporal visual field. Therefore, when the red glass is placed before the right eye, the false image, which is the farthest temporally of the two images, becomes colored and is thereby identified. In general, for the cardinal directions of gaze the image that is deviated farthest from the center of the visual field is referable to the eye with the paretic muscle.

The compensatory movements made by the head and neck and by other eye muscles in cases of nerve injury and diplopia should be mentioned. For example, when nerve IV is injured and the superior oblique muscle is paralyzed, the unopposed action of the inferior oblique muscle extorts the eye. The appearance that this injury gives the patient appears to be the origin of "nerf pathetique," the French term for nerve IV. To compensate for the extorsion deviation the patient tilts his or her head. In the case of the right superior oblique muscle the patient tilts the head to the left (opposite) shoulder. This rotation of the head is equivalent to extorting the left eye. To compensate for this extorsion, the left eye intorts. This intorsion is the conjugate movement required to match the extorsion deviation in the right eye and to restore fusion of the images from each eye.

Central control of eye movements: mechanisms in the performance of basic eye movements

The neurophysiological problem of moving the eyes, with varying degrees of conjugate and convergent activity, is one of adjusting the impulses to the twelve extraocular muscles to produce fusion of the images from each eye, to maintain fixation, and to maintain a constant orientation of the horizontal meridian of the visual field with respect to the gravitational field. Voluntary and reflex control mechanisms are used to adjust the impulses to the eye muscles. A complete description of the activities of brainstem neurons used in performing these movements has not been achieved even for what appears to be the simplest situation, conjugate lateral gaze in the horizontal plane. A tentative diagram of the brainstem pathways mediating lateral gaze, based largely on the clinical effects of lesions in disrupting gaze, is shown in Fig. 8-40. Each

half of the pons can be considered to have a center for lateral gaze, which is near the nucleus of nerve VI, although some studies have questioned the existence of this center as an entity apart from the nucleus of nerve VI. The center receives input from the contralateral cortex, probably largely from the frontal lobe eye fields, which are in the premotor cortex, largely in Brodmann's area 8. The pontine center influences the motoneurons of the ipsilateral nucleus of nerve VI and the motoneurons of the contralateral nucleus of nerve III that innervate the medial rectus muscle of the contralateral eye.

Stimulation of the frontal eye field cortex produces deviation of the eyes to the contralateral side of the body. A lesion of this cortex results in an inability to look toward the opposite side of the body, or an inability to look at the half of the visual field represented in that hemisphere. Because of the unopposed activity of the contralateral frontal lobe eye field, the eyes are deviated toward the side of the lesion. Therefore, a lesion of the right motor and premotor cortex will produce a hemiparesis of the left side of the body, with the eyes deviated to the right.

A lesion of the pons, damaging the pontine center for lateral gaze, produces an inability to look toward the side of the lesion. Therefore, a lesion of the right side of the pons that damages the right corticospinal tract and the pontine gaze center will produce a

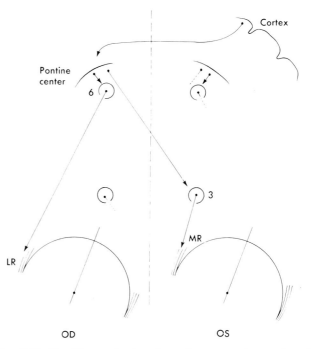

Fig. 8-40. Possible mechanism for voluntary conjugate lateral gaze. *3, 6,* nuclei of nerves III and VI; *LR, MR,* lateral and medial rectus muscles; *OD, OS,* right and left eyes.

hemiparesis of the left side of the body, with the eyes deviated to the left, that is, to the same side of the body as the weakness.

The center for vertical gaze appears to be coextensive with some part of the pretectal region. Tumors in the area of the pineal gland that compress the pretectal region can produce paralysis of upward gaze, which is one feature of Parinaud's syndrome. Although unilateral stimulation of the frontal and occipital eye fields will produce horizontal and oblique eye movements, pure vertical eye movements can be evoked only by bilateral cortical stimulation.

A number of motor activities occur simultaneously during convergence; collectively these are called the near reflex. This consists of convergence, contraction of the ciliary muscle to produce accommodation of the lens for near vision, and pupilloconstriction. How the integration of somatic motor and parasympathetic activity occurs is not known.

Mention should be made here of some aspects of the pupillomotor system. Afferents from the retina appear to synapse on interneurons in the pretectal area, which project to the parasympathetic neurons of the oculomotor nerve complex. The pupil constricts and dilates with increased and decreased retinal illumination respectively, in an attempt to keep the illumination of the retina constant. There is a certain amount of oscillation of the pupillary response (alternate constriction and dilation) in response to a step change in illumination. Oscillation of pupillary diameter, when clinically marked, is called hippus (Gk. *hippos*, galloping of a horse). Lesions in the pretectal area can produce loss of the light reflex (pupilloconstriction to light).

The pathways producing pupilloconstriction in the near reflex do not appear to go through the pretectal area. This seems to be the basis, in certain diseases, of a loss of reflex pupillary constriction to light, with preservation of pupilloconstriction during accommodation. These characteristics and an irregular, miotic pupil comprise the Argyll Robertson pupil, which is found in some cases of neurosyphilis and in some other brain diseases.

Although little is known about the cellular neurophysiology of conjugate and convergence movements, information has been obtained about some of the characteristics of voluntary and reflex control of these movements. The types of eye movements frequently made during normal daily activities are saccadic eye movements and smooth-pursuit movements, which are particular types of movement in which the conjugate and convergence mechanisms are used. Saccadic eye movements are step displacements of the eyes, such as the short jumps the eyes make when a person is reading. Saccadic eye movements can be evoked by a step displacement of a fixation point. Once a saccadic movement is initiated by a step displacement of a fixation point (target), the eye will not respond to a further change in the position of the target for about 100 to 200 msec. It should be mentioned that small involuntary movements of the eyes, which have been called physiological nystagmus, and small saccadic eye movements occur even when the eyes are fixated on a target, with the result that the image of a target point is projected onto a small and constantly changing area of the retina and not on a retinal point. Such small saccadic movements are important for normal vision; if the image of a target point is stabilized on a retinal point, which can be accomplished with optical-mechanical devices that compensate for the eye movements, visual perception of the target will fade.

In the case of smooth-pursuit or tracking movements, the visual input appears to be sampled continuously and motor output modified continuously during the movement. Cells in the frontal motor cortical eye fields have been found to fire preferentially with the occurrence of either saccadic or tracking movements, suggesting that there are control systems for each of these two types of movement.

The ability of object movement in the visual field to evoke eye movement is so strong that it has the characteristics of a reflex, in the sense of an involuntary sensory control of motor activity.

If a series of moving objects passes in front of the eyes, such as telephone poles seen from the window of a moving train or a series of vertical stripes on a rotating drum, the eyes fixate on one of the objects in the series, follow it to the mechanical limit of tracking movement, and then make a rapid return movement to be in position to track the next object in the series. This is called optokinetic nystagmus. This response may be disturbed after various brain lesions.

The other main sources of sensory (reflex) control of eye movements are vestibular and proprioceptive.

Vestibular-ocular reflexes, which are very powerful, can be divided into tonic and phasic effects. Maintaining the horizontal meridian of the visual field at right angles to the gravitational field can be described as a tonic effect. The utricle-otolith receptors are thought to be most important for this effect, which also involves compensatory movements of the head, neck, and body.

Making compensatory movements that are opposite to acceleratory movements of the head, especially rotatory movement, thereby maintaining fixation, is a phasic effect that is mediated by the semicircular canals.

The vestibular nerve projections to the vestibular nuclei of the brainstem are described in Chapter 7. The semicircular canals probably project largely to the superior and medial vestibular nuclei. The ascending projections to the MLF come largely from these two nuclei. The ascending projections of the superior vestibular nucleus are uncrossed. The descending projections to the MLF come largely from the medial vestibular nucleus, and the other major descending vestibular projection, the lateral vestibulospinal tract, comes from the lateral vestibular nucleus.

The neurophysiological details of how vestibular impulses act on motoneurons of the eye muscles are still poorly known.

Destruction and stimulation of the peripheral vestibular apparatus produce patterns of eye movement of considerable clinical importance. Destruction of a labyrinth or injury of a vestibular nerve results in unopposed activity of the contralateral labyrinth. The unopposed activity of one labyrinth produces rhythmic, slow, conjugate deviation of the eyes to the contralateral side of the body, with a quicker movement that returns the eyes to the ipsilateral side of the body. This oscillatory movement of the eyes is called nystagmus (nodding). Although it is somewhat confusing, the direction of the nystagmus, for example, to the right or to the left, is named after the direction of the quick component. Therefore, destruction of the right labyrinth will produce a nystagmus to the left, with a slow component to the right. The clinical naming of the direction of the nystagmus, not in terms of the direction of the slow component, which is the active component caused by unbalanced vestibular activity, but in terms of the quick, or compensatory, component, is probably because nystagmus usually becomes more pronounced when the patient moves his or her eyes in voluntary lateral gaze to the side of the quick component. In some cases nystagmus will be apparent only on lateral gaze. To summarize, destruction of the right labyrinth produces nystagmus with a slow component to the right and a quick component to the left, which will be intensified on left lateral gaze; this is termed nystagmus to the left.

Nystagmus is a common finding in brainstem lesions and may also be produced by disturbances of the proprioceptive input from neck muscles.

The integrity of brainstem vestibular pathways can be tested clinically by stimulating the semicircular canals and observing the eye movements produced. Movement of the cilia of the hair cell receptors of the ampullae of the semicircular canals can be produced with a physiological or natural type of stimulus by rotating the patient in Bárány's chair. However, nonsimultaneous testing of the vestibular apparatus of each ear is desirable, and vestibular testing is usually performed clinically with caloric testing, in which the eardrum is irrigated with cold or warm water, thereby producing convection currents in the endolymph of the semicircular canals. Each of the three semicircular canals can be tested individually by placing the patient's head in the position where the canal to be tested is vertical. The maximal convection current will develop in the canal that is placed in the vertical position because cold water sinks and warm water rises. The eye movements evoked by stimulation of each of the canals are in the same plane as the canal stimulated (Flourens' law). Stimulation of the horizontal canal produces horizontal nystagmus, and this canal is usually selected for the testing of the integrity of vestibulo-ocular reflexes.

To test the horizontal canal the patient is placed in a supine recumbent position, with the head flexed 30° forward. The eardrum is examined with an otoscope to be certain that it is intact. The external canal is then irrigated with cold (30° C) or warm (44° C) water (7° below or above body temperature), or with ice water. Ice water is most frequently used for quick testing, as it is a powerful stimulus.

The mechanism of production of nystagmus in caloric testing is as follows. Cold water irrigation chills the promontory of the semicircular canal and produces an endolymph convection current in the canal. If warm water is used the endolymph current will be reversed, and all of the reactions described below will be in the opposite direction.

As discussed in Chapter 7, the hair cells of the ampulla are morphologically and functionally polarized. The vestibular neurons normally have a steady rate of discharge with the head at rest, firing at a rate of about 90/sec in the monkey. Movements of the endolymph that cause the stereocilia to be bent toward the kinocilium result in an increase in the resting rate of discharge; opposite movements reduce the rate of discharge. For the horizontal canal, movement of the cupula in the direction of the position of the utricle increases the rate of discharge of the vestibular fibers from the horizontal canal. The endolymph current set up in the horizontal canal by cold-water irrigation is in such a direction as to bend the cupula away from the direction of the utricle and to reduce the firing of the vestibular neurons. Because the right and left canals work together, the effect of the contralateral unirrigated canal on eye movement becomes preponderant, producing nystagmus with the slow component away from the side of the preponderant canal.

If caloric testing is carried out by irrigating the external auditory canal with 10 ml of ice water in

10 seconds, the response occurs with a latency of about 40 seconds and has a duration of about 30 seconds.

When the right ear, for example, is irrigated with cold water, the following responses occur:

1. Vertigo, which is a sensation of the rotation of the external world around the individual. The external world appears to move in the direction of the endolymphatic current. When the right ear is irrigated, the patient has the sensation that the external world is moving to the right.
2. Past-pointing to the right.
3. Falling to the right.
4. Nystagmus, with the slow component to the right and the quick component to the left (nystagmus to the left).

The essential effects are those that are produced by turning the head to the left, with compensatory movement of the eyes to the right to maintain fixation. These effects would also be produced by stimulation of the left horizontal semicircular canal by irrigation of the left external auditory canal with warm water.

Quantitative caloric testing can be carried out using methods devised by Hallpike. In addition, the responses of the eyes can be recorded with electronystagmography. A small voltage exists between the cornea and the retina. This potential can be recorded by electrodes applied temporally and frontally. Movement of the eye produces a fluctuation in the voltage recorded. With the use of quantitative testing methods and sensitive recording techniques, the effects of lesions of cortical areas on the vestibulo-ocular reflexes can be detected by the changes they produce in the patterns of response to caloric stimulation.

BIBLIOGRAPHY
Motor systems

Abdelmoumene, M., Besson, J. M., and Aleonard, P.: Cortical areas exerting presynaptic inhibitory action on the spinal cord in cat and monkey, Brain Res. 20:327-329, 1970.

Asanuma, H., and Sakata, H.: Functional organization of a cortical efferent system examined with focal depth stimulation in cats, J. Neurophysiol. 30:35-54, 1967.

Bard, P.: Studies on the cerebral cortex. I. Localized control of placing and hopping reactions in the cat and their normal management by small cortical remnants, Arch. Neurol. Psychiatr. 30:40-74, 1933.

Bates, J. A. V.: The individuality of the motor cortex, Brain 83:654-667, 1960.

Brookhart, J. M., Mori, S., and Reynolds, P.: Postural reactions to two directions of displacement in dogs, Am. J. Physiol. 218:719-725, 1970.

Brookhart, J. M., and Zanchetti, A.: The relation between electrocortical waves and responsiveness of the corticospinal system, Electroencephalogr. Clin. Neurophysiol. 8:427-444, 1956.

Brooks, V., and Stoney, D., Jr.: Motor mechanisms; the role of the pyramidal system in motor control, Ann. Rev. Physiol. 33:337-392, 1971.

Chase, M. H., and McGinty, D. J.: Modulation of spontaneous and reflex activity of the jaw musculature by orbital cortical stimulation in the freely-moving cat, Brain Res. 19:117-126, 1970.

Deecke, L., Scheid, P., and Kornhuber, H. H.: Distribution of readiness potential, pre-motion positivity, and motor potential of the human cerebral cortex preceding voluntary finger movements, Exp. Brain Res. 7:158-168, 1969.

DeLong, M. R.: Activity of pallidal neurons during movement, J. Neurophysiol. 34:414-427, 1971.

Denny-Brown, D.: The cerebral control of movement, Liverpool, 1966, Liverpool University Press.

Evarts, E. V.: Pyramidal tract activity associated with a conditioned hand movement in the monkey, J. Neurophysiol. 29:1011-1027, 1966.

Gillingham, F. J., and Donaldson, I. M. L., editors: Third symposium on Parkinson's disease, Edinburgh, 1969, E. & S. Livingstone.

Gilman, S., and Ebel, H. C.: Fusimotor neuron responses to natural stimuli as a function of prestimulus fusimotor activity in decerebellate cats, Brain Res. 21:367-384, 1970.

Granit, R.: The basis of motor control, New York, 1970, Academic Press, Inc.

Grigg, P., and Preston, J. B.: Baboon flexor and extensor fusimotor neurons and their modulation by motor cortex, J. Neurophysiol. 34:428-436, 1971.

Grillner, S., Hongo, T., and Lund, S.: The origin of descending fibres monosynaptically activating spinoreticular neurones, Brain Res. 10:259-262, 1968.

Holmes, G.: The cerebellum of man, Brain 62:1-30, 1939.

Hongo, T., and Jankowska, E.: Effects from the sensorimotor cortex on the spinal cord in cats with transected pyramids, Exp. Brain Res. 3:117-134, 1967.

Hornykiewicz, O.: Dopamine (3-Hydroxytyramine) and brain function, Pharmacol. Rev. 18:925-963, 1966.

Humphrey, D. R.: Re-analysis of the antidromic cortical response. I. Potentials evoked by stimulation of the isolated pyramidal tract, Electroencephalogr. Clin. Neurophysiol. 24:116-129, 1968.

Ito, M., Kawai, N., and Udo, M.: The origin of cerebellar-induced inhibition of Deiters' neurones. III. Localization of the inhibitory zone, Exp. Brain Res. 4:310-320, 1968.

Kennedy, D., Evoy, W. H., Dane, B., and Hanawalt, J. T.: The central nervous organization underlying control of antagonistic muscles in the crayfish. II. Coding of position by command fibers, J. Exp. Zool. 165:239-248, 1967.

Kuypers, H. G.: The descending pathways to the spinal cord, their anatomy and function. In Eccles, J. C., and Schadé, J. P., editors: Progress in brain research, vol. XI, Organization of the spinal cord, Amsterdam, 1964, Elsevier Publishing Co.

Lassek, A. M.: The pyramidal tract, Springfield, Ill., 1954, Charles C Thomas, Publisher.

McCouch, G. P., Deering, I. D., and Ling, T. H.: Location of receptors for tonic neck reflexes, J. Neurophysiol. 14:191-195, 1951.

McCouch, G. P., Liu, C. N., and Chambers, W. W.: Descending tracts and spinal shock in the monkey (Macaca mulata), Brain 89:359-376, 1966.

McLennan, H., and York, D. H.: The action of dopamine on neurones of the caudate nucleus, J. Physiol. (Lond.) 189:393-402, 1967.

Moyes, P. D.: Longitudinal myelotomy for spasticity, J. Neurosurg. 31:615-619, 1969.

Muybridge, E.: The human figure in motion, New York, 1955, Dover Publications, Inc.

Nathan, P. W., and Smith, M. C.: Long descending tracts in man. I. Review of present knowledge, Brain 78:248-303, 1955.

Nyberg-Hansen, R.: Further studies on the origin of corticospinal fibers in the cat; an experimental study with the Nauta method, Brain Res. 16:39-54, 1969.

Penfield, W., and Welch, K.: The supplementary motor area of the cerebral cortex, Arch. Neurol. Psychiatr. 66:289-317, 1951.

Phillips, C. G.: Motor apparatus of the baboon's hand; the Ferrier Lecture, Proc. R. Soc. Lond. [Biol.] 173:141-174, 1969.

Rondot, P.: Syndromes of central motor disorder. In Vinken, P. J., and Bruyn, G. W., editors: Disturbances of nervous function, vol. I, Handbook of clinical neurology, Amsterdam, 1969, North-Holland Publishing Co.

Stark, L.: Neurological control systems, New York, 1968, Plenum Publishing Corp.

Stern, G.: The effects of lesions in the substantia nigra, Brain 89:449-478, 1966.

Stewart, D. H., Jr., and Preston, J. B.: Functional coupling between the pyramidal tract and segmental motoneurons in cat and primate, J. Neurophysiol. 30:453-465, 1967.

Thach, W. T.: Discharges of cerebellar neurons related to two maintained postures and two prompt movements. II. Purkinje cell output and input, J. Neurophysiol. 33:537-547, 1970.

Vallbo, A. B.: Impulse patterns in muscle nerve during voluntary contraction in man, Acta Physiol. Scand. 69:123-124, 1967.

Willis, W. D., and Magni, F.: The properties of reticulospinal neurons. In Eccles, J. C., and Schadé, J. P., editors: Progress in brain research, vol. XII, Physiology of spinal neurons, Amsterdam, 1964, Elsevier Publishing Co.

Wilson, V. J., and Yoshida, M.: Comparison of effects of stimulation of Deiters' nucleus and medial longitudinal fasciculus on neck, forelimb, and hindlimb motorneurons, J. Neurophysiol. 32:743-758, 1969.

Reticular formation

Berman, A. L.: The brain stem of the cat; a cytoarchitectonic atlas with stereotaxic coordinates, Madison, 1968, University of Wisconsin Press.

Bowsher, D.: Reticular projections to lateral geniculate in cat, Brain Res. 23:247-249, 1970.

Brodal, A.: The reticular formation of the brain stem; anatomical aspects and functional correlations, Edinburgh, 1957, Oliver & Boyd Ltd.

Buser, P., Richard, D., and Lescop, J.: Control of mesencephalic reticular cells through sensorimotor cortex, Exp. Brain Res. 9:83-95, 1969.

Magni, F., and Willis, W. D.: Subcortical and peripheral control of brainstem reticular neurons, Arch. Ital. Biol. 102:434-448, 1964.

Magoun, H. W.: The waking brain, ed. 2, Springfield, Ill., 1963, Charles C Thomas, Publisher.

Nauta, W. J. H., and Kuypers, H. G. J. M.: Some ascending pathways in the brainstem reticular formation. In Jasper, H., and others, editors: Reticular formation of the brain, Henry Ford Hospital Symposium, Boston, 1958, Little, Brown and Co.

Olszewski, J.: The cytoarchitecture of the human reticular formation. In Delafresnaye, J. F., editor: Brain mechanisms and consciousness, Oxford, 1954, Blackwell Scientific Publications Ltd.

Ramon-Moliner, E., and Nauta, W. J. H.: The isodendritic core of the brainstem, J. Comp. Neurol. 126:311-336, 1966.

Segundo, J. P., Takenaka, T., and Encabo, H.: Electrophysiology of bulbar reticular neurons, J. Neurophysiol. 30:1194-1220, 1967.

Shute, C. C. D., and Lewis, P. R.: The ascending cholinergic reticular system; neocortical, olfactory and subcortical projections, Brain 90:497-520, 1967.

Sousa-Pinto, A.: The cortical projection onto the paramedian reticular and perihypoglossal nuclei (nucleus praepositus hypoglossi, nucleus intercalatus and nucleus of Roller) of the medulla oblongata of the cat; an experimental-anatomical study, Brain Res. 18:77-91, 1970.

Valverde, F.: Reticular formation of the pons and medulla oblongata; a Golgi study, J. Comp. Neurol. 116:71-99, 1961.

Cerebellum

Allen, G. I., Korn, H., Oshima, T., and Toyama, K.: Time course of pyramidal activation of pontine nuclei cells in the cat, Brain Res. 19:291-294, 1970.

Bloedel, J. R., and Roberts, W. J.: Action of climbing fibers in cerebellar cortex of the cat, J. Neurophysiol. 34:17-31, 1971.

Brodal,: P.: The corticopontine projection in the cat. I. Demonstration of a somatotopically organized projection from the primary sensorimotor cortex, Exp. Brain Res. 5:210-234, 1968.

Conde, H., and Angaut, P.: An electrophysiological study of the cerebellar projections to the nucleus ventralis lateralis thalami in the cat. II. Nucleus lateralis, Brain Res. 20:107-119, 1970.

Crill, W. E.: Unitary multiple-spiked responses in cat inferior olive nucleus, J. Neurophysiol. 33:199-209, 1970.

Dow, R. S., and Moruzzi, G.: The physiology and pathology of the cerebellum, Minneapolis, 1958, University of Minnesota Press.

Eccles, J. C., Ito, M., and Szentagothai, J.: The cerebellum as a neuronal machine, New York, 1967, Springer Publishing Co., Inc.

Fox, C. A., Hillman, D. E., Siegesmund, K. A., and Dutta, C. R.: The primate cerebellar cortex; a Golgi and electron microscopical study. In Fox, C. A., and Snider, R., editors: Progress in brain research, vol. 25, Amsterdam, 1967, Elsevier Publishing Co.

Granit, R., and Phillips, C. G.: Excitatory and inhibitory processes acting upon individual Purkinje cells of the cerebellum in cats, J. Physiol. (Lond.) 133:520-547, 1956.

Larramendi, L. M. H.: Morphological characteristics of extrinsic and intrinsic nerve terminals and their synapses in the cerebellar cortex of the mouse. In Fields, W. S. and Willis, W. D., Jr., editors: The cerebellum in health and disease, St. Louis, 1970, Warren H. Green, Inc.

Llinas, R., editor: Neurobiology of cerebellar evolution and development, Chicago, 1969, American Medical Association.

Maisson, J.: The mammalian red nucleus, Physiol. Rev. 47:383-436, 1967.

Mugnaini, E., and Walberg, F.: An experimental electron microscopical study on the mode of termination of cerebellar corticovestibular fibers in the cat lateral vestibular nucleus (Deiters' nucleus), Exp. Brain Res. 4:212-236, 1967.

Obata, K., Takeda, K., and Shinozaki, H.: Further study on pharmacological properties of the cerebellar-induced inhibition of Deiters' neurons, Exp. Brain Res. 11:327-342, 1970.

Oscarsson, O.: Functional organization of the spino- and cuneocerebellar tracts, Physiol. Rev. **45**:495-522, 1965.

Sasaki, K., Kawaguchi, S., Shimono, T., and Prelevic, S.: Electrophysiological studies of the pontine nuclei, Brain Res. **20**:425-438, 1970.

Tsukahara, N., and Bando, T.: Red nuclear and interposate nuclear excitation of pontine nuclear cell, Brain Res. **19**:295-298, 1970.

Uno, M., Yoshida, M., and Hirota, I.: The mode of cerebello-thalamic relay transmission investigated with intracellular recording from cells of the ventrolateral nucleus of cat's thalamus, Exp. Brain Res. **10**:121-139, 1970.

Basal ganglia

Carman, J. B.: Anatomic basis of surgical treatment of Parkinson's disease, N. England. J. Med. **279**:919-930, 1968.

Carpenter, M. B., and McMasters, R. E.: Lesions of substantia nigra in the rhesus monkey; efferent fiber degeneration and behavioral observations, Am. J. Anat. **114**:293-320, 1964.

Dahlstrom, A., and Fuxe, K.: Evidence for the existence of monoamine-containing neurons in the central nervous system. I. Demonstration of monoamines in the cell bodies of brain stem neurons, Acta Physiol. Scand. **62**(Suppl. 232):1-55, 1964.

Frigyesi, T. L., and Machek, J.: Basal ganglia–diencephalon synaptic relations in the cat. I. An intracellular study of dorsal thalamic neurons during capsular and basal ganglia stimulation, Brain Res. **20**:201-217, 1970.

Gebbink, T. B.: Structure and connections of the basal ganglia in man, Assen, The Netherlands, 1967, Royal Van Gorcum Ltd.

Goswell, M. J., and Sedgwick, E. M.: An electrophysiological study of a topographical relationship between the caudate nucleus and the substantia nigra of the cat, Brain Res. **23**:112-116, 1970.

Hökfelt, T., and Ungerstedt, U.: Electron and fluorescence microscopical studies on the nucleus caudatus putamen of the rat after unilateral lesions of ascending nigro-neostriatal dopamine neurons, Acta Physiol. Scand. **76**:415-426, 1969.

Hornykiewicz, O.: Dopamine (3-hydroxytyramine) and brain function, Pharmacol. Rev. **18**:925-964, 1966.

Kemp, J. M.: The termination of strio-pallidal and strio-nigral fibers, Brain Res. **17**:125-128, 1970.

Leblanc, F. E., and Cordeau, J. P.: Modulation of pyramidal tract cell activity by ventrolateral thalamic regions; its possible role in tremorogenic mechanisms, Brain Res. **14**:255-270, 1969.

Locke, S.: Connexions between caudate and pallidum of man, Brain **92**:419-422, 1969.

Malliani, A., and Purpura, D.: Intracellular studies of the corpus striatum; patterns of synaptic activities in lenticular and entopeduncular neurons, Brain Res. **6**:341-354, 1967.

Nauta, W. J. H., and Mehler, W. R.: Projections of the lentiform nucleus in the monkey, Brain Res. **1**:3-42, 1966.

Olivier, A., Parent, A., Simard, H., and Poirier, L. J.: Cholinesterasic striatopallidal and substantia nigral efferents in the cat and the monkey, Brain Res. **18**:273-282, 1970.

York, D. H.: Possible dopaminergic pathway from substantia nigra to putamen, Brain Res. **20**:233-249, 1970.

Oculomotor system

Bach y Rita, P., and Collins, C. C., editors: The control of eye movements, New York, 1971, Academic Press, Inc.

Bizzi, E.: Discharge of frontal eye field neurons during saccadic and following key movements in unanesthetized monkeys, Exp. Brain Res. **6**:69-80, 1968.

Cogan, D. G.: Neurology of the ocular muscles, ed. 2, Springfield, Ill., 1956, Charles C Thomas, Publisher.

Goldberg, J. M., and Fernandez, C.: Physiology of peripheral neurons innervating semicircular canals of the squirrel monkey. I. Resting discharge and response to constant angular accelerations, J. Neurophysiol. **34**:635-660, 1971.

Rothstein, T. L., and Alvord, E. C.: Posterior internuclear ophthalmoplegia, Arch. Neurol. **24**:191-202, 1971.

Schlag, J., and Schlag-Rey, M.: Induction of oculomotor responses by electrical stimulation of the prefrontal cortex in the cat, Brain Res. **22**:1-13, 1970.

Yarbus, A. L.: Eye movements and vision, New York, 1967, Plenum Publishing Corp.

CHAPTER 9

Central autonomic control

This chapter is concerned with the regulation of visceral function by the central nervous system. The subject is very broad, encompassing much of physiology and pathophysiology. Consequently, the emphasis here is restricted to a few topics of particular concern in the clinical disciplines of the neurosciences.

A highly important topic not treated in this text is the regulation of the endocrine glands by the nervous system. The final common pathway for neuroendocrine control is through the neurosecretory neurons of the hypothalamus. These either secrete hormones directly into the circulation from terminals within the neurohypophysis or affect the hormonal activity of the adenohypophysis by means of releasing and inhibitory factors that reach the pituitary gland by way of its portal system. A subject of great future interest will be the organization of the neural pathways that modulate the activity of the hypothalamic neurosecretory neurons.

Surprisingly little is known about the details of the central neural mechanisms involved in autonomic regulation. This is undoubtedly because of both the complexity of the regulatory systems and the experimental difficulties in studying them.

The autonomic regulatory systems resemble in many of their features the somatic regulatory systems described in previous chapters. Furthermore, most visceral functions are controlled through complex mechanisms in which both visceral and somatic structures play a role. The autonomic regulatory systems are thus highly integrative.

Information on which the regulatory systems act is fed into the central nervous system by afferent fibers connected with receptor organs. In some cases the receptors lie within the central nervous system, although most receptors are located in the periphery. The centrally located receptors are generally near the ventricular system or are adjacent to capillaries where the normal blood-brain barrier is defective; that is, where the blood-brain barrier is more permeable than in other places in the brain (see Chapter 5). The cerebral receptors are therefore in an advantageous position to detect intravascular and intracranial chemical changes that might affect brain function. The output of the autonomic regulatory systems involves both the peripheral autonomic (sympathetic and parasympathetic; see Chapter 3) and the somatic outflow. Effector organs include muscle (smooth, cardiac, and skeletal) and glands. The central mechanisms of the regulatory systems include relatively simple reflex arcs at either the spinal cord or brainstem level and more complex long circuit pathways operating through higher centers of the brain, including the reticular formation, hypothalamus, and limbic areas. It now appears that the cerebellum also plays an important role in autonomic regulation.

The suprasegmental portions of the autonomic regulatory systems are often essential to the systems' proper function, especially the portions of the systems that lie in the reticular formation of the medulla. The collective term often applied to a population of neurons involved in a particular regulatory function and located in a specific region of the central nervous system is center. There are a number of such centers in the medullary reticular formation that regulate cardiovascular function and respiration (Fig. 9-1). These have been termed the vital centers, because interference with their operation may lead rapidly to death. Other centers in the pontine and mesencephalic reticular formation, in the diencephalon, and in limbic

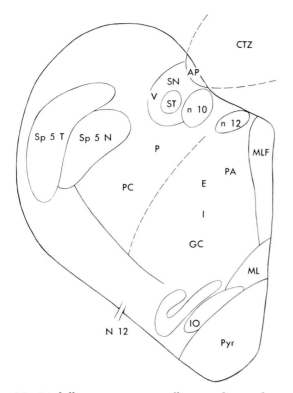

Fig. 9-1. Medullary centers controlling cardiovascular and respiratory activities. Transverse section of the medulla of the cat, rostral to the obex. Abbreviations: *V*, vomiting center; *CTZ*, chemoreceptor trigger zone; *E*, expiratory center; *I*, inspiratory center; *P*, vasopressor area; *AP*, area postrema; *SN, ST*, solitary nucleus and tract; *n 10*, dorsal motor nucleus of the vagus nerve; *n 12*, hypoglossal nucleus; *N 12*, exiting axons of the hypoglossal nerve; *PA*, paramedian reticular area; *GC*, gigantocellular reticular area; *PC*, parvicellular reticular area; *MLF*, medial longitudinal fasciculus; *ML*, medial lemniscus; *IO*, inferior olivary nucleus; *Pyr*, pyramid; *Sp 5 T, Sp 5 N*, spinal trigeminal tract and nucleus.

structures are responsible for the additional control of autonomic functions. There is a suggestion of duality of function in the diencephalon that is related to the parasympathetic-sympathetic divisions of the autonomic nervous system. The preoptic-septal areas are related to activities such as micturition and erection, in which the parasympathetic nervous system has a predominant role. The hypothalamus is related to activities such as rage and heat conservation, in which sympathetic discharge has a prominent role. No obvious duality appears in the limbic structures, whose function is highly integrative (see Chapter 10).

The descending spinal pathways that mediate most autonomic activities are the reticulospinal fibers of the anterolateral quadrants of the spinal cord.

CARDIOVASCULAR CONTROL SYSTEM

Function. The cardiovascular system is designed to deliver blood to various organs at the proper rate. The

nervous system helps to regulate blood flow through organs largely by the control of blood vessel diameter and, to a lesser extent, by changes of heart rate. The medullary vasomotor center provides the tonic excitation of the sympathetic outflow that maintains normal resting systolic blood pressure at about 120 mm Hg in young adults. If the cervical spinal cord is transected, separating the vasomotor center from the preganglionic sympathetic neurons in the intermediate column of the thoracic spinal cord, sympathetic discharge decreases and the systolic blood pressure falls to about 80 to 100 mm Hg. It is largely by modulation of the vasomotor center by the baroceptor reflexes and by descending influences that cardiovascular adjustments are made to optimize the delivery of blood to different organs during changes of activity, such as during the change from a recumbent to an erect posture.

Afferent inputs. The most important afferent input to the cardiovascular control system is from the baroceptors (pressure receptors) of the carotid sinus and aortic arch, because these receptors act as transducers in a negative feedback system for the regulation of arterial blood pressure. (The carotid sinus is the dilatation of the common carotid artery where it bifurcates into internal and external carotid arteries.) Other peripheral inputs affecting cardiovascular function can be regarded as means for altering the properties of the control system. These include other baroceptors, the arterial chemoreceptors, the lung inflation receptors, and a variety of somatic, visceral, and special sensory receptors (Fig. 9-2).

Output. The motor output of the cardiovascular control system is through the sympathetic and parasympathetic nervous systems. The intrinsic rhythm of the heart is modulated by neural control. Sympathetic action causes an increase in heart rate and in force of contraction (positive inotropic [influencing muscle] effect), whereas parasympathetic action mediated by the vagus nerve causes the opposite effects. Blood vessel diameter is regulated by a combination of factors whose importance varies with the particular vascular bed. Vasoconstriction is generally produced by sympathetic activity. Vasodilatation may be produced by inhibition of sympathetic vasomotor drive, by the activity of parasympathetic (for example, nervi erigentes to genital erectile tissue) or sympathetic vasodilator fibers (to skeletal muscle, for example), or by nonneural means, such as the production of local metabolites. Another way in which the nervous system can exert control over cardiovascular function is through the release of catecholamines from postganglionic cells in the adrenal medulla by sympathetic preganglionic fiber discharge.

Carotid sinus reflex. As mentioned above, the most important reflex in the cardiovascular control system

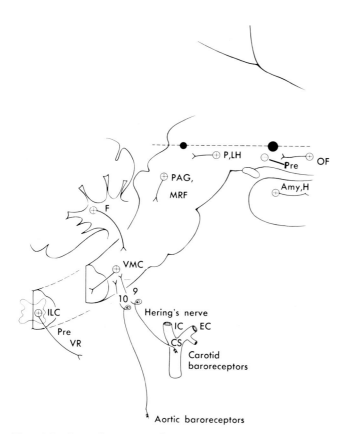

Fig. 9-2. Central areas and peripheral structures involved in cardiovascular control. Sagittal section of the brain. Sites where stimulation produces an increase of blood pressure are indicated with a plus sign; sites where stimulation or increased firing rate of a projection produces a fall of blood pressure are indicated with a minus sign. Abbreviations: *ILC,* sympathetic preganglionic neuron in the intermediate column of the thoracic spinal cord; *Pre VR,* preganglionic axon exiting in ventral root; *VMC,* medullary vasomotor center; *IC, EC,* internal and external carotid arteries; *CS,* carotid sinus; *9,* glossopharyngeal nerve; *10,* vagus nerve; *F,* fastigial nucleus; *PAG,* periaqueductal gray; *MRF,* midbrain reticular formation; *P, LH,* posterior and lateral hypothalamus; *Pre,* preoptic area; *OF,* orbital frontal cortex; *Amy,* amygdaloid nucleus; *H,* hippocampal formation.

is triggered by the systemic arterial baroceptors. The greatest amount of information about baroceptor function has been derived from studies of the carotid sinus reflex by Heymans and others. The carotid sinus reflex is normally elicited by changes in systemic arterial blood pressure. The baroceptors are slowly adapting and maintain a resting afferent discharge at normal levels of blood pressure. When the pressure within the carotid sinus is elevated, the discharge rate of the baroceptor afferents increases. This causes a reflex decrease in sympathetic discharge, a fall of blood pressure toward its original value, and an increase in the discharge of the parasympathetic fibers of the vagus nerve, which produces a decreased heart rate. Manual compression of the carotid sinus can stimulate the

carotid sinus nerve and can trigger reflex hypotension and bradycardia. These can be severe enough to produce hypoperfusion of the brain and loss of consciousness.

Reducing the carotid sinus pressure produces an abrupt rise in systemic arterial pressure. If the common carotid arteries are cross clamped, reducing the pressure within the carotid arteries at the sinus to near zero, and if the aortic baroceptors are made nonfunctional by cutting the vagi, the resultant reflex increase in sympathetic discharge will raise the systemic systolic blood pressure to 250 to 300 mm Hg in a few seconds.

The carotid sinus nerve therefore exerts a tonic inhibitory action over the vasomotor center neurons of the medulla. The site and mechanism of this inhibitory effect has not been completely clarified.

Afferent fibers of the carotid sinus nerve branch and terminate within the wall of the carotid sinus as free endings. The adequate stimulus that excites the afferents appears to be stretch of the receptor endings. The afferents include both myelinated and unmyelinated fibers that travel to the medulla in the glossopharyngeal nerve. The afferents appear to synapse both in the nucleus of the tractus solitarius and in the medullary reticular formation, particularly in the paramedial reticular area (Fig. 9-1). The activity of neurons of the nucleus of the tractus solitarius is probably then relayed into the reticular formation. The neurons involved are different from those signalling taste (see Chapter 7). One of the areas of the medullary reticular formation that seems to be involved is coextensive with the vasodepressor center, a region that when stimulated electrically causes a reduction in systemic arterial blood pressure.

Other cardiovascular reflexes. There are a number of other receptors in addition to the carotid sinus and aortic baroceptors that play a role in the cardiovascular regulatory system. These include special mechanoreceptors and chemoreceptors, as well as many nonspecific receptors in the skin and in muscle. Many of the reflex adjustments triggered by these receptors involve not only cardiovascular responses but also respiratory and other responses. For a detailed consideration of these reflexes, the student should refer to a textbook of cardiovascular physiology.

Cardiovascular centers. There are several sets of neurons in the medullary reticular formation that play a major role in cardiovascular regulation. These are called the medullary cardiac and vasomotor centers and are included among the vital centers. Different sets of neurons produce either excitation or inhibition of the heart (cardioaccelerator and cardioinhibitory centers) and either a reduction or an increase in blood pressure (vasodepressor and vasopressor centers). The actions of these centers are mediated by way of the autonomic nervous system through reticulospinal connections to the sympathetic preganglionic neurons in the upper thoracic spinal cord and by short local connections to the vagal preganglionic neurons in the dorsal motor nucleus or to cells in or near the nucleus ambiguus.

In addition to the input from peripheral receptors already discussed, the neurons of the cardiovascular centers receive important descending control from a number of higher centers (Fig. 9-2). These include the periaqueductal gray area, posterior and lateral hypothalamus, preoptic area, forebrain limbic structures, orbitofrontal cerebral cortex, and the fastigial nucleus of the cerebellum.

Clinical applications. There are a great many important clinical considerations related to the cardiovascular control system. Most of these fall outside the scope of this discussion. The ones that are mentioned here are the Cushing response, cerebellar tonsillar coning, essential hypertension, and orthostatic hypotension.

The Cushing response has been discussed in relationship to the problem of an increased intracranial pressure (see Chapter 5). The response consists of an elevation in systemic arterial blood pressure and bradycardia.

The terminal events in many individuals suffering from an increased intracranial pressure can sometimes be related to shifts in brain structures against bone or dura. Common pathological findings at autopsy in such cases are coning of the cerebellar tonsils into the foramen magnum or notching of the uncus by the tentorium. It is possible that associated with cerebellar coning there may be compression of the medullary vital centers and loss of their function, leading to death.

The cause of essential hypertension, the commonest form of hypertension, is not known, but it is possible that hyperactivity of the central vasomotor system plays a role. Methods of treatment of hypertension have utilized chemical blocking of the sympathetic ganglia to produce vasodilatation and reduce the systemic blood pressure. A recent approach to the treatment of hypertension makes use of the carotid sinus reflex as a device for lowering the blood pressure. Electrodes are implanted for long periods in the region of the carotid sinus to allow continuous stimulation of the baroceptor afferents by a device similar to a cardiac pacemaker.

Orthostatic hypotension refers to the condition resulting from a failure of compensatory baroceptor regulation of blood flow and pressure that normally occurs on assuming the standing position. Orthostatic

hypotension can be produced by sympathectomy and by the administration of sympathetic-ganglion blocking agents. Orthostatic hypotension may also be present in individuals who have sustained damage to the anterolateral quadrants of the cervical or thoracic spinal cord or both, because the descending tracts from the vasomotor centers descend with the reticulospinal fibers in the anterolateral quadrants of the cord.

RESPIRATION

Function. The respiratory system provides for the exchange of oxygen and carbon dioxide between the atmosphere and body tissues. Because the gases are transported by the blood, the control of respiration is closely linked to that of the cardiovascular system.

Although a discussion of respiratory control is commonly included in a consideration of autonomic regulation, it should be pointed out that the neuromuscular apparatus for respiration is really more akin to the somatic system. The respiratory motoneurons are not autonomic, and the muscles are skeletal in type. Furthermore, respiration is subject to a considerable degree of voluntary control. However, the close relationship between cardiovascular and respiratory function makes it convenient to discuss these systems together.

Respiratory muscles. The movement of air into the lungs is dependent on muscular activity. The chief muscle concerned with inspiration is the diaphragm. When it contracts, its dome is lowered toward the abdominal cavity, thus increasing the volume of the thoracic cage. A pressure gradient is established between the air outside the body and that in the lungs. Air flows along this gradient into the lungs through the air passages. The external intercostal muscles contribute to inspiration by elevating the anterior margins of the ribs and thus increasing the volume of the thorax. However, they are not essential to inspiration, provided that the diaphragm functions normally. During severe exercise other muscles, including the scalene and sternomastoid muscles, contribute.

Expiration during normal respiration is passive. The elastic recoil of the chest is sufficient to expel the inspired air when the muscles of inspiration relax. However, during respiratory distress, active expiration may be initiated. The main expiratory muscles are those lining the abdominal wall and the internal intercostal muscles.

Afferent inputs. There are a number of sensory receptors that provide information that can alter respiration. These include stretch receptors located within lung tissue and respiratory muscles and the chemoreceptors of the carotid and aortic bodies. There are also chemoreceptors within the medulla. Other receptors less specific to the respiratory system can also have important effects. The afferent fibers from the stretch receptors of the lungs are carried in the vagus nerves. Those from stretch receptors in the respiratory muscles are in the appropriate thoracic nerves. The afferents from the chemoreceptors are in cranial nerves IX (carotid body) and X (aortic body).

Output. The motor drive to the respiratory muscles is from motoneurons located within the ventral horn of the spinal cord. Both gamma and alpha motoneurons are involved, inasmuch as the respiratory muscles contain muscle spindles in addition to the extrafusal muscle fibers (see Chapter 2 for a discussion of muscle spindles). The diaphragm is innervated by the phrenic nerves, which arise from cervical segments 3 to 5. The intercostal muscles are supplied by branches of the intercostal nerves.

Reflexes at the spinal cord level. There are a large number of reflexes that include a respiratory component. Some of these operate at the spinal cord level and others at the brainstem level. Two are discussed here: the stretch reflex in the intercostal muscles mediated by muscle spindles and autogenic inhibition from Golgi tendon organs. The gamma loop has been found to provide an important facilitatory pathway for the discharge of alpha motoneurons to the external intercostal muscles, which assist in inspiration (see Chapter 4 for a discussion of the stretch reflex and gamma loop mechanisms). It seems likely that the diaphragm is also controlled in part by a stretch reflex.

Pontomedullary respiratory centers. Respiration cannot be maintained by spinal mechanisms alone. If the spinal cord is transected above C3, respiration

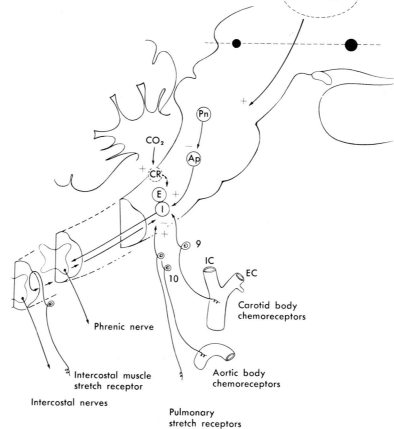

Fig. 9-3. Central areas and peripheral structures involved in control of respiration. Diagram and abbreviations as in Fig. 9-2. Sites where stimulation or activation of projections produces an increase in rate and depth of inspiration are shown with a plus sign; sites where stimulation produces a decrease are shown with a minus sign. Other abbreviations: *E, I,* expiratory and inspiratory portions of the medullary respiratory center; *CR,* presumed central chemoreceptors for CO_2; *Ap,* apneustic center; *Pn,* pneumotaxic center.

ceases. On the other hand, respiration is essentially normal if the brainstem is transected above the pons and if the cerebellum is removed. Evidently, respiration is coordinated by neurons located in the medulla and pons. A variety of experiments involving lesions, stimulation, and recordings have led to the conclusion that there are three respiratory centers in the lower brainstem: the medullary center, the apneustic center, and the pneumotaxic center (Fig. 9-3).

The medullary center can produce inspiration and expiration, although not in a normal pattern without interaction with the pontine centers. The medullary center can be subdivided into an inspiratory and an expiratory center. Electrical stimulation of the inspiratory center causes maximal inspiration; stimulation of the expiratory center results in maximal expiration. It is thought that there is a reciprocal inhibitory linkage between neurons of these two centers.

The apneustic center is in the lower two thirds of the pons. Its action can be demonstrated by destruction of the pneumotaxic center and section of the vagus nerves. When unrestrained, the apneustic center causes a prolonged inspiration. This effect is mediated through the inspiratory center of the medulla.

The pneumotaxic center is in the upper third of the pons, near the locus ceruleus. It causes an increase in the rate of respiration when stimulated electrically. The main effect is through the promotion of expiration. The function of the pneumotaxic center appears to be to provide a periodic inhibition of the apneustic center.

Inflation reflex. Stretch receptors within lung tissue, probably in bronchi and bronchioles, are activated as the lung inflates during inspiration. The afferent activity is carried to the brainstem by way of the vagus nerves. Reflex connections made by the vagal afferents by way of the nucleus solitarius and reticular formation cause an inhibition of neurons in the inspiratory and apneustic centers. Thus, distension of the lungs activates a negative feedback mechanism that limits the amount of distension. The inflation reflex (one of the Hering-Breuer reflexes, named after their codiscoverers) has a comparable effect to that of the pneumotaxic center.

Chemoreceptor reflexes. There appear to be two sets of chemoreceptors that function in respiration: the peripheral and the central chemoreceptors. The peripheral chemoreceptors are the carotid and aortic bodies. The carotid body is located at the bifurcation of the common carotid artery into the internal and external carotid arteries. The aortic body lies between the arch of the aorta and the pulmonary artery. The afferent fibers from the carotid body travel to the brainstem in the glossopharyngeal nerve, whereas those

from the aortic body are in the vagus nerve. The chemoreceptors receive a rich arterial blood supply. The details of the structure of the chemoreceptors are still under investigation. In addition to afferent fibers, the carotid body contains efferents that appear to end on granule-containing parenchymal or glomus cells. The functional relationships of the various components of the carotid body are not yet known.

The afferent fibers from the carotid and aortic bodies appear to respond to a decrease in arterial oxygen tension and also to an increase in arterial carbon dioxide tension (or to the lowered pH associated with this). The reflex effects of these chemoreceptors include an increase in both the volume of air inspired during each breath and an increase in the frequency of breathing. There are also important cardiovascular adjustments. It seems likely that an effective chemoreceptor reflex from the carotid and aortic bodies occurs clinically only with rather severe hypoxia. A role for this reflex in normal respiration has not been established.

In addition to the peripheral chemoreceptors, there are centrally located chemoreceptors. These seem to be particularly sensitive to changes in the carbon dioxide tension (or lowered pH) in arterial blood but not to lowered oxygen tension. The precise identification of the receptors has not yet been accomplished. It used to be thought that the neurons of the medullary respiratory centers were themselves the receptors. However, there is now evidence that the receptors are separate and that they detect alterations in the carbon dioxide tension of the cerebrospinal fluid as well as of the blood.

The reflex effects of an increase in carbon dioxide tension that are mediated by the central chemoreceptors include an increase in the rate and depth of respiration. Unlike the peripheral chemoreceptor reflexes, there is little effect on the cardiovascular system. A chronic increase in carbon dioxide tension may decrease the sensitivity of the respiratory centers, interfering with their responsiveness to the reflex action of the chemoreceptors.

Other respiratory reflexes. Other reflexes that affect the respiratory system include the deflation reflex (the second Hering-Breuer reflex), the response to pain and to intense cold, and many others. An alteration in respiration is the basis for several important complex reflex or voluntary acts, including vomiting, coughing, sneezing, sniffing, sighing, yawning, hiccuping, snoring, performing Valsalva's maneuver, and talking. Furthermore, respiration must be coordinated with swallowing.

Effects of higher centers. A powerful drive to respiration is produced by alertness or consciousness. The locus of origin of this drive is not clear, but it probably

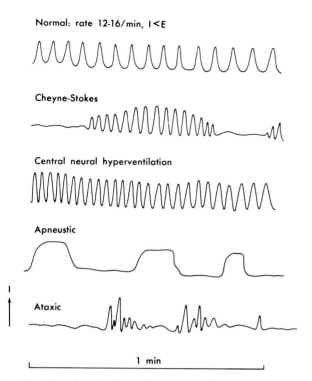

Normal: rate 12-16/min, I<E

Cheyne-Stokes

Central neural hyperventilation

Apneustic

Ataxic

1 min

Fig. 9-4. Normal and abnormal patterns of respiration. (After Plum and Posner, 1966.)

arises from thalamocortical mechanisms. Carbon dioxide and alertness are the two major drives to respiration. When an alert individual voluntarily hyperventilates about ten deep breaths and lowers arterial Pco_2 by about 10 mm Hg to about 30 mm Hg, there is a period of posthyperventilation apnea that lasts about 10 seconds, after which spontaneous respiration starts again. In the unconscious or anesthetized patient the period of apnea following lowering of Pco_2 is greatly prolonged. Another way of stating this is that the arterial Pco_2 must rise to higher than normal levels to stimulate respiration. (See the discussions below on Cheyne-Stokes respiration and undine syndrome.)

Clinical applications. Neurogenic disturbances of respiration produce changes in the depth, rate, and pattern of inspiration. The normal respiratory rate is about 12 to 16 inspirations per minute, with a tidal volume of 300 to 500 ml (Fig. 9-4). Hypoventilation caused by a decreased tidal volume may be found in patients with spinal injury, poliomyelitis, or amyotrophic lateral sclerosis, in which motoneurons, including the respiratory ones in the bulbar forms of these diseases, may die. Hypoventilation may also result from a disturbance of the respiratory centers. For instance, depressant drugs, such as barbiturates, or local anesthetics administered into the cerebrospinal fluid

for spinal anesthesia, can compromise the functioning of the respiratory centers. Changes in rate and pattern of respiration have been correlated with lesions of various levels of the neuraxis by Plum and his co-workers. Cheyne-Stokes respiration consists of trains of rapid inspirations (hyperpnea) of gradually increasing and then decreasing depth, interspersed with periods of apnea. It is seen in patients with bilateral hemispheric or internal capsule lesions in which there is a depression of consciousness. The periods of apnea appear to be the posthyperventilation apnea seen when the respiratory drive of alertness is removed.

Central neurogenic hyperventilation is a pattern of regular hyperventilation, which can be seen in patients who have midbrain lesions and who are comatose.

In apneustic breathing there are inspiratory spasms of varying length, often lasting several seconds. It is found in patients with lesions of the lower pons.

Ataxic breathing is gasping, highly irregular in rate and depth, and without order; it is also called Biot's breathing. It is seen in patients with medullary lesions. The respiratory centers are thought to be damaged in such cases, and it is usually a preterminal event.

Two types of disturbances of respiration can be produced by cervical spinal cord injury and bilateral anterolateral cervical cordotomy, in which the spinothalamic tracts are destroyed for pain relief and the reticulospinal tracts have sustained damage as well. Hypoventilation can be produced by such lesions. However, bilateral cervical cordotomy can also produce sleep apnea, or undine syndrome (undine, a water spirit; a mortal who loved an undine was punished by losing the ability to breathe when he fell asleep). The cause of sleep apnea is not completely clear. In this condition the normal hyperventilatory response to CO_2 is much reduced. When the stimulus to respiration produced by wakefulness is also removed during sleep, apnea results. The condition is often self-limited, but in some cases it may be fatal.

VOMITING

Function. Vomiting is a protective reflex that produces rapid emptying of the stomach through a contraction of abdominal muscles, coupled with a relaxation of the cardiac sphincter. The studies of S. C. Wang and his co-workers have shown that vomiting is essentially a modulated respiratory act that, like respiration, is under peripheral sensory and central chemoreceptor control.

Afferent input. Sensory receptors that induce vomiting are found in the region of the pharynx. They are supplied by the glossopharyngeal and vagus nerves. In addition, there are centrally located chemoreceptors in the medullary chemoreceptor trigger zone (CTZ) that respond to chemical agents in the bloodstream. The CTZ lies adjacent to the vomiting center proper. The CTZ is coextensive with the area postrema of the medulla, one of the regions of the brain where the blood-brain barrier is highly permeable to substances in the blood (Fig. 9-1). Visceral sensory stimuli and chemical stimuli in the bloodstream are each adequate stimuli for triggering vomiting. CTZ-mediated vomiting presumably developed as a means of emptying the stomach of harmful ingested substances before their concentration in the bloodstream reaches a dangerous level; it can be readily induced by the intravenous injection of various drugs, notably apomorphine.

Output. The motor supply includes both the somatic innervation of the abdominal muscles and the autonomic innervation of the stomach and its cardiac sphincter. The latter is inhibited.

Vomiting center. The vomiting response is organized by a center located in the lateral medulla adjacent to the solitary tract and nucleus (Fig. 9-1). Afferent impulses that trigger vomiting enter this area through the solitary tract and from the CTZ. Autonomic and somatic motor activities are integrated by this center, in an as yet unknown way, to produce vomiting. The lower esophagus and the gastroesophageal junction, the cardia, relax. There is then a strong descent of the diaphragm and passive compression of the stomach, which empties through the relaxed esophagus. It appears that neurons of the respiratory center in the medial reticular formation and the motor nuclei of the vagi are switched into a new, integrated pattern of activity by the lateral reticular formation neurons that comprise the vomiting center.

Clinical applications. Vomiting is an important response clinically, both as a protective mechanism and as a hazard. It is often useful to induce vomiting to help eliminate ingested substances, such as drugs. However, vomiting in a comatose or anesthetized patient can be life threatening. Vomiting in certain disease states, such as hyperemesis gravidarum, can be controlled by drugs that are thought to depress the vomiting center. Surgical destruction of the CTZ has been carried out in a few cases to control intractable vomiting.

SWALLOWING

Function. The mechanism of swallowing (deglutition) serves to introduce food and drink into the digestive system while automatically excluding these substances from entry into the respiratory tract or refluxing into the nasopharynx. The reflexes that occur during swallowing are complex.

The movement of a bolus of food or of a drink during swallowing is accomplished by the following sequence of actions. The base of the tongue is elevated and the oral cavity compressed, pushing the food to the pharynx. After the food enters the pharynx, muscular contractions of its wall push the food into the esophagus, which then propels its contents to the stomach. The cardiac sphincter relaxes to allow entry of the material into the stomach. During the passage of substances through the pharynx, the glottis is closed and covered by the epiglottis. The nasopharynx is occluded by elevation of the palate.

Afferent input. Swallowing is triggered by tactile stimulation of the mucosa of the palate, pharynx, and epiglottis. The sensory receptors involved may be free endings of myelinated nerve fibers. The most important afferents are carried in the glossopharyngeal nerve and in the superior laryngeal branch of the vagus nerve, although some are also in the trigeminal nerve. The afferents enter the medulla and synapse in the nucleus solitarius. The role of proprioceptive afferents from the muscles involved in swallowing is not clear.

Output. The motoneurons responsible for swallowing include several sets. Trigeminal and facial motoneurons are mostly involved in chewing rather than in swallowing. The hypoglossal nucleus contains the motoneurons that operate the tongue. The nucleus ambiguus contains the motoneurons that activate the palatal, pharyngeal, and esophageal musculature (it is not clear whether this holds true also for the smooth muscle of the esophagus, or whether this is supplied by the dorsal motor nucleus of the vagus).

Swallowing center. The act of swallowing is thought to be coordinated by a swallowing center located in the medullary reticular formation. The center ensures bilateral activity and the proper sequencing. The process appears to be initiated by a combination of reflex and volitional processes, neither of which trigger swallowing in itself.

Clinical applications. Difficulty with swallowing (dysphagia) is a characteristic of diseases affecting the functioning of bulbar motoneurons. In addition to an inability to propel a bolus of food down the esophagus, patients with dysphagia may complain of a reflux of food or drink into the nasopharynx or of these substances entering the larynx and even the lower respiratory tree. Pneumonia can result from the latter and may be the cause of death in people with bulbar palsy. Pseudobulbar palsy refers to dysphagia and dysarthria (difficulty in articulating speech) caused by damage to motor tracts descending to the bulbar motoneurons (see Chapters 8 and 12).

FEEDING

Function. The process of feeding involves the generation of hunger and thirst drives, food gathering and preparation, salivation, chewing, swallowing, and gastrointestinal and digestive activity. The setting into motion of these activities in response to sensory stimuli from the gastrointestinal tract and in response to changes in the chemical content of the blood appears to be in large part carried out by hypothalamic nuclei. However, psychological control of eating and drinking, presumably mediated by the cortex, is important both in humans and in animals.

Afferent input. Hunger sensations are in part the sensations produced by contractions of the stomach, which are transmitted by nerve X (vagus). Inhibition of feeding is produced in part by sensations of distention of the stomach. The gastric stretch receptors are very slowly adapting and continue to signal as long as the stomach is distended. Satiety is also produced by the sensations of eating and drinking. Sensations of dryness of the mucous membranes of the mouth and throat, transmitted by nerves V, IX, and X, form part of the sensation of thirst. Decreased salivary output, which occurs in response to increased tonicity of the blood, is an important factor in producing the sensations of dryness and thirst.

In addition to peripheral receptors, activation of central receptors appears to play a role both in generating sensations of hunger and thirst and in activating eating and drinking behavior. There is some evidence for receptors in the hypothalamus that respond to changes in the level of blood glucose. A fall in blood glucose will activate the motor nuclei of the vagi and produce gastric contractions. However, even when the vagi are cut, a fall in blood glucose can produce a sensation of hunger.

There are also hypothalamic receptors that respond to osmolarity of the blood. Increasing blood osmolarity stimulates these receptors and leads to decreased salivary output, a sensation of thirst, and drinking.

The activity of central receptors therefore appears both to trigger eating and drinking behavior and to produce states of intraoral and gastrointestinal activity that are sensed by peripheral receptors that in themselves trigger eating and drinking.

Output. The activities of salivation, chewing, and swallowing appear to be organized in the brainstem. Salivation is mediated by cranial parasympathetic fibers that pass through nerve IX to the parotid gland and nerve VII to the submaxillary and sublingual glands. Chewing is an automatic, rhythmic activity mediated by nerve V.

Hypothalamic eating and drinking centers. The lateral hypothalamus contains an eating center. Direct electrical or chemical stimulation here produces eating; destruction produces aphagia. The ventromedial hypothalamus contains a satiety center, which appears to inhibit the laterally placed eating center. Destruction of the ventromedial hypothalamus produces marked hyperphagia, and animals with such lesions become very obese. The satiety center is probably under both central and peripheral control.

The anterior hypothalamus contains a drinking center; destruction here produces adipsia.

Animals and humans who are deprived of certain substances in their diet, such as salt, can develop a specific hunger for these substances and will preferentially eat foods containing them. The mechanism of the development of these specific hungers is not understood.

Clinical applications. Obesity is caused by eating in excess of energy expenditure (or, simply, by overeating) in the great majority of cases and appears to be the result of psychogenic causes. Very obese persons will eat whether they are hungry or not.

Psychogenic polydipsia also occurs, although there is no particular relationship to obesity in this condition. Individuals with psychogenic polydipsia have a large urinary output. Unlike patients with true diabetes insipidus, who have a lack of hypothalamic-posteropituitary antidiuretic hormone (ADH), patients with psychogenic polydipsia can concentrate their urine when water is withheld or when various drugs are used to stimulate ADH secretion.

Certain sympathomimetic amines, such as amphetamine, can be used to suppress appetite. Their site of action appears to be the lateral hypothalamic eating center. Similarly effective drugs to stimulate appetite have not been developed.

Anorexia nervosa is an uncommon condition, generally occurring in young women, in which there is abhorrence of eating, and vomiting if feeding is forced. The condition appears to be of psychogenic origin.

REGULATION OF TEMPERATURE

Function. Body temperature in humans is maintained at quite close to 98.6° F (37° C). This refers to body core temperature, which can be regarded as heart blood temperature. Esophageal temperature can also be taken as core temperature. Rectal and oral temperatures are used as convenient approximations to core temperature. Skin temperature is usually 6 to 8 degrees cooler than core temperature.

There is no specific core temperature that is normal, and body temperature undergoes cyclic variation both during the day and over longer periods of time, as during the menstrual cycle. Some individuals have higher average body temperatures than others; however, the body temperature of most healthy individuals generally lies between 96.8° and 100.4° F (36° to 38° C). The means by which body temperature is regulated include alterations in both autonomic and somatic functions. The precision of temperature regulation in any individual is a quite remarkable example of biological negative feedback mechanisms.

Afferent inputs. Information about temperature is provided by peripheral and central thermal receptors. Cutaneous cold and warm receptors signal the temperature at the body surface (see Chapter 2), whereas thermodetectors in the central nervous system, specifically in the anterior hypothalamus, sense the core body temperature. The central thermodetector neurons have been demonstrated by the use of small thermal probes inserted into the hypothalamus.

Output. The nervous system can lower body temperature by evaporative heat loss through respiration and sweating and radiation of heat from blood in the cutaneous circulation. Heat is conserved by preventing these processes from being effective, by piloerection to improve surface insulation (vestigial in humans, accounting for "gooseflesh"), and by increased muscular activity (extreme is shivering).

Heat loss and heat conservation centers. The control of thermal balance is regulated by the hypothalamus. The anterior part of the hypothalamus appears to contain a set of neurons that coordinate the heat loss mechanisms. These neurons are, collectively, the heat loss center. Stimulation in this region produces panting, vasodilatation, and cessation of shivering; lesions here abolish the ability of the animal to lose heat. Similar experiments suggest that a heat conservation center is located in the posterior hypothalamus. Its action would be to evoke piloerection and shivering and to oppose the actions of the heat loss center.

The operation of the hypothalamic centers is dominated by the action of the central thermodetectors. The peripheral thermoreceptors provide information that is useful for eliciting local changes, such as shifts in blood flow within the skin.

Clinical applications. There are numerous important clinical considerations concerning temperature regulation. For instance, anesthesia tends to suppress the ability of mammals to regulate their temperature; it is not uncommon for the body temperature to fall during surgery. Hypothermia is used deliberately in cases in which a lowered metabolic rate is advantageous, such as during procedures when cerebral blood flow is likely to be marginal. The body is externally cooled, after induction of anesthesia, to a core temperature of about 28° to 30° C for moderate hypothermia. At temperatures below 27° C cardiac fibrilla-

tion occurs, and for deep hypothermia, to 15° C, special techniques must be used.

A rise in temperature is common with infections and many other disease states. The manner in which fever is produced in various diseases is not completely clear. Some substances, such as certain polysaccharide compounds, when injected into the bloodstream are pyrogens, which produce a rise in body temperature. Presumably these substances act directly or indirectly on the hypothalamus to inhibit the heat loss center or activate the heat conservation center or both. Often, fever commences with constriction of vessels in the skin, producing decreased skin temperature and a sensation of a chill, followed by shivering. The cutaneous vasoconstriction prevents heat loss and the shivering increases core temperature, producing the fever. The subsiding of fever is often accompanied by peripheral vasodilatation and sweating, which release heat from the body core. The mechanism of action of drugs that are commonly used to reduce fever, such as aspirin, is not understood.

MICTURITION

Function. Periodic and complete emptying of the urinary bladder is an important control function of the central nervous system. The act of micturition involves a combination of visceral and somatic activity. About 50 ml of urine per hour normally enters the bladder and progressively stretches the detrusor muscle. Despite increasing distention by urine, the intravesical pressure normally remains fairly constant until micturition is initiated, either voluntarily or reflexly (Fig. 9-5). Central inhibition of detrusor muscle tone appears to be an important aspect of the control of micturition, although little is known of how this inhibition is carried out.

Afferent input. The bladder wall contains stretch receptors that appear to be arranged in series with

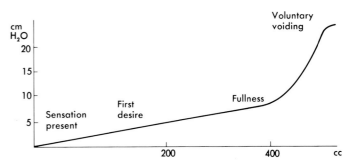

Fig. 9-5. Normal cystometrogram. Intravesical pressure as a function of volume of fluid in the bladder. Temperature sensation normally is present when the fluid first enters the bladder. The first desire to void occurs when the bladder contains about 175 ml. Fullness is felt at about 400 ml. Voiding (detrusor contraction) occurs at 400 to 500 ml.

the smooth-muscle cells. Firing occurs when the bladder stretches or when it contracts. The afferent fibers from the stretch receptors travel in the pelvic nerves to the sacral spinal cord (S2 to 4). Somatic afferents to the sacral cord also contribute information that affects bladder control (Fig. 9-6).

Output. Bladder emptying is produced by the contraction of the detrusor muscle and muscles of the

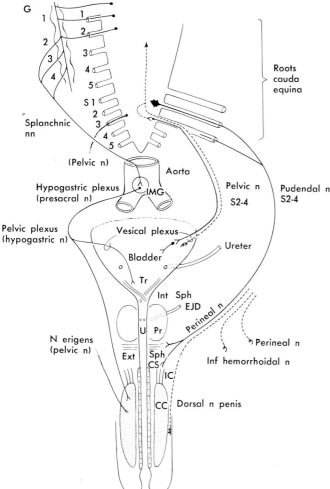

Fig. 9-6. Innervation of the bladder and the male genitals. The parasympathetic and the somatic motor and sensory innervation are shown on the right side of the diagram (with the exception of the pelvic nerve [parasympathetic nerve] supply to the genitals, which is shown, for clarity, on the left side of the diagram). The sympathetic innervation is shown on the left side of the diagram. Efferent axons, solid lines; afferent axons, broken lines. Abbreviations, sympathetic innervation: *L*, lumbar spinal cord, segments, and roots; *G*, paravertebral sympathetic ganglia; *IMG*, inferior mesenteric ganglia. Parasympathetic innervation: *S*, sacral spinal cord. Pelvic structures: *Tr*, trigone of bladder; *Int Sph*, internal sphincter of bladder; *EJD*, ejaculatory duct; *U*, urethra; *Pr*, prostate gland; *Ext Sph*, external sphincter; *CS*, corpus spongiosum of penis; *CC*, corpus cavernosum; *IC*, ischiocavernosus muscle.

abdominal wall, coupled with relaxation of the internal (smooth muscle) and external (skeletal muscle) sphincters of the bladder.

The motor supply of the detrusor muscle is provided by the sacral parasympathetic nervous system by means of the pelvic nerve. The preganglionic neurons are located in the intermediate gray matter of the spinal cord at sacral segments 2 to 4 (generally only two of these segments in a given individual). The third sacral root is generally the most important root for bladder function. The sacral parasympathetic fibers, which exit from the conus medullaris through sacral roots 2, 3, and 4, travel in the cauda equina, exit through the foramina of the sacrum, and then combine on each side of the body to form the right and left pelvic nerves respectively (Fig. 9-6). The synaptic connections with postganglionic parasympathetic neurons are made in ganglia located on or in the bladder wall. Stimulation of the pelvic nerve produces a powerful contraction of the detrusor muscle.

Sympathetic nerve fibers also supply the bladder, particularly in the area of the trigone, where the ureters enter the bladder. The preganglionic sympathetic neurons lie in the intermediate gray matter of the spinal cord, probably at T12, L1, and L2. They send their preganglionic axons through the upper lumbar paravertebral sympathetic ganglia into the splanchnic nerves, probably to the sympathetic ganglia that lie around the aortic bifurcation, such as the inferior mesenteric ganglia. The postganglionic neurons descend as the hypogastric plexus (presacral nerve), which divides into right and left pelvic plexuses (hypogastric nerves).

The pelvic plexuses and the vesical plexus are composed of a mixture of all types of nerves going to and from the bladder. The function of the sympathetic supply to the bladder is not clear. There is evidence that transmission through parasympathetic ganglia of the viscera is inhibited by stimulation of the sympathetic nerves innervating the viscera. Sympathetic stimulation has been reported to inhibit bladder contraction. There is some clinical evidence that contraction of the internal sphincter is under sympathetic control. However, micturition is not disturbed by sympathectomy, although sexual function is, as is discussed in the last section of this chapter.

The somatic motor innervation of the striated muscles of the perineal floor, including the external sphincter, comes from motoneurons that lie in sacral segments 2, 3, and 4. Their axons, after exiting from the sacral foramina, combine to form the pudendal nerve. Stimulation of the pudendal nerve constricts the external sphincter and compresses the urethra. During micturition the motoneurons of the pudendal nerve are inhibited and the external sphincter relaxes.

The mode of opening of the internal sphincter in micturition is not clear. Relaxation or opening of the bladder neck may be produced by the arrangement of detrusor muscle fibers around the bladder neck. The bladder neck appears to be pulled open when the detrusor muscle contracts under parasympathetic stimulation. It also has been suggested that relaxation of sympathetic tone is involved in opening of the internal sphincter.

Reflex emptying of the bladder. There is a sacral spinal cord reflex pathway that allows at least partial emptying of the bladder. However, the normal process of micturition involves either a long reflex loop through the brainstem or a very powerful descending facilitation of the sacral reflex. As the bladder fills, stretch receptors provide an increasing afferent input that facilitates contraction of the bladder wall. When contraction begins to occur, the stretch receptor input is enhanced, because the receptors are in series with the muscle fibers. Thus a positive feedback loop is put into operation, resulting in a complete emptying of the bladder, which then silences the stretch receptor afferents. A number of additional reflexes have also been described that facilitate detrusor contraction, such as the flow of urine through the urethra.

Micturition centers. The normal reflex operation of micturition appears to be coordinated by several centers. There is a powerful facilitatory center in the pontine reticular formation (Barrington's center). A number of other central areas have been reported to have either a facilitatory or inhibitory effect on micturition. Stimulation of the preoptic area in the cat produces powerful bladder contractions, which in unanesthetized animals are accompanied by the appropriate somatic posture for micturition. The descending motor pathways for controlling micturition lie in the anterolateral quadrants of the spinal cord. They are apparently intermingled with other reticulospinal pathways that mediate respiratory and cardiovascular activity.

Clinical applications. The functional state of the human bladder can be evaluated in detail through the use of a cystometrogram, which involves introducing a catheter through the urethra into the bladder, introducing sterile saline at either a constant rate or in fixed increments, and recording the intravesical (bladder) pressure. Observations can be made of bladder sensation, bladder capacity, and the threshold for reflex bladder contractions.

Lesions of the central nervous system, especially spinal cord lesions involving the anterolateral quadrants bilaterally, can result in the loss of function of the long pathways between the sacral spinal cord and the brainstem that normally are responsible for triggering bladder emptying. For a time after such an injury, the bladder may be atonic, not emptying of its own accord, and urine must be drained with a urethral catheter or suprapubic cystostomy. However, at a later stage the bladder may empty spontaneously, although not completely, as long as the sacral reflex pathway is intact. There may even be a lowered threshold for reflex bladder contraction (uninhibited neurogenic bladder).

If the external sphincter is weak, there may be spontaneous loss of urine (urinary incontinence). In some cases this occurs in combination with failure of detrusor muscle contraction. In such cases the bladder distends with urine until there is a moderately high intravesical pressure, at which point overflow incontinence occurs. The principal concern clinically in impaired emptying of the bladder is the likelihood of urinary tract infections caused by urinary stasis. However, the management of incontinence of urine is also a problem. One technique for control of timing of bladder contraction is the administration of cholinergic agents, such as urecholine, to induce bladder emptying.

Attempts are currently being made to develop bladder stimulators to allow emptying the bladder without the use of indwelling catheters in individuals with spinal cord injury and other causes of bladder dysfunction. This has proved to be a more difficult technical problem than the development of indwelling cardiac pacemakers. Electrical stimulation of the sacral nerve roots has not proved successful because of simultaneous activation of the detrusor muscle and the external sphincter, which closes the urethra. Implantation of electrodes directly on the detrusor muscle has met with initial success but with eventual failure of detrusor contraction caused by scarring around the electrodes.

DEFECATION

Function. Defecation serves to eliminate the solid wastes of the digestive process from the body. The control of defecation involves both visceral and somatic structures.

Afferent input. The act of defecation is triggered by stretch receptors in the wall of the rectum. The receptors appear to be arranged in series with smooth-muscle fibers, as in the bladder. Thus the stretch receptors are activated both by distension of the rectum and by contraction of the musculature. Tactile receptors of the skin and anus and the bladder stretch receptors help facilitate defecation.

Output. The muscles that produce defecation include the smooth muscle lining the rectum. In addition, the contraction of the diaphragm and abdominal wall, coupled with closure of the glottis, raises the pressure in the body cavities, thus assisting evacuation. A forced expiration against a closed glottis is called Valsalva's maneuver. The pelvic diaphragm contracts simultaneously, preventing rectal prolapse, and the internal (smooth muscle) and external (skeletal muscle) sphincters relax. The actions of the rectum and internal anal sphincter during defecation are controlled by the parasympathetic nervous system. The preganglionic fibers arise from neurons in sacral segments 2 to 4, and the postganglionic neurons are in ganglia of the pelvic plexus. The external anal sphincter is supplied by motoneurons of the sacral spinal cord through the pudendal nerve.

Defecation reflex. The process of defecation is normally initiated in response to rectal distension by feces. A series of progressively incrementing rectal contractions occurs, accompanied by relaxation of the internal anal sphincter. The organization of this reflex appears similar to that for micturition.

Higher centers. Defecation can be elicited by stimulation of regions of the diencephalon and telencephalon. A cerebral cortical influence can be either facilitatory or inhibitory. Voluntary suppression of defecation is mediated by contraction of the pelvic diaphragm and external anal sphincter.

Clinical applications. Spinal cord injuries or brain lesions may interfere with defecation, leading to fecal impaction. This is one of the management problems common to patients with neurological disease. However, it is much less serious than the problem of the neurogenic bladder.

SEXUAL FUNCTION

Function. In lower mammals the occurrence of sexual activity is largely under hormonal control. In the female in many species, the changes in the level of the gonadal hormones, estrogen and progesterone, which are associated with ovulation, induce estrous behavior and stimulate the production of various sensory cues that indicate that the female is receptive to intromission. These sensory cues trigger sexual activity in the male. In contrast, human sexual activity is largely under psychological control and is much less dependent on cyclic hormonal activity than is the sexual activity of lower mammals.

The presence of at least a basic level of circulating sex hormones is, however, necessary for libido (pleasure), or the drive to sexual activity, in both humans and lower animals. The central site of action of sex hormones in producing libido is thought to be in the hypothalamus and possibly in forebrain limbic structures as well. The relationship between levels of specific female and male sex hormones and the pattern of sexual activity exhibited (female or male, heterosexual or homosexual) is still unclear. The extent that patterns of sexual behavior are determined genetically, by the influence of gonadal hormones on the developing nervous system, or by early experience and learning is also unclear.

In a restricted sense sexual function can be regarded as those activities essential to reproduction. In the male this activity can be divided into two stages: erection and ejaculation, which consist of the phase of glandular secretion of seminal fluid and the phase of ejaculation (to cast out) and the sensations of orgasm. The process of sexual arousal and orgasm can be considered homologous in the female. Although there is no ejaculation, there is a phase of vulval glandular secretion that probably is controlled in the same way in which the periurethral glands in the male secrete the seminal fluid.

Afferent input. The nerve supply to the genital organs in the female and male follow essentially the same pattern. The clitoris and vagina and the penis are supplied by branches of the pudendal nerve, which arises from sacral segments 2, 3, and 4 (Fig. 9-6). The reflex center for erection and ejaculation to which these afferents project appears to be in the sacral segments. Both the parasympathetic and somatic motoneurons are involved. In addition the participation of the sympathetic neurons of the lower thoracic and upper lumbar cord appears to be essential for normal sexual function.

Some sensory fibers probably run with both the parasympathetic and the sympathetic nerves to the genitalia.

Output. The response to sexual arousal, produced by psychological means and by genital stimulation, can be regarded as essentially similar in both the female and the male. In initial stage of erection, or engorgement, the vessels of the genital erectile tissue of the clitoris and of the penis (the paired corpora cavernosa and the periurethral corpus spongiosum) become engorged with blood. The mechanism of engorgement (called potency in the male) is not definitely known. The vascular engorgement appears to be in part mediated by the parasympathetic neurons of sacral segments 2, 3, and 4, which pass through the pelvic nerve and then to the genitals (nervus erigentes, erecting). However, the somatic motoneurons of the same sacral segments, which innervate the bulbocavernous and ischiocavernous muscles through branches of the pudendal nerve, also appear to aid in engorgement by compressing the venous outflow from the erectile tissue. Finally, the sympathetic nervous system plays a role, although the nature of the action of the sympathetic nerves is not completely clear. The course of sympathetic fibers to the genital organs is similar to that taken by sympathetic fibers to the bladder (Fig. 9-6). In a large percentage of males with bilateral thoracolumbar sympathectomy there will be a decrease or loss of erection and ejaculation. Less is known about the effect of sympathectomy on sexual function in the female.

As indicated above, the reflex center for erection appears to be in the sacral spinal cord, with possibly a sympathetic center involved in the thoracic cord. It is likely that the reflex functions of these centers are not dependent on the circulating level of sex hormones, as erection can occur in the infant. The influence of the sex hormones appears to be on libido, or the psychogenic drive to sexual activity, which engages or drives these centers by means of pathways that lie in the anterolateral quadrants of the spinal cord.

The phase of ejaculation also appears to involve integration of parasympathetic, sympathetic, and somatic motor activity. The emission of prostatic and vesicular fluid appears to be stimulated by sympathetic discharge. The smooth muscles of the ductus deferens, seminal vesicles, and ejaculatory ducts, which constrict in peristaltic activity to propel semen, also appear to be under sympathetic control. It is likely that distention of the urethra with semen is a stimulus for ejaculation. The internal sphincter of the bladder is thought to constrict during ejaculation. It is not definitely known if this activity is under sympathetic or parasympathetic control. In orgasm, the striated muscles of the pelvic floor contract spasmodically, and these contractions in the male are part of the mechanism of ejaculation.

Little is known of the central mechanisms that control sexual arousal. Electrical stimulation of the preoptic and septal areas in the monkey can produce penile erection. Increased sexual activity has been reported to be produced by bilateral amygdaloid nucleus lesions and by lesions of the adjacent piriform cortex (see Chapter 10).

Clinical applications. Damage to the sacral spinal cord, the pelvic nerves, or the lower thoracic and upper lumbar sympathetic outflow will interfere with potency and ejaculation. The damage must generally be bilateral to produce complete loss of function. In cases of such damage a neurogenic bladder is generally also present.

Loss of erection, or at least of psychogenically driven erection, is an early sign of spinal cord compression. Bilateral anterolateral quadrant cordotomy can also produce loss of potency by damaging descending reticulospinal projections. Nevertheless, erec-

tion can occur in the presence of transection of the spinal cord. In acute cervical spinal cord injury, acute spontaneous erection may occur, lasting many hours (priapism). It is not known if this is a release or an irritative phenomenon. In men with long-standing transection of the spinal cord at the cervical or upper thoracic levels, reflex erection and ejaculation can occur.

Retrograde ejaculation, or orgasm without external emission of semen (the semen enters the bladder), is seen in some patients, who usually exhibit some additional disturbances of bladder and sexual function, generally on the basis of a neuropathy, such as diabetic neuropathy, affecting the pelvic nerves. In retrograde ejaculation it is thought that the internal sphincter of the bladder fails to close during ejaculation, allowing semen to enter the bladder.

BIBLIOGRAPHY
General

Appenzeller, O.: The autonomic nervous system, Amsterdam, 1970, North-Holland Publishing Co.
Hess, W. R.: The functional organization of the diencephalon, New York, 1957, Grune & Stratton, Inc.
Monnier, M.: Functions of the nervous system, vol. 1, General physiology, autonomic functions, Amsterdam, 1968, Elsevier Publishing Co.

Cardiovascular control system

Enoch, D. M., and Kerr, F. W. L.: Hypothalamic vasopressor and vesicopressor pathways. II. Anatomic study of their course and connections, Arch. Neurol. **16**:307-320, 1967.
Folkow, B., Heymans, C., and Neil, E.: Integrated aspects of cardiovascular regulation. In Circulation, vol. 3, Handbook of physiology, sect. 2, Washington, D.C., 1965, American Physiological Society.
Korner, P. I.: Integrative neural cardiovascular control, Physiol. Rev. **51**:312-367, 1971.
Miura, M., and Reis, D. J.: The paramedial reticular nucleus; a site of inhibitory interaction between projections from fastigial nucleus and carotid sinus nerve acting on blood pressure, J. Physiol. (Lond.) **216**:441-460, 1971.
Pickering, G.: High blood pressure, ed. 2, New York, 1968, Grune & Stratton, Inc.

Respiration

Andersen, P., and Sears, T. A.: Medullary activation of intercostal fusimotor and alpha motoneurones, J. Physiol. (Lond.) **209**:739-755, 1970.
Biscoe, T. J.: Carotid body; structure and function, Physiol. Rev. **51**:437-495, 1971.
Cohen, M. I.: How respiratory rhythm originates; evidence from discharge patterns of brainstem respiratory neurons. In Porter, R., editor: Ciba Foundation Hering-Breuer Centenary Symposium; breathing, London, 1970, J. & A. Churchill.
Comroe, J. H.: Physiology of respiration, Chicago, 1965, Year Book Medical Publishers, Inc.
Fencl, V., Heisey, S. R., Held, D., and Pappenheimer, J. R.: Role of cerebrospinal fluid in the respiratory response to CO_2 as studied in unanesthetized goats. In Brooks, C. McC., Kao,

F. F., and Lloyd, B. B., editors: Cerebrospinal fluid and the regulation of respiration, Philadelphia, 1965, F. A. Davis Co.

Plum, F., and Alvord, E. C., Jr.: Apneustic breathing in man, Arch. Neurol. **10**:101-112, 1964.

Vomiting

Borison, H. L., and Wang, S. C.: Functional localization of central coordinating mechanism for emesis in the cat, J. Neurophysiol. **12**:305-313, 1949.

Roth, G. I., Walton, P. L., and Yamamoto, W. S.: Area postrema; abrupt EEG synchronization following close intra-arterial perfusion with serotonin, Brain Res. **23**:223-233, 1970.

Swallowing

Doty, R. W.: Neural organization of deglutition. In Alimentary canal, vol. 4, Handbook of physiology, sect. 6, Washington, D.C., 1968, American Physiological Society.

Feeding

Anand, B. K., and Pillai, R. V.: Activity of single neurones in the hypothalamic feeding centres; effect of gastric distention, J. Physiol. (Lond.) **192**:63-77, 1967.

Andersson, B.: Thirst—and brain control of water balance, Am. Sci. **59**:408-415, 1971.

Davenport, H. W.: Physiology of the digestive tract, Chicago, 1961, Year Book Medical Publishers, Inc.

Eliasson, S. G.: Central control of digestive function. In: Neurophysiology, vol. 2, Handbook of physiology, sect. 1, Washington, D.C., 1960, American Physiological Society.

Grossman, S. P.: A neuropharmacological analysis of hypothalamic and extrahypothalamic mechanisms concerned with the regulation of food and water intake, Ann. N. Y. Acad. Sci. **157**:902-917, 1969.

Kerr, F. W. L., and Preshaw, R. M.: Secretomotor function of the dorsal motor nucleus of the vagus, J. Physiol. (Lond.) **205**:405-415, 1969.

Mason, G. R., and Nelsen, T. S.: Gastric secretory and motor responses to anterior hypothalamic stimulation, Am. J. Physiol. **217**:1771-1775, 1969.

Vincent, J. D., and Hayward, J. N.: Activity of single cells in the osmoreceptor-supraoptic nuclear complex in the hypothalamus of the waking rhesus monkey, Brain Res. **23**:105-108, 1970.

Regulation of temperature

Atkins, E.: Pathogenesis of fever, Physiol. Rev. **40**:580-646, 1960.

Hardy, J. D., Hellon, R. F., and Sutherland, K.: Temperature sensitive neurones in the dog's hypothalamus, J. Physiol. (Lond.) **175**:242-253, 1964.

Hayward, J. N., and Baker, M. A.: A comparative study of the role of the cerebral arterial blood in the regulation of brain temperature in live mammals, Brain Res. **16**:417-440, 1969.

Keefer, C. S., and Leard, S. E.: Prolonged and perplexing fevers, Boston, 1955, Little, Brown and Co.

Strom, G.: Central nervous regulation of body temperature. In: Neurophysiology, vol. 2, Handbook of physiology, sect. 1, Washington, D.C., 1960, American Physiological Society.

Tachibana, S.: Relation between hypothalamic heat production and intra- and extracranial circulatory factors, Brain Res. **16**:405-416, 1969.

Micturition and defecation

Barrington, F. J. F.: The component reflexes of micturition in the cat. III. Brain **64**:239-243, 1941.

Bors, E., and Comarr, A. E.: Neurological urology, Baltimore, 1971, University Park Press.

De Groat, W. C., and Ryall, R. W.: Reflexes to sacral parasympathetic neurones concerned with micturition in the cat, J. Physiol. (Lond.) **200**:87-108, 1969.

Kuru, M.: Nervous control of micturition, Physiol. Rev. **45**:425-494, 1965.

Ruch, T. C.: Central control of the bladder. In: Neurophysiology, vol. 2, Handbook of physiology, sect. 1, Washington, D.C., 1960, American Physiology Society.

Sexual function

Beach, F. A.: A review of physiological and psychological studies of sexual behavior in mammals, Physiol. Rev. **27**:240-307, 1947.

Chhina, G. S., and Anand, B. K.: Responses of neurones in the hypothalamus and limbic system to genital stimulation in adult and immature monkeys, Brain Res. **13**:511-521, 1969.

Green, J. D., Clemente, C. D., and DeGroot, J.: Rhinencephalic lesions and behavior in cats; an analysis of the Klüver-Bucy syndrome with particular reference to normal and abnormal sexual behavior, J. Comp. Neurol. **108**:505-545, 1957.

Harris, G. W.: Hormonal differentiation of the developing central nervous system with respect to patterns of endocrine function, Philos. Trans. R. Soc. Lond. [Biol. Sci.], **259**:165-178, 1970.

Kinsey, A. C., Pomeroy, W. B., Martin, C. E., and Gebhard, P. H.: Sexual behavior in the human female, Philadelphia, 1953, W. B. Saunders Co.

MacLean, P. D., and Ploog, D. W.: Cerebral representation of penile erection, J. Neurophysiol. **25**:29-55, 1962.

Masters, W. H., and Johnson, V.: Human sexual response, Boston, 1966, Little, Brown and Co.

Limbic structures

The term limbic lobe was used by the French physician P. Broca to designate the structures on the limbus, or margin, of the neocortex. These structures lie in a C-shaped arc on the medial and basilar surface of the cerebral hemispheres, surrounding the lateral ventricles (Figs. 10-1 to 10-4).

Limbic cortical areas have reciprocal connections with medially and ventrally located diencephalic and mesencephalic structures: the anterior and medial dorsal thalamic nuclei, the preoptic area, the hypothalamus, and the midline nuclei of the midbrain.

There are physiological as well as anatomical facts that make it logical to discuss these areas together and to treat them as a group of related systems, while not ignoring the interdependence of limbic structures on other parts of the brain.

The rostral and ventral portions of the limbic cortex developed as a sensory cortex for olfaction in primitive vertebrates. However, only a small portion of limbic cortical and subcortical structures receive direct olfactory input in higher mammals. The larger, nonolfactory portions of the limbic structures appear to modulate sympathetic and parasympathetic activity by affecting hypothalamic and mesencephalic neurons that also control autonomic activity. The type of modulation exerted appears to be an integration of autonomic and somatic motor activity into complex behavior that we recognize as emotional behavior. Sexual activity and expression of aggression appear to be particularly related to limbic structures. Limbic structures also appear to be important in some parts of the process of learning and memory.

ANATOMICAL ORIENTATION

The anatomy of the limbic structures is particularly complex. Several approaches have been used to attempt to classify limbic structures and to relate them to each other according to a general principle, such as evolutionary development, relationship to olfaction, or their connections. In this section the structures usually classified as limbic are enumerated; in the following sections they are related to each other according to the major projections. The major limbic structures are as follows:

1. Olfactory bulb
2. Olfactory tract, medial and lateral olfactory striae, anterior olfactory nucleus
3. Anterior perforated substance, diagonal band region
4. Rostral parahippocampal gyrus, uncus, prepiriform cortex, and periamygdaloid cortex
5. Amygdaloid nucleus: corticomedial and basolateral nuclei; stria terminalis, and ventral amygdalofugal pathways
6. Parahippocampal gyrus, subiculum (entorhinal cortex)
7. Hippocampal formation: dentate gyrus, Ammon's horn, fornix, hippocampal commissure

At the rostral and basal portion of the skull the fibers of the olfactory nerve enter the olfactory bulb (see Chapter 7). The olfactory tract is composed largely of the efferent axons of the mitral cells of the olfactory bulb. The olfactory tract passes caudally in

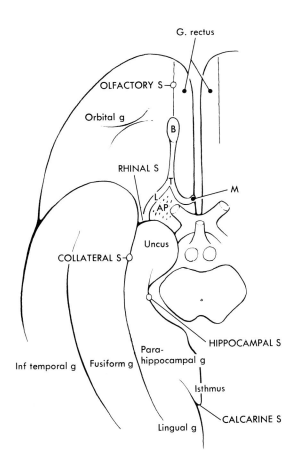

the olfactory sulcus (Figs. 10-1 and 10-2). At the level of the anterior perforated substance the olfactory tract divides into lateral and medial striae; an intermediate stria can be seen in some brains. The area of the anterior perforated substance in humans is thought to be homologous with the olfactory tubercle of lower mammals.

Posterior and lateral to the anterior perforated substance, the lateral olfactory tract enters the rostral portion of the parahippocampal gyrus. (This gyrus is sometimes called the hippocampal gyrus, a term that tends to confuse it with the hippocampus proper, described on p. 374.) The cortex of the rostral part of the parahippocampal gyrus has connections different from those in the cortex of the more caudal part of the gyrus; the lateral part is called the gyrus ambiens, and the medial part is called periamygdaloid cortex, near the uncus. The gyrus ambiens and the gray matter over the lateral olfactory stria together constitute

Fig. 10-1. Frontal and temporal lobe structures at the base of the brain. Right cerebral hemisphere. Abbreviations: *g,* gyrus; *S,* sulcus; *AP,* anterior perforated substance; *B,* olfactory bulb; *T,* olfactory tract; *L, M,* lateral and medial olfactory striae.

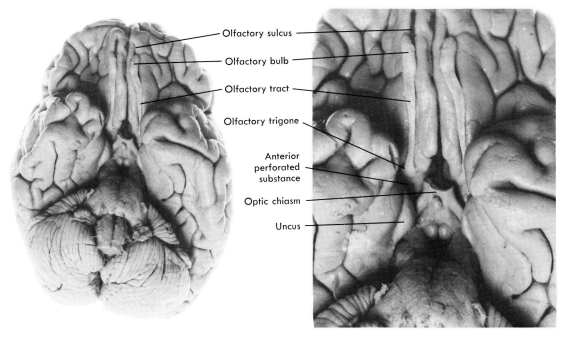

Fig. 10-2. Olfactory structures of the basal telencephalon, shown in two enlargements of the base of the brain. The olfactory bulb and tract are indicated. The olfactory tract splits into the lateral and medial olfactory striae at the olfactory trigone. Part of the olfactory receiving area of the cerebral cortex is in the anterior perforated substance, and part is adjacent to the uncus. Other olfactory tract connections are to the parolfactory and paraterminal gyri, which are just rostral to the lamina terminalis and the anterior commissure, deep to the optic chiasm.

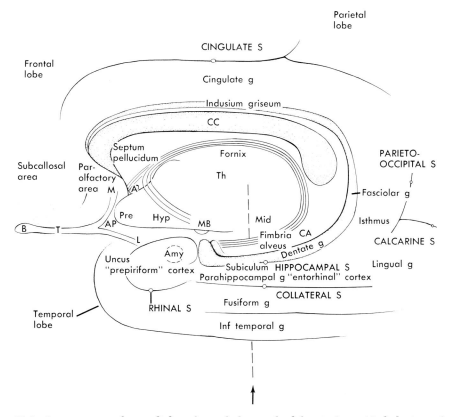

Fig. 10-3. Structures on the medial surface of the cerebral hemisphere. Medial view of the right hemisphere. The vertical line *(arrow)* indicates the plane of the transverse section shown in Fig. 10-9. The term prepiriform area can be used in a more restricted sense to apply to the gray matter along the lateral olfactory stria in the posterior orbital cortex–sphenoidal area. This cortex blends into the cortex of the rostral parahippocampal gyrus, adjacent to the hook of the uncus, which some authors term piriform area. Abbreviations: *g,* gyrus; *S,* sulcus; *CA,* cornu Ammon, covered by the fibers of the fimbria and the alveus; *CC,* corpus callosum; *A,* anterior commissure; *Amy,* amygdaloid nucleus; *Th,* thalamus; *Pre,* preoptic area; *Hyp,* hypothalamus; *MB,* mamillary body; *Mid,* midbrain; *B,* olfactory bulb; *T,* olfactory tract; *L, M,* lateral and medial striae; *AP,* anterior perforated substance.

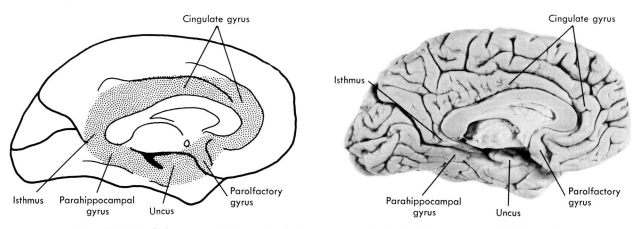

Fig. 10-4. Medial aspect of the cerebral hemisphere with the brainstem removed. The gyri belonging to the limbic lobe are indicated. These gyri include the cingulate gyrus, the parahippocampal gyrus, and the uncus. The region that bridges between the cingulate and parahippocampal gyri is termed the isthmus.

the prepiriform cortex. The gyrus ambiens is continuous caudally with the entorhinal area of the parahippocampal gyrus. The prepiriform cortex, periamygdaloid cortex, and entorhinal area together are equivalent to the piriform (pear-shaped) lobe of lower mammals. The piriform lobe is prominent in macrosmatic animals, those having a well-developed olfactory sense. The rostral parahippocampal gyrus is separated from the orbitofrontal cortex by the rhinal sulcus. The rostromedial part of the gyrus is

hook shaped and is therefore called the uncus. The uncus lies at the edge of the tentorium adjacent to the midbrain. In cases of expanding masses of the cerebral hemispheres the uncus may herniate through the tentorium, compressing the midbrain (see Chapter 12). The uncus is frequently mentioned in neuropathology, although very little is known about its normal function.

The amygdaloid (almond-shaped) nucleus lies beneath the cortex of the uncus, slightly rostral to the

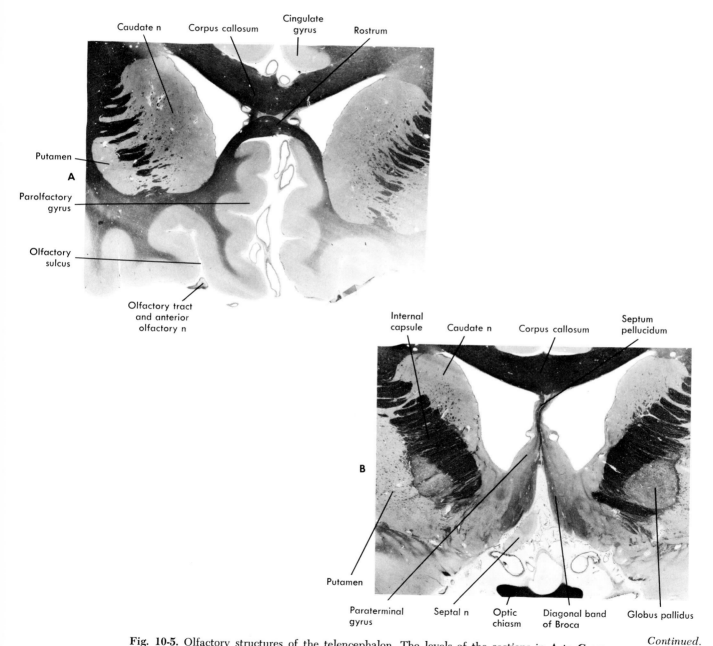

Fig. 10-5. Olfactory structures of the telencephalon. The levels of the sections in **A** to **C** are shown on the brain in **D**. The olfactory regions shown include the olfactory tract and anterior olfactory nucleus, the parolfactory gyrus, the paraterminal gyrus and diagonal band of Broca, and the amygdaloid nucleus.

Continued.

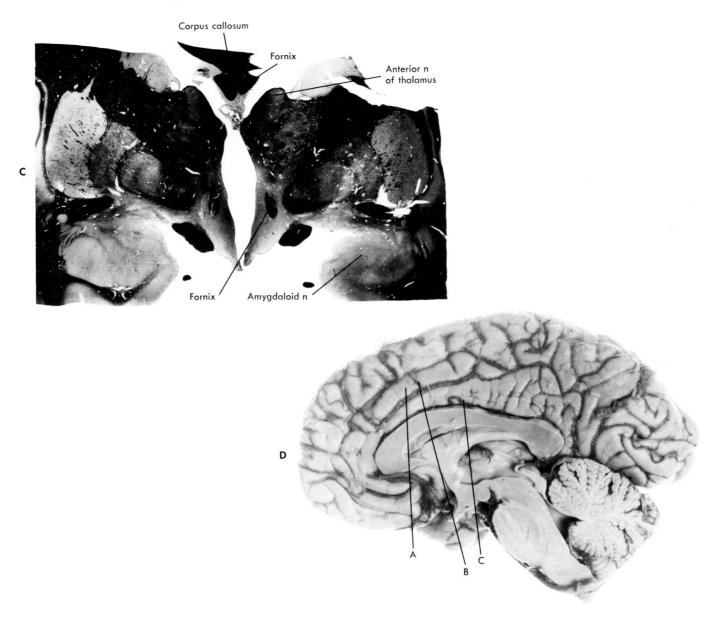

Corpus callosum

Fornix

Anterior n
of thalamus

C

Fornix   Amygdaloid n

D

A

B

C

Fig. 10-5, cont'd. For legend see p. 371.

hippocampal formation and to the tip of the temporal horn of the lateral ventricle. The amygdaloid nucleus can be divided into corticomedial and basolateral groups of nuclei. The corticomedial groups receive olfactory input. The efferent projection of the amygdaloid nucleus is through the stria terminalis and ventral amygdalofugal pathways. The stria terminalis arches around the ventricular system in a course that is similar to that taken by the efferent projection of the hippocampus, the fornix. However, the stria terminalis lies in the lateral wall of the ventricle in the groove at the medial edge of the caudate nucleus, whereas the fornix lies medially and superiorly in the

roof of the ventricle below the corpus callosum for most of its trajectory (Fig. 10-5).

The medial olfactory stria passes medially along the anterior perforated substance and merges with the parolfactory gyrus and the paraterminal gyrus. The parolfactory gyrus is a continuation of the cingulate gyrus beneath the genu and rostrum of the corpus callosum (Fig. 10-5, *A*). The paraterminal gyrus, or precommissural septum, is a zone of primitive cortex found along the rostral margin of the lamina terminalis and the anterior commissure (Fig. 10-5, *B*). It is comparable in part to the septal region in lower mammals.

Between and caudal to the lateral and medial olfactory striae is the anterior perforated substance. The name is derived from the numerous branches of the middle and anterior cerebral arteries, which enter the brain through this region. The caudal margin of the anterior perforated substance is formed by the diagonal band of Broca, which runs along the edge of the optic tract. The diagonal band courses between the periamygdaloid cortex and the par021 paraterminal gyrus.

The foregoing structures related directly to olfaction can properly be called rhinencephalic, although this term is often used in a wider sense to refer to all limbic structures.

The major portion of the parahippocampal gyrus, the part that is often referred to as the hippocampal gyrus, is called the entorhinal area. It does not receive direct olfactory input but receives fibers from the area of the uncus. The collateral sulcus is the lateral border of the parahippocampal gyrus, which separates it from the occipitotemporal (fusiform) gyrus.

The hippocampal sulcus is the medial border of the parahippocampal gyrus, which separates it from the hippocampal formation. The latter can be considered to have only three cell layers (archicortex). The parahippocampal gyrus has a transitional structure (paleocortex) that is like six-layered cortex in the lateral part of the gyrus and tends toward three-layered cortex in the medial part of the gyrus. (Archicortex and paleocortex equal the allocortex, in contrast to isocortex or neocortex.) The medial portion of the parahippocampal gyrus is called the subiculum (a layer). Afferents enter the hippocampal formation through it.

The hippocampal formation consists of the dentate gyrus and Ammon's horn (Fig. 10-3). Ammon's horn (CA, cornu ammonis) is itself often called the hippocampus. Some authors include the subiculum as part of the hippocampal formation. The dentate gyrus and CA are cortical gyri that are interlocked in a complex manner. Their structure is described in the section on the hippocampal formation. The dentate gyrus is continuous with the fasciolar (little band) gyrus, which is continuous with the supracallosal gyrus (indusium griseum, gray undergarment). This is a vestigial gyrus in humans; in rodents, however, which are much used in research on limbic structures, a considerable portion of the hippocampal formation lies above the corpus callosum. The growth of the neocortex and the corpus callosum in primates and humans appears to relegate the hippocampal formation to a largely ventral, medial, and temporal position. The gray matter of the cortex of CA is covered by axons that are largely efferent, although there are

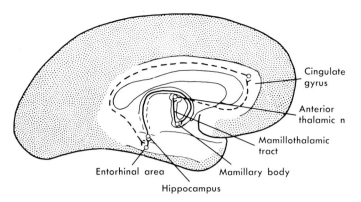

Fig. 10-6. Limbic circuit involving the hippocampus. The hippocampus is shown to receive input from the entorhinal area. Its output is through the fornix and in part to the mamillary body. One of the projections of the mamillary body is to the anterior thalamic nucleus, which in turn is connected with the cingulate gyrus. The cingulate gyrus has a return path to the entorhinal area through the cingulum. Other connections are made by each of the components of the circuit.

afferents as well, which in different portions of their trajectories are called the alveus and the fimbria. The axons finally collect into a thick bundle, the fornix (arch). The fornix arches over the roof of the third ventricle to terminate in part at the level of the anterior commissure in precommissural and postcommissural areas and then passes through the hypothalamus to end largely in the mamillary nuclei (Fig. 10-6). The fornix also contains afferent fibers to the hippocampal formation.

The hippocampal formations of each hemisphere are connected by a fiber bundle, the hippocampal commissure, or psalterium, which lies under the caudal part of the fornix.

The telencephalic limbic structures are related to the following areas:

Neocortex: the cingulate gyrus and the cortex at the junction of the orbital, insular, and medial anterior temporal gyri. The uncinate fasciculus connects the orbitofrontal cortex with the temporal cortex.
Diencephalon: in the thalamus, the anterior and the medial dorsal nuclei.
Hypothalamus: the preoptic, anterior hypothalamic, ventromedial hypothalamic, lateral hypothalamic, and mamillary nuclei. In humans the septum pellucidum is a thin structure with an insignificant number of neurons; however, in lower mammals the septum is thicker and receives limbic projections.
Midbrain: the habenular, interpenduncular, and raphe nuclei, the tegmental nuclei of Gudden, the periaqueductal gray matter.

OLFACTORY PROJECTIONS

The olfactory pathways of the limbic system are summarized in Fig. 10-7. Olfactory hair cells project

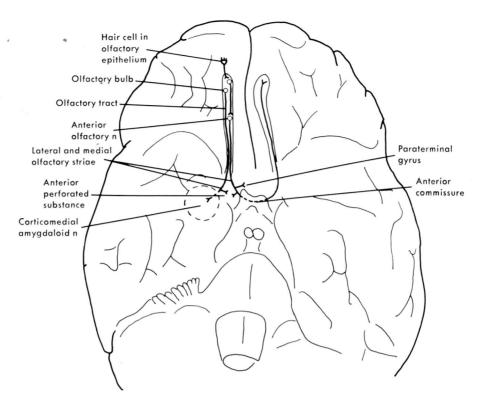

Fig. 10-7. Olfactory pathways. The connection of an olfactory hair cell with the olfactory bulb is shown. Mitral and tufted cells project caudally along the olfactory tract, as indicated, with either a direct connection with the olfactory cortex or with a relay in the anterior olfactory nucleus. The lateral olfactory stria projections terminate in the anterior perforated substance, prepiriform cortex, and corticomedial amygdaloid nucleus. The medial olfactory stria projects to the anterior perforated substance and the paraterminal gyrus; some fibers also decussate in the anterior commissure and turn rostrally into the contralateral olfactory tract.

through the olfactory nerves to the olfactory bulb. The output from the olfactory bulb is by way of the axons of mitral and tufted cells. For details about the interconnections within the olfactory bulb, see Chapter 7. The axons pass caudally in the olfactory tract. Some axons synapse on neurons within the olfactory tract that form the anterior olfactory nucleus; other axons continue directly to synapse in the primary olfactory receiving areas. Axons from the anterior olfactory nucleus also project to the olfactory cortex. The olfactory tract splits into lateral and medial olfactory striae. Fibers in the lateral olfactory stria end in the lateral part of the anterior perforated substance, the prepiriform cortex, and the corticomedial part of the amygdaloid nucleus. The entorhinal area does not get direct olfactory projections, but relayed olfactory information; it is thus an olfactory association area. Olfactory axons in the medial olfactory stria terminate in the anterior perforated substance and probably also in the paraterminal gyrus (precommissural septum). Some cross in the anterior commissure and turn rostrally in the contralateral olfactory tract to

end in the anterior olfactory nucleus and the olfactory bulb. It is of interest that the olfactory system is the one sensory pathway that does not utilize a thalamic relay.

HIPPOCAMPAL FORMATION
Structure

The hippocampal formation consists of the dentate gyrus and Ammon's horn (CA), or the hippocampus (Table 10-1). The term Ammon's horn derives from Amon (Amun), the Egyptian deity who was especially

Table 10-1. Structure of the hippocampal formation

Dentate gyrus	Ammon's horn
Molecular layer	Molecular layer
	Tangential fibers
	Stratum lacunosum fibers
Granular layer	Pyramidal layer
	Stratum radiatum
	Stratum pyramidale, or lucidum
Polymorphic layer	Polymorphic layer, or stratum oriens

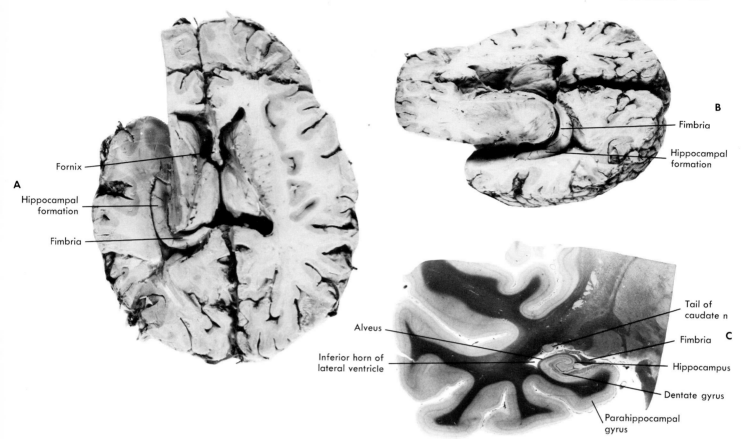

Fig. 10-8. Hippocampal formation. The gross specimens in **A** and **B** show the hippocampus as a ridge in the floor of the temporal horn of the lateral ventricle. The section in **C** shows the way in which the hippocampal formation is related to other portions of the temporal lobe.

venerated at Thebes and whose symbol was a ram with curled horns. The dentate gyrus, or fascia dentata, is so named because of its toothed appearance, which is caused in part by a series of perforating arteries that arise from the anterior and posterior choroidal arteries and penetrate the gyrus along its length. The hippocampus is named after its resemblance to a seahorse.

The hippocampus can be demonstrated grossly by a dissection that removes the brain overlying the temporal horn of the lateral ventricle (Fig. 10-8). The floor of the ventricle in the temporal lobe is formed by a layer of white matter, the alveus, which covers the gray matter of the hippocampus. The fimbria is a structure that runs along the medial wall of the temporal horn. It is composed of axons that collect together from the alveus, and caudally the fimbria becomes continuous with the fornix.

In cross section, the cortex of the dentate gyrus and the cortex of CA can be visualized as two interlocking U-shaped cortices (Figs. 10-8 to 10-10). The efferent neuron of each of these cortices is a pyramidal neu-

ron. In the dentate gyrus these are rather stunted pyramids called granule cells. In CA there is a stratum of well-developed pyramidal neurons. The pyramidal neurons of the pyramidal layer of CA are arranged so that the apical dendrites of the cells are facing toward the inside of the interlocking U shapes. Therefore, when CA is penetrated with an electrode from the ventricular surface, the basilar dendrites of pyramidal neurons are approached before the somata.

Different parts of the hippocampus have been labeled hippocampal fields CA1 through CA4 (in another terminology, fields H1 through H5), largely on the basis of the cytoarchitecture of the pyramidal neurons. In humans, field CA1 lies nearest to the temporal horn of the lateral ventricle. Field CA4 lies closest to the hippocampal sulcus and is that part of the U of CA that interlocks with the U of the dentate gyrus. The pyramidal neurons of CA1 are highly sensitive to anoxia and ischemia. In this area, known to the neuropathologist as Sommer's sector, the pyramidal neurons may show degenerative changes in cases of cerebral ischemia and in some cases of

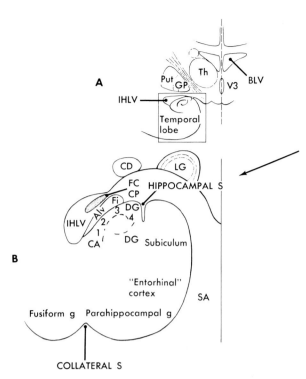

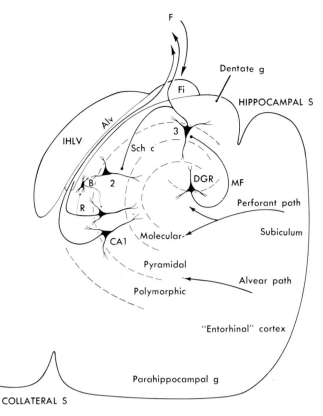

Fig. 10-9. Hippocampal formation and parahippocampal gyrus. Transverse section through the right cerebral hemisphere, anterior-posterior view. The arrow indicates the direction of view of Fig. 10-3. **A,** Section showing the position of the hippocampal formation on the medial aspect of the temporal lobe. Abbreviations: *BLV,* body of lateral ventricle; *IHLV,* inferior horn of lateral ventricle; *Put,* putamen; *GP,* globus pallidus; *Th,* thalamus; *V₃,* third ventricle. **B,** Enlarged view of hippocampal formation slightly caudal to section **A.** Abbreviations: *Alv,* alveus; *Fi,* fimbria; *CA,* cornu Ammon, fields 1 through 4; *DG,* dentate gyrus; *FC,* choroid fissure (lead line extends to the choroid plexus in the choroid fissure); *CP,* choroid plexus of the inferior horn of the lateral ventricle; *SA,* subarachnoid space; *CD,* tail of the caudate nucleus; *LG,* lateral geniculate nucleus.

Fig. 10-10. Structure and conduction pathways of hippocampal formation. *CA,* cornu Ammon pyramidal cells shown in fields 1 through 3. The orientation of their somata and processes in the molecular, pyramidal, and polymorphic layers of CA are shown. Their axons are shown projecting through the alveus *(Alv)* and fimbria *(Fi)* to the fornix *(F).* A pyramidal neuron of CA3 is shown giving off a Schaffer collateral *(Sch c).* A recurrent collateral *(R)* of a CA pyramidal cell is shown going to a basket cell *(B)* in the polymorphic layer. The basket cell axon is shown synapsing on a pyramidal cell soma. The dentate granule cell *(DGR)* is shown giving off a mossy fiber *(MF)* projecting to CA. The afferent perforant and alvear pathways are shown. (Based largely on data from lower mammals.)

temporal lobe epilepsy. Degenerative neuronal changes, which may be found in patients with psychomotor seizures, are more widely distributed than in field CA1 of the hippocampus; cerebellar, amygdaloid, thalamic, and cortical changes are found. In the hippocampus, changes are also found in the dentate gyrus and in the end-folium, or Bratz's sector, corresponding to fields CA3 and CA4.

The pyramidal neurons of CA3 are very large, and their axons give off prominent recurrent collateral fibers called Schaffer collaterals. Recurrent collaterals are also given off by axons of the pyramidal neurons in other fields.

In addition to pyramidal neurons, the dentate gyrus and CA contain other neurons and afferent fibers arranged so that each of these cortices has a three-layered appearance (Table 10-1). In the dentate gyrus

the first layer on the outside of the U is the molecular layer; the second layer is the granular layer of pyramidal cells; the third layer is a layer of polymorphic cells.

In CA the first layer on the inside of the U is the molecular layer. It contains a layer of tangential fibers and a fiber layer called the stratum lacunosum. The second layer is the pyramidal layer, which has the row of pyramidal cells. The portion of the pyramidal layer containing the apical dendrites of these cells is the stratum radiatum. The somata of the cells lie in the stratum pyramidale, or the stratum lucidum, which is best developed in field CA3. The third layer is the polymorphic layer, also called the stratum oriens.

Basket cells lie at the junction of the pyramidal and polymorphic layers. Some authors consider them to be modified pyramidal cells. The axons of the basket cells loop back through the pyramidal layer and form a plexus around the bodies of the pyramidal cells.

Afferents to the hippocampal formation go to both the dentate gyrus and to CA. A very important feature of the afferents to CA pyramids is that afferents from different sources synapse on the CA pyramids in distinct strata. Another important feature is that there is a considerable degree of topographic specificity, or point-to-point organization, of the intrahippocampal connections.

Afferents to the hippocampal formation enter from three sources: the entorhinal cortex, the fornix, and the hippocampal commissure, from the contralateral hippocampus. There are two main pathways from the entorhinal cortex, the alvear (medial entorhinal) pathway and the perforant (lateral entorhinal) pathway (Fig. 10-10). The alvear pathway passes deep in the subiculum and distributes in part to the polymorphic layer of field CA1 to synapse on basal dendrites of pyramidal neurons that extend into the polymorphic layer. The perforant pathway passes across the subiculum more superficially and distributes in part to fields CA1 and CA2 to the apical dendrites of pyramidal neurons and also to granule cells of the dentate gyrus.

The efferent projection of the hippocampal formation is from the pyramidal neurons of CA. Their axons collect in the alveus (trough) and fimbria (fringe) and are distributed largely through the fornix and the hippocampal commissure.

The intrinsic connections of the hippocampal formation have been partially clarified. The axons of the granule cells of the dentate gyrus are called mossy fibers. These project in part to field CA3 to the proximal apical dendrites of CA3 pyramidal neurons. The axons of CA3 pyramidal neurons give rise to recurrent axons, the Schaffer collaterals, which project largely to CA1 to synapse with apical dendrites of CA1 pyramidal cells.

Limbic pathways involving the hippocampus

Only some of the pathways involving the hippocampus will be described; the details of the connections within the hippocampal formation will be discussed in the next section. A scheme of the main projection pathway is shown in Fig. 10-6. Neurons within the entorhinal area project into the hippocampus. The output of the hippocampus is through the fornix. Axons from the hippocampus project through the fornix to the mamillary body, where they synapse on neurons that project through the mamillothalamic tract to the anterior nuclei of the thalamus (see Fig.

6-13). The anterior nuclei are specific relay nuclei that project to the cingulate gyrus. Neurons of the cingulate gyrus connect with the entorhinal area through the cingulum. Thus, a closed circuit is formed. However, there are many points along the pathway at which axons connect with other structures outside this circuit. For instance, the hippocampus on one side is connected with that on the other side through the hippocampal commissure, which is formed by axons crossing from one fornix to the other. The fornix distributes not only to the mamillary body but also to the precommissural septum, to the preoptic and anterior hypothalamic nuclei, and directly to the anterior nuclei of the thalamus. The mamillary bodies have tegmental connections. The cingulate gyrus projects to the brainstem reticular formation as well as to the entorhinal area. Thus, activity in the hippocampus can reach widely distributed regions of the brain rather directly.

Electrophysiology of hippocampal neurons

Because of the more accessible location of the hippocampal pyramidal neurons in fields CA2 and CA3, intracellular recording, largely in these cells in the cat, has shown that they are similar in some respects to pyramidal neurons of the neocortex. The input resistance and time constant of hippocampal pyramidal neurons are generally slightly greater than those of the larger pyramidal neurons of the motor cortex. When efferent axons of hippocampal pyramidal cells are excited by stimulating the fornix, antidromic invasion of the cell soma occurs in the same manner as in motor cortex pyramidal cells (see Fig. 6-30). In addition excitation of afferent fibers in the fornix evokes EPSPs in hippocampal pyramidal cells. Stimulation of the perforant pathway evokes longer lasting, more asynchronous EPSPs. IPSPs of hippocampal pyramidal cells, like those of neocortical neurons, are of very long duration.

Some electrophysiological activities of hippocampal pyramidal neurons are, however, quite different from those of neocortical pyramidal cells. Brief depolarizing potentials that are several millivolts in amplitude and several milliseconds in duration, and that appear to be unitary events rather than graded responses like EPSPs, are frequently recorded in hippocampal pyramidal neurons. Spike responses often appear to arise from these fast prepotentials (FPPs). The FPPs have been interpreted as spikes generated at sites in the dendritic tree and recorded at reduced amplitude by the micropipette in the cell soma. FPPs are particularly likely to be seen when the cell is under intense synaptic bombardment, as during a seizure. Spike generation in dendrites occurs in injured chromatolysing neurons and may occur in cerebellar Purkinje cells. However, dendritic spike generation rarely, if ever, occurs in normal neocortical neurons.

Hippocampal pyramidal neurons also exhibit depolarization shifts and oscillations of membrane potential rather like those of neocortical neurons during experimental seizure activity (see Chapter 6 and p. 379). How much of this is caused by intrinsic properties of the neurons and how much is caused by the circuitry of the hippocampus is not clear.

In lightly anesthetized or unanesthetized animals hippocampal neurons exhibit spontaneous rhythmic fluctuation of membrane potential of up to 10 mV, in theta range (4 to 7 Hz). These potentials appear to be the source of the hippocampal theta rhythm, which can be recorded from the hippocampus with a gross electrode.

Electrophysiology of intrinsic hippocampal connections

The hippocampus has been important as a model system for understanding relationships between anatomical structure and electrophysiological activity. The laminar organization of the hippocampus, with segregation of synaptic inputs on different portions of vertically oriented pyramidal cells, makes it a model system for attempting to understand the interactions of different types of input on a cell and for correlating the structure of synapses with their electrophysiological activity. Considerations of this sort led Renshaw, Forbes, and Morrison to perform the original microelectrode studies of the hippocampus.

Intracellular and field potential recordings have provided evidence that there is a powerful set of intrinsic inhibitory neurons within the hippocampus that are synaptically activated by pyramidal neuron discharge. The evidence for this is that the fornix is cut and time is allowed for the afferents in it to degenerate (deafferentated fornix preparation); the fornix is then stimulated, and intracellular recording in CA pyramids records antidromic spikes followed by IPSPs in some pyramidal neurons. Because no

afferents to the CA pyramidal neurons have been stimulated, the IPSPs must be caused by a recurrent pathway from CA pyramidal neurons. The latency of the IPSP indicates that there is at least one interneuron in the pathway. If the extracellular field potential generated by the IPSP is plotted to reveal its sinks and sources within the layers of the hippocampus, the extracellular positivity corresponding to the intracellular hyperpolarization of the IPSP is maximal at the level of the somata of CA pyramids. Inasmuch as the basket cell axons terminate around the somata of CA pyramids, it is thought that they mediate the IPSP and form a widely ramifying inhibitory system in the hippocampus. Recordings have been made from hippocampal interneurons, which discharge at high frequencies during the IPSP of pyramidal neurons, like the Renshaw cells of the spinal cord; although they have not been anatomically identified as basket cells, they probably are. Synapses with elongated vesicles that end on the somata of pyramidal neurons may possibly be basket cell inhibitory synapses. The structural arrangement and presumed inhibitory activity of these cells have been likened to the basket cell–Purkinje cell system of the cerebellum. However, there still is considerable controversy about the locus of inhibitory synapses on hippocampal cells.

In addition to evidence for recurrent inhibition in the hippocampus, similar evidence exists for recurrent excitation.

Electrophysiological and anatomical evidence has suggested the above pathway as one of the basic hippocampal circuits, the pathway by which impulses entering the hippocampal formation sequentially activate its cells. In this circuit the perforant pathway–mossy-fiber–Schaffer collateral pathway is thought of as extending across the hippocampal formation (Fig. 10-10) in a series of rows, producing a beam of excitation similar to the beam of excitation produced in the cerebellum by exciting the parallel fibers of a folium.

In addition, CA pyramidal neuron discharge is

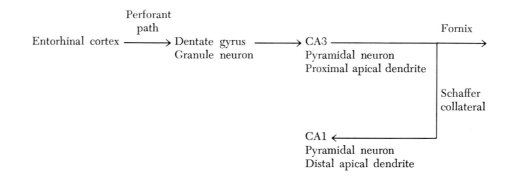

thought of as producing recurrent excitation of basket cells, which then inhibit adjacent CA pyramidal neurons as follows:

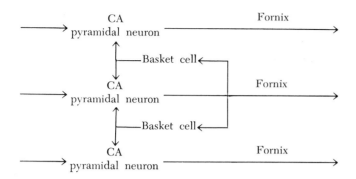

Therefore, the beam of excitation extending across a slice of hippocampus would be surrounded by zones of relatively less excited cells.

The relationship between hippocampal neuronal activity and behavior remains obscure. However, knowledge of the circuitry has thrown light on the important clinical problem of temporal lobe epilepsy.

Generation of epileptic activity in the hippocampal formation

Hippocampal pyramidal neurons appear to be more prone than neocortical neurons to develop repetitive discharge and paroxysmal depolarization following strong afferent stimulation. When the intact fornix is stimulated repetitively, discharging both afferent fibers and firing CA pyramidal cells antidromically, the pyramidal neurons discharge repetitively and undergo a large sustained depolarization so that their membrane potential has a mean value of about 30 mV. Small spike potentials are generated in the depolarized cells. Recording from the surface of the hippocampus with a gross electrode shows epileptiform activity. The seizure activity is terminated by a hyperpolarization of the cell, which appears to be an IPSP. This type of seizure activity is like that of neocortical neurons (see Chapter 6).

However, a different type of seizure, which can be called an inhibitory seizure, can be observed in hippocampal neurons. This type of seizure can be induced by stimulating the deafferentated fornix. Antidromic firing of CA pyramidal cells then occurs, followed by recurrent inhibition and recurrent excitation of pyramidal cells. The majority of the CA pyramids become hyperpolarized under these conditions. However, potentials recorded from the surface of the hippocampus show epileptiform activity.

A model has been proposed by Dichter and Spencer to explain these findings. In this model, recurrent excitation of a small number of CA pyramidal neurons

sets up an excitatory focus, or pacemaker. At the same time, recurrent activation of the more powerful and widespread system of inhibitory interneurons produces a surrounding zone of hyperpolarized pyramidal follower cells. The hyperpolarized surround limits the spread of the seizure activity in the hippocampus. The interplay of the excitatory pacemaker and the inhibitory follower cells produces the surface recording pattern of interictal spiking seen in epileptogenic foci. However, if the inhibitory interneurons are fired at high frequencies for too long, they will be inactivated. CA pyramids will then be disinhibited; that is, there will be unopposed recurrent excitation of these cells, and the seizure will spread. The model therefore also gives an explanation of the mechanism of transition of interictal spiking into a generalized seizure.

Although hippocampal neurons can be easily driven into epileptic activity, there is only a weak tendency in experimentally evoked hippocampal seizures for the seizure activity to spread from the hippocampal projections into the nonspecific or specific thalamic systems and to their neocortical projections. The tendency of hippocampal seizure activity to remain localized to limbic structures is probably the reason why psychomotor or temporal lobe seizures remain partial seizures in some cases and do not produce a generalized seizure with loss of consciousness.

AMYGDALOID NUCLEUS
Limbic pathways involving the amygdaloid nucleus and the septal region

Several important pathways in the limbic system relay in the amygdaloid nucleus, the septal region, or both. In humans, this includes the precommissural septum (paraterminal gyrus). The olfactory connections to the corticomedial amygdaloid nucleus have already been mentioned. The basolateral cell groups of the amygdala are nonolfactory and are particularly large in primates and humans. The main input to the basolateral amygdaloid nuclear groups is from the prepiriform and periamygdaloid cortexes. Their main output is through the stria terminalis and the ventral amygdalofugal pathway (Fig. 10-11). The stria terminalis terminates in the preoptic and anterior hypothalamic nuclei and in the septal region. The ventral amygdalofugal pathway distributes to several structures, including the medial dorsal nucleus of the thalamus, parts of the hypothalamus, and the midbrain reticular formation. The medial dorsal nucleus of the thalamus is a specific relay nucleus that projects to the orbitofrontal cortex. A circuit is then formed by connections from the orbitofrontal cortex back to the prepiriform and periamygdaloid cortexes.

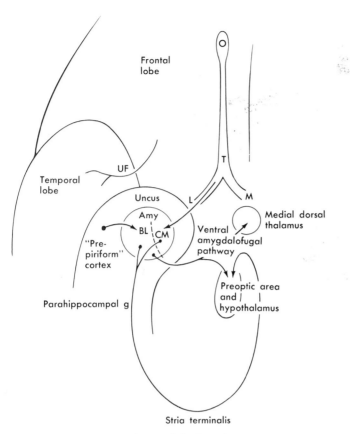

Fig. 10-11. Projections of amygdaloid nucleus. Abbreviations: *Amy*, amygdaloid nucleus; *BL, CM,* basolateral and cortico-medial cell groups; *O,* olfactory bulb; *T,* olfactory tract; *L, M,* lateral and medial striae; *UF,* uncinate fasciculus.

An important descending pathway from the septal region is through the stria medullaris to the habenula (Fig. 10-12). The habenula projects through the fasciculus retroflexus (of Meynert) to the interpeduncular nucleus of the midbrain. The interpeduncular nucleus is in turn connected with more caudal nuclei of the brainstem tegmentum. Other descending connections from the limbic system to the midbrain tegmentum are from the preoptic anterior hypothalamic nuclei through the medial forebrain bundle.

There are also ascending connections from the brainstem to the limbic structures of the diencephalon and telencephalon. Among these are projections from monoamine-containing cells, including the serotonergic neurons of the midbrain raphe nuclei (see below).

The full extent of the limbic projections are much more complex than the connections indicated here. Although some of the connections appear to form closed loops, it is not known if these loops actually function as circuits and, if so, what their functions are.

NEUROTRANSMITTERS

Substances that are putative neurotransmitters are found in high concentration in brainstem limbic projections. The loci of these substances have been studied largely in rodents and cats. These cell groups lie in the midbrain reticular formation adjacent to the red nucleus, the substantia nigra, and the interpeduncular nucleus. The homologies of these cell groups with the cytoarchitectural divisions of the human reticular formation, based on Nissl-stained material, are un-

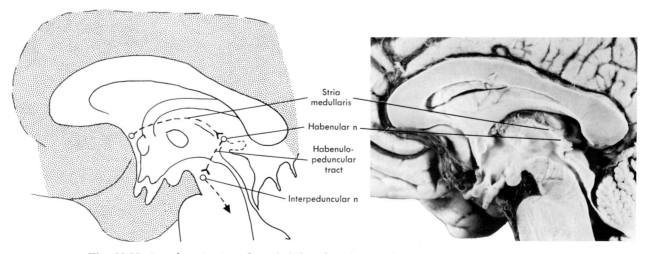

Fig. 10-12. Septal projections through habenula. The septal region projects to the habenular nuclei through the stria medullaris. The habenula, in turn, is connected to the interpeduncular nucleus of the midbrain through the habenulopeduncular tract (fasciculus retroflexus of Meynert). The interpeduncular nucleus has descending projections to the brainstem tegmentum.

known. The neurons of the raphe nuclei contain either 5-hydroxytryptamine (5-HT, serotonin) or a very closely related substance. The axons of these neurons project strongly to the anterior hypothalamus and preoptic areas.

Dopamine- and norepinephrine-containing neurons of the ventral tegmental area, which are located a little more laterally in general than the 5-HT neurons, project to the preoptic and diagonal band area and to the hypothalamus.

There are moderate amounts of dopamine, norepinephrine 5-HT, and acetylcholine (ACh) in the hippocampal formation. The sites of origin of the axons containing these substances are not definitely known. Some of the dopamine, norepinephrine and 5-HT axons appear to come from the limbic midbrain. Some of the ACh may be in more caudally originating reticular formation projections reported to go to the hippocampus.

ROLE OF LIMBIC STRUCTURES IN BEHAVIOR

The role of limbic structures in behavior has been inferred from studies of the effects of stimulation and of ablation of limbic structures and from observations of patients with temporal lobe epilepsy and with infarctions and other lesions of limbic structures.

Stimulation studies

Stimulation of limbic structures evokes autonomic, somatic, motor, and sensory responses that are qualitatively rather similar when evoked from various structures. For the sake of brevity the responses are discussed without reference to particular structures, although some of the responses may be evoked with greater frequency or intensity in some areas than in others.

Autonomic responses that are predominantly evoked by limbic stimulation are salivation, changes in gastrointestinal tract motility, and changes in blood pressure.

The somatic motor activities evoked by limbic stimulation often have a repetitive or rhythmic character. Some of these responses are related to eating, such as chewing, licking, and sniffing. This is not surprising in view of the olfactory connections of limbic structures. Stimulation can also evoke contraversive movements and posturing that can be interpreted as attack, defense, or flight movements. Fully developed patterns of activity can also be evoked, such as grooming and searching, or orienting, behavior.

Prepiriform and periamygdaloid electrical stimulation in humans can evoke olfactory sensations. The odors generally have an unpleasant quality, like that of burning rubber. Limbic stimulation may also evoke visceral sensations and feelings of vertigo.

A remarkable finding by Olds and his collaborators was that animals will work, performing bar pressing or other tasks, for long periods of time if the activity is followed by electrical stimulation of limbic areas. Stimulation of the area of the medial forebrain bundle is particularly effective in evoking self-stimulating behavior. Similar behavior has been found in humans studied with depth electrodes implanted in subcortical areas for the purpose of localizing sites of seizure discharge or for localizing structures prior to psychosurgery. The anatomical sites of stimulation are not known precisely in most of the human studies, but they appear to be within the thalamus and within limbic structures. In general, two types of emotional responses have been evoked in humans by limbic stimulation. One type of response is a feeling of pleasure, which is not well described. Patients state that the stimulation feels good, and self-stimulation can be evoked from brain loci yielding this type of response. The other type of response evoked is of fear or terror, which does not lead to self-stimulation behavior.

Studies of endocrine function have shown numerous changes in blood hormone levels following limbic stimulation. These neuroendocrine effects are, however, beyond the scope of this chapter.

Not surprisingly, the activities that can be produced by electrical stimulation are frequently observed in patients with temporal lobe seizures.

Ablation studies

The general character of the effects produced by telencephalic limbic ablations in the primate can be seen after bilateral anterior temporal lobectomy, which removes the major telencephalic limbic structures. The syndrome seen after such extirpations was described by Klüver and Bucy, and includes decreased emotional responsiveness; increased sexual activity; increased manipulation of objects, especially oral manipulation; and visual agnosia, or difficulty in recognizing objects. It is not clear which anatomical structures are most involved in different aspects of the syndrome. Bilateral destruction of the amygdaloid nucleus produces a reduction of aggressive behavior, both in species that are predatory and in aggressive individuals of particular species. Increased sexual activity is also produced. Surgical destruction of the amygdaloid nucleus has been carried out in humans in attempts to control severe aggressive behavior. There are some differences in the behavioral effects produced by amygdaloidectomy and other limbic ablations in different species.

Ablations of the thalamic or neocortical areas or both to which the telencephalic limbic structures send ascending projections produce largely a decrease in emotional responsiveness. There are also many other effects on mental processes following such ablations, particularly if the anterior portions of the frontal lobes are removed bilaterally. Such changes include a decreased attention span and unconcern about various socially conditioned forms of behavior, such as maintenance of personal appearance and inhibition of emotional expression. However, the most consistent features of ablation of thalamic and neocortical areas to which telencephalic limbic structures project are a reduction in emotional responsiveness and a decrease in emotionally driven motor behavior. Various structures have been ablated in humans for the purpose of relieving incapacitating anxiety and agitated behavior. These so-called psychosurgical procedures have included stereotaxic destruction of the AV and MD thalamic nuclei; cingulumotomy, or destruction of the fiber tract of the cingulate gyrus; frontal leukotomy, or cutting the fiber tracts of the frontal lobes just anterior to the frontal horns of the lateral ventricles, which interrupts thalamofrontal connections; topectomy, or removing portions of the cortex of the frontal lobes; and frontal lobotomy, in which the interruption of the frontal lobe fiber tracts is carried out, as in a leukotomy, but with removal of the frontal lobes anterior to the ventricular system as well. All of these procedures are more effective when performed bilaterally rather than unilaterally. It is a reasonable hypothesis that the common factor in the effect of these procedures in reducing emotional responsiveness is interruption of the ascending telencephalic limbic projections and that the exact site of interruption may not be as important as the fact of interruption of the circuits. At the present time only cingulumotomy and frontal leukotomy are being used to any extent as therapeutic procedures, because they are easier to perform and have less morbidity and other undesirable side effects than the other procedures.

The tranquilizing and mood-elevating drugs have rather similar effects on emotional behavior as psychosurgical procedures. Most of these drugs are central antagonists of catecholamines or serotonin, putative neurotransmitters in limbic structures.

The behavioral effects of ablation of descending projections of telencephalic limbic structures are particularly difficult to analyze in terms of what their limbic role may be, because hypothalamic and mesencephalic structures serve as parts of many regulatory systems. Animals with lesions in these areas may show a wide variety of deficits in autonomic regulation.

An important effect that should be mentioned is that destruction of the midbrain raphe nuclei produces severe disturbances of sleep, with almost continual wakefulness (see Chapter 11). Changes in the rhythms of hippocampal potentials have been found in sleep and wakefulness. Hippocampal synchronization (theta rhythm) is seen when animals are aroused, at the same time that the EEG of the neocortex becomes desynchronized. The exact behavior that hippocampal synchronization is related to is still somewhat controversial. It appears to be most closely related to an alert state and is found when animals appear to be preparing for a movement.

Limbic ablations and memory deficits are discussed below.

Function in emotion

The results of stimulation and ablation experiments strongly suggest that limbic structures are involved in the generation of sensations of emotion. The olfactory connections of limbic structures are interesting in this respect, as are the ascending pathways emphasized by Papez in "A Proposed Mechanism of Emotion," in which he discussed the possible role of limbic circuits in emotion. It is a common experience that odors are powerful in evoking emotions and memories. A striking description of this is given in the opening section of Proust's *Remembrance of Things Past*.

The persistence of emotional states, or moods, over long periods of time implies a long-lasting corresponding neural state. Some authors have suggested that reverberating circuits could serve to sustain the neural events that must persist over long periods of time as the neural substrates of emotion or of memory. As discussed above, it is not known whether such circuits actually exist. The recurrent excitation and inhibition that appear to be involved in hippocampal seizure activity comprise a reverberating circuit; however, the time scale of the activity of the actual circuit is less than a second. Nevertheless, the interictal epileptiform activity it produces may last for some hours. Such mechanisms therefore may be found to be involved in the generation of long-lasting neural activity.

Function in memory

A number of patients who have had bilateral damage to the hippocampal formation have been carefully observed. The fact that some of these patients have also had other brain injuries has complicated the interpretation of the data. However, most of these patients with hippocampal injury have exhibited difficulty with memory. Memory for recent events was more affected than for events that occurred long before the time of brain injury. Memory for emotionally charged events appeared to become more disturbed than for emotionally neutral events, and memory appeared to be more impaired when the patients were emotionally upset. It is generally agreed that the memory trace, or engram, is not stored or laid down in the hippocampus. As well as can be determined at present, storage of information is a function of the brain as a whole. The hippocampus, however, may be involved in the processes of sorting and supplying information that is to be stored and may similarly be involved in the process of recall of the information.

Patients with Korsakoff's syndrome, which is observed in some cases of chronic alcoholism, also show memory loss and intellectual impairment. The lesions in the brain usually include hippocampal lesions but are more widespread, with degeneration in the mamillary nuclei and in the medial dorsal thalamus and periaqueductal gray matter.

Changes in hippocampal potentials recorded with implanted electrodes have been reported in learning situations in animals. The appearance of synchronization (theta waves) seems most closely related to arousal and goal-directed motor activity in these situations.

The importance of emotional activity and motivation in the learning process is clear, even if the neurophysiological mechanisms are not. It seems that sensory information that is perceived as emotionally significant or that is associated with the generation of strong emotions is selected for memory and that the hippocampal formation is involved in these processes.

Clinical aspects

Clinically noticeable changes in olfactory sensation are almost always caused by damage to the olfactory receptors or to the olfactory nerve, bulb, or tract. Processes that damage only the cortical receptive areas for olfaction without producing concomitant damage of the olfactory tracts are quite uncommon. Attempts have been made to develop quantitative olfactory testing and to study the disturbances that may be produced by damage to the olfactory receptive areas.

Nonolfactory limbic structures

Disturbances in personality, in affect, and in memory can suggest frontal lobe and anterior temporal lobe damage. However, the normal functioning of nonolfactory limbic structures cannot be tested in ways comparable to the testing of sensory or motor systems. The normal emotional states and drives of patients can be described and quantitated to some extent, but individual differences in personality and drive cannot at present be related to the functional state of particular brain structures. Some differences in the EEG recorded from temporal leads have been reported in patients with personality disturbances and aggressive in be-

havior. Some patients who have attacks of temporal lobe seizure activity accompanied by behavioral outbursts of rage have also been studied with depth-recording electrodes. These findings have interesting implications for the understanding of normal function. However, whether limbic activity determines the fundamental personality structure of individuals and to what extent limbic activity contributes to or determines or modulates consciousness and mental processes is unknown.

Further, the presumed limbic role in integration of memory process and in generation of emotions is the type of activity that is implied in the psychiatric construct of the unconscious. One of the most important of Freud's achievements was his recognition of processes occurring within the individual that do not enter consciousness but that nevertheless are powerful in determining behavior. Much effort has been expended in trying to find organic correlates of psychiatric constructs. Perhaps the language of psychiatry cannot be reduced to the language of neurophysiology. This is the mind-body problem restated. Nevertheless, the unconscious processes appear to be occurring somewhere (perhaps everywhere) in the brain, and eventually there may be some way of describing them.

BIBLIOGRAPHY

Adey, W. R.: Studies of hippocampal electrical activity during approach learning. In Delafresnaye, J. F., editor: Brain mechanisms and learning, Springfield, Ill., 1961, Charles C Thomas, Publisher.

Andersen, P., Eccles, J. C., and Løyning, Y.: Location of postsynaptic inhibitory synapses on hippocampal pyramids, J. Neurophysiol. 27:592-607, 1964.

Andersen, P., and Lømo, T.: Control of hippocampal output by afferent volley frequency. In Adey, W. R., and Tokizane, T., editors: Structure and function of the limbic system; progress in brain research, vol. 27, Amsterdam, 1967, Elsevier Publishing Co.

Andy, O. J., and Stephan, H.: The septum of the cat, Springfield, Ill., 1964, Charles C Thomas, Publisher.

Ballantine, H. T., Cassidy, W. L., Flanagan, N. B., and Marino, R., Jr.: Stereotaxic anterior cingulumotomy for neuropsychiatric illness and intractable pain, J. Neurosurg. 26:488-495, 1967.

Blackstad, T. W.: Studies on the hippocampus; methods of analysis. In Brazier, M. A. B., editor: The interneuron, Berkeley, Calif., 1969, University of California Press.

Broca, P.: Anatomie comparée circonvolutions cérébrales; le grand lobe limbique et la scissure limbique dans la série des mammifères, Rev. Anthropol. Series 2 1:385-498, 1878.

Cooper, J. R., Bloom, F. E., and Roth, R. H.: The biochemical basis of neuropharmacology, ed. 2, New York, 1974, Oxford University Press, Inc.

De Jong, R. N., Itabashi, H. H., and Olsen, J R.: Memory loss due to hippocampal lesions, Arch. Neurol. 20:339-348, 1969.

De Vito, J. L., and White, L. E., Jr.: Projections from the fornix to the hippocampal formation in the squirrel monkey, J. Comp. Neurol. 127:389-398, 1966.

Dichter, M., and Spencer, W. A.: Penicillin-induced interictal discharges from the cat hippocampus. I. Characteristics and topographical features, J. Neurophysiol. **32**:649-662, 1969.

Domesick, V. B.: Projections from the cingulate cortex in the rat, Brain Res. **12**:296-320, 1969.

Douglas, R. J.: The hippocampus and behavior, Psychol. Bull. **67**:416-442, 1967.

Dreifuss, J. J., Murphy, J. T., and Gloor, P.: Contrasting effects of two identified amygdaloid efferent pathways on single hypothalamic neurons, J. Neurophysiol. **31**:237-248, 1968.

Fernandez de Molina, A., and Hunsperger, R. W.: Organization of the subcortical system governing defense and flight reactions in the cat, J. Physiol. (Lond.) **160**:200-213, 1962.

Freeman, W., and Watts, J. W.: Psychosurgery, ed. 2, Springfield, Ill., 1950, Charles C Thomas, Publisher.

Gastaut, H., and Lammars, H. J.: Anatomie du rhinencéphale. In Alajouanine, T., editor: Les grandes activities du rhinencéphale, vol. 1, Paris, 1961, Masson & Cie, Editeurs.

Green, J. D.: The hippocampus, Physiol. Rev. **44**:561-608, 1964.

Heimer, L.: Synaptic distribution of centripetal and centrifugal nerve fibers in the olfactory system of the rat, J. Anat. **103**:413-432, 1968.

Heimer, L., and Nauta, W. J. H.: The hypothalamic distribution of the stria terminalis in the rat, Brain Res. **13**:284-297, 1969.

Ito, M., and Olds, J.: Unit activity during self-stimulation behavior, J. Neurophysiol. **34**:263-273, 1971.

Kaada, B. R.: Somato-motor, autonomic, and electrocorticographic responses to electrical stimulation of "rhinencephalic" and other structures in primates, cat and dog, Acta Physiol. Scand. **24** (Suppl. 83), 1951.

Kaada, B. R., Andersen, P., and Jansen, J.: Stimulation of the amygdaloid nuclear complex in unanesthetized cats, Neurol. **4**:48-64, 1954.

Kandel, E. R., and Spencer, W. A.: Electrophysiology of hippocampal neurons. II. After-potentials and repetitive firing, J. Neurophysiol. **24**:243-259, 1961.

Kandel, E. R., Spencer, W. A., and Brinley, F. J.: Electrophysiology of hippocampal neurons. I. Sequential invasion and synaptic organization, J. Neurophysiol. **24**:225-242, 1961.

Klüver, H., and Bucy, P. C.: "Psychic blindness" and other symptoms following bilateral temporal lobectomy in Rhesus monkeys, Am. J. Physiol. **119**:352-353, 1937.

Kreindler, A., and Steriade, M.: Desynchronizing and synchronizing electrical reactions induced by stimulating dorsal and ventral levels of the amygdaloid complex, Acta Physiol. Acad. Sci. Hung. **26**:157, 1965.

Laatsch, R. H., and Cowan, W. M.: Electron microscopic studies of the dentate gyrus of the rat. I. Normal structure with special reference to synaptic organization, J. Comp. Neurol. **128**:359-396, 1966.

Lewis, P. R., and Shute, C. C. D.: The cholinergic limbic system; projections to the hippocampal formation, medial cortex, nuclei of the ascending cholinergic reticular system and the subfornical organ and supraoptic crest, Brain **90**:521-540, 1967.

Lorente de Nó, R.: Studies on the structure of the cerebral cortex. II. Continuation of the study of the ammonic system, J. Psychol. Neurol. **46**:113-177, 1934.

Margerison, J. H., and Corsellis, J. A. N.: Epilepsy and the temporal lobes, Brain **89**:499-530, 1966.

Mettler, F. A.: Selective partial ablation of the frontal cortex; a correlative study of its effects on human psychotic subjects, New York, 1949, Hoeber.

Millhouse, O. E.: A Golgi study of the descending medial forebrain bundle, Brain Res. **15**:341-363, 1969.

Mishkin, M.: Preservation of central sets after frontal lesions in monkeys. In Warren, J. M., and Akert, K., editors: The frontal granular cortex and behavior, New York, 1964, McGraw-Hill Book Co.

Moniz, E.: Tentative opératoires dans le traitement de certaines psychoses, Paris, 1936, Masson & Cie, Editeurs.

Nauta, W. J. H.: Hippocampal projections and related neural pathways to the midbrain in the cat, Brain **81**:319-340, 1958.

Nauta, W. J. H.: Fibre degeneration following lesions of the amygdaloid complex in the monkey, J. Anat. **95**:515-531, 1961.

Olds, J., and Milner, P.: Positive reinforcement produced by electrical stimulation of septal area and other regions of the rat brain, J. Comp. Physiol. Psych. **47**:419-427, 1954.

Papez, J. W.: A proposed mechanism of emotion, Arch. Neurol. Psychiat. **38**:725-743, 1937.

Pigache, R. M.: The anatomy of "paleocortex"; a critical review, Ergebn. Anat. Entwicklungsgesch **43**:1-62, 1970.

Pribram, K. H., Wilson, W. A., and Conners, J.: Effects of lesions of the medial forebrain on alternation behavior of rhesus monkeys, Exp. Neurol. **6**:36-47, 1962.

Purpura, D. P., McMurtry, J. G., Leonard, C. F., and Mailliani, A.: Evidence for dendritic origin of spikes without depolarizing prepotentials in hippocampal neurons during and after seizure, J. Neurophysiol. **29**:954-979, 1966.

Raisman, G.: The connexions of the septum, Brain **89**:317-348, 1966.

Raisman, G., Cowan, W. M., and Powell, T. P. S.: An experimental analysis of the efferent projection of the hippocampus, Brain **89**:83-108, 1966.

Renshaw, B., Forbes, A., and Morrison, B. R.: Activity of isocortex and hippocampus; electrical studies with microelectrodes, J. Neurophysiol. **3**:74-105, 1940.

Robinson, B. W., and Mishkin, M.: Alimentary responses to forebrain stimulation in monkeys, Exp. Brain Res. **4**:330-366, 1968.

Sem-Jacobsen, C. W.: Depth electrographic stimulation of the human brain and behavior; from fourteen years of studies and treatment of Parkinson's disease and mental disorder with implanted electrodes, Springfield, II., 1968, Charles C Thomas, Publisher.

Smythies, J. R.: Brain mechanisms and behavior, New York, 1970, Academic Press, Inc.

Spencer, W. A., and Kandel, E. R.: Electrophysiology of hippocampal neurons. III. Firing level and time constant, J. Neurophysiol. **24**:260-271, 1961.

Spencer, W. A., and Kandel, E. R.: Electrophysiology of hippocampal neurons. IV. Fast prepotentials, J. Neurophysiol. **24**:272-285, 1961.

Valverde, F.: Studies on the piriform lobe, Cambridge, 1965, Harvard University Press.

Westrum, L. E., and Blackstad, T. W.: An electron microscopic study of the stratum radiatum of the rat hippocampus (Regio Superior, CA$_1$) with particular emphasis on synaptology, J. Comp. Neurol. **119**:281-309, 1962.

Yokota, T., Reeves, A. G., and MacLean, P. D.: Differential effects of septal and olfactory volleys on intracellular responses of hippocampal neurons in awake, sitting monkeys, J. Neurophysiol. **33**:96-107, 1970.

Higher functions

In this chapter the psychological processes that are often called higher functions are discussed in relationship to physiological activities in the human brain. The reasons for discussing these processes separately from specific brain areas described in previous chapters are twofold. First, the neural substrates of these processes are still very poorly known; second, the participation and interaction of many brain areas appear to be involved in most of these processes. In agreement with the evidence of widespread participation of cortical and subcortical areas in these processes is the fact that many of the higher functions, such as consciousness, attention, and perception, are intimately interrelated.

CONSCIOUSNESS

Consciousness (awareness) can be thought of as the background or field in which sensations are experienced and in which mental processes occur; it can also be thought of as awareness of sensation and of self. Attention and perception are closely related to consciousness. That one is conscious of something implies sensation and perception of something. Thinking and the use of language occur within the field of consciousness.

How consciousness depends on the activity of the brain is unknown. The mind-body problem has long been a subject of speculation, and various views have been taken about the relationship of mind and matter (brain). One view is to regard mind as a thing or substance in itself that interacts with matter. A version of this idea is that of Descartes, who conceived of the soul (a unitary thing) acting on the pineal gland (a single, unpaired portion of the brain). Another viewpoint is to regard mind and brain as two separate but parallel phenomena. In the present century the view has been developed that the appearance of a mind-body problem is caused by improper analysis of our sense data and improper use of language. In any event, we can describe our sense data, including the sensation of our state of awareness, sensations of our motor activity, and sense data obtained from observation of instruments measuring the activity of our own nervous systems, and we can correlate these observations.

Our knowledge of another person's state of consciousness is an inference based on observation of his or her motor activity. Inasmuch as depressed and altered states of consciousness are of great medical importance, an operational definition of states of consciousness based on observation of motor activity is clinically useful. The most useful behavioral indications of the state of consciousness are speech and the pattern of somatic and eye movements. The states of motor behavior can be correlated with states of consciousness, as indicated on p. 386.

The intermediate stages of consciousness between full alertness and coma (unconsciousness) are often called stuporous or semicomatose states. A somewhat different grouping of speech and somatic motor criteria could also be chosen to illustrate the same point of the correlation of the psychological state of consciousness and motor behavior. Furthermore, as is discussed below, there can be some variability in this correlation, depending on the size of the lesion in the brain causing the disturbance of consciousness. Loss of the psychological state of consciousness probably occurs at about motor stage 5 in the following classification.

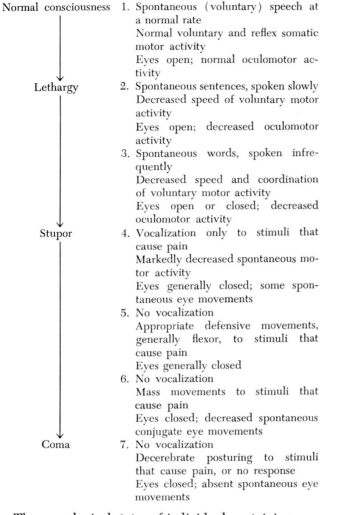

Normal consciousness
1. Spontaneous (voluntary) speech at a normal rate
Normal voluntary and reflex somatic motor activity
Eyes open; normal oculomotor activity

Lethargy
2. Spontaneous sentences, spoken slowly
Decreased speed of voluntary motor activity
Eyes open; decreased oculomotor activity
3. Spontaneous words, spoken infrequently
Decreased speed and coordination of voluntary motor activity
Eyes open or closed; decreased oculomotor activity

Stupor
4. Vocalization only to stimuli that cause pain
Markedly decreased spontaneous motor activity
Eyes generally closed; some spontaneous eye movements
5. No vocalization
Appropriate defensive movements, generally flexor, to stimuli that cause pain
Eyes generally closed
6. No vocalization
Mass movements to stimuli that cause pain
Eyes closed; decreased spontaneous conjugate eye movements

Coma
7. No vocalization
Decerebrate posturing to stimuli that cause pain, or no response
Eyes closed; absent spontaneous eye movements

The neurological status of individuals sustaining progressive brain damage, such as that caused by an expanding intracranial hematoma due to bleeding into the subdural space (see Chapter 5), can often be observed to go downward through the motor stages in the above-mentioned classification. Furthermore, the neurological status of individuals who are recovering from severe brain injury may frequently be observed to progress upward through these stages. The clinical observation that progressive cerebral damage, first involving the cortex and then the thalamus and brainstem, can lead to progressive depression of consciousness and motor activity suggests an interplay of cortical and subcortical areas in consciousness. A similar interplay exists in the control of sensory and motor systems (see Chapters 7 and 8). The neural substrates of consciousness are discussed further below.

Consciousness may be altered, rather than depressed, in some conditions. Sleep is the most familiar type of alteration of consciousness. Other altered states, such as hypnotic states, delirium, and exaltation, can be produced by psychological means and by drugs.

The state of electrocortical activity, which depends on interactions between the cortex, thalamus, and reticular formation, can be correlated with behavioral stages of consciousness. The normal electrocortical rhythms recorded with gross surface or scalp electrodes have been described in Chapter 6. Normal electrocortical activity in patients who are awake fluctuates between bilaterally synchronized rhythms at the alpha (8 to 12 Hz) frequency and lower voltage, faster desynchronized activity. Low-voltage fast activity can also be produced by sensory stimulation. The same stimuli can also result in behavioral arousal. With depression of consciousness there generally is slowing and disruption of synchronization, or disorganization, of electrocortical activity. However, the correspondence between states of consciousness and electrocortical activity recorded with gross electrodes is not exact. There can be considerable disorganization of the electroencephalogram without disturbances of consciousness, and there can be synchronized activity in comatose and anesthetized patients. Abnormal patterns of activity in thalamocortical systems can produce disruptions of consciousness. An example is the loss of consciousness seen in generalized seizures, including the prolonged losses of consciousness in major (grand mal) and the briefer losses of consciousness in minor (petit mal) seizures. Clouding and distortions of consciousness can occur in psychomotor seizures (see Chapter 6).

Consciousness appears to depend on the interaction of wide areas of the cerebral cortex with subcortical areas, particularly the thalamus, the periventricular hypothalamus, and the reticular formation. Sensory input to these areas is very important in activating them, or putting them into a state in which consciousness occurs.

There are two major types of brain damage that produce loss of consciousness. The first is the apallic (without a pallium or cortex) state. This refers to widespread severe damage to the cerebral hemispheres, with less damage to basal ganglia, thalamic structures, and brainstem structures. The apallic state can be produced by head injury and by cerebral anoxia. The electroencephalogram is disorganized, slowed, or even isoelectric in the apallic state.

The second type of brain damage that produces coma is damage to the thalamus and reticular formation of the brainstem. A number of well-studied cases of brainstem damage caused by localized arterial occlusions, hemorrhages, or both, have indicated that the thalamus and the pontine-mesencephalic reticular formation are necessary substrates for consciousness in humans. Destruction of either or both of these areas produces coma. Destruction of the caudal thalamus and of the rostral reticular formation, the mesencephalic reticular formation, appears to produce behavioral coma, with electroencephalographic disorganization and slowing.

In a case of mesencephalic reticular formation destruction studied by Ingvar and Sourander, in which the damage extended into the caudal thalamus, hypothalamus, and the rostral pons, the EEG showed severe generalized slowing, with the dominant frequencies in the delta band (less than 4 Hz). Cerebral blood flow and oxygen uptake were found to be severely depressed. The cerebral blood flow and oxygen uptake were about one fifth of their normal values of 50 ml of blood ± 5/100 g (SD) of brain tissue per minute and 3.3 ml O_2 ± 0.8/100 g of brain tissue per minute. The depression of cerebral blood flow and oxygen uptake in this case of decreased cerebral activity caused by coma was similar to the depression of blood flow and oxygen uptake produced by general anesthetic agents, although the depression measured in this case was even more severe than that produced in the surgical stage of anesthesia, where these parameters are usually reduced to about half their normal rates.

In contrast damage to the pontine reticular formation in humans appears to produce behavioral unconsciousness, with an electroencephalographic pattern resembling that of a quietly resting awake patient. The EEG shows alpha activity (8 to 12 Hz) in the posterior portions of the cerebrum. In a case of pontine damage studied by Wilkus and others, the electroencephalogram also showed transitions to a pattern of slow-wave sleep, with activity in the 4- to 7-Hz range, bursts of 14-Hz sleep spindles, and slow transients resembling K-complexes. Photically evoked cortical potentials were normal in form, latency, and amplitude, but no rhythmic after-activity followed the evoked response. Cortical potentials were not evoked by sound, because the ascending auditory pathways had been destroyed in the pons.

Damage to reticular nuclei rather than to the ascending sensory pathways appears to be the common anatomical lesion in the cases of human brainstem damage resulting in coma. Which reticular nuclei are essential for consciousness is not known. The presence of a normal resting electroencephalographic pattern in some cases of coma does not mean that electrocortical activity is normal in such cases, because the EEG is only a crude indicator of the degree of thalamocortical synchrony. It is probable that the reticular projections necessary for consciousness are those that go to the diencephalon and that play a role in thalamocortical interactions.

There may be some species differences in the importance of reticular nuclei in consciousness. The gigantocellular pontine reticular area can be destroyed in the rat without producing coma. A staged, gradual destruction of reticular nuclei in the cat can produce an apathetic state but not unconsciousness.

The foregoing discussion of consciousness has emphasized the interrelationships of different levels of the neuraxis in consciousness and the correlations between consciousness, motor activity, and electrocortical activity, each of which depends on the functioning of several levels of the neuraxis. Because of the participation of different levels of the neuraxis in each of these spheres, it is not surprising that the behavioral and electrocorticographic characteristics of loss of consciousness produced by lesions of different levels of the neuraxis may be different. One of the interesting variants of the comatose state is coma vigil, also called akinetic mutism. These terms describe a state in which the patient lies quietly, with no spontaneous speech or movement and no response to verbal stimuli. However, the patient's eyes are open. Various oculomotor, somatomotor, and autonomic reflexes can be evoked. Coma vigil is produced by brainstem lesions. The reason for the eyes being open rather than closed is not clear, but probably relates to the sparing of certain motor pathways by the lesion.

A large number of disease states can produce coma. In addition, coma can be produced by various drugs, including those that are classed as anesthetic agents.

Plum and Posner studied the cause of coma in 386 patients admitted to a general hospital while in coma. About half of the patients had intracranial disease. The most common intracranial pathological condition was vascular occlusion or hemorrhage; somewhat less common conditions were intracranial mass lesions, including brain tumors and head trauma. Other intracranial causes of coma were infection (meningitis, brain abscess) and postictal (postseizure) coma. Approximately half of the patients admitted to the hospital while in coma did not have primary intracranial pathological conditions. These patients had taken overdoses of drugs or had severe systemic metabolic disturbances. The way in which metabolic disturbances, such as severe hepatic failure, uremia, hypoglycemia, and diabetic acidosis, produce coma is unknown.

Coma produced by trauma to the head is of considerable clinical importance and theoretical interest. The term cerebral concussion (cerebral commotion in the older medical terminology) refers to a loss of consciousness produced by a blow to the head, without gross structural brain damage. Unconsciousness in concussion lasts from a few seconds to about half an hour. There is often peripheral vasoconstriction and tachycardia during the period of unconsciousness. Focal seizures, generalized seizures, or both, at the time of concussion, or during the course of coma are produced in a small percent of closed-head injuries (those in which the brain is not penetrated by a foreign body or by a piece of fractured skull). There may be some small hemorrhages in the brain in such cases. The actual pathological condition of concussion in human clinical cases is unknown because such patients recover promptly unless injuries to other organs have occurred. In concussion electrocortical activity is generally slowed and disorganized during the period of unconsciousness.

The mechanism of coma in concussion is unknown. A blow to the head is much more likely to produce coma if the head and neck are either extended or flexed by the blow. This has long been known by boxers, who try to keep their chins tucked in and their necks rigid to prevent their heads from being snapped backwards by a blow. It is likely that sudden flexure and stretching of the brainstem produces dysfunction of reticular nuclei, leading to coma.

A much more violent blow is required to produce coma if the head is rigidly supported. A strong blow to a rigidly supported head will produce relative movement of the brain and the skull, with compression of the brain against the skull both at the site of injury (coup injury) and at the point opposite to the site of the blow (contrecoup injury). Various rotatory and translational movements of the cerebral hemispheres relative to the brainstem are also produced and it is likely that these distortions of brain tissue are important in producing coma after a blow to the rigidly supported head, as well as in the case in which the head is unsupported and the brainstem is flexed.

Anesthetic agents are defined as drugs that produce a loss of consciousness that is dose related and is predictable and controllable in duration and depth. In addition, the drugs that are classed as anesthetics have a good factor of safety in that they produce a much greater depression of consciousness than of cardiovascular and respiratory function.

For some of the clinically used gaseous (inhalation) anesthetic agents, four stages of anesthesia are commonly recognized, in which there is progressive depression of electrocortical activity and of spontaneous motor and reflex activity as the concentration of the anesthetic agent in the brain is increased. Consciousness is lost between the first stage (stage of analgesia or of induction) and the second stage (stage of delirium or of excitement). The third stage is the stage of surgical anesthesia, in which there is sufficient depression of reflex activity so that painful stimuli do not produce somatomotor and autonomic reflexes, such as the eye blink, and in which there is relaxation of muscle tone. However, medullary respiratory and cardio-

vascular reflexes are not seriously depressed. In the fourth stage these medullary functions are depressed.

The mechanism of action of general anesthetics in producing loss of consciousness is not definitely known. The majority of general anesthetic drugs produce a greater depression of transmission of activity in multisynaptic pathways than in monosynaptic pathways. Sensory-evoked activity in the reticular formation appears to be particularly depressed. The effect of the barbiturate general anesthetics in producing synchronization of the electrocorticogram (barbiturate spindles) and in blocking the desynchronizing effect of sensory stimulation is rather similar to the effect of a large lesion of the pontine reticular formation.

SLEEP

Sleep is an altered state of consciousness. The brain in sleep is not unconscious, that is, unaware. That perceptual mechanisms function in sleep is shown by the ability of sounds that are significant, such as a child's cry, to awaken a sleeping individual, whereas much louder but insignificant sounds, such as traffic noises, will not produce awakening. The working in of stimuli, particularly of sounds, into the content of dreams also demonstrates the activity of perceptual mechanisms in sleep. Sleep, like many other bodily functions, is a cyclic, or circadian (L. *circa*, about; *dies*, a day), phenomenon. The length of the period of the cycle is probably related to the 24-hour period of rotation of the earth and the resulting light-dark cycles. Probably as a result of evolutionary development many circadian activities are controlled endogenously, although they can be reset by environmental stimuli.

Behaviorally and physiologically characterized sleep occurs in reptiles, but sleep is more developed and complex in birds and mammals. It is not clear if reptiles have rapid eye movement (REM) sleep. Lower mammals generally appear to sleep more and to have a slightly smaller proportion of REM sleep to total sleep than do humans. The biological significance of sleep is still unclear.

In people, normal sleep is marked by a progression of stages that can be characterized in several ways: behaviorally, by means of the level of somatic and autonomic motor activity and by the intensity of stimuli required for awakening; electroencephalographically; and psychologically, by awakening sleepers and obtaining reports of their sensations and dreams, if any. By using behavioral, electroencephalographic, and psychological data one can distinguish two major sleep states, non-REM sleep and REM sleep. These terms are defined further below. Non-REM sleep is also called slow-wave sleep because of

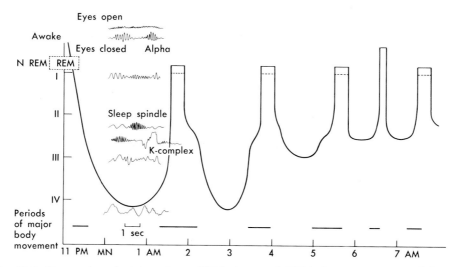

Fig. 11-1. Progression of states of non-REM sleep and REM sleep in a young adult. The electroencephalographic activity that characterizes stages 1 through 4 of non-REM sleep is illustrated.

Table 11-1. Sleep states

Stage	Percent of sleep (young adults)	Behavior	EEG
Non-REM			
1	5	Drowsy Rolling eye movements	7 to 10 Hz (theta-alpha) of fluctuating frequency and low voltage
2	50	Light sleep Readily aroused	3 to 7 Hz low-voltage, plus bursts of 12 to 14 Hz sleep spindles K-complexes
3		Moderate-depth sleep Blood pressure reduced Heart slowed	1 to 2 Hz (delta) waves of high volatge, few sleep spindles
	20	Pupils miotic Slightly depressed monosynaptic reflexes	
4		Deep sleep	1 to 2 Hz (delta) waves of high voltage
REM			
	25	Bursts of eye movement Increased and irregular autonomic activity	Low-voltage fast activity

the progressive slowing of the EEG potentials as the behavioral depth of sleep increases. REM sleep has been called paradoxical sleep, because the EEG shows low-voltage fast activity, similar to that in arousal. The progression of behavioral and EEG changes in a typical night's sleep in young adults is shown in Fig. 11-1. The sleep pattern is characterized by a fairly rapid transition from drowsiness to deep sleep in the early portion of the night. Deep sleep is then punctuated by periods of progressive lightening of sleep, which become slightly more frequent toward the end of the sleep period. There are usually four to six cycles of lightening of sleep per night. During the periods of lightening, the state of sleep usually undergoes a transition to a period of REM sleep. The periods of REM sleep lasts about 20 minutes and occur with a 90-minute interval.

The characteristics of non-REM and REM sleep states can now be further defined. Dement and Kleitman have classified the four stages of the non-REM sleep state, as indicated in Table 11-1.

In non-REM sleep there is some tone in the postural muscles, such as the antigravity muscles (extensors) of the neck, although tone is less pronounced than in the waking state. The monosynaptic reflexes are not markedly inhibited. The threshold for limb movement evoked by motor cortex stimulation is raised. There are no pronounced episodes of autonomic activity, and the pupils are miotic. Certain neuroendocrine events are also related to sleep states; growth hormone, for example, is released in sleep stages 3 and 4.

In contrast, REM sleep is characterized by a low-voltage high-frequency (20 to 30 Hz) EEG pattern that is remarkably similar to that during arousal. The behavioral events that occur during REM sleep may be subdivided into phasic and tonic activities. The most striking phasic events are the bursts of 50 to 60 eye movements per minute for which this form of sleep is named. However, muscular twitching is not confined to the eye muscles. In animals such as the cat, for example, twitchings of the vibrissae and tail are also prominent. The REM movements are associated with high-voltage potentials in the pons, lateral geniculate nucleus, and occipital cortex (PGO waves). They occur in clusters at a rate of about 60/min. The REM and PGO phenomena appear to mimic the processes of waking visual activity. Among the tonic events is a loss of tension in the postural muscles, particularly the neck extensors. There is a marked inhibition of brainstem and spinal cord reflexes. Autonomic responses include irregular respiration, a maintained reduction in arterial blood pressure interrupted by short-lasting episodes of hypertension during the bursts of eye movements, and signs of sexual arousal, including erection in the male.

Dreaming occurs largely during REM sleep periods. Nightmares are associated with REM periods. However, dreams can also occur in non-REM sleep. The incubus (to lie on; a demon that lies on a sleeping person's chest), which is an oppressive type of nightmare accompanied by a suffocating feeling and terror without much specific dream imagery, occurs in stage 4 of non-REM sleep.

REM sleep is not to be considered a variant of light, stage 1 sleep. Thresholds for auditory arousal in REM sleep are generally equivalent to those in stage 2 sleep.

Sleep states appear to be produced, at least in part, by changes in activity of neurons in the brainstem reticular formation and hypothalamus. Theories of the changes of activity of these neurons fall into two categories, which may be called passive (fatigue state) and active theories of sleep.

The modern version of the passive theory of sleep is based on the description of the reticular activating system as the neural mechanism that determines the level of arousal. Because the reticular system is activated by afferent input from the various sense organs as well as from the cerebral cortex, it is conceivable that sleep results from the reduction in sensory input that would be expected to occur under the external conditions conducive to sleep.

The active theories of sleep invoke a neural triggering mechanism that causes the development of the sleep states. The reticular activating system may be inhibited, or the triggering system may operate at a higher level of the nervous system in competition with the reticular activating system. Present evidence favors the concept of an active rather than a passive sleep mechanism.

There is now evidence that monoaminergic neurons in the brainstem are involved in the sleep mechanism. Destruction of the serotoninergic neurons in the raphe nuclei of the brainstem causes almost continuous wakefulness (insomnia) in cats, whereas the administration of drugs that elevate brain serotonin levels causes an increase in the amount of slow-wave sleep and reduces the amount of REM sleep. Changes in brain catecholamines also affect sleep. For instance, if a precursor of catecholamines is administered, sleep is suppressed. The details of how the monoaminergic pathways of the brain fit into the neural mechanisms for sleep are, however, unknown. It is likely that the groups of reticular formation neurons that are essential for both sleep and consciousness are somewhat different. The presence of sleeplike transitions in the EEG pattern of patients in coma was discussed in the section on consciousness.

Sleeplessness is associated with deterioration of psychological performance and with minor neurological changes such as tremor, nystagmus, dysarthria, and weakness of neck flexion.

Narcolepsy is a relatively uncommon condition that is characterized by attacks of sleep and by profound loss of muscle tone (cataplexy). In addition, there may be sleep paralysis, an inability to move that occurs in the drowsy state, and hypnagogic hallucinations, which are similar to dream states. Narcoleptic attacks may be attacks of REM sleep, that is, sleep initiated with a REM state instead of stage 1 non-REM sleep as is normal.

ATTENTION

Attention can be defined, in psychological terms, as directing perceptual mechanisms to stimuli in the field of consciousness. Attention can also be defined behaviorally by the occurrence of orienting of sensory receptors to a stimulus. Orienting is usually produced by a change of stimulus level, by the presentation of a novel stimulus, or by a stimulus that the organism has learned is a signal for reward or punishment. Attention is related to the process of arousal. Electrophysiological signs of the process of paying attention to stimuli can be observed by recording sensory-evoked potentials from the cerebral cortex. When a quietly resting animal whose electrocorticogram shows synchronized high-voltage rhythmic activity in the alpha (8- to 12-Hz) frequency band is presented with a stimulus, such as a click, a primary evoked potential will be evoked in the auditory cortex, and secondary responses of longer latency will be recorded over wide areas of the cerebral cortex. If the stimulus arouses the animal, the animal will usually orient to the stimulus, and the dominant rhythm of the neocortical electrocorticogram will generally shift to faster frequencies of lower voltage (electrocortical arousal). In contrast, the electrical activity of the hippocampal formation may exhibit trains of rhythmic synchronized potentials of large amplitude in the theta (4- to 7-Hz) range (see Chapters 6 and 10). However, with repetitive presentations, the stimulus becomes ineffective in producing arousal and orientation. As this occurs, the amplitude of the sensory-evoked primary response decreases, and the stimulus will not evoke electrocortical arousal. This process is an example of habituation.

Restoration of the behavioral and electrical signs of attention to the stimulus can be produced by changing the character of the stimulus or by making it significant to the animal. This process is called dishabituation. It is not yet clear whether dishabituation is merely a reversal of the processes of habituation or whether it is a different type of process.

Changes in the amplitude of sensory-evoked potentials during the processes of habituation and dishabituation have been most thoroughly studied in the auditory pathways. The appropriate increases and decreases of amplitude of potentials associated with behavioral signs of attention and habituation have been found at all levels of the auditory pathway, from the cochlear receptors to the auditory cortex, in some but not all of the studies done to investigate this problem. It is thought that descending systems, originating at least in part in the cortex, mediate these changes in afferent input and act as a control system that modulates and directs sensory input.

Expectancy is a psychological state closely related to attention. An expectancy state can be produced by an experimental situation in which paired stimuli are used and in which the first stimulus is followed after a short period of time by a second stimulus that is made significant by being associated with reward or punishment. In such situations a negative potential, with a time course of seconds, can be recorded from wide areas of the cerebral cortex on presentation of the first stimulus. This potential has been termed the contingent negative variation (CNV). The CNV is generally maximal over the vertex of the skull.

In addition to the process of activation of attention, other neural mechanisms appear to be necessary for maintaining attention. In primates these mechanisms appear to be located in the frontal lobes of the brain, in the rostral frontal cortex (see Chapter 6). Removal of this cortex in the monkey and in humans produces a markedly reduced attention span. Although individuals with such lesions will attend to the presentation of novel stimuli, they are not able to maintain their attention for more than brief periods of time. Other aspects of frontal lobe lesions are discussed in Chapter 10. Bilateral lesions of the caudate nuclei, which receive extensive projections from the frontal cortex as well as from the rest of the neocortex, have also been reported to produce a reduced ability to perform tasks that require delayed responses and maintained attention to stimuli.

PERCEPTION

The process of perception presupposes the activities of consciousness and attention. Perception also implies cognition, or recognition and judgment of sensory stimuli. Sensory experience and learning during development appear to play a role in forming the perceptual mechanisms of adult animals. Deprivation of visual experience has been shown to result in malformation of a proportion of the dendritic spines of visual cortex neurons in the mouse, although some spines develop normally in the absence of vision. Visual deprivation also produces changes in the shapes of the receptive fields of cat visual cortex neurons.

Many of the psychophysiological studies of perception have been directed to understanding the manner in which the physical characteristics of stimuli are encoded by neural activity. Most stimuli have the psychological attributes of intensity, quality, and position in space. The manner in which these attributes of the stimulus are encoded by the receptors, as well as the transformations in the neural activity at each relay station in the sensory pathway, has been extensively studied in the somatosensory system (see Chapter 7).

A related type of psychophysical study is the description of laws relating the physical property of the intensity of the stimulus to the psychological property of the intensity of the percept. It has long been known that this is a nonlinear relationship in which the intensity of a series of stimuli must increase in an exponential manner to produce equally spaced increments of sensation. Studies by Stevens have shown that a power function best describes the transformation of stimulus energy to the intensity of the percept. The relationship is described by the equation

$$\text{Sensation} = k \times \text{stimulus}^B$$

The exponent B for the sensation of brightness is about one third. Much of this transformation appears to occur at the level of the sensory receptors. This transformation gives the sensory systems an immense range of responsiveness to stimuli.

An important property of visual perception is constancy of the percepts. Size constancy is an example of this phenomenon. For example, a chair observed from a distance of 10 feet does not look twice as large as a chair observed from a distance of 20 feet, even though its retinal image is twice as large in the first case. Learning no doubt plays a role in the development of the constancies, which contribute to our sensation of the stability of the external world and are important in our being able to manipulate the world around us.

Another important aspect of perception that is closely related to learning and memory is the recognition of objects. This aspect of perception is related to the problem of the knowledge of universals, in the terminology of classical philosophy. For example, we can recognize (classify) a particular object, such as a chair, that we have never seen before as an example of a class of objects (chairs) even when the object is presented to us in novel spatial orientations, such as upside down.

Perceptual mechanisms tend to group objects into patterns. The visual illusions have been used, especially by the Gestalt (configuration) school of psychologists, to study the organizational properties of perceptual mechanisms. For example, on initial viewing of a perspective drawing of a cubic form (the Necker cube), the viewer sees the cube as if he were either looking slightly down at it or slightly up at it. On prolonged fixation the viewer's perspective point suddenly shifts to the other possible viewpoint. The visual illusions suggest that certain central states of activity on which perception depends are more stable than others. It is not known to what extent such organizational tendencies in perception are innate and to what extent they are learned.

There may be a considerable degree of inherent, or "prewired," organization of responses to particular types of stimuli built into the nervous system. Recording from single neurons at various levels of the visual system in amphibia and in mammals has revealed the presence of neurons that act as detectors for certain properties of the stimulus, such as motion detectors, edge detectors, or contour detectors. There are, however, many difficulties both in carrying out and in interpreting these experiments. Another property that appears to be at least partially inherent in the nervous system is that of surround inhibition, in which a peripheral stimulus produces a patch of excited cells in relay nuclei and in sensory cortices, surrounded by a zone of inhibited cells. It is thought that surround inhibition is a mechanism for increasing sensory discrimination that operates by increasing the contrast between the stimulated and nonstimulated points of the receptive surfaces of the body.

The visual illusions also indicate that critically spaced and timed stimuli can induce neural activities that are interpreted as physical stimuli. An example of this is the "phi" phenomenon, in which a viewer in a dark room sees first one light go on and off and then another light, at some distance from the first, blink on and off. If the distances and the timing of the light flashes are correctly adjusted, a light will appear to jump from the position of the first light to the position of the second light. The sensation of movement produced by cinematography is a similar phenomenon.

The primary corticosensory areas have major roles in the perception of most sensations. The role in perception of the association cortex adjacent to the primary sensory cortical areas is less well understood. Ablation of the primary sensory cortices in humans has shown that the severity of the perceptual deficit associated with lesions of primary receptive cortex is greatest for the visual cortex. Damage to the primary visual cortex produces blindness in corresponding portions of the contralateral visual fields (see Chapter 7). Direct electrical stimulation of the visual cortex with long-term implanted electrodes in a person who lost vision in adult life has produced visual sensations of small spots of light in what corresponds to appropriate contralateral portions of the former visual field of the patient. Stimulation of the cortex adjacent to the primary visual cortex has been reported to produce visual sensations of various formed images, often colored and exhibiting motion, in either the contralateral or ipsilateral visual fields.

Lesions of the primary somatosensory cortex produce an impaired sense of touch and impaired two-point discrimination, point localization, and position sense in the corresponding contralateral parts of the body. There is raising of the threshold for these sensations in the hand after ablation of the hand area. However, there can be some residual perception of these modalities.

In some individuals there can also be a deficit in point localization in the ipsilateral hand after destruction of the hand area of the somatosensory cortex. Direct stimulation of the somatosensory cortex produces contralateral paresthesias rather than sensations of touch or position.

Auditory cortex lesions have been less thoroughly studied. Little effect on the sensation of hearing with the contralateral ear is produced by unilateral primary auditory cortex lesions. However, there is evidence that the auditory cortex of each hemisphere preferentially receives input from the contralateral ear by way of the crossed auditory pathway. Input from the ipsilateral ear through the uncrossed pathway can, however, also be used by each auditory cortex. In animals, bilateral auditory cortex removal does not appear to result in loss of hearing (intensity and tone discrimination) but does interfere with recognition of timbre (harmonics) and temporal patterns of sounds. Direct electrical stimulation of the human auditory cortex produces buzzing and other noiselike sounds, often referred to the contralateral ear.

Direct electrical stimulation of the somatosensory cortex has shown that to produce a sensory perception the cortex must be excited for a definite period of time, approximately half a second. This observation suggests that the initial positive-negative waves of the sensory-evoked response merely signal the entry of afferent activity to the cortex and that it is the elaboration of activity occurring over about the next half second that is associated with perception. In agreement with this concept is the fact that although stimulation of Ia afferent fibers can evoke a primary evoked response with a short latency in the sensorimotor cortex of the cat, this response does not appear to be associated with any perception of sensation. The exact amount of neural tissue that must be activated to provide sensation is not known. Perhaps about a cubic millimeter of cortex must be activated; undoubtedly corticothalamic and corticocortical projections are secondarily activated by direct cortical stimulation, which produces sensation.

The role of parietotemporo-occipital association cortex, surrounding the primary sensory, auditory, and visual cortices respectively, appears to be the elaboration or interpretation of information received by the primary receptive areas. However, little is known with certainty about the function of association cortex in perception. Damage to the parietal lobe, without damage to the primary receptive sensory area, does not result in difficulty in tactile recognition of objects with the contralateral hand, according to carefully carried out studies in humans. However, it is possible that combined somatosensory cortex and parietal lobe association cortex lesions may produce a more severe tactile recognition deficit than that produced by a primary somatosensory cortex lesion alone.

Disturbances of identification, recognition, discrimination, or classification are called agnosias (without knowledge of). There is considerable uncertainty about agnosias. It is not clear to what extent patients with agnosias in each of the various sensory spheres (largely somatosensory, auditory, and visual) have deficits of reception of the primary data of sensation of intensity, quality, and position in space. The term agnosia is used to indicate clinically a loss of the ability to classify stimuli that is out of proportion to the loss of perception of the existence of stimuli being presented. For example, a patient with visual agnosia

is unable to identify an object in the visual field as a chair, although visual fields and visual acuity are normal. The agnosias are related to the disconnection syndromes (see the section on cerebral dominance) and to aphasia (see the section on language). Agnosias can be produced by lesions of the association cortex of the parietotemporo-occipital area, which lies between the primary receptive cortices for somatic sensation, audition, and vision.

A type of inattention to contralateral somatosensory and visual stimuli, called the extinction phenomenon, can be recognized in patients with parietal and parieto-occipital lobe lesions respectively. In patients with such lesions, simultaneous stimulation of corresponding points on each side of the body or of corresponding points in right and left visual fields (double simultaneous stimulation) results in a failure to perceive the application of the stimulus on the side of the body contralateral to the lesion.

Hallucinations and illusions are disorders of perception and are discussed in relationship to psychomotor seizures in Chapter 6.

LEARNING

The process of learning is generally thought of as producing a structural or electrophysiological change in the brain. This change has been called the memory trace. This term can be used without implying any particular type of localization or mechanism of memory storage.

In addition to the processes that produce the memory trace, there are also processes for gaining access to the trace, for recalling it to consciousness, and for producing motor activity.

To study these processes, various models of learning situations have been developed. The conditioned reflex studied extensively by Pavlov is one of these paradigms. An unconditioned stimulus (US) is presented, which produces a reflex, or natural unconditioned response (UR). In his early studies Pavlov used a piece of meat as the US that produced the UR of salivation. The US is then paired temporally with a conditioned stimulus (CS), such as a tone. After a variable number of presentations the CS will evoke the response, which is then termed the conditioned response (CR). The CR can differ from the UR in some ways. This sequence can be shown as:

$$US \longrightarrow UR$$
$$US + CS \longrightarrow UR$$
$$CS \longrightarrow CR$$

It is important to note that the unconditioned stimulus often has the characteristics of a reward (food) or punishment (a shock, for example) in this type of experiment. This model of learning is also called classical conditioning.

Another paradigm of learning is instrumental, or operant, conditioning, in which an animal learns to respond to a stimulus with a motor activity, such as pressing a bar, when the motor activity is rewarded or reinforced by gratification of a drive or by brain stimulation in certain limbic structures (see Chapter 10).

These models of learning indicate the importance of drives, emotion, the generation of visceral activity, and the satiety of visceral activity in producing learning. Some relationships of limbic structures to such activities and to memory are discussed in Chapter 10. One role of drives in learning may be to produce the exploratory motor and mental activities of making responses and of "rehearsing" responses that are necessary for learning.

Studies of learning in mammals, using such models of the learning process, have indicated that there is no single brain area in which learning and memory are represented. The ability to learn and remember appears to be a function of the total amount of cerebral tissue functioning. The hippocampus, however, appears to have a role in assembling recent experiences into memory, although the trace is not uniquely stored in the hippocampus (see Chapter 10).

In its broadest sense, learning can be thought of as plasticity, or modifiability, of synaptic function. A simple model of plasticity of synaptic function that has been carefully studied is the process of habituation (see section on attention). A recent important development in neurobiology has been the use of simple systems, largely invertebrate preparations, to study habituation and other plastic processes. Habituation of the gill withdrawal reflex of the mollusc *Aplysia* (the sea hare) has been studied intensively by Kandel and his associates. This process depends on only a limited number of sensory neurons and a few motoneurons. All of the neurons controlling the reflex behavior can be identified, and their connections and electrophysiological activity can be specified. Stimulation of the body that gives rise to gill withdrawal evokes EPSPs in the motoneurons controlling gill withdrawal. By means of intracellular recording during habituation, it has been shown that habituation is associated with a decrement of the EPSP produced by stimulating the body surface. This reduction in synaptic efficacy can be attributed to presynaptic changes.

Another example of modifiability of synaptic function by prior activity is posttetanic potentiation, in which a conditioning period of high-frequency firing of a presynaptic terminal results in hyperpolarization of the terminal and a greater release of transmitter substance to testing stimuli for a variable period of time.

These are essentially short-term changes in synaptic function. How such short-term changes might be converted into long-term changes lasting for years is not known.

It is likely that there is more than one kind of neural mechanism in learning, at least in mammals, and that the different paradigms of learning emphasize the use of various mechanisms.

The transfer and storage of perceptual experience into memory also appears to consist of several processes in mammals. The following model of memory is currently being widely studied. Sense data appear to be initially put into short-term storage. This storage has a finite capacity to absorb information over specific periods of time. For example, recall of digits presented in a random order (nonmeaningful pattern) is limited to about seven digits at a time. The storage for purely visual information is much greater than for linguistic information (symbols). Materials can be recalled from this storage for varying periods of time. Unless there is a very strong emotional significance to the sensory data or unless it is rehearsed, after a short period of time it cannot be recalled voluntarily (forgetting), although it can often be recognized for a longer time as experienced material. Transfer of experience to long-term or permanent storage occurs over a finite period of time, perhaps several hours, after the material enters short-term storage. This process is called consolidation. Consolidation is particularly susceptible to disruption. A mechanism is also required for gaining access to storage. The only known anatomical correlates of these presumed mechanisms are the hippocampal formation and temporal lobe, which appear to function in the control of storage or recall or both, perhaps by selecting items for storage and recall.

Penfield and his associates have shown that direct electrical stimulation of the cortex of the temporal lobe with gross electrodes in awake patients undergoing craniotomy evokes or recalls memory sequences that continue to "unroll" as long as the stimulation is maintained. This does not mean that the memories are stored in the temporal lobe. The minimal explanation of these findings appears to be that recall mechanisms are being activated.

Change in synaptic function during learning and memory implies either growth of new synaptic connections or a change in the functional effectiveness of synapses. In either event, changes in the metabolic activity and possibly in the configuration of molecules of the membranes in the presynaptic and postsynaptic membranes would not be unexpected. There is therefore reason to believe that metabolic activity, perhaps of protein synthesis in particular, might be important in learning and in memory. Attempts to test this hypothesis have been made by studying the effect on learning of inhibition of brain protein synthesis produced by administration of various drugs. These experiments are subject to many technical and theoretical difficulties. However, the recent studies of Baronedes and his associates suggest that inhibition of protein synthesis in the mouse brain affects the transfer of short-term memory to memory storage. Inhibition of protein synthesis during or immediately after training results in a situation where the animal can learn a task but remembers it for only about 3 hours. The same drugs do not produce loss of consolidated memories.

Amnesia refers to a disturbance of memory. Amnesia can occur as part of rather generalized brain disorders, as described in the discussion of dementia. However, of greater interest in terms of memory mechanisms is amnesia produced by cerebral concussion or generalized seizures, particularly those produced by electroconvulsive therapy. Concussion and seizures appear particularly to affect consolidation, resulting in a loss of the experiences that were stored in the period immediately prior to the insult (retrograde amnesia) and for a period after the insult (anterograde amnesia).

CEREBRAL DOMINANCE

Cerebral dominance refers to the predominant control of certain motor and psychological activities by one of the cerebral hemispheres. The psychomotor activities in which one hemisphere is most clearly dominant are in the use of the hands (handedness), language functions, and in visualization of spatial relationships. Cerebral dominance has not been studied very extensively in lower forms. Certain individuals of other species, such as monkeys and cats, tend to preferentially use one forelimb for manipulation. However, the general motor dominance of the left cerebral hemisphere appears to be largely a human feature.

The preferential use of one hand for skilled activities develops during the latter half of the first year of life. About 90% of all people are right handed, although the figure varies slightly in different countries. The remainder are either clearly left handed or, in a small number of cases, are ambidextrous. There is some tendency to inheritance of handedness. The corticospinal system, as discussed in Chapter 8, plays a major role in the performance of skilled hand movements. Therefore, the corticospinal system of the left hemisphere is used preferentially in most individuals in skilled hand movement early in childhood and may be considered to receive more training as the child develops. However, the left hand and the corticospinal system originating in the right cerebral hemisphere are capable of being trained to perform highly skilled movements. Conversely, children who are predominantly left handed can be taught to write and perform other skilled acts with their right hand.

The motor expression of language and the understanding of spoken and written language are also controlled by the left cerebral hemisphere in over 90% of all people (language is discussed later in this chapter). The association of skilled control of the hand and of language function in the same cerebral hemisphere in the majority of persons is undoubtedly not fortuitous but must represent some type of efficient neural mechanism that had survival value. However, in left-handed persons (with right hemisphere motor dominance) language function is still generally represented in the left hemisphere. Left-handed persons do tend to have less complete dominance of language by the left hemisphere than do right-handed persons; that is, a left-handed person with destruction of the speech areas of the left hemisphere is more likely to have some speech function remaining than a right-handed person with a similar lesion.

The effects of lesions of the right cerebral hemisphere indicate that in most persons the right temporal lobe contains mechanisms for the storage of tone memories and that the right parieto-occipital area is important for the perception and visualization of spatial relationships.

There is no fine-structural or electrophysiological basis known for the dominance of one hemisphere; however, some differences in structure of the left hemisphere compared with the right have been correlated with language function. The superior margin of the left temporal lobe (see the section on language) is about 1 cm longer than the right in about 65% of brains.

The evidence for cerebral dominance has come largely from the study of persons with brain lesions. A method of producing transient and reversible depression of function of a cerebral hemisphere by injecting a short-acting anesthetic agent such as Amytal, a barbiturate compound, into an internal carotid artery was described by Wada. The test is often performed in conjunction with carotid arteriography, carried out for the localization and diagnosis of brain lesions (see Chapter 5). The anesthetic produces brief dysfunction of the territory supplied by the injected carotid artery. Hemispheric depression is manifested by a transient weakness of the contralateral side of the body. During this period the level of consciousness and production of speech are tested. Reception of speech and memory can also be tested. Knowledge of the localization of language function to the right or left hemisphere is of clinical importance in cases in which epilepsy, usually with a psychomotor component, can be shown to be caused by an area of epileptic discharge in or adjacent to the temporal lobe (see Chapters 6 and 10). In about one third to one half of such cases in which the seizures cannot be suppressed by anticonvulsant drugs, excision of the affected temporal lobe will alleviate the seizures. If the affected hemisphere can be demonstrated not to be dominant for language, the surgeon knows that the amount of temporal and inferior frontal lobe tissue that can be resected without producing disturbances of language is greater than if the resection were performed on the dominant side of the brain.

Communication between the right and left hemispheres is carried out largely through the corpus callosum. In an ingenious experiment Myers cut the optic chiasm and the corpus callosum in adult cats and monkeys (Fig. 11-2). Each hemisphere of such a

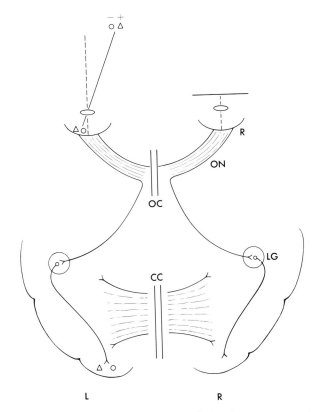

Fig. 11-2. Split-brain preparation used for demonstrating the role of the corpus callosum in interhemispheric transfer of information. Abbreviations: *R,* retina; *ON,* optic nerve; *OC,* optic chiasm (cut); *CC,* corpus callosum (cut); *LG,* lateral geniculate nucleus; *L, R,* left and right visual cortices. A mask has been placed over the right eye. The left hemisphere is being trained to discriminate between a triangle and a circle.

split, or bisected, brain can be trained to respond to visual stimuli presented in the ipsilateral nasal field from which it can still receive visual input. The left hemisphere can be trained to respond positively to a triangle and not to a circle, whereas the right hemisphere can be taught the opposite task. Additional experiments by Sperry, Myers, Gazzaniga, and others showed that information received by one hemisphere is transferred through the corpus callosum to the contralateral hemisphere.

The general class of intellectual deficits produced by cutting of the cerebral commissures has been called disconnection syndromes. Commissurotomy has been performed in humans to attempt to prevent the spread of seizures from one hemisphere to the other. The most striking effects of disconnection are related to the dominance of the hemispheres for specific functions. For example, a patient with a disconnection syndrome can recognize an unseen object, such as a key, placed in the *right* hand (tactile recognition dependent on the left postcentral gyrus) and can describe it verbally as a key. However, the same patient cannot verbally describe the object when it is placed in the *left* hand, because the tactile information from the object goes to the right hemisphere, which is disconnected from the speech mechanism of the left hemisphere. The apparent lack of effect of commissurotomy on general intellectual and behavioral performance in adults is caused by the fact that both hemispheres have already been trained to respond to most situations. Ipsilateral sensory pathways and the number of ways in which one hemisphere can utilize cues, such as orienting responses, as a signal of activity in the other hemisphere also appear to be responsible for the ability of the commissurotomized patient to function fairly normally on many tasks.

After damage to one hemisphere, the remaining hemisphere can assume the functions of the damaged hemisphere to some degree. This effect is greatest in the very young individual. After hemispherectomy performed for relief of intractable seizures or after massive cerebral damage caused by cerebral infarction in infancy, normal motor dominance (ability to perform skilled movements) and language function can be assumed by the remaining hemisphere.

LANGUAGE

Language functions are frequently divided clinically into motor (expressive) speech functions and sensory (receptive) hearing and reading functions. However, these functions are closely related in the development of language and in the production of speech. Speech can be severely disrupted by preventing an individual from hearing words as they are uttered. This can be shown by electrically recording speech as it is uttered and playing it back through earphones to the individual after a very brief delay. As indicated in the preceding section, the left cerebral hemisphere contains the language mechanisms in the great majority of persons. In the remainder of individuals both hemispheres contribute to language functions, and in a few individuals there is a definite right hemisphere dominance.

Localization of language function has largely been a result of the study of the effects of brain lesions that produce speech disturbances, which are called aphasias (speechlessness). Aphasias are a very complex and still incompletely understood subject. In general, damage to the left inferior frontal gyrus, in the area of the ascending and horizontal rami of the lateral fissure (Figs. 5-12 and 11-3), results in an inability to produce speech, or an expressive aphasia. The term expressive aphasia should probably be limited to describe loss of fluency of speech. The correlation of speech expression with the left inferior frontal gyrus was made by Broca, and the area is often called by his name. In expressive aphasia, in this limited sense, patients are able to think of the words they wish to say, may be able to write them, and can understand their meaning when they hear or see them, to varying degrees. There is, however, a much more profound disturbance of the ability to articulate speech than of understanding speech. The deficit varies in severity

from a total inability to articulate words (although sounds can be made) to some hesitancy of speech. After lesions of Broca's area there is generally some compensation or reorganization of speech function, particularly in young individuals, and some degree of normal speech will often be attained.

Broca's area lies immediately rostral to the area of the primary motor cortex (Ms1) where the vocal musculature is represented (Fig. 8-3). Electrophysiological evidence of the participation of Broca's area in articulation of speech has recently been obtained. Nonpolarizable electrodes and direct-current amplifiers (see Appendix I) are used for recording from the scalp over Broca's area. A slow negative potential of several seconds' duration can be recorded over Broca's area with word production. The onset of the potential begins up to 1 second prior to uttering words. These slow potentials are similar to the readiness potentials (RP) that are found over the motor cortex prior to making a movement of the contralateral body musculature. The RP differs from the CNV potential (see the section on attention) by being more focally localized to the motor areas related to the muscles making the movement.

Receptive aphasia is produced by damage to the area of the supramarginal and angular gyri of the left parietal lobe and to the posterior portion of the superior temporal gyrus (Wernicke's area) (Fig. 11-3). Wernicke's area is adjacent to the auditory cor-

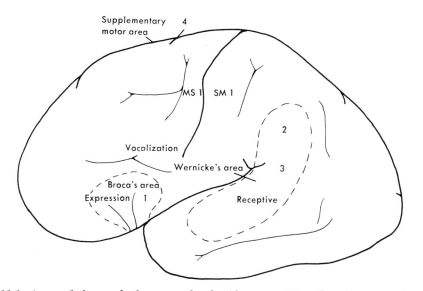

Fig. 11-3. Areas of the cerebral cortex related to language. Note that these areas lie in the left hemisphere in the majority of persons. *SM 1, MS 1,* primary somatic sensory and motor cortices. The numbers *1* to *4* indicate cortical sites where electrical stimulation produces disruption of speech. Site 4 is on the medial surface of the hemisphere, just in front of the motor foot area. Areas where vocalization is produced by direct electrical stimulation are near the face area of MS 1 and in the supplementary motor area, which lies on the medial surface of the hemisphere.

tex (the transverse temporal gyrus of Heschl; see Chapter 7). In receptive aphasia the patient has a disturbance of comprehension of language. As a result the expression of language may also be disturbed, with the production of jargon, substitutions of words (paraphasia), and other expressive disturbances; speech, however, is generally fluent.

Most severe and lasting aphasias are caused by damage to the parietotemporal speech areas.

Damage to the left cerebral hemisphere in the area of the junctions of the parietal, occipital, and temporal lobes can also produce disturbances in reading (dyslexia), writing (dysgraphia), and in the ability to calculate.

As indicated in the section on cerebral dominance, language is represented, at least in terms of the effects of lesions of the hemispheres, in the left hemisphere. Only about 1% of right-handed persons with aphasia will have a right hemisphere lesion. Of left-handed persons with aphasia, about 40% have a right hemisphere lesion. As might be expected, language disturbances can be produced by lesions of subcortical fibers and by disturbances of function of the specific thalamic nuclei that have connections with cortical speech areas.

INTELLIGENCE

Intelligence (to choose between, to discriminate) is a term that indicates the quality of the entire range of mental abilities of an individual. Psychologists have tended to regard intelligence as an underlying ability or power that makes itself manifest in the ability to classify, to understand relationships, and to reason. In addition to the quality of general intelligence, individuals manifest more specialized primary abilities, such as verbal ability, arithmetical ability, and ability to perceive spatial relationships. The quality of the primary abilities is generally positively correlated with general intelligence. However, some individuals may have considerable verbal ability and little mathematical ability, and so on.

The ability to learn and to remember is also closely related to the level of general intelligence of an individual but is not in itself equivalent to general intelligence. Individuals use their ability to perceive relationships, to reason, and to solve problems; and problem-solving tests can be used as a measure of general intelligence.

General intelligence appears to some degree to be an inherited trait. It appears reasonable to believe that general intelligence depends on brain structure. However, no specific anatomical or electrophysiological features of the brain have yet been associated with intelligence. In humans there is no known relationship between brain size or weight and intelligence, provided that the brain is grossly normally developed and is within the normal range of brain weight (see Chapter 5).

Certain specialized abilities in animals, such as the ability to learn mazes, can be selected and bred for, resulting in progeny with high or low levels of these abilities (maze-bright or maze-dull progeny). The inheritance of specific structures of portions of the brain has also been demonstrated. Mutant mice that have distinctive features of the hippocampus (cornu ammonis, or CA) have been recognized. These anatomical features of CA are transmitted according to mendelian laws. However, little is yet known about the behavioral correlates of these hereditarily transmitted anatomical features of the brain.

Gross mental retardation, or the failure to develop mental abilities within the normal range of intelligence, is frequently associated with gross malformation of the brain. Various factors, such as disorders of amino acid or lipid metabolism, perinatal anoxia, and intrauterine infection, have been identified that produce maldevelopment of the brain. However, little has yet been done to characterize the fine structure of the maldevelopment in various types of mental retardation, largely because not enough is known about the normal structure and function of specific brain areas to be able to specify clearly the changes that have occurred in the "wiring diagrams" of the areas.

Dementia refers to a severe deterioration of intelligence. Senile dementia is associated with neuropathological evidence of severe aging of the brain. Anatomical changes include degeneration of neurons and the formation of senile plaques and neurofibrillar tangles, which are microscopic structures composed of degenerated neurons and other material. The chemistry and ultrastructure of such areas of degeneration in senile dementia are now undergoing intensive investigation. Individuals in the early stages of progressive senile dementia generally exhibit a patchy loss of mental abilities. There may be quite severe loss of some types of intellectual ability, with relative sparing of other abilities until quite late in the course of deterioration. Recent memory is, however, impaired in most cases early in the disease.

INSTINCTIVE BEHAVIOR AND DRIVES

The term instinctive behavior is used to designate complex behavior, generally involving integration of autonomic and somatic motor activity, that is largely concerned with obtaining food and with reproduction. The neural substrates or central programs for these activities appear to be inherent in the nervous system, although sensory experience and learning are necessary for their proper development. Locomotor behavior and speech can be regarded as instinctive behavior. However, what is generally meant by instinctive behavior in animals is the integration of autonomic and motor behavior into more complex activities, such as hunting and killing, courtship, and reproductive behavior.

Complex visceral activities are generally associated with these activities. The sensations of emotion consist in part of the sensations of these visceral activities. These and other visceral sensations, such as hunger, appear to act as drives or stimuli to produce motor behavior. In addition, as discussed in Chapter 10, mental processes that are not represented in consciousness can determine behavior. The goal of much drive-induced motor activity is to maintain or to restore a particular visceral state, such as the state of satiety after eating. The term conation (to attempt) has been used to describe the drive toward fulfillment of unconscious desire, or the putting forth of effort to reach goals. The central neural mechanisms that integrate drives and instinctive behavior are not understood, although the importance of limbic structures such as the amygdaloid nuclei in sexual and attack behavior and the ventromedial hypothalamic nuclei in feeding behavior has been established (see Chapters 9 and 10).

The stimuli for activating the neural mechanisms generating drive and instinctive behavior are both sensory (from exteroceptors and interoceptors) and hormonal. Many of the studies of the adequate stimuli for triggering instinctive behavior, such as mating behavior, have been made in lower vertebrates such as fish and birds. These studies have revealed that some instinctive behavior is triggered by complex and prolonged patterns of sensory stimulation, such as the proportion of light to darkness in a 24-hour period. Such patterns of stimulation can activate the hypothalamo-pituitary axis and result in release of hormones from the pituitary gland. The hormones secreted by the pituitary gland act on target glands and stimulate their hormonal output. These hormones then act on the brain and result in particular patterns of behavior.

MENTAL DISORDERS

Disorders of mental functioning can be divided into those that have a known organic basis, such as the acute and the chronic brain syndromes caused by trauma, metabolic disturbances, increased intracranial pressure, and degenerative diseases, and those disorders that have no known organic cause and are considered psychogenic in origin. The psychogenic disturbances can be divided into psychoses, psychophysiological autonomic disturbances, psychoneuroses, and personality disturbances. Psychoses are severe forms of disorganization of mental activity and are medical problems of major significance. They can be divided into the affective (manic-depressive), schizophrenic, and paranoid reactions. The point that is emphasized here is that psychoses are characterized by disturbances of emotional reactivity, by disturbances of thinking, and by disturbances of perception. Disturbances of these mental functions occur in varying degrees in each type of psychotic disorder.

Various lines of evidence suggest that psychotic disorders have specific organic causes. These lines of evidence are the difficulty of explaining psychotic behavior in the psychodynamic terms that appear to explain psychoneurotic behavior; the induction of psychoticlike states with drugs that affect central synaptic function; the alteration of psychotic behavior with other drugs, such as lithium, which suppresses manic behavior; and changes in blood and urine levels of metabolites of various putative neurotransmitters in patients with psychotic disorders. However, it cannot be said that any firm foundation of understanding an organic basis for mental illness has been achieved.

BIBLIOGRAPHY
Consciousness

Ayer, A. J.: Language, truth and logic, London, 1951, Victor Gollancz Ltd.

Chase, T. N., Moretti, L., and Prensky, A. L.: Clinical and electroencephalographic manifestations of vascular lesions of the pons, Neurology (Minneap.) **18**:357-368, 1968.

Eccles, J. C., editor: Brain and conscious experience, New York, 1966, Springer Publishing Co., Inc.

Ingvar, D. H., and Sourander, P.: Destruction of the reticular core of the brainstem, Arch. Neurol. **23**:1-8, 1970.

Lashley, K. S.: Persistent problems in the evolution of mind, Q. Rev. Biol. **24**:28-42, 1949.

Plum, F., and Posner, J. B.: The diagnosis of stupor and coma, Philadelphia, 1966, F. A. Davis Co.

Wilkus, R. J., Harvey, F., Ojemann, L. M., and Lettich, E.: Electroencephalogram and sensory evoked potentials; findings in an unresponsive patient with a pontine infarct, Arch. Neurol. **24**:538-544, 1971.

Sleep

Chase, M. H., and McGinty, D. J.: Somatomotor inhibition and excitation by forebrain stimulation during sleep and wakefulness; orbital cortex, Brain Res. **19**:127-136, 1970.

Dement, W. C., and Kleitman, N.: Cyclic variations in EEG during sleep and their relation to eye movements, body motility and dreaming, Electroencephalogr. Clin. Neurophysiol. **9**:673-690, 1957.

Jouvet, M.: Neurophysiology of the states of sleep, Physiol. Rev. **47**:117-177, 1967.

Jouvet, M.: Biogenic amines and the states of sleep, Science **163**:32-41, 1969.

Noda, H., and Adey, W. R.: Firing of neuron pairs in cat association cortex during sleep and wakefulness, J. Neurophysiol. **33**:672-684, 1970.

Rechtschaffen, A., and Dement, W. C.: Narcolepsy and hypersomnia. In Kales, A., editor: Sleep; physiology and pathology; a symposium, Philadelphia, 1969, J. B. Lippincott Co.

Roffwarg, H. P., Muzio, J. N., and Dement, W. C.: Ontogenetic development of the human sleep-dream cycle, Science 152:604-619, 1966.

Sassin, J. F.: Neurological findings following short-term sleep deprivation, Arch. Neurol. 22:54-56, 1970.

Attention

Hernandez-Peon, R.: Reticular mechanisms of sensory control. In Rosenblith, W. A., editor: Sensory communication, New York, 1961, John Wiley & Sons, Inc.

Milner, B.: Some effects of frontal lobectomy in man. In Warren, J. M., and Akert, K., editors: The frontal granular cortex and behavior, New York, 1964, McGraw-Hill Book Co.

Milner, P. M.: Physiological psychology, New York, 1970, Holt, Rinehart & Winston, Inc.

Thompson, R. F., and Spencer, W. A.: Habituation; a model phenomenon for the study of neuronal substrates of behavior, Psychol. Rev. 73:16-43, 1966.

Perception

Cassinari, V., and Pagni, C. A.: Central pain; a neurosurgical survey, Cambridge, 1969, Harvard University Press.

Corkin, S., Milner, B., and Rasmussen, T.: Somatosensory thresholds; contrasting effects of postcentral-gyrus and posterior parietal lobe excisions, Arch. Neurol. 23:41-58, 1970.

Critchley, M.: The parietal lobes, Baltimore, 1953, The William & Wilkins Co.

Gibson, E. J.: Principles of perceptual learning and development, New York, 1969, Appleton-Century-Crofts.

Köhler, W.: Gestalt psychology, New York, 1929, Liveright.

Mishkin, M.: Visual mechanisms beyond the striate cortex. In Russell, R. W., editor: Frontiers in physiological psychology, New York, 1966, Academic Press, Inc.

Semmes, J., Weinstein, S., Ghent, L., and Teuber, H. L.: Somatosensory changes after penetrating brain wounds in man, Cambridge, 1960, Harvard University Press.

Stevens, S. S.: Neural events and the psychophysical law, Science 170:1043-1050, 1970.

Teuber, H. L., Battersby, W. S., and Bender, M. B.: Visual field defects after penetrating missile wounds of the brain, Cambridge, 1960, Harvard University Press.

Valverde, F.: Rate and extent of recovery from dark rearing in the visual cortex of the mouse, Brain Res. 33:1-12, 1971.

Learning

Baronedes, S. H., and Cohen, H. D.: Comparative effects of cyclohexamide and puromycin on cerebral protein synthesis and consolidation of memory in mice, Brain Res. 4:44-51, 1970.

Griffith, J. S.: The transition from short- to long-term memory. In Horn, G., and Hinde, R. A., editors: Short-term changes in neural activity and behavior, Cambridge, 1970, Cambridge University Press.

Kandel, E. R., and Spencer, W. A.: Cellular neurophysiological approaches in the study of learning, Physiol. Rev. 48:65-134, 1968.

Pribram, K. H., editor: On the biology of learning, New York, 1970, Harcourt Brace Jovanovich, Inc.

Russell, W. R.: The traumatic amnesias, New York, 1971, Oxford University Press, Inc.

Spencer, W. A., and April, R. S.: Plastic properties of monosynaptic pathways in mammals. In Horn, G., and Hinde, R.

A., editors: Short term changes in neural activity and behavior, Cambridge, 1970, Cambridge University Press.

Whitty, C. W. M., and Zangwill, O. L., editors: Amnesia, London, 1966, Butterworth & Co. (Publishers) Ltd.

Young, J. Z.: A model of the brain, New York, 1964, Oxford University Press, Inc.

Cerebral dominance

Ebner, F. F., and Myers, R.: Corpus callosum and the interhemispheric transfer of tactual learning, J. Neurophysiol. 25:380-391, 1962.

Fedio, P., and Weinberg, L. K.: Dysnomia and impairment of verbal memory following intracarotid injection of sodium amytal, Brain Res. 31:159-167, 1971.

Gazzaniga, M. S.: The bisected brain, New York, 1970, Appleton-Century-Crofts.

Lehman, R. A. W.: Hand preference and cerebral predominance in 24 rhesus monkeys, J. Neurol. Sci. 10:185-192, 1970.

Milner, B.: Laterality effects in audition. In Mountcastle, V. B., editor: Interhemispheric relations and cerebral dominance, Baltimore, 1962, The Johns Hopkins Press.

Mountcastle, V. B., editor: Interhemispheric relations and cerebral dominance, Baltimore, 1962, The Johns Hopkins Press.

Zangwill, O.: Cerebral dominance and its relation to psychological function, Springfield, Ill., 1960, Charles C Thomas, Publisher.

Language

Geschwind, N.: The organization of language and the brain, Science 170:940-944, 1970.

Luria, A. R.: Traumatic aphasia, The Hague, 1969, Mouton Publishers.

McAdam, D. W., and Whitaker, H. A.: Language production; electroencephalographic localization in the normal human brain, Science 172:499-502, 1971.

Milner, B.: Brain mechanisms suggested by studies of temporal lobes. In Darley, F. L., editor: Brain mechanisms underlying speech and language, New York, 1967, Grune & Stratton, Inc.

Neilsen, J. M.: Agnosia, apraxia, aphasia; their value in cerebral localization, ed. 2, New York, 1962, Hafner Publishing Co., Inc.

Penfield, W., and Roberts, L.: Speech and brain mechanisms, New York, 1966, Atheneum Publishers.

Intelligence

Gordon, E. B., and Sim, M.: The EEG in presenile dementia, J. Neurol. Neurosurg. Psychiatry 30:285-291, 1967.

Lashley, K. S.: Brain mechanisms and intelligence, Chicago, 1929, University of Chicago Press.

Spearman, C., and Wynne-Jones, L. L.: Human abilities, London, 1950, The Macmillan Co.

Tomlinson, B., Blessed, G., and Roth, M.: Observations on the brains of non-demented old people, J. Neurol. Sci. 7:331-356, 1968.

Wimer, R. E., Wimer, C. C., and Roderick, T. H.: Genetic variability in forebrain structures between inbred strains of mice, Brain Res. 16:257-264, 1969.

Instinctive behavior and drives

Black, P., editor: Physiological correlates of emotion, New York, 1970, Academic Press, Inc.

Chi, C. C., and Flynn, J. P.: Neural pathways associated with hypothalamically elicited attack behavior in cats, Science **171:**703-706, 1971.

Hebb, D. O.: The organization of behavior, New York, 1949, John Wiley & Sons, Inc.

Pribram, K. H., and Melges, F. T.: Psychophysiological bases of emotion. In Vinken, P. J., and Bruyn, G. W., editors: Handbook of clinical neurology, vol. 3, Amsterdam, 1969, North-Holland Publishing Co.

Thorpe, W. H.: Learning and instinct in animals, London, 1956, Methuen & Co., Ltd.

Mental disorders

Himwich, H. E., Kety, S. S., and Smythies, J. R., editors: Amines and schizophrenia, New York, 1967, Pergamon Press, Inc.

Kolb, L. C.: Modern clinical psychiatry, ed. 8, Philadelphia, 1973, W. B. Saunders Co.

Schildkraut, J. J.: The catecholamine hypotheses of affective disorders; a review of supporting evidence, Am. J. Psychiatry **122:**509-522, 1965.

Smythies, J. R.: Biological psychiatry; a review of recent advances, Berlin, 1968, Springer-Verlag, New York, Inc.

CHAPTER 12

Principles of application of anatomy and physiology in neurological diagnosis

The process of diagnosing a neurological illness involves two distinct steps: (1) determination of the anatomical site of the lesion in the nervous system, and (2) determination of the pathological condition of the lesion and its cause.

The *method* used in this process is the correlation of information obtained from the patient's history, from the neurological examination, and from special diagnostic studies, such as skull and spine x-ray films, angiography, ventriculography, myelography, electroencephalography, electromyography, nerve conduction time, spinal fluid examination, and biochemical tests.

The *process of diagnosis* (anatomical localization and the formulation of a differential diagnosis of possible lesions and their causes) and the application of *the principal methods of diagnosis* (history taking and neurological examination) are discussed separately here. In practice these activities are carried out nearly simultaneously by a clinician as a result of experience in examining patients with neurological diseases. However, it is useful for the student initially to consider these two aspects of diagnosis separately.

PROCESS OF NEUROLOGICAL DIAGNOSIS

The first step in the process of anatomical localization of a lesion is to determine the site of the lesion in the longitudinal plane in the nervous system (Fig. 12-1). This involves determining if the lesion is situated at one or more of the following levels of the neuraxis: receptor (sense organ) or effector (muscle, usually), peripheral nerve, spinal roots, spinal cord, brainstem, cerebellum, or cerebrum. When a hypothesis is formed about the longitudinal level of the lesion, the lesion is localized in the horizontal plane, that is, in a transverse section of the neuraxis (Fig. 12-1). This involves determining if the lesion is located at one or more of the following sites of the section: left side, right side, dorsal, ventral, central, or peripheral. Most lesions of the nervous system are single lesions (single tumors, infarctions, hemorrhages, and so on), and an attempt is always made to account for the findings of the neurological examination on the basis of a single lesion. Only when the neurological findings cannot be explained by a single lesion should the lesion be considered to involve multiple sites. For example, a patient is found to have weakness of the right arm and leg (right-sided hemiparesis) and intention tremor (terminal ataxia) of the right arm and leg. These findings could be produced by two lesions: a lesion of the left motor cortex, producing hemiparesis, and a lesion of the right cerebellum, producing ataxia. However, these neurological signs can be explained more economically by a single lesion that involves the posterior limb of the left internal capsule (corticospinal fibers) and the left ventrolateral thalamic nucleus (cerebellocortical projection). Another site at which a single lesion will produce hemiparesis and terminal ataxia of the contralateral limbs is the pons, where the corticospinal tract and the cerebellar peduncles are contiguous. Inability to explain a constellation of neurological signs by a single lesion that damages

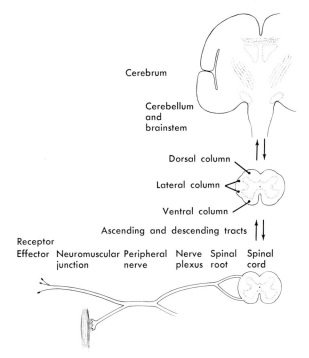

Fig. 12-1. Longitudinal and transverse levels of the nervous system.

a number of contiguous structures is an important indicator of the cause of disease. Multiple sites of damage to the nervous system are frequently produced by metastatic tumors, multiple vascular occlusions, or various types of demyelinating disease (most frequently by multiple, or disseminated, sclerosis).

Following the processes of anatomical localization of the lesion, the second step in the process of diagnosis is to formulate a list of the probable causes of the lesion. A list of probable causes and the reasons for assigning a ranking of probabilities is called a differential diagnosis. A differential diagnosis is arrived at by first considering the possible types of pathological lesions that can occur at the particular site in the nervous system to which the lesion has been localized. The various classes of pathological lesions of the nervous system are:

1. Congenital malformations
2. Neoplasms
3. Vascular disease
4. Infections: bacterial, fungal, protozoal, helminthic, viral
5. Inflammatory or granulomatous disease of a noninfectious or unknown cause
6. Metabolic disease and toxic and deficiency disorders
7. Demyelinating disease (diseases of immunological mechanisms?)
8. Degenerative diseases of unknown cause
9. Structural or metabolic alteration secondary to trauma

Certain pathological conditions occur more frequently than others in particular sites in the nervous system,

and knowledge of their probability of occurrence aids in formulating a differential diagnosis.

The age of the patient is another factor considered in formulating a differential diagnosis. For example, in children tumors of the cerebellum are more common than vascular occlusions of blood vessels of the cerebellum.

The temporal progression of symptoms and signs is also considered. A hemiparesis that develops slowly is likely to be caused by a slowly developing lesion, such as a tumor, whereas a rapid onset of hemisparesis is more likely to be caused by a vascular occlusion. There can be multiple causes of symptoms, such as vascular hemorrhage in a necrotic tumor.

METHODS OF NEUROLOGICAL DIAGNOSIS

The methods of clinical investigation of the nervous system are history taking, neurological examination, and special diagnostic studies.

History taking

The history of the patient's illness is of primary importance in the investigation of neurological disease. It cannot be emphasized too strongly that history taking is an active process during which hypotheses about the locus and cause of the lesion are formulated, and questions are designed to test these hypotheses. It has been said that it should be possible to determine the locus and cause of the lesion in the majority of cases of neurological disease on the basis of the history alone. Perhaps this is an overstatement; but a hypothesis about the site of the lesion, a differential diagnosis, and a plan of neurological examination should be developed by the examiner while taking the patient's history.

Hypotheses about the possible locus of the lesion are based on knowledge of the association of certain neurological findings that occur as parts of constellations of symptoms and signs. The association of particular neurological signs is based on the contiguity of anatomical structures and the physiological consequences of certain lesions. For example, if a patient is found to have weakness of the left facial muscles, the lesion must be somewhere in the motor pathway that passes from the right motor cortex through the internal capsule to the brainstem nucleus of the left facial nerve and along the left facial nerve to the left facial muscles. Therefore, the patient is questioned about and examined for the presence of lesions of structures that lie in contiguity with the possible loci of the lesion. In particular, because nerves VII and VIII lie together in the internal acoustic meatus, the function of nerve VIII is examined, and because the genu of nerve VII runs around the nucleus of nerve VI in the brainstem, the function of nerve VI is examined.

The finding of an anatomically and physiologically consistent constellation of neurological abnormalities is used not only for localizing the site of lesions but also for weighing the significance of particular abnormal findings. For instance, a small number of people who have no neurological disease will exhibit pathological reflexes such as Babinski's sign (dorsiflexion of the great toe and fanning of the toes when the sole is stroked firmly) instead of the normal plantar flexion of the toes. However, when this sign is present in persons who have a neurological disease that has damaged the corticospinal projections, there is almost always a change in the myotatic reflexes of the muscles of the same leg. Therefore, the presence of Babinski's sign as an isolated finding does not have the same significance as its presence as part of a constellation of signs that includes hyperactive myotatic reflexes, decreased rapid-succession movements, weakness of leg muscles that is more marked in the distal dorsiflexors than in the proximal leg muscles, and circumabduction of the leg when walking. Descriptions of some of the common constellations of signs found in nerve, spinal cord, brainstem, and cerebral lesions are given in the final sections of this chapter.

Neurological examination

The following order of examination of the nervous system is one that is often useful:

1. Cranial nerves
2. Motor system
3. Somatosensory system
4. Reflexes (which involve both sensory and motor systems)
5. Mental status

This order of examination is particularly useful in patients who are seriously ill or obtunded, because the maximum degree of information about seriously ill patients can usually be obtained most quickly by examination of the cranial nerves, particularly of the optic fundi, and by examination of the motor system. Nevertheless, the examination should be individualized. It is often best to examine the area of the patient's complaints first. This also enables the clinician to reexamine the major area after a time to see if the findings are consistent.

The following format for recording the history and the findings of the physical and neurological examinations is reasonably complete and simple and indicates the type of information collected during the examination.

A. History
   1. Chief complaint
   2. Present illness
   3. Family history
   4. Social history
   5. Past medical history
   6. Review of systems
B. Examination
   1. Physical examination
     a. Skull: tenderness, swelling, lacerations
     b. Neck: suppleness, muscle spasm, tenderness
     c. Spine: mobility, spasm, tenderness
     d. Pulses and bruits: carotid, supraclavicular, ocular
     e. Complete examination of systems (cardiac, pulmonary, and so on)
   2. Neurological examination
     a. Cranial nerves
     b. Motor systems
     c. Sensory systems
     d. Reflexes
     e. Mental status
C. Summary of history and positive findings of the physical and neurological examinations
D. Formulation of differential diagnosis
   1. Site of lesion
   2. Differential diagnosis

The neurological examination form is presented in detail on p. 405.

It should be emphasized that, just as in taking a history, the neurological examination is an active process in which the examiner tests hypotheses about the site of the lesion.

Description of the specific techniques used for carrying out the neurological examination is beyond the scope of this book. These techniques are well described in a number of texts listed in the Bibliography (p. 428).

Special diagnostic studies

The formulation of the history and the differential diagnosis is the basis of selecting the special diagnostic studies. Such tests are best regarded as aids clarifying the differential diagnosis and not as the primary method of making a diagnosis. In some cases of neurological disease none of the methods of diagnosis may yield enough information to identify the disease. Even the most complete radiological and biochemical studies and direct visualization and biopsy of lesions of the nervous system at surgery may not provide unambiguous evidence of the cause of an illness. Therefore, it is important to formulate clearly the differential diagnosis for the patient's medical record so that the patient's clinical course can be followed with the appropriate range of examinations over a period of time, during which the cause of the illness will often become apparent.

NEUROLOGICAL EXAMINATION

A. Cranial nerves

  I. Olfactory
  II. Optic (OD, OS)
    a. Visual acuity (uncorrected and corrected for errors of refraction)
    b. Visual fields
    c. Fundi
    d. Light reflexes, direct and consensual
  III. Oculomotor (OD, OS)
    a. Pupillary size
    b. Lids
  III, IV, VI. Oculomotor, trochlear, abducens (OD, OS)
    a. Movements
    b. Diplopia
    c. Nystagmus
  V. Trigeminal (right, left)
    a. Sensory
    b. Motor
  VII. Facial (right, left)
    a. Face
      (1) Upper
      (2) Lower
    b. Platysma
    c. Taste
  VIII. Vestibulocochlear (AD, AS)
    a. Auditory
      (1) Air conduction
      (2) Bone conduction
      (3) Weber test (sound lateralized to right or left ear)
    b. Vestibular
  IX, X. Glossopharyngeal, vagus (right, left)
    a. Swallowing
    b. Phonation
    c. Movement of palate and uvula
    d. Pharyngeal reflex
  XI. Accessory (right, left)
    a. Sternocleidomastoid and trapezius
  XII. Hypoglossal (right, left)
    a. Movement, atrophy, fibrillation of tongue

B. Motor systems (note right or left handed)

  1. Patterned movement
    a. Gait
    b. Station and equilibrium
    c. Rapid-succession movements
    d. Movement requiring terminal control (finger to nose, heel to shin)
    e. Handwriting
  2. Muscle testing (right, left)
    a. Muscle weakness (specify paralysis or marked, moderate, or slight weakness, or normal strength)
      (1) Arm
      (2) Trunk
      (3) Leg
    b. Muscle status (specify atrophy, fasciculations, tone, tenderness)
      (1) Arm
      (2) Trunk
      (3) Leg
    c. Autonomic motor systems
      (1) Sweating
      (2) Skin temperature
      (3) Trophic changes

C. Somatosensory systems (right, left)

  1. Nerve tenderness
  2. Primary modalities
    a. Light touch
    b. Muscle sense
    c. Joint position
    d. Vibration
    e. Cutaneous pain
    f. Deep pain
    g. Temperature
  3. Complex modalities
    a. Two-point discrimination
    b. Stereognosis
    c. Palm writing
    d. Simultaneous recognition
  4. Trophic changes

D. Reflexes (right, left)

  1. Myotatic
    a. Arm
    b. Leg
  2. Superficial
    a. Abdominal
    b. Cremasteric
    c. Plantar
  3. Sphincteric
    a. Anal
    b. Bulbocavernous

E. Mental status

  1. Behavior and appearance
  2. Stream of talk: overproductive, underproductive
  3. Emotional state
  4. Mental content: illusions, hallucinations
  5. Intellectual status
    a. Orientation: time, place, identity
    b. Memory: remote, recent, immediate recall
    c. Insight and judgment
  6. Body image, right-left orientation
  7. Receptive disturbances
    a. Visual agnosia
    b. Auditory agnosia
    c. Tactile agnosia
    d. Comprehension of speech
    e. Comprehension of writing
  8. Expressive disturbances
    a. Speech
    b. Writing
    c. Reading

COMMON NEUROLOGICAL SYNDROMES

A syndrome is a consistent group of symptoms and signs produced by a similar pathological process in different individuals. There are a large number of neurological syndromes, but only some of the commonest patterns of neurological signs can be discussed here.

Signs produced by lesions of various levels of the neuraxis are described here separately from the discussions of the anatomy and physiology of these areas, presented in previous chapters, for the following reasons. A major objective of clinical neurology is localization of lesions. The presence of certain neurological signs can be used to accurately localize a lesion to a part of the nervous system, yet the exact structures and physiological mechanisms that produce the signs may not be known. In addition, the appearance of certain signs is not always uniquely related to lesions of particular brain areas. Damage to different structures can produce rather similar symptoms. For example, a decrease in the rapidity of performance of skilled movements or rapid alternating movements can be produced both by cerebellar and motor cortex lesions, even though other signs may appear in cerebellar and cerebral lesions that will characterize the site of the lesion. The motor system and other neurological systems act as a whole, with interaction between their parts.

Peripheral, segmental, and suprasegmental representation of somatic sensation and movement

To localize lesions in the nervous system it is necessary to know the distribution of the muscular and cutaneous branches of peripheral nerves, the courses that nerve fibers take in the brachial and lumbosacral nerve plexuses, the muscular and cutaneous distribution of the ventral and dorsal roots of spinal segments respectively, and the central course of spinal and suprasegmental sensory and motor pathways.

Nerve fibers from the skin join sensory and motor fibers from muscles to form a mixed peripheral nerve (Fig. 12-2). The cutaneous distribution of peripheral nerves is not necessarily closely related to the muscles they supply. In the thoracic area the sensory and motor fibers of thoracic nerves enter and come from the spinal cord directly through the dorsal and ventral roots respectively. However, the nerves from the arm and from the leg join to form the brachial and lumbosacral plexuses respectively, through which nerve fibers are distributed to and from the spinal cord. The plexuses can be divided, as shown in Figs. 12-3 to 12-5, into cords, divisions, trunks, and roots. Sensory fibers from the cutaneous distribution of a nerve may

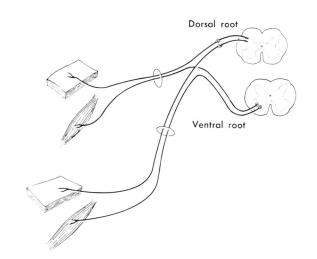

Fig. 12-2. Passage of cutaneous and muscular peripheral nerve fibers into peripheral nerves, and their distribution through a nerve plexus, into different segments of the spinal cord.

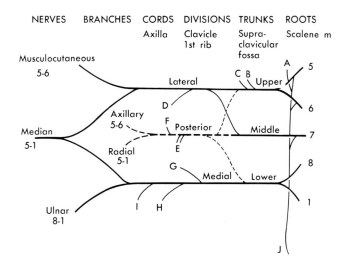

Fig. 12-3. Brachial plexus and nerves arising directly from its roots, trunks, and cords. Anterior divisions, solid lines; posterior divisions, broken lines. The three posterior divisions join to form the posterior cord (heavy broken line). Upper plexus: *A*, dorsal scapular n (levator scapulae, rhomboid m); *B*, subclavian n (subclavius m); *C*, suprascapular n (supraspinatus and infraspinatus m); *D*, lateral anterior thoracic n (pectoral m). Middle plexus: *E*, subscapular n (subscapular and teres major m); *F*, thoracodorsal n (latissimus dorsi m). Lower plexus: *G*, medial anterior thoracic n (pectoral m); *H*, medial cutaneous n of arm; *I*, medial cutaneous n of forearm. Upper and middle plexus: *J*, long thoracic n (serratus anterior m).

be distributed through cords, divisions, and trunks to enter the spinal cord through several roots (for example, ulnar nerve, C8 and T1 roots; musculocutaneous nerve, C5 and C6 roots). In a similar manner axons of ventral horn motoneurons of a cord segment may be distributed through the plexuses to several

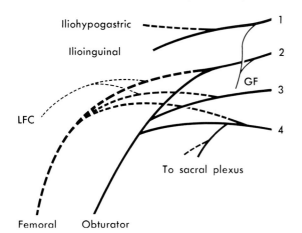

Fig. 12-4. Lumbar plexus. Anterior divisions, solid lines; posterior divisions, broken lines. Abbreviations: *GF*, genitofemoral n; *LFC*, lateral femoral cutaneous n.

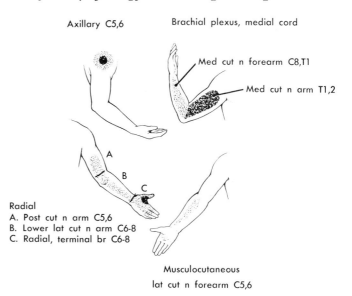

Fig. 12-6. Cutaneous distribution of nerves that supply the skin of the arm, the forearm, and part of the dorsum of the hand. The area of isolated supply of the axillary and radial nerves is indicated by the dense stippling.

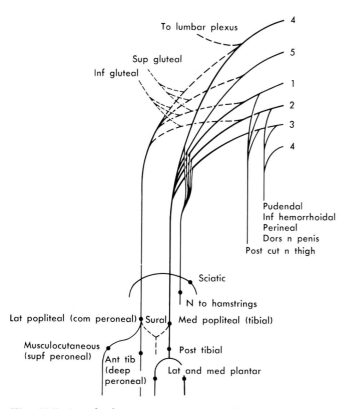

Fig. 12-5. Sacral plexus and origins and distribution of the branches of the sciatic nerve. Anterior divisions of plexus, solid lines; posterior divisions, broken lines.

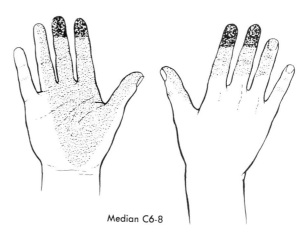

Median C6-8

Fig. 12-7. Cutaneous distribution of the median nerve. The area of isolated supply is indicated by the dense stippling.

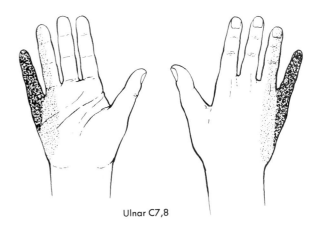

Ulnar C7,8

Fig. 12-8. Cutaneous distribution of the ulnar nerve. The area of isolated supply is indicated by the dense stippling. The major root supply is from C8. A contribution may come from C7 or T1 in some cases.

Table 12-1. Muscular distribution of major nerves

Nerve	Muscle	Root	Nerve	Muscle	Root
Brachial plexus°			*Brachial plexus—cont'd*		
Nerves arising directly from roots, trunks, and cords of the brachial plexus			Ulnar		
			From medial cord	Flexor carpi ulnaris	7,8†
				Flexor digitorum profundus 3 and 4	**8,1**
From upper plexus				Abductor digiti minimi‡	8,1
Dorsal scapular	Levator scapulae	4,5†		Opponens digiti minimi‡	8,1
	Rhomboid			Adductor pollicis‡	8,1
Suprascapular	Supraspinatus	**5**		Flexor pollicis brevis‡	8,1
	Infraspinatus			First palmar interosseous‡	8,1
From middle plexus				First dorsal interosseous‡	8,1
Subscapular	Subscapular	5,6	*Lumbar plexus°*		
	Teres major		Femoral	Iliopsoas	1,2,3§
Thoracodorsal	Lattissimus dorsi	6,7,8		Sartorius	**2,3**
From upper and middle plexus				Quadriceps femoris	**2,3,4**
Long thoracic	Serratus anterior	5,6,7		Rectus femoris, vastus lateralis, vastus intermedius and vastus medialis	
From all roots			Obturator	Anterior	
Lateral and medial anterior thoracic	Pectoral			Gracilis	**2,3,4**
	Clavicular part	5,6,7,8		Adductor longus	**2,3,4**
	Sternal part	6,7,8,1		Posterior	
Axillary (circumflex)				Adductor magnus	**2,3,4**
From posterior cord	Deltoid	**5,6**			
Musculocutaneous			*Sacral plexus°*		
From lateral cord	Biceps	5,6	Sciatic		
Radial			Nerve to hamstring‖	Semitendinous	4,**5**,S1,2
From posterior cord	Triceps	7,8		Biceps femoris, long head	4,**5**,S1,2
	Brachioradialis	5,6		Semimembranous	4,**5**,S1,2
	Extensor carpi radialis longus	6,7	Medial popliteal (tibial) division	Gastrocnemius	S1,2
	Supinator	5,6,7		Posterior tibial	4,5
	Extensor digitorum communis	7,8	Posterior tibial branch	Flexor digitorum longus	S1,2
	Extensor carpi ulnaris	7,8		Flexor hallucis longus	S1,2
	Abductor pollicis longus	7,8	Medial and lateral plantar branches of posterior tibial branch	Abductor hallucis#	S1,2
	Extensor pollicis longus	7,8		Abductor digiti minimi#	S1,2
	Extensor pollicis brevis	7,8		Fourth dorsal interosseous#	S1,2
	Extensor indicis	7,8		First dorsal interosseous#	S1,2
Median			Lateral popliteal (common peroneal) division		
From lateral (roots 6,7) and medial (roots 8,1) cords of plexus	Pronator teres	**6,7**			
	Flexor carpi radialis	6,7,8	Anterior tibial branch (deep peroneal)	Anterior tibial	4,**5**
	Flexor digitorum superficialis	7,8,1		Extensor digitorum longus	**5**,S1
	Flexor pollicis longus	8,1		Extensor hallucis longus	**5**,S1
	Flexor digitorum profundus 1 and 2	8,1		Extensor digitorum brevis#	S1
	Abductor pollicis brevis‡	8,1	Musculocutaneous branch (superficial peroneal)	Peroneus longus	**5**,S1
	Flexor pollicis brevis‡	8,1		Peroneus brevis	**5**,S1
	Opponens pollicis‡	8,1	Inferior gluteal	Gluteus maximus	5,S1
	Lumbricals 1 and 2‡	8,1	Superior gluteal nerve	Gluteus medius and minimus	4,5,S1
				Tensor fasciae latae	4,5,S1

°Major muscles that are tested are listed in order of the origin of the branches to them, proximal to distal. The major root supply is in boldface type.

†Root 1, thoracic; roots 4 to 8, cervical.

‡Intrinsic hand muscle.

§Lumbar unless specified; S, sacral.

‖Often considered to be part of the medial popliteal division.

#Intrinsic foot muscle.

Table 12-2. Testing of cord segments

Segment	Muscles
C2	Extensors of neck
C3,4	Trapezius, diaphragm
C5	Deltoid, rhomboids, infraspinatus
C6	Biceps, brachioradialis
C7	Triceps, extensor carpi ulnaris, extensor digitorum
C8	Flexor carpi ulnaris
C8 to T1	Intrinsic hand muscles
L2,3	Iliopsoas, adductors of thigh
L4	Quadriceps
L5	Tibialis anterior, extensor hallucis longus
S1	Gastrocnemius
S2	Intrinsic foot muscles

peripheral nerves (for example, the C8 segment sends fibers to the median, radial, and ulnar nerves).

Table 12-1 gives the distribution of muscular branches of the major peripheral nerves and the major spinal motor segment related to each muscle. Table 12-2 presents the major muscular distribution of spinal cord motor segments.

The cutaneous areas innervated by the major nerves of the arm and leg are shown in Figs. 12-6 to 12-10. Fig. 12-11 illustrates the cutaneous areas, called dermatomes, supplied by each cord segment.

Variations in the patterns of innervation of muscle and skin by nerves and cord segments can occur. The variability in the innervation of the intrinsic hand muscles by the median and ulnar nerves is of some clinical importance. In addition, various texts may differ by one segment in assigning a particular cord segment to a dermatome or in assigning a segment as the major motor supply to a particular muscle.

Peripheral nerve syndromes

A mixed peripheral nerve contains somatic motor, autonomic motor, and sensory fibers. The signs of a peripheral nerve injury depend on the cause of the injury, the severity of the injury, and the extent to which different types of fibers in the nerve are damaged. Crushing or cutting injuries tend to damage all types of fibers in a nerve. In some metabolic diseases of nerves, as in diabetic neuropathy, the largest nerve fibers, which carry proprioceptive and muscle spindle information, are damaged earlier than the smaller fibers. Gradual compression of nerve tissue, as by a tumor invading a nerve plexus, also tends to impair large-fiber function early in the course of the disease, and muscle weakness and loss of proprioceptive information may be produced, whereas pain sensation is not as noticeably affected.

Damage to the somatic motor fibers of peripheral nerves (or to the ventral horn motoneurons) produces

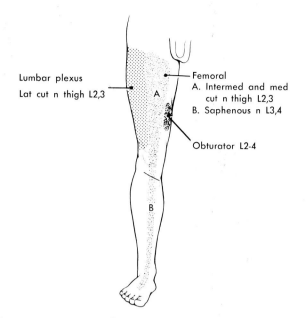

Fig. 12-9. Cutaneous distribution of nerves to the leg, arising from the lumbar plexus, which supply the skin of the anterior thigh and part of the skin of the anterior lower leg.

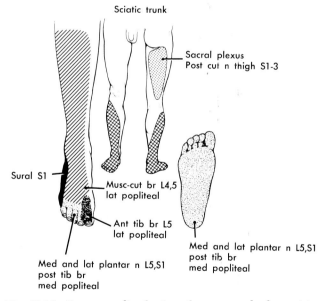

Fig. 12-10. Cutaneous distribution of nerves to the leg, arising from the sacral plexus, which supply the skin of the posterior thigh and the major portion of the lower leg and the foot. The area of supply of the sciatic nerve is double hatched; the distributions of individual cutaneous branches of the sciatic nerve within this area are indicated in the drawings of the lower leg and of the foot: the sural nerve, the musculo-cutaneous branch of the lateral popliteal nerve, the anterior tibial branch of the lateral popliteal nerve, and the medial and lateral plantar nerves, which are the terminal branches of the posterior tibial branch of the medial popliteal nerve.

ILLUSTRATIVE CASE HISTORY
Neuromuscular disease

Mr. B. T., age 66

1. **History**
   a. Chief complaint: Drooping of the right eyelid
   b. Present illness: Seven years prior to admission the patient had diplopia and unsteadiness of gait for 8 months. Diplopia was most marked on downward left lateral gaze. Three weeks prior to the present admission the patient noted drooping of the right eyelid. This is more marked at the end of the day.

2. **Examination**
   a. Physical examination: BP 150/90, P 84 regular, T 98°. Results of the physical examination normal.
   b. Neurological examination: Cranial nerves: 50% ptosis of right eyelid, questionable ptosis of left eyelid. Patient compensated for ptosis by wrinkling the forehead and elevating the eyebrows. Subjective diplopia on left lateral gaze, but eye movements appeared normal to the examiner. However, testing of the oculomotor muscles revealed weakness of the right medial rectus muscle. Facial asymmetry with drooping of the left side of the face, but no definite facial weakness. Motor: slight weakness of the dorsiflexors of the left wrist. Sensory: normal. Reflexes: normal.

3. **Summary**
   Two episodes of diplopia 7 years apart and a 3-week history of ptosis of the right eyelid. Neurological deficits: moderate ptosis of the right eyelid and slight weakness of the right medial rectus muscle, slight weakness of left wrist dorsiflexors, and drooping of left side of face.

4. **Formulation**
   a. Site of lesion:

   (1) Oculomotor nerve, or neuromuscular junction to levator muscle of eyelid and medial rectus muscle.
   (2) Possible lesion of corticospinal tract, right cerebrum.
   b. Differential diagnosis:
   (1) Infarction of right midbrain affecting right nerve III and corticospinal tract.
   (2) Infarction of right nerve III.
   (3) Compression of right nerve III by aneurysm of the carotid artery or by a tumor at the base of the skull.
   (4) Defect in neuromuscular transmission (myasthenia gravis).

5. **Laboratory data**
   Blood count, blood chemistries and urinalysis normal.
   Chest and mediastinal x-ray films normal.

6. **Course in hospital**
   The following special diagnostic studies were performed. Skull x-ray films normal. Results of visual field examinations normal. Audiometry revealed a bilateral hearing loss for tones above 2,000 cycles. A Tensilon test was performed. Tensilon (edrophonium chloride) is a short-acting anticholinesterase that reverses neuromuscular blockage produced by curarelike drugs at the neuromuscular synapse. After 10 mg of Tensilon was injected intravenously, the ptosis of the right eyelid disappeared and the strength of the dorsiflexors of the left wrist improved. The test was repeated 2 days later, first giving a control injection of saline. There was no improvement of strength with saline; but when the dose of Tensilon was injected, the muscular weakness disappeared. The patient was treated with Mestinon, a long-lasting anticholinesterase, which improved his ptosis and weakness.

7. **Diagnosis**
   Disease of neuromuscular transmission (myasthenia gravis).

---

flaccidity and loss of tonus of the muscles they innervate and weakness of muscular contraction on voluntary effort. The weakness is roughly in proportion to the number of motoneurons damaged. Trophic changes are also produced. The most clinically apparent trophic changes are fibrillation, the repetitive discharge of single muscle fibers, which can be detected by electromyography (see Chapter 3), and atrophy of muscle fibers. Disuse will also produce atrophy of normally innervated muscles. However, the degree of muscle atrophy that is produced by lesions of peripheral nerves or motoneurons (lower motoneuron lesions) is usually much greater than that produced by immobilization or by lesions of descending motor pathways (upper motoneuron lesions). The atrophy caused by nerve lesions is also generally more focal, corresponding to the muscular distribution of the nerve distal to the lesion, whereas lesions of the descending motor pathways tend to produce weakness of muscles of the entire half of the body distal to the lesion. Small lesions of the motor cortex can produce focal weakness in an extremity or in the face. However, there is a strong tendency in lesions of the motor cortex or descending motor pathways for the distal muscles of the limbs to be weaker than the proximal and limb girdle muscles and for the dorsiflexors of the wrist and foot to be weaker than the plantar flexors. The patterns of change in muscle strength that are produced by lesions of descending motor pathways are therefore usually more extensive and have a different distribution than those produced by lesions of nerves in limbs.

Damage to the sensory fibers of peripheral nerves produces hypesthesia (reduced sensation) or anesthesia (loss of sensation) in the cutaneous area supplied by the nerve. As indicated above, touch, vibration and position sense, and pain and temperature sensation can be reduced to different degrees, depending on the cause and the pathological condition of the nerve damage. When there is incomplete damage to a nerve, the patient may experience hyperesthesia (increased awareness of sensation) or hyperpathia (increased awareness of sensation, with an unpleasant quality to the sensation). There often appears to be a relatively greater destruction of large than of small fibers in such cases, although this point requires more investigation. In these cases normal cutaneous stimulation, such as touching or stroking, has an unpleasant quality, and there may be a subjective impression of a lower than normal threshold to touch or pain stimuli. However, when sensory thresholds are carefully measured in such cases, they are generally found to be increased for all modalities, and the hyperesthetic and hyperpathic qualities appear to be caused by changes

in central transmission of sensory impulses produced by the different pattern of sensory input to the spinal cord (see the section on somatic sensory mechanisms in Chapter 7).

There is considerable overlap of the cutaneous areas of supply of individual nerves, so the area of loss of sensation after nerve or dorsal root section is usually rather small. The overlap of sensory innervation on the trunk is so extensive that for a truncal dermatome (Fig. 12-11) to be anesthetized by dorsal root section, the root above it and below it must also be sectioned. Some limb nerves, however, do have a rather consistent though small area of isolated cutaneous innervation that can be detected clinically after nerve

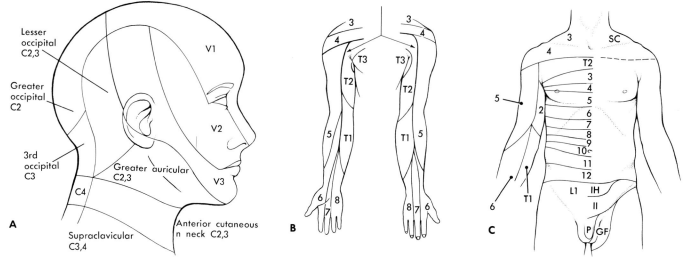

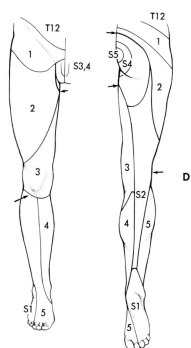

Fig. 12-11. Cutaneous distribution of spinal dorsal roots (dermatomes) and of the three divisions of the trigeminal cranial nerve (V 1 to 3) to the face. **A,** Face, head, and neck. **B,** Arm. Areas of distribution of cervical roots shown by numbers 3 through 8. Thoracic root distribution prefixed by the letter T. A narrow band of skin over the biceps (adjacent to the T2 dermatome) may be supplied by the C6 root, as indicated by the upper 6 in the anterior view of the right arm. **C,** Trunk. Lumbar root distributions prefixed by the letter L. *SC,* area of distribution of supraclavicular nerves; *IH,* iliohypogastric nerve; *Il,* ilioinguinal nerve; *P,* dorsal nerve of penis, a terminal branch of the pudendal nerve; *GF,* genitofemoral nerve (the ventral portion of the scrotum is supplied by a perineal branch of the pudendal nerve). **D,** Leg. Lumbar root distributions shown by numbers 1 to 5. Sacral root distributions prefixed by the letter S. Note: The arrows indicate contiguous cutaneous boundaries of roots whose spinal origins are not contiguous; for example, C6 and T2 in the arm.

ILLUSTRATIVE CASE HISTORY
Peripheral nerve disease

Mr. S. F., age 21

1. History

    a. Chief complaint: Numbness and weakness of the left hand.

    b. Present illness: The patient stated that he has been taking one injection of heroin intravenously daily for the past year until 2 months prior to admission, when he went to work in a camp outside of the city. He had severe withdrawal symptoms for a week and was nauseated and unable to eat. He then felt well until 2 weeks prior to admission, when he noted the onset of progressive malaise, anorexia, and dark-colored urine. He returned from the country on the day prior to admission. He was unable to eat. In the early evening he went to a friend's house. He then took a double shot of heroin intravenously in a vein in the left antecubital fossa. After the injection he got high and then passed out for a few minutes. He went home and went to bed. In retrospect, he states that he slept with his arms hanging over the sides of the bed. He awoke at about 4:00 A.M. and noted that his left arm was numb from the fingers to the shoulder, but mostly in the area of the left thenar eminence. He also noted that he could not raise his arm. He noted fasciculations of the muscles of the left arm and of the muscles of the right arm to a lesser degree. He felt feverish and came to the hospital.

2. Examination

    a. Physical examination: BP 100/70, P 84 regular, T 100.8°. Results of physical examination unremarkable.

    b. Neurological examination: Cranial nerves: pupils pinpoint. Motor: gait slightly ataxic. Rapid, coarse fasciculations in the left deltoid, biceps, and branchioradialis muscles. There was approximately 25% of normal strength in the left deltoid, biceps, triceps, and wrist extensors. There was approximately 75% of normal strength in the left wrist flexors. The intrinsic hand muscles were strong. There was approximately 75% of normal strength in the right deltoid muscle. The other muscles of the right arm were normal in strength. There was slight ataxia on finger-nose testing with the right arm, but marked ataxia, caused by weakness, on testing the left upper extremity. Sensory: hypesthesia in the

C5 to 6 dermatome distribution on the left. Reflexes: deep-tendon reflexes absent in the upper extremities. Patellar reflexes and Achilles reflexes were obtainable but hypoactive. There were no pathological reflexes.

3. Summary

Acute onset of weakness and fasciculations in proximal muscles of the arms, left more marked than right. The muscles most affected are supplied by the axillary, radial, and musculocutaneous nerves, by the posterior (axillary and radial nerve) and lateral (musculocutaneous nerve) cords of the brachial plexus, and by the C5,6,7 ventral roots and cord segments. Mild sensory deficit in the left arm over the radial side of the forearm in skin supplied by the radial nerve and the C5,6 roots. Fever, malaise, abnormal liver chemistries, and positive results of serological study.

4. Formulation

    a. Site of lesion:

        (1) Upper and middle brachial plexus.

        (2) C5 to 7 spinal roots.

    b. Differential diagnosis:

        (1) Compression lesion of brachial plexus sustained by stretching of arm over side of bed.

        (2) Rule out infection of central nervous system.

5. Laboratory data

Blood count and urinalysis normal. Blood chemistries showed mild abnormalities of liver function. Results of blood serological study abnormal.

Chest x-ray film normal.

6. Course in hospital

The following special diagnostic studies were performed. Cervical spine films normal. Lumbar puncture normal: opening pressure 150 mm CSF crystal-clear fluid, protein 28 mg/100 ml, glucose 100 mg/100 ml, and 1 WBC. Results of serological study normal.

The muscular weakness rapidly improved over a course of 2 days.

7. Diagnosis

    a. Bilateral upper branchial plexus compression.

    b. Resolving serum hepatitis.

    c. Abnormal results of serological study to be investigated.

---

injury. Some of these areas are illustrated in Figs. 12-6 to 12-10.

Damage to the sympathetic autonomic fibers of nerves produces a decrease of sweating in the cutaneous supply of the nerve. The skin may be warm because of vasodilatation produced by interruption of sympathetic vasoconstrictor fibers. Vasodilatation is usually most apparent for a few days or weeks after an acute injury to a nerve. There is also loss of pilomotor activity, resulting in the loss of the gooseflesh seen in response to cold.

Interruption of parasympathetic fibers in cranial and sacral nerves produces impaired activity of the muscular and glandular structures they supply (see the section on the autonomic nervous system in Chapter 3).

Changes that occur in the texture of the skin after nerve injury are called trophic changes. These changes are atrophy, loss of elasticity of the skin, and loss of hair. The skin appears thin, glossy, and tightly stretched. Healing of skin injuries is poor, and skin ulcers often develop. Trophic changes develop to a variable degree after nerve injury and are most marked in the hand and to a lesser degree in the foot. The cause of trophic changes is poorly understood. Impaired sympathetic innervation probably plays a part. However, sensory denervation also appears to be important in the causation of trophic changes.

The patterns of muscular weakness and sensory deficits produced by a nerve injury are used to differentiate peripheral nerve lesions from central lesions and to identify the nerve injured and the locus of injury along the course of the nerve. For example, weakness of dorsiflexion of the wrist could be caused by a lesion of peripheral nerves, spinal roots, spinal motoneurons, descending motor pathways, or the motor cortex. To investigate the site of the lesion, the muscles that dorsiflex the wrist are tested: the extensor carpi radialis longus (C6,7), the extensor carpi ulnaris (C7,8), and the extensor digitorum (C7,8). All of these muscles are supplied by the radial nerve. If these muscles are weak, it can be hypothesized that the radial nerve has been injured. The functions of other radial-innervated muscles in the forearm are then tested: the supinator (C6), the abductor pollicis longus (C8), and extensors pollicis longus and brevis (C8). If all of these muscles are also weak, a radial nerve lesion is also suggested; if only the muscles with a major innervation from root 6 or 7 are weak and those with a major innervation from the C8 root are stronger, a C7 root lesion is suggested. Other C7 root–innervated muscles can then be examined to test the hypothesis of C7 root injury. The triceps is innervated both by radial nerve and the C7 root, so that weakness of this muscle in itself cannot differentiate between a nerve and root lesion. However, if the triceps is strong, a C7 root lesion is unlikely; the radial nerve, however, could be injured in the arm distal to the point of exit of the branches to the triceps. Any sensory deficit associated with the weakness is then tested to determine if the sensory loss follows a pattern of a radial nerve injury (diminished sensation over the web space between the thumb and index finger, which is supplied by the C6 root) or if the sensory loss is in the C7 root distribution (middle finger and palm, dorsal and palmar surfaces of hand). The tendon jerk reflexes in the arm are then tested, with the object of determining if they are decreased in radial-innervated muscles (triceps, C7) or in cord segments (biceps, C6; triceps, C7; finger flexion, C8) or if there is a generalized decrease or increase in the reflex activity of all of the muscles, which would suggest a suprasegmental lesion. The ability to perform patterned movements of the fingers and the limb is then tested to determine if there are deficits in the suprasegmental control of the limb muscles. Therefore, by

a series of tests of hypotheses it can be determined if the deficit produced by the lesion is most consistent with a nerve, plexus, root, or central lesion. Nerves commonly injured are the radial nerve at the humerus, the ulnar nerve at the wrist, and the lateral popliteal nerve in the leg. Description of the signs of these injuries is beyond the scope of this book, but are described in the texts listed in the references.

Spinal cord syndromes

In most cases of spinal cord disease a single longitudinal level of the spinal cord is damaged. The damage usually involves one to three cord segments but can be more extensive. Localization of the longitudinal level of a cord lesion is usually not difficult if the lesion is complete. Localization is made by finding the dermatome levels at which various sensory modalities are impaired and the motor segmental levels at which weakness is found. However, if the lesion is caused by a progressive process that affects a greater transverse area of the cord over time, only part of the somatic muscular and sensory representation at the longitudinal level of the lesion may be found to be affected at the time of examination. For example, in gradual compression of one side of the cervical cord by the growth of an extrinsic tumor, such as meningioma, initial compression of the most lateral fibers, which represent the lumbosacral area in the corticospinal tract and in the spinothalamic tract, can produce motor and sensory changes initially detectable only at a lumbar level.

When cord lesions are regarded in the transverse plane, many lesions can be classified either as lateral lesions, which largely affect the white matter of one side of the cord, or as central lesions, which largely damage the gray matter of the cord.

The signs of a complete lateral lesion of the cord, produced by hemisection of the cord, were described in the nineteenth century by the French neurologist Brown-Séquard. Many cases of spinal cord injury, particularly those caused by direct trauma or by tumors, exhibit at least a part of the Brown-Séquard syndrome. Hemisection of the spinal cord in the thoracic and cervical areas produces, below the level of the lesion:

1. Ipsilateral loss of voluntary movement
2. Ipsilateral loss of discriminative touch, position, and vibration sensation, but preservation of crude touch
3. Contralateral loss of pain and temperature sensations

The dermatome level of the loss of pain is usually one or two segments lower than the level of the spinal cord lesion. The anatomical basis of the syndrome, illustrated in Fig. 12-12, is that cord hemisection interrupts:

1. Fibers mediating voluntary movement, the lateral corticospinal tract in the lateral column and the reticulospinal and other motor projections in the anterolateral column, which are distributed ipsilaterally to ventral horn motoneurons.
2. Fibers mediating discriminative touch and position sensations, the gracile and cuneate tracts, which arise from ipsilateral dorsal root ganglion cells and ascend in the ipsilateral dorsal column.
3. Fibers mediating pain and temperature, the spinothalamic tract, which arise in contralateral spinal gray neurons that receive contralateral dorsal root ganglion cell projections. The axons of the second-order neurons of the pain pathway decussate in the ventral white commissure of the cord and then ascend in the anterolateral column.

In contrast to the type of sensory loss produced by peripheral nerve transection, in which all modalities of somatic sensation are lost together in the anesthetized area, in the Brown-Séquard syndrome each half of the body exhibits a dissociated sensory loss, in which there is loss of some of the sensory modalities without loss of the other. The presence of a dissociated sensory loss suggests injury of sensory pathways in the spinal cord or brainstem, where pathways mediating different sensory modalities are segregated to some degree.

The second major pattern of transverse cord injury is that of the central cord lesion. The lamination of the posterior columns, of the lateral corticospinal tract, and of the spinothalamic tract places the fibers representing the lumbosacral area peripherally and the cervical fibers centrally, or closest to the gray matter in all of these tracts. This lamination is most fully developed in the cervical cord. A central cervical cord injury can be produced by damage to the anterior spinal artery, resulting in infarction of the central gray matter of the cervical spinal cord. This will produce a flaccid weakness (lower motoneuron type of weakness) of the muscles supplied by the ventral horn motoneurons of the infarcted segments. Fibers in the white matter adjacent to the central gray will be affected to varying degrees. However, patients with this type of injury are usually able to feel touch and pain in the lumbar and sacral areas (sacral sparing) and are able to move their legs to some extent because of sparing of the lumbar fibers in the peripheral white matter of the cord.

In contrast to the signs produced by a central lesion, progressive damage of the thoracic or cervical cord, spreading from the periphery to the center of the cord, produces motor and sensory loss starting in the lumbosacral area. The level of the deficits ascends to thoracic and cervical areas over time, as discussed above.

Damage to specific levels of the spinal cord. Because lower lumbar and sacral cord segments are crowded together in the conus medullaris, lesions of the conus can produce extensive weakness and sensory loss in the legs and sensory loss in the perineum. A small conus lesion can initially produce weakness of the lumbar, pelvic, and thigh musculature, supplied by upper lumbar segments, resulting in a waddling gait and only mild disturbances of bowel, bladder, and sexual function. An enlarging lesion may produce increasing weakness of lumbar-innervated proximal muscles, as well as weakness of sacral segment–innervated distal leg muscles and severe impairment of bowel, bladder, and sexual functions. The loss of these functions is produced both by damage to descending autonomic tracts of the anterolateral columns and by damage to parasympathetic preganglionic neurons in the sacral segments of the spinal cord.

Because of the small area of the conus, lesions of the conus generally extensively damage both gray and white matter. Hemisection of the conus does not usually produce a complete Brown-Séquard syndrome with a definite dissociation of touch and pain. In-

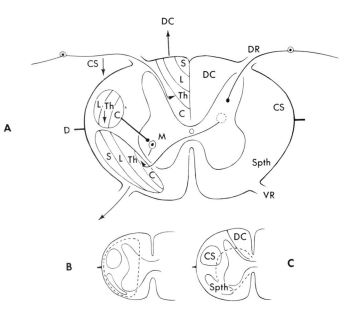

Fig. 12-12. **A,** Laminar arrangement of fibers in the dorsal columns, corticospinal tract, and spinothalamic tract, illustrated for a transverse section of the cervical spinal cord. **B,** Laterally placed lesion of the spinal cord, illustrated here as an almost total right-sided hemisection, which produces a Brown-Séquard syndrome. **C,** Central cord lesion, which produces a central cord syndrome.

stead, touch and pain are often lost ipsilateral to the hemisection because of interruption of entering dorsal root fibers subserving all sensory modalities.

Injuries of the cervical and lumbar spine often produce injury to both the spinal cord proper and the spinal roots. Such injuries can produce complex neurological signs because of the difference in the motor and sensory representations of the roots and the intrinsic spinal cord segments lying opposite each vertebral body level (see Chapter 4). For example, a dislocation of the cervical spine at the level of the fifth and sixth cervical vertebrae can crush the C6 roots that exit between the C5 and C6 vertebrae, producing pain, numbness, and weakness in the C6 distribution (sensory loss in the radial border of the hand and forearm; weakness of the biceps muscles). This injury can also crush the C8 cord segment that lies opposite the C6 vertebral body, producing lower motoneuron weakness in the distribution of the C8 segment (flaccid weakness of intrinsic hand muscles). C8 segment damage can also result in loss of voluntary movement below the C8 level, caused by damage to descending motor pathways. The injury can also produce sensory loss in the C8 dermatome (ulnar border of the hand and forearm) and below it, caused by damage to ascending dorsal column and anterolateral column sensory pathways. Lumbar injuries or tumors of the conus medullaris and of the cauda equina can also produce similarly complex neurological findings by injuring both the spinal cord and the nerve roots of the cauda equina.

Progression of motor and reflex signs after cord injury. Motor and sensory effects of lesions of the spinal cord have been described by the terms weakness and sensory loss. The clinical characteristics of the weakness and sensory deficits produced by cord lesions are, however, related to the structures injured, to the temporal course of production of the lesion, and to the age of the lesions. The effect of gradually compressive lesions in producing ascending sensory and motor levels has already been mentioned.

An acute lesion of the cord that completely interrupts descending motor pathways, particularly the corticospinal tract, produces flaccid paralysis of somatic musculature below the level of the lesion. All voluntary and reflex movement is lost in the acute phase of the injury. In this respect the initial signs of lesions of the descending motor pathways (upper motoneuron lesions) resemble the signs produced by damage to ventral horn motoneurons (lower motoneuron lesions). However, following complete destruction of ventral horn motoneurons, voluntary movement and reflexes are lost permanently, whereas even in complete lesions of the descending motor pathways,

myotatic reflexes (muscle-stretch or tendon-jerk reflexes) and superficial reflexes (evoked by skin stimulation) below the level of the lesion will return in a variable period of time. In some patients flexion of a limb to painful stimuli may occur a few hours after cord injury, but in other patients the return of reflexes does not occur for days. The superficial reflexes evoked after several days or weeks following cord injury often differ from normal reflexes in two important ways. The first difference is that the motor response may be aberrant. Such aberrant responses are called pathological reflexes. The most important pathological reflex is the plantar, or toe sign, described by the French neurologist Babinski. Normally the toes plantar-flex when the sole of the foot is stroked from the heel toward the third and fourth toes. The stimulus for evoking the response should not be so strong as to be painful, but should be strong enough to be slightly unpleasant. Following injury of the descending motor pathways, stroking the sole evokes extension (dorsiflexion) of the great toe and fanning, extension, or flexion of the other toes. Another change in superficial reflexes found after injury of descending motor pathways is the loss of reflex contraction of the cremasteric and abdominal muscles, which can normally be evoked by scratching the skin adjacent to them. A second major difference in the reflexes after cord injury is that the cutaneous areas from which reflexes can be evoked may become larger than normal.

The myotatic reflexes also undergo progressive changes after lesions of the descending motor pathways. After 2 to 3 weeks the myotatic reflexes generally become hyperactive. Muscles that have increased myotatic reflexes also generally exhibit increased resistance to stretching. Such muscles are called spastic.

If the lesion of the descending motor pathways is not complete, there may be some voluntary movement of muscles. Impaired voluntary movement is called paresis, in contrast to the absence of movement, or paralysis.

Muscles can be both spastic and weak in varying degrees following the return of voluntary movement after incomplete lesions of descending motor pathways. In some cases of injury to descending motor tracts, the limb muscles, particularly the proximal muscles of the upper arm and of the thigh, are quite strong but are also very spastic. When this happens there is impairment of the ability to rapidly contract and relax antagonistic limb muscles alternately (impaired rapid-succession movements). Therefore, although the limb may be strong, it may not be useful to the patient.

It is likely that in spinal cord injury, damage to the corticospinal tract produces the immediate loss of movement. How much coexisting damage to other descending motor pathways modifies the immediate signs of corticospinal tract injury is not known. The return of both reflex activity and voluntary activity probably depends on any residual corticospinal tract axons that regain function and also on the activity of other descending motor pathways. The vestibulospinal and reticulospinal tracts are probably quite important in humans for recovery of motor function after corticospinal tract injury. Recovery of voluntary movement of proximal limb muscles can occur after complete corticospinal tract lesions, although fine and rapid movements of distal muscles (especially finger movement) remain impaired. The variability in the time and quality of recovery of reflexes and voluntary movement in humans after lesions of the descending motor pathways sustained at various levels of the neuraxis is probably related to the varying degrees of

---

ILLUSTRATIVE CASE HISTORY
Spinal cord disease

Mr. L. W., age 58

1. **History**
   a. Chief complaint: Difficulty in walking.
   b. Present illness: Eight months prior to admission the patient noted difficulty in walking. Several weeks later he noted dragging of the left leg and stumbling. This became progressively more pronounced. He noted weakness of the right leg 3 months prior to admission. He noted weakness of the left arm in the past month. In the past 3 months he has noted fasciculations of shoulder, arm, and thigh muscles. No change in his voice, no dysphagia, no urinary or sexual changes, no sensory changes.

2. **Examination**
   a. Physical examination: BP 120/70, P 80 regular, T 99°. Abdomen: cholecystectomy and hernia repair incisional scars. Scar of pilonidal cyst surgery at base of spine.
   b. Neurological examination: Motor: right handed. Spastic hemiparetic gait, with the left side much more affected than the right. Decreased left arm swing. Fasciculations of deltoid, biceps, trapezius, and quadriceps muscles bilaterally. Moderate atrophy of all muscles of shoulder girdle, upper arm, forearm, and intrinsic hand muscles; left greater than right. Moderate atrophy of hamstrings, gastrocnemius, quadriceps, and foot dorsiflexors; left greater than right. Right arm muscles were 75% of normal strength; proximal and distal muscles affected equally. Left arm muscles were 50% of normal strength. In the right leg the dorsiflexors of the foot were 75% of normal strength. In the left leg, dorsiflexors of the foot were 50% of normal strength. Both quadriceps were 75% of normal strength. Equilibratory tests were well performed. Rapid-succession movements were decreased on the left side. Reflexes: myotatic reflexes were hyperactive in the arms and legs. Babinski's sign was present bilaterally. No sensory abnormalities or cranial nerve abnormalities were found.

3. **Summary**
   Progressive weakness of arms and legs, more marked on the left than the right side. Limb muscle atrophy and fasciculations more marked in the arms than the legs. Hyperactive myotatic reflexes and the presence of pathological reflexes.

4. **Formulation**
   a. Site of lesion:
      (1) Cervical spinal cord: bilateral damage to ventral horn motoneurons and to descending motor pathways.
      (2) Lumbar spinal cord: probable bilateral damage to ventral horn motoneurons.
   b. Differential diagnosis:
      (1) Degenerative disease of motoneurons (amyotrophic lateral sclerosis).
      (2) Possible compression of cervical spinal cord by an extrinsic mass ventral to the spinal cord.

5. **Laboratory data**
   Blood count, urinalysis, and blood chemistries normal.
   Chest x-ray film normal, with the exception of minimal bilateral basal pleural thickening.

6. **Course in hospital**
   The following special diagnostic studies were performed. Cervical spine films revealed minimal reversal of the normal cervical lordotic curve, associated with narrowing of the intervertebral disc spaces C5-6 and C6-7. There were anterior and posterior osteophytes projecting in relation to the narrowed disc spaces, with narrowing of the spinal canal at the level of the C6 to 7 vertebrae. However, these findings on x-ray films were minimal and would not be capable of producing the atrophy or the fasciculations seen in the deltoid muscles (C5 root).
   Lumbar puncture with a No. 18 needle at L5-S1 revealed an opening pressure of 180 mm CSF and a closing pressure of 120, after 12 ml of crystal-clear fluid were removed. CSF examination: 2 WBC/mm³, protein 53 mg/100 mg, glucose 74 mg/100 ml. Manometrics indicated an open spinal subarachnoid space with no block.
   Electromyography revealed fibrillation potentials in many muscles, indicating widespread denervation of muscle fibers in the arms and legs.
   Spastic quadriparesis, wasting of muscles, muscle fasciculation, hyperactive reflexes, the presence of Babinski's sign, and no sensory changes, combined with normal CSF chemistries, the findings on electromyography that suggested motoneuron damage at numerous cord levels, normal manometrics, and essentially normal cervical spine x-ray studies except for minimal osteoarthritic changes suggest the diagnosis of a primary degenerative disease of ventral horn motoneurons and of descending motor pathways.

7. **Diagnosis**
   Degenerative disease of motoneurons (amyotrophic lateral sclerosis).

damage to all of the motor systems. Both the transverse extent and the longitudinal level of the lesion will affect the proportion of fibers of each of the motor systems that are damaged by the lesion.

There is still only a limited understanding of the changes that occur in the electrophysiological activity of anterior horn motoneurons and in the pathways projecting to them during the processes of recovery of reflex activity and of voluntary activity following lesions of descending motor pathways.

CRANIAL NERVES

From a clinical viewpoint the cranial nerves are thought of in numerical order, and the various peripheral functions subserved by each nerve are tested individually. A unified presentation of the cranial nerves is therefore desirable (Table 12-3). However, in order to appreciate the central connections of the cranial nerves and their contribution to the structure of the brainstem and to sensory and motor systems, the nerves should be studied according to their component nuclei and to a classification by their major functions. The brainstem loci of the cranial nerve nuclei are discussed and illustrated in Chapter 6. The following section on cranial nerve examination should be read in conjunction with the appropriate section of Chapter 6 and as a background for the more detailed presentation of sensory aspects of cranial nerves I, II, V, VII, VIII, IX, and X as part of sensory systems in Chapter 7 and of the presentation of cranial nerves III, IV, and VI as part of the oculomotor system in Chapter 8.

Cranial nerve testing

Although the cranial nerves are tested clinically generally in numerical order, in some instances a functionally related group of nerves is tested together. A battery of clinical tests of cranial nerve function is available, but many of the tests are not used in the routine neurological examination. The most commonly employed tests used in office or bedside examination are mentioned here. For those nerves that contain several types of fibers (particularly nerves V, VII, VIII, and X), knowledge of the points along the anatomical course of the nerve at which particular fibers enter and leave the nerve, and the finding of a loss of one type of function with the preservation of other functions, can be used to identify the anatomical site at which the nerve was injured. The reader is referred to textbooks of neurological diagnosis for such detailed cranial nerve anatomy and for further details about other available techniques of examination.

The olfactory nerve as well as the remainder of the olfactory pathway is tested for each side separately by having the patient identify the smell of various substances while the opposite nostril is occluded. Commonly available stimuli include coffee grounds, tobacco, or perfume. Substances that might irritate the pain receptors of the nasal mucosa supplied by the trigeminal nerve should be avoided. Quantitative testing of olfactory sensation has been carried out for research purposes but is not generally used clinically.

The fundus of the eye and the appearance of the optic nerve head, or optic disc, should always be examined by ophthalmoscopy. Among the various changes that may occur in pathological states, a particularly important one for neurological diagnosis is the presence of papilledema. Papilledema produces an enlargement of the blind spot, caused by swelling of the optic nerve head, and a decrease in visual acuity. Visual acuity is usually tested through the use of a standardized stimulus (Snellen's chart). Visual fields are tested at the bedside by the confrontation method. For more detailed examination a tangent screen or a perimeter is used.

The oculomotor, trochlear, and abducens nerves are examined together by determining if the operation of the extrinsic eye muscles is normal. Abnormalities include ptosis, strabismus, and diplopia. In addition, the parasympathetic component of the oculomotor nerve is examined by determining if the pupil is of normal size and if it reacts appropriately to light and to accommodation. Two pathological changes of the pupillary responses that are not caused by oculomotor damage but by damage to the pretectal area of the midbrain and by damage to the sympathetic innervation to the eye respectively are the Argyll Robertson sign (absence of light reflex with preservation of pupillary constriction during accommodation) and Horner's syndrome (miosis, partial ptosis, vasodilatation in the facial skin, anhidrosis, and enophthalmos).

The trigeminal nerve has both a sensory and a motor component. The sensory component to the skin of the face is often tested along with the sensory examination of the skin of the body. Stimuli used include mild tactile (cotton wisp), moderate pressure (blunt part of safety pin) and painful (pinprick) gradations of mechanical stimuli and thermal stimuli (tubes filled with cool and warm water). Of particular importance is the use of comparable stimuli to the two sides of the body. The corneal reflex (blinking of both eyes when the edge of the cornea is touched by a wisp of cotton) also serves as a test of trigeminal sensory function, because the afferents of the reflex travel in the ophthalmic division. The motor limb is in the facial nerve (orbicularis oculi muscle), which is thus tested simultaneously with the sensory component.

Table 12-3. Cells of origin, fiber components, and functions of cranial nerves

Nerve	Cells of origin	Major branches	Somatic afferent	Visceral afferent	Somatic efferent	Visceral efferent
I Olfactory Smell*	Olfactory epithelial hair cells	Olfactory filaments		Smell (special)		
II Optic Vision*	Retinal ganglion cells	Optic nerves–chiasm–optic tracts	Vision (special)			
III Oculomotor Pupilloconstriction* Accommodation*	Edinger-Westphal nucleus	Oculomotor nerve–ciliary ganglion–ciliary nerves				Intrinsic eye muscles Pupilloconstrictor of iris Accommodation—ciliary muscle (general)
Lid elevation* Upward, medial, downward eye movement*	Third nucleus	Oculomotor nerve			Extraocular muscles Levator palpebrae Superior rectus Medial rectus Inferior rectus Inferior oblique	
IV Trochlear Downward, medial eye movement*	Fourth nucleus	Trochlear nerve			Superior oblique	
VI Abducens Lateral eye movement*	Sixth nucleus	Abducens nerve			Lateral rectus	
V Trigeminal Facial and cranial sensation*	Gasserian ganglion, sensory root (portio major)	Ophthalmic (V_1) branch Maxillary (V_2) branch Mandibular (V_3) branch	Sensation, anterior one half of scalp, facial skin and mucosa, anterior two thirds of tongue, dura of anterior and middle fossa (general)			
Jaw muscle sensation*	Mesencephalic fifth nucleus	Motor root	Proprioception, muscles of mastication (general)			
Jaw movement*	Motor fifth nucleus	Motor root (portio minor)				Muscles of mastication Temporalis, masseter, pterygoid, digastric (special)

Nerve / Function	Ganglion or nucleus	Branch	Modality	Structures
VII Facial				
Sensation, part of external ear	Geniculate ganglion	Nervus intermedius–ramus of vagus to ear	Sensation, part of external ear (general)	
Taste*	Geniculate ganglion	Nervus intermedius–chorda tympani–lingual nerve		Taste, anterior two thirds to tongue (special)
Deep facial sensation	Geniculate ganglion	Nervus intermedius		Sensation, deep facial (general)
Facial movement*	Seventh motor nucleus	Temporofacial branch; Cervicofacial branch		Muscles of facial expression, scalp muscles, auricular muscles, stylohyoid, posterior belly of digastric, stapedius (special)
Salivation	Superior salivatory nucleus	Nervus intermedius–chorda tympani–lingual nerve–submaxillary ganglion		Salivation Submaxillary and sublingual glands (general)
Tearing	Superior salivatory nucleus	Nervus intermedius–greater superficial petrosal nerve–sphenopalatine ganglion		Tearing Lacrimal glands, mucous membrane of nasopharynx (general)
VIII Statoacoustic				
Vestibular*	Vestibular ganglion	Vestibular nerve	Vestibular (special)	
Hearing*	Spiral ganglion of cochlea	Cochlear nerve	Hearing (special)	
IX Glossopharyngeal				
Sensation, part of external ear	Superior ganglion	Ramus of vagus to ear	Sensation, part of external ear (general)	
Taste	Petrosal (inferior) ganglion			Taste, posterior third of tongue (special)
Carotid reflexes		Carotid sinus nerve		Carotid sinus and body, baroceptors and chemoreceptors (special)
Pharyngeal sensation*	Petrosal ganglion	Pharyngeal branch		Sensation, pharyngeal and posterior third of tongue (general)

*Major functions commonly tested.

Table 12-3. Cells of origin, fiber components, and functions of cranial nerves—cont'd

Nerve	Cells of origin	Major branches	Somatic afferent	Somatic efferent	Visceral afferent	Visceral efferent
Gag reflex Swallowing	Nucleus ambiguus	Lingual branch Pharyngeal plexus (with vagus)				Muscle of pharynx: stylopharyngeal muscle (special)
Salivation	Inferior salivatory nucleus	Tympanic nerve—lesser superficial petrosal nerve—otic ganglion				Salivation Parotid gland (general)
X Vagus Sensation, part of external ear	Jugular ganglion		Sensation, part of external ear, dura of posterior fossa (general)			
Visceral sensation, afferent, pharynx, thoracic and abdominal viscera	Nodose ganglion				Aortic arch baroceptors, chemoreceptors, pulmonary inflation receptors (special) Sensation—pharynx, thorax, abdomen (general)	
Swallowing* Gag reflex* Phonation*	Nucleus ambiguus	Pharyngeal plexus Laryngeal nerves, especially recurrent				Muscles of pharynx (special) Muscles of larynx (special)
Cardiac slowing Bronchoconstriction	Dorsal tenth motor nucleus					Branches to smooth muscles, glands of thoracic and abdominal viscera, and heart (general)
Gastric secretion Peristalsis	?Inferior salivatory nucleus					
XI Accessory Swallowing	Nucleus ambiguus	Cranial root				Muscles of pharynx (vagal innervation more important) (special)
Turn head to contralateral side* Elevate shoulder	Ventral horn C1 to 5 segments	Spinal root				Sternocleidomastoid muscle (and C$_2$ ventral root branch) Trapezius muscle (and C$_{3,4}$ ventral root branch) (special)
XII Hypoglossal Tongue movement*	Twelfth nucleus	Hypoglossal nerve		Muscles of tongue: hypoglossus, genioglossus, and styloglossus		

An important cranial nerve syndrome is the superior orbital fissure syndrome. The third, fourth, and sixth nerves and the first division of nerve V enter the orbit through the superior orbital fissure of the sphenoid bone (see Fig. 5-2). A pathological process such as inflammation or tumor growth at that point can produce various degrees of ophthalmoplegia (ocular muscle paralysis) and anesthesia of the forehead and cornea.

Motor function of the trigeminal nerve can be examined by inspection of the integrity and action of the muscles of mastication. The masseter and temporal muscles contract during jaw closure, and inequalities of their contraction on the right and left sides of the face can be palpated. The digastric and pterygoid muscles contract during jaw opening. The pterygoid muscles of each side of the jaw pull the lower jaw toward the midline of the face, so that in a case of unilateral weakness of the pterygoid muscles the resultant muscle imbalance causes the lower jaw to deviate to the side of the weak muscle. The masseter reflex (contraction of masseters following a blow to the chin by reflex hammer) serves to check the status of the stretch reflex of this cranial nerve.

The main function of the facial nerve that is routinely tested is its innervation of the muscles of facial expression. The other motor function of the nerve, its parasympathetic supply of salivary and other glands, is considered in particular when there is weakness of the facial muscles and when it is important to determine the point along the course of the facial nerve at which the nerve has been injured. The parasympathetic fibers of the nerve, as well as the taste fibers, leave the nerve in the temporal bone proximal to the point at which the facial motor fibers leave the skull through the stylomastoid foramen. The corneal reflex has been mentioned. The sensory functions of the facial nerve are generally not tested routinely. However, in special cases the sense of taste may be examined by applying substances to restricted areas of the anterior part of the tongue.

Cranial nerve VIII is examined for both its acoustic and vestibular functions. Hearing may be roughly examined using a watch. The tuning fork tests of Rinne (air versus bone conduction) and of Weber (lateralization of sound from tuning fork in midline of forehead) may be used. Audiometry can determine degrees of hearing loss and the distribution of loss in various regions of the auditory spectrum. The vestibular apparatus is tested in part during the examination of the motor system (maintenance of posture, coordination) and in part in the examination of the oculomotor nerves (nystagmus). In addition, special tests may be used, including caloric testing (introduction of cold or warm water into the external auditory canal). The battery of audiometric and vestibular tests has become highly developed, and the reader should consult audiological texts for details.

Glossopharyngeal nerve function is examined along with that of the vagus nerve. The contribution of fibers of the glossopharyngeal nerve to pharyngeal sensation is probably slightly greater than that of the vagus, and that of the vagus is greater in swallowing and in palatal movement. However, the upper rootlets of the complex of nerves IX to X can be cut unilaterally without producing much loss of pharyngeal sensation or movement. Sensory and motor functions of these nerves are tested by evoking the gag reflex or by stroking the soft palate, the pillars of the tonsils, or the posterior pharyngeal wall. The normal response is retraction of the palate and the uvula, as well as of the base of the tongue. In unilateral paralysis of the motor component of the vagus, contraction of the normally innervated muscles of the pharynx pulls the uvula toward the normal side. This can often be seen without evoking a gag reflex, merely by observing the normal retraction of the palate during phonation, as in saying "ah."

The motor function of the vagus is examined by determining the ability of the patient to swallow normally, without regurgitation. The movements of the vocal cords may, in addition, be examined by laryngoscopy. The quality of the voice (phonation) is also determined. Unilateral vagal injury usually produces hoarseness.

The spinal root of the accessory nerve is tested mainly by study of the action of the sternocleidomastoid muscles. The sternocleidomastoid muscle runs from the sternum and clavicle to the mastoid process of the skull, which lies behind the center of rotation of the head. Contraction of the sternocleidomastoid pulls and rotates the head and neck to the opposite side of the body. In unilateral weakness of the sternocleidomastoid muscle the head can be rotated only weakly to the opposite side of the body. The spinal root of nerve XI also supplies part of the innervation of the trapezius muscle (also supplied by C3,4 ventral roots), which elevates (shrugs) the shoulder.

The hypoglossal nerve is tested by examination of the mobility and appearance of the tongue. Hemiatrophy of the tongue or fasciculations may be noted as a result of hypoglossal injury. The tongue is protruded largely by the genioglossus muscle (chin to tongue), which essentially pulls the tongue forward. In the case of unilateral hypoglossal damage and weakness of the genioglossus muscle of one side, the muscular imbalance results in deviation of the tip of the tongue to the side of the weak muscle.

These tests are summarized in Table 12-4.

Table 12-4. Clinical tests of cranial nerve function

Cranial nerve	Fiber component	Clinical test
I	Olfactory afferents	Odor applied in one nostril
II	Visual pathway	Visual acuity (Snellen's chart), visual fields (confrontation, tangent screen, perimeter), fundus (ophthalmoscopy)
III, IV, VI	Motor to extrinsic eye muscles	Eye and lid movements
	Parasympathetic	Pupillary response to light and accommodation
V	Somatic sensory fibers	Sensation of skin of face; corneal reflex
	Motor fibers	Muscles of mastication, masseter reflex
VII	Sensory fibers	Taste, anterior two thirds of tongue
	Motor fibers	Muscles of facial expression, corneal reflex
VIII	Auditory component	Qualitative test of hearing (watch ticking), Rinne and Weber tuning fork tests, audiometry
	Vestibular component	Posture and coordination, caloric tests, oculonystagmography
IX, X	Motor component	Voice, swallowing, gag reflex
	Sensory component	Gag reflex, pharyngeal sensation
XI	Motor fibers	Sternocleidomastoid and trapezius function
XII	Motor fibers	Tongue function

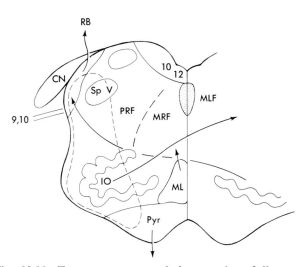

Fig. 12-13. Transverse section of the rostral medulla. Some structures from adjacent levels have been included to indicate their relative positions. A lesion that damages the corticospinal tract, cerebellar projections, and cranial nerve fibers passing through the brainstem is indicated. Abbreviations: *CN*, cochlear nucleus; *IO*, inferior olive; *ML*, medial lemniscus; *MLF*, medial longitudinal fasciculus; *Pyr*, pyramid; *RB*, restiform body; *MRF*, magnocellular portion of reticular formation; *PRF*, parvicellular portion of reticular formation; *SpV*, spinal tract and nucleus of trigeminal nerve; *9,10*, sites of exit of cranial nerves IX and X; *10,12*, dorsal motor nucleus of cranial nerve X and nucleus of nerve XII.

Brainstem syndromes

The brainstem consists of cranial nerve nuclei and their emerging nerves, nuclei associated with ascending and descending axons, and ascending and decending pathways. Many lesions of the brainstem can be classified either as lateral or central lesions. The pattern of blood supply to the brainstem is related to the development of these patterns of brainstem injury, because the brainstem is supplied by lateral branches and shorter medial branches of the basilar and vertebral arteries. Specific sites of tumor growth are also responsible for lateral or medial brainstem syndromes. Tumors of the cerebellopontine angle, including nerve VIII tumors (acoustic tumors), tend to produce signs of a lateral brainstem lesion. Intrinsic tumors of the brainstem (gliomas, syrinxes) tend to produce signs of medial, or central, lesions.

Lateral brainstem lesions frequently damage the cerebellar peduncles, producing ataxia of the ipsilateral limbs. Nerves V, VII, and VIII and their nuclei are located laterally in the brainstem and are also frequently damaged by lateral lesions.

The nuclei of nerves III, IV, and VI and the medial longitudinal fasciculus are located medially in the brainstem, and disturbances of eye movement are typically seen in medial lesions. The medial lemniscus, the pyramids, and the descending corticospinal tract in the pons may also be damaged by medially placed lesions.

A constellation of signs following lesions on one side of the brainstem in which there is usually a mixture of lateral and medial injury is:

1. Ipsilateral disturbances of cranial nerve function
2. Contralateral somatic muscular weakness, with or without contralateral loss of touch, position, and pain sensations

The anatomical basis of these signs, shown in Fig. 12-13 is:

1. Damage to brainstem cranial nerve nuclei and to their exiting axons.
2. Damage to the corticospinal tract above the level of its decussation at the spinomedullary junction. If the medial lemniscus is also damaged rostral to the point of decussation of its axons, which arise in the gracile and cuneate nuclei, there will

ILLUSTRATIVE CASE HISTORY
Brainstem disease

Miss C. E., age 12

1. History
   a. Chief complaint: Left facial weakness, double vision, and falling.
   b. Present illness: A 3-week history of weight loss of 10 pounds, with severe anorexia but no nausea or vomiting. Ataxic gait with tendency to fall to the left. Left facial weakness, and diplopia on left lateral gaze.

2. Examination
   a. Physical examination: BP 100/60, P 100 regular, T 99.2°.
   b. Neurological examination: A small thin girl, with marked wasting of the face. Cranial nerves: a left nerve VI palsy, with diplopia on left gaze. Nystagmus present on right and left lateral gaze. Weakness of the muscles supplied by nerve VII on the left. Decreased auditory acuity on the left. Motor: right handed. Ataxic gait and ataxia of the left arm. Decreased rapid succession movements of the left hand. Sensory: normal. Reflexes: normal.

3. Summary
Rapid progression of impaired function of left nerves VI, VII, and VIII and ataxia and impairment of control of rapid movement of the left hand.

4. Formulation
   a. Site of lesion: Brainstem, at the level of the midpons. Left lateral and central brainstem with damage to cerebellar peduncles, nerves VII and VIII, and nerve VI.
   b. Differential diagnosis:
     (1) Intrinsic (intraaxial) lesion of the brainstem; probably a tumor (low-grade astrocytoma, brainstem glioma).
     (2) Possible tumor extrinsic to the brainstem, compressing the brainstem.
     (a) Tumor of cerebellum.
     (b) Cerebellopontine angle tumor.

5. Laboratory data
Blood count, urinalysis, and blood chemistries normal.

Skull and chest x-ray films normal.
Spinal fluid: Protein 35 mg/100 ml, glucose 71 mg/100 ml, WBC 1, RBC 1, results of serological study normal.

6. Course in hospital
The following special diagnostic studies were performed. Caloric testing of the vestibular nerve and audiometric studies indicated impairment of function of the cochlear division of nerve VIII on the left. Electroencephalogram was interpreted as normal for her age group. There was no evidence of increased intracranial pressure on lumbar puncture: opening pressure was 70 mm CSF, closing pressure 35 mm CSF. A pneumoencephalogram was performed. A total of 35 ml of air was injected through the lumbar subarachnoid space. The fourth ventricle was distorted and rotated to the right. Air filled the right cerebellopontine angle. The left angle did not fill. In the frontal projection the third ventricle was seen in the midline position. The lateral ventricles were normal.

The pneumoencephalographic findings were most consistent with the diagnosis of a surgically resectable tumor extrinsic to the brainstem that was compressing the brainstem. The neurological signs were most consistent with an intrinsic brainstem tumor. Because of the possibility of a lesion that could be treated by excision, exploration of the posterior fossa was recommended.

The patient underwent a suboccipital craniectomy and exploration of the posterior fossa. The left cerebellopontine angle was explored, nerves IX and X identified, and nerve VII stimulated electrically, which produced contraction of the left facial musculature. No tumor was seen in the cerebellopontine angle. The left cerebellar hemisphere was then retracted to expose the brainstem, and the obex and floor of the fourth ventricle were seen. The brainstem appeared to be swollen, and rotated slightly to the right. The impression was of a brainstem glioma on the left. The lesion could not be excised. The tumor was subsequently treated with radiotherapy.

7. Diagnosis
Intraaxial tumor of pons (brainstem glioma).

---

be contralateral impairment of touch and position sense. If there also is damage to the lateral spinothalamic tract, which is more laterally placed in the brainstem than is the medial lemniscus, there will also be contralateral impairment of pain and temperature sensation, because the spinothalamic tract arises from contralateral neurons of the spinal gray matter.

This type of brainstem lesion therefore produces an ipsilateral cranial nerve impairment and a contralateral somatic motor impairment. This constellation of signs is called an alternating hemiplegia.

A brainstem syndrome that combines signs of Horner's syndrome and a lateral brainstem syndrome is the Wallenberg syndrome. The basis of these signs is also shown in Fig. 12-13.

1. Ipsilateral weakness of palatal, pharyngeal, and vocal cord muscles and ipsilateral facial analgesia
2. Ipsilateral Horner's syndrome
3. Ipsilateral limb ataxia
4. Contralateral loss of pain and temperature sensation on body

The usual cause of the Wallenberg syndrome is occlusion of the posterior inferior cerebellar artery (see Chapter 5), resulting in lateral medullary and cerebellar damage to:

1. Cranial nerves IX and X and trigeminal spinal tract and nucleus
2. Reticulospinal tracts to sympathetic preganglionic neurons
3. Cerebellar peduncles and the cerebellum
4. Spinothalamic tract

Cerebellar syndromes

Cerebellar lesions produce impaired control of voluntary movement, of posture, and of equilibratory adjustments necessary to maintaining an upright posture. The effects of cerebellar lesions on movements are quite complex. The effects can be seen during the performance of a variety of different types of movements made by limb and head and trunk muscles, and a number of different terms are used to describe these abnormalities of movement. There are also some differences in the signs produced by lesions of the hemispheres of the posterior lobe, of the vermis of the posterior lobe, and of the anterior and the flocculonodular lobes in general. However, the majority of clinically significant cerebellar lesions affect rather large areas of the cerebellum, including the deep nuclei. Most patients therefore have signs of impaired functioning of several cerebellar systems. Patients with cerebellar disease generally exhibit (1) cerebellar ataxia, (2) decomposition of movement and asynergia, (3) hypotonia of muscles, and (4) difficulty in maintaining equilibrium.

Cerebellar ataxia is impaired muscular coordination of the limbs when performing a movement. The ataxia is most marked when voluntary movements are made to bring a limb to a particular point in space. Normally the extremity of the limb is carried smoothly along a path to the desired target. In cerebellar disease, as the extremity of the limb is carried toward the target, the limb oscillates around the center of the path of movement. The oscillation is more marked as the limb approaches the target. This is referred to as terminal ataxia and resembles that of a defective pursuit device that overshoots when it homes in on its target. This type of movement is also called intention tremor, because it is a tremor that appears on voluntary movement. The error in bringing the limbs to a desired position is called dysmetria. Some authors differentiate between ataxia (incoordinated movements in a general sense) and intention tremor. Other authors subsume tremor, decomposition of movement, and asynergia under ataxia.

Lesions of the hemispheres produce ataxia in the ipsilateral limbs, with less effect on truncal muscles. Lesions of the vermis produce largely a truncal ataxia, which results in unsteadiness and tremor of the trunk, neck, and head. Limb ataxia, at least, is probably largely produced by neocerebellar lesions that interfere with cerebellar–dentate–ventrolateral thalamus–motor cortex projections.

An impaired ability to check movements (rebound phenomenon) is probably caused by the same mechanism that produces ataxia, as well as by muscular hypotonia.

Disturbances in the rhythm of speech (scanning speech) may also be a form of ataxia.

Nystagmus, particularly nystagmus that appears on lateral gaze, may in some cases be another form of ataxia. Nystagmus may also be produced by damage to the flocculonodular lobe, where it appears to be related to impaired control of vestibulo-ocular reflexes.

Decomposition of movement and asynergia mean that a complex act involving a number of movements at different joints is performed in a series of steps instead of synchronously. The term asynergia has been used to describe the failure of groups of muscles to act together normally. The inability to perform rapidly alternating movements can be considered to be a form of asynergia. These effects are probably caused by impairment of cerebellar–motor cortex projections.

In hypotonia of muscles the limbs may be pendulous. This is most easily seen in the legs after testing the knee jerk. The leg may swing back and forth at the knee instead of coming to rest after the quadriceps contracts and relaxes. Hypotonia is probably caused by damage to cerebellar–motor cortex projections.

Difficulty in maintaining equilibrium is caused by damage to the flocculonodular lobe, which receives a heavy vestibular projection. Children with medulloblastoma, an intrinsic tumor that often first appears in this area of the cerebellum, may exhibit unsteadiness as the earliest sign of the tumor.

Lesions of the cerebellar projections in the brainstem can produce signs similar to those of direct cerebellar injury.

Remarkable improvement in the neurological deficits produced by cerebellar lesions can occur over a period of months after an acute injury. Almost complete recovery from the effects of hemispheric lesions can occur if the deep nuclei are not damaged.

Cerebral syndromes

Cerebral lesions can be divided into those that are purely subcortical, those in which the gyri of a lobe are injured, and those in which both the gyri and the subcortical structures are damaged. Because of the concentration of neurons related to the entire cortex in the internal capsule and thalamus, a single small subcortical lesion in these areas can produce severe sensory and motor deficits, which, if produced by lesions of gyri, could be produced only by larger lesions located in several lobes. A common clinically apparent subcortical lesion is an infarction of the posterior limb of the internal capsule, with some damage to the adjacent thalamus and subcortical white matter. When the internal capsule fibers related to the precentral and post-central gyri are damaged, the neurological deficit consists of a contralateral hemiparesis and a contralateral hemisensory deficit (see Fig. 8-3). Light touch and position sensation are usually more impaired than pain sensation.

When the most posterior portions of the internal capsule and corona radiata are damaged, injuring the lateral geniculate–calcarine fissure visual system projections, a defect in relatively congruous portions of the contralateral visual field of both eyes is produced. When all of the geniculocalcarine fibers of one hemisphere are damaged, vision is lost in the contralateral half of the visual field of both eyes. This condition is called homonymous hemianopsia.

Subcortical lesions interrupting fibers from cortical areas controlling speech and other complex functions (see Chapter 11) can produce language disturbances and interfere with other higher functions.

The neurological deficits that are most apparent after focal damage to the cortex itself are hemiparesis (frontal motor cortex), hemisensory deficits (parietal somatosensory cortex), hemianopsia (occipital visual cortex), and aphasia (frontal opercular cortex, temporoparietal cortex). Deficits in certain other neurological functions may not be very apparent following focal lesions of lobes unless special examinations are carried out. A hearing deficit, for example, is not grossly apparent after unilateral damage to the temporal auditory cortex. The reason probably is that some of the neurons of the cochlear nuclei decussate in the brainstem, and auditory information from each ear is projected bilaterally.

Focal lesions of the parietal lobes can produce difficulties in interpretation of stimuli, particularly of somatosensory information, although the perception of touch, vibration, pain, and temperature in themselves is not affected to as great a degree.

Lesions of the frontal lobes can produce changes in attention span, social behavior, and mood.

Lesions of the limbic lobe can produce rather similar changes. The effects of limbic lesions, including memory deficits produced by hippocampal lesions, are discussed in Chapter 10.

Dementia, or marked deterioration of many aspects of mental functioning, is generally associated with widespread degenerative changes in the cortex.

A syndrome of considerable clinical importance is that of compression of a cerebral hemisphere by a tumor or by a subdural or epidural hematoma of suffi-

cient size to produce downward herniation of the medial portion of the temporal lobe through the tentorial notch, causing compression of the brainstem. Herniation of the temporal lobe through the tentorial incisura is often called uncal herniation. However, the entire length of the parahippocampal gyrus and the dentate gyrus can herniate, in addition to the uncal tip of the parahippocampal gyrus. The signs produced by uncal herniation are:

1. Ipsilateral pupillary dilatation
2. Contralateral hemiparesis
3. Deterioration in the state of consciousness

The basis of the signs is:

1. Compression of the ipsilateral nerve III, as it passes through the tentorial notch, by the herniating temporal lobe. Compression of the brainstem and changes in descending autonomic activity may also play a role in the pupillary dilatation.
2. Compression of the ipsilateral cerebral peduncle by the herniating temporal lobe. The contralateral hemiparesis may also be produced by damage to the motor systems in the ipsilateral cerebrum by the pathological process producing the herniation. In some cases, however, there is a hemiparesis that is ipsilateral to both the side of herniation and to the dilated pupil. The most reliable sign of the side of herniation is the ipsilateral pupillary dilatation. The mechanism of hemiparesis ipsilateral to the herniation is thought to be compression of the contralateral cerebral peduncle against the contralateral tentorial edge.
3. Deterioration in the state of consciousness is probably a result of a number of factors, including compression of the thalamus and brainstem and raised intracranial pressure.

If the signs of cerebral herniation are recognized early in their course, and if the pathology producing the herniation is relieved promptly, irreversible vascular damage to the midbrain, resulting in coma and eventual death, may be avoided.

The following case histories, illustrate neurological deficits of increasing complexity produced by cerebral lesions: a progressive hemiparesis associated with focal seizures, and a hemiparesis associated with apraxia and deficits in interpretation of somatic sensory stimuli.

ILLUSTRATIVE CASE HISTORY
Cerebral disease

Mr. G. E., age 65

1. History
a. Chief complaint: Weakness and numbness of the right leg and arm.

b. Present illness: One year prior to admission the patient noted cramping pains in the right leg. These cramps have become more severe and at times are associated with jerking movements of the leg. Four months prior to admission numbness of the right foot and dragging of the right leg developed. He was admitted to a hospital, where a lumbar puncture showed protein of 103 mg/100 ml and 3 WBC. Myelography was performed and reported as showing multiple lumbar disc protrusions into the lumbar subarachnoid space. Six weeks prior to the present admission he noticed weakness and clumsiness of the right hand. He denies having bowel or bladder symptoms, headaches, vomiting, or visual disturbances.

2. Examination
a. Physical examination: BP 200/90, P 68 regular, T 98.6°. Protuberance of the skull in the midparietal area on the left side of the sagittal suture. Scoliosis in the thoracic region with concavity to the right; varicose veins of the legs.

b. Neurological examination: Right handed. Cranial nerves: normal. Motor: hemiparetic gait, with the right leg rotated outward, dragging of the right foot, and diminished right arm swing. Approximately 25% atrophy of the muscles of the right leg, more marked distally than proximally; approximately 50% weakness of the muscles of the right leg, more marked distally, with a partial foot drop on the right. Approximately 25% weakness of the muscles of the right arm, including the deltoids, triceps, biceps, wrist extensors and flexors, and hand muscles. Terminal ataxia of the right arm on finger-to-nose testing. Sensory: marked diminution of light touch, vibration, and position sense in the right leg. Vibration sense was diminished in the right arm. Pain sensation was diminished in the right leg below the knee. Reflexes: deep-tendon reflexes more active in the right than the left leg. Babinski's sign was present on the right. Hoffmann's sign present on the right.

3. Summary
A 1-year history of progressive spastic hemiplegia and hemisensory deficits, more marked in the leg than in the arm and not involving the face. Episodes that, on the basis of the history, appear to be focal motor seizures of the right foot.

4. Formulation
a. Site of lesion: Left precentral frontal (motor) cortex, involving the medial surface of the cortex (leg area) more than the lateral surface of the cortex, and involving the postcentral parietal area.

b. Differential diagnosis:
(1) Parasagittal extra-axial (extrinsic) tumor; meningioma.
(2) Intra-axial (intrinsic) tumor; astrocytoma.

5. Laboratory data
Blood count, urinalysis, and blood chemistries normal.
X-ray films of chest: healed apical fibrotic tuberculosis.
Electrocardiogram: normal.
Spinal fluid: protein 124 mg/100 ml, glucose 64 mg/100 ml, WBC 1, results of serological tests normal.

6. Course in hospital
The following special diagnostic studies were performed. Skull x-ray films showed thickening of the skull in the left parietal area. The EEG was mildly abnormal with intermittent low-voltage slow activity in the left parietal area. A left common carotid anteriogram showed an egg-sized tumor stain, typical of a meningioma, lying in the frontal parietal area in a parasagittal location. The blood supply was derived partially from the external carotid circulation, which is typical of meningeal tumors. The superior sagittal venous sinus was not occluded by the tumor.

While in the hospital the patient was observed to have what he had called a cramp of the right leg. This was a typical focal motor seizure involving the muscles of the right leg. The patient was placed on a regimen of anticonvulsant medication. Because the tumor appeared to be a benign and resectable tumor, craniotomy and excision of the tumor was recommended.

A free bone flap was turned in the parietal area. The tumor was found to have invaded dura and bone. When the dura was opened a soft, highly vascular tumor was found attached to the falx in the frontal parietal area. The major portion of the tumor and its attachment to the falx were removed. Some tumor that was invading the superior sagittal sinus was not removed.

Postoperatively, the right hemiparesis was more marked for a few days and then began to improve. The patient was discharged 3 weeks after the surgery, with improvement in strength and sensory perception in the right arm and leg.

7. Diagnosis
Left parasagittal parietal meningioma.

ILLUSTRATIVE CASE HISTORY
Cerebral disease

Mr. K. T., age 50

1. History
   a. Chief complaint: Weakness of the left leg, difficulty in dressing.
   b. Present illness: On the day prior to admission the patient arose from bed and then fell because of weakness of the legs. Shortly thereafter he had severe headache and his neck became stiff. He got up and noted that his left leg was weak. On the day of admission he noted an inability to put his shirt on correctly. He could not decide where the arms went with respect to the sleeves of the shirt. He was unable to put his pants on in the normal manner. He finally dressed by putting his pants on the floor and first putting one leg in and then the other. The weakness of the left leg persisted, and he came to the hospital.

2. Examination
   a. Physical examination: BP 140/90, P 80 regular, T 99.6°. The results of a general physical examination were unremarkable.
   b. Neurological examination: Cranial nerves: normal. Motor: right handed. Gait: drags the left lower extremity and neglects it, bumping into objects; station, unsteady with eyes open and closed. Generalized weakness of the left arm and leg, particularly in dorsiflexion of the foot. Sensory: decreased position sense in fingers of left hand and toes of left foot. Shows extinction of left arm and face on double stimulation. Makes errors in palm writing. Reflexes: plantar reflex upward on the left. Tendon jerks increased on left. Mental status: patient exhibits a marked apraxia in trying to dress. He also exhibits a partial neglect of the left side. He was unable to construct figures correctly. He was able to read and speak correctly.

3. Summary
Acute onset of weakness of left arm and leg, neglect of the left side of the body and motor apraxia.

4. Formulation
   a. Site of lesion: Right parietal cortex, producing changes in sensation and interpretation of sensory stimuli and either extending subcortically to the corticospinal tract fibers in the internal capsule or extending frontally to the precentral cortex, to produce hemiparesis.
   b. Differential diagnosis: The sudden onset of headache and stiff neck suggest intracranial hemorrhage.

   (1) Arteriovenous malformation, parietal cortex.
   (2) Aneurysm, middle cerebral artery.
   (3) Hemorrhage into an intra-axial tumor (metastatic tumor or glioma).

5. Laboratory data
Blood count, blood chemistries, and laboratory data normal. Chest x-ray film normal.

6. Course in hospital
On the day after admission the patient complained of worsening headache and stiffness of the neck, and he became confused and lethargic. He was not febrile and did not have a leukocytosis. The following special diagnostic studies were done. Skull x-ray films: normal. EEG: mildly and diffusely abnormal, with more marked slow activity in the right temporal and occipital areas. Lumbar puncture: opening pressure 330 mm CSF. The fluid was bloody, with a xanthochromic supernatant. RBC 20,000/mm³, WBC 45/mm³, 70% polymorphonuclear cells, 30% lymphocytes, protein 96 mg/100 ml, glucose 50 mg/100 ml, results of serological study normal. On the second day that the patient was in the hospital a right common carotid arteriogram was performed. Prominent superficial parietal branches of the middle cerebral artery were seen, which extended into the posterior parietal area to supply dilated arterial channels. There was very rapid filling of large draining veins. Displacement of vessels indicated a moderate-sized intracerebral hematoma associated with the arteriovenous malformation, which had obviously bled. Evacuation of the intracerebral hematoma and resection of the malformation was recommended. On the third day a right parieto-occipital craniotomy was performed, and the arteries feeding the malformation were occluded with metallic clips. The intracerebral hematoma was removed. The veins draining the malformation were occluded with clips and coagulated, and the malformation was removed. The patient's neurological status improved progressively after removal of the lesion. Three weeks after the operation his gait was normal. There was still a decrease in rapid-succession movements in the left leg. Sensory examination was normal. Deep-tendon reflexes were still hyperactive in the left leg. The constructional apraxia had disappeared, and he was able to dress himself. His mental status was normal.

7. Diagnosis
Ruptured arteriovenous malformation of the right posterior parietal area, with intracerebral hemorrhage.

BIBLIOGRAPHY

Bateman, J. E.: Trauma to nerves in limbs, Philadelphia, 1962, W. B. Saunders Co.

Bender, M. B., editor: Approach to diagnosis in modern neurology, New York, 1967, Grune & Stratton, Inc.

Bickerstaff, E. R.: Neurological examination in clinical practice, ed. 3, Philadelphia, 1973, J. B. Lippincott Co.

Brain, W. R.: Clinical neurology, ed. 4, revised by R. Bannister, New York, 1973, Oxford University Press, Inc.

Brodal, A.: The cranial nerves; anatomy and anatomicoclinical correlations, ed. 2, Philadelphia, 1965, J. B. Lippincott Co.

Brodal, A.: Neurological anatomy in relation to clinical medicine, ed. 2, New York, 1969, Oxford University Press, Inc.

Brown-Séquard, C. E.: Course of lectures on the physiology and pathology of the central nervous system. Delivered at the Royal College of Surgeons of England in May, 1858, Philadelphia, 1860, Collins.

Charcot, J. M.: Lectures on the localisation of cerebral and spinal diseases. Delivered at the Faculty of Medicine of Paris. Translated and edited by W. B. Hadden, London, 1883, The New Sydenham Society.

Chusid, J. G.: Correlative neuroanatomy and functional neurology, ed. 16, Los Altos, Calif., 1976, Lange Medical Publications.

Cogan, D. G.: Neurology of the visual system, Springfield, Ill., 1974, Charles C Thomas, Publisher.

Critchley, M.: The parietal lobes, Baltimore, 1953, The Williams & Wilkins Co.

De Jong, R.: The neurologic examination, incorporating the fundamentals of neuroanatomy and neurophysiology, ed. 3, New York, 1967, Hoeber.

Denny-Brown, D.: Handbook of neurological examination and case recording. Cambridge, 1957, Harvard University Press.

Elliot, F. A.: Clinical neurology, ed. 2, Philadelphia, 1971, W. B. Saunders Co.

Fisher, C. M.: A lacunar stroke; the dysarthria–clumsy hand syndrome, Neurology **17**:614-617, 1967.

Gilroy, J., and Meyer, J. S.: Medical neurology, ed. 2, New York, 1975, The Macmillan Co.

Haymaker, W.: Bing's local diagnosis in neurological diseases, ed. 15, St. Louis, 1969, The C. V. Mosby Co.

Haymaker, W., and Schiller, F., editors: The founders of neurology, ed. 2, Springfield, Ill., 1970, Charles C Thomas, Publisher.

Haymaker, W., and Woodhall, B.: Peripheral nerve injuries, ed. 2, Philadelphia, 1953, W. B. Saunders Co.

Holmes, G. M.: Introduction to clinical neurology, ed. 3, revised by B. Matthews, Edinburgh, 1968, E. & S. Livingstone.

Jennett, W. B.: An introduction to neurosurgery, ed. 2, St. Louis, 1970, The C. V. Mosby Co.

Lance, J. W., and McLeod, J. G.: Physiological approach to clinical neurology, London, 1975, Butterworth & Co. (Publishers) Ltd.

Locke, S.: Neurology, Boston, 1966, Little, Brown and Co.

McDowell, F., and Wolff, H. G.: Handbook of neurological diagnostic methods, Baltimore, 1960, The Williams & Wilkins Co.

Merritt, H. H.: A textbook of neurology, ed. 5, Philadelphia, 1973, Lea & Febiger.

Monrad-Krohn, G. H., and Refsum, S.: The clinical examination of the nervous system, ed. 12, New York, 1964, Hoeber.

Norris, F. H.: The EMG; a guide and atlas for practical electromyography, New York, 1963, Grune & Stratton, Inc.

Parker, H. L.: Clinical studies in neurology, Springfield, Ill., 1969, Charles C Thomas, Publisher.

Plum, F., and Posner, J. B.: The diagnosis of stupor and coma, ed. 2, Philadelphia, 1972, F. A. Davis Co.

Pritchard, E. A. B.: Aids to neurology, ed. 2, London, 1959, Baillière, Tindall & Cox.

Purves-Steward, J., and Worster-Drought, C.: The diagnosis of nervous diseases, ed. 10, London, 1952, Edward Arnold (Publishers) Ltd.

Schadé, J. P.: The peripheral nervous system, Amsterdam, 1966, Elsevier Publishing Co.

Spillane, J. D.: An atlas of clinical neurology, ed. 2, New York, 1975, Oxford University Press, Inc.

Stookey, B.: Surgical and mechanical treatment of peripheral nerves, Philadelphia, 1922, W. B. Saunders Co.

Sunderland, S.: Nerves and nerve injuries, Edinburgh, 1968, E. & S. Livingstone.

Tilney, F., and Riley, H. A.: The form and functions of the central nervous system: an introduction to the study of nervous diseases, New York, 1921, Hoeber.

Toole, J. F., editor: Special techniques for neurologic diagnosis, Philadelphia, 1969, F. A. Davis Co.

Tyrer, J. W. H., and Sutherland, J. M.: Exercises in neurological diagnosis, Edinburgh, 1967, E. & S. Livingstone.

Vick, N. A.: Grinker's neurology, ed. 7, Springfield, Ill., 1976, Charles C Thomas, Publisher.

Walker, A. E.: Somatotopic localization of spinothalamic and secondary trigeminal tracts in mesencephalon, Arch. Neurol. Psychiatry **48**:884-889, 1942.

Walsh, F. B., and Hoyt, W. F.: Clinical neuro-ophthalmology, ed. 3, Baltimore, 1969, The Williams & Wilkins Co.

Walshe, F. M. R.: Further critical studies in neurology and other essays and addresses, New York, 1965, Longman, Inc.

Walshe, F. M. R.: Diseases of the nervous system, described for practitioners and students, ed. 11, Edinburgh, 1970, E. & S. Livingstone.

White, J. C., and Sweet, W. H.: Pain and the neurosurgeon; a forty-year experience, Springfield, Ill., 1969, Charles C Thomas, Publisher.

Wolf, J. K.: The classical brain stem syndromes, Springfield, Ill., 1971, Charles C Thomas, Publisher.

Wyke, B. D.: Principles of general neurology; an introduction to the basic principles of medical and surgical neurology, New York, 1969, American Elsevier Publishing Co., Inc.

Techniques in neuroanatomy and neurophysiology

NEUROANATOMICAL TECHNIQUES
Stains

Nissl stain. A very useful staining procedure for demonstrating neuronal cell bodies and proximal dendrites was introduced by Franz Nissl. This staining technique was based on the observation that clumps of material within the cytoplasm of neurons take up basic aniline dyes, such as cresyl-fast violet, thionine, or toluidine blue (Fig. I-1). The areas involved have been named Nissl bodies, or Nissl substance, and have been shown to be rich in RNA. The nucleus also stains, both in neurons and in neuroglia. The axon and axon hillock do not contain Nissl bodies and do not stain. On a section of nervous tissue, it is easy to see clumps of neurons forming nuclei; hence, many students of the cytoarchitecture of nervous tissue have employed Nissl stains as their primary technique. A careful analysis of the patterns of distribution of Nissl substance and the fineness of grain of the Nissl bodies has assisted neuroanatomists in distinguishing between neuronal cell types in adjacent or overlapping nuclei. Retrograde chromatolysis has been studied by using Nissl-staining procedures. In experimental work, it is often possible to produce clear-cut chromatolysis in very young animals, whereas results in adult animals may be equivocal; this is the basis of the Gud-den technique. The axons forming a particular pathway are interrupted, and a search is conducted of various nuclei stained by the Nissl technique to locate the neurons giving rise to the pathway.

Horseradish peroxidase technique. A new anatomic procedure that is rapidly replacing retrograde chromatolysis for the identification of the cell bodies of origin of nervous pathways is the horseradish peroxidase technique, adapted for use in the central nervous system by LaVail and LaVail. The marker enzyme is injected into the vicinity of synaptic terminals. The terminals take up the enzyme, which is then tranported by retrograde axoplasmic flow to the cell bodies of the neurons giving rise to the synaptic endings (Fig. I-2). The neurons can then be identified by a histochemical staining procedure. Horseradish peroxidase can also be transported in the anterograde direction, but confusion of this with retrograde transport can be avoided by careful interpretation of the histological sections and by modification of the details of the procedure. The advantages of the approach over retrograde chromatolysis are that it depends on a physiological mechanism rather than on a pathological process; cells of all sizes can be identified, whereas chromatolysis is difficult to detect in small neurons; the timing for optimal results is short; and the labelling is produced following injection near the synaptic terminals, whereas chromatolysis is best when the axon is damaged near the cell body. The technique is a major advance in neuroanatomy and is widely used; it will provide a substantial alteration in our knowledge of neural pathways.

Myelin sheath stains. Many procedures have been described for staining the myelin sheaths of peripheral and central nervous system axons. One such technique involves staining with osmic acid. Others include the Weigert, luxol-fast blue, and a variety of other pro-

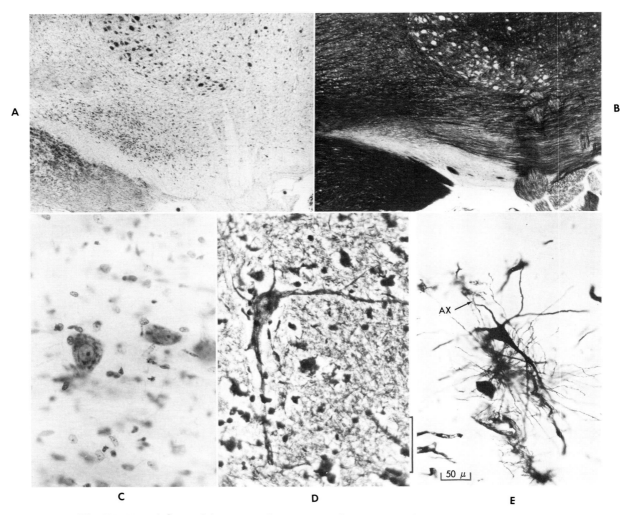

Fig. I-1. Use of dye and heavy metal stains to study the morphology of a brainstem nucleus. A low-power photomicrograph in **A** shows a sagittal section through the junction of the pons *(left side of figure)* and mesencephalon *(right side of figure)* in the cat. The stain is for Nissl substance and demonstrates the cytoarchitecture of part of the substantia nigra and of the red nucleus. An adjacent section, **B**, shows the myeloarchitecture of this area as stained with iron-hematoxylin. **C** through **E** are high-power photomicrographs of large neurons of the zona compacta of the substantia nigra. Nissl substance is stained in **C** with cresyl-fast violet; neurofibrils in **D** with Bielschowsky's silver method; and the entire neuron in **E** with silver dichromate by a rapid Golgi method.

cedures and modifications. Students of the myeloarchitectonics of nervous tissue have used myelin sheath stains to observe the patterns of distribution of myelinated fibers. Myelin sheath stains are very useful also for the demonstration of areas lacking myelin. The contrast between regions containing myelin and those lacking myelin is helpful in neuropathological demonstrations, for example, of demyelinating diseases or of damage that interrupts long myelinated pathways. The course of myelination during development can be followed by using myelin sheath stains on specimens of different ages. The diameters of axons are

generally measured using a myelin sheath stain and including the myelin sheath in the measurement.

Marchi stain. During the course of wallerian degeneration, the myelin sheath fragments and is removed. As the myelin breaks down, its chemical composition changes. The Marchi stain takes advantage of this. The procedure stains only the degenerating fragments of myelin, which become black against the light background formed by normal fibers. Unfortunately, the stain is somewhat capricious, because artifacts often occur that can be confused with degeneration. However, if used with care this approach can give useful

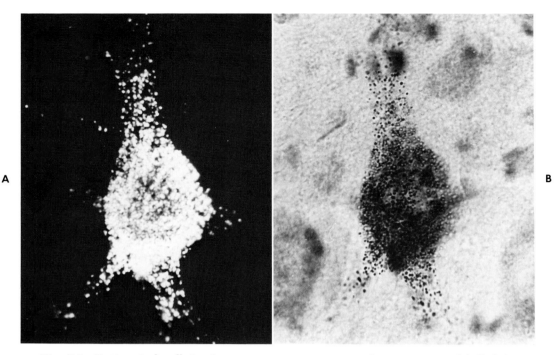

Fig. I-2. Corticospinal cell in the cat sensorimotor cortex. The neuron was labelled by retrograde axoplasmic transport of horseradish peroxidase injected into the lumbosacral enlargement of the spinal cord. In **A** the photograph was made using dark-field illumination; in **B** the peroxidase reaction product is demonstrated with bright-field illumination. (Courtesy Dr. J. D. Coulter.)

results. The major drawback of the Marchi stain is that by definition it cannot show the terminals of fibers, which are generally unmyelinated, nor can it demonstrate degenerating unmyelinated fibers.

Heavy-metal stains. A large number of procedures have been developed by which heavy metals are deposited along the membranes or within neurons or neuroglia. Usually, silver or gold is the metal used. The heavy-metal stains include various Cajal stains, the Bodian stain, and many others. It is likely that the stain is associated with neurofilaments and microtubules in the cytoplasm. Because these organelles are present in the cell body, dendrites, and the axon, all of these structures may be demonstrated. When neurofilaments are present in synaptic boutons, a heavy-metal stain may cause the bouton to look like a small ring. Sometimes synaptic endings have instead a solid, dark appearance. By suitable modifications, neuroglia of various kinds can be stained preferentially. This approach was used particularly successfully by Pio del Río Hortega.

Golgi stain. One particular type of heavy-metal stain merits special emphasis. This is the Golgi stain, named after its originator. There are many modifications of this stain. Basically, the procedure results in the complete staining in black of a small fraction,

generally 1% to 2%, of the neurons in a section. The rest of the neurons and the neuroglia take on a yellow to orange coloration, which provides good contrast with the stained neurons. Sometimes counterstains are used to bring out the structure of unstained neurons better. In young animals the axon often stains, although this is less readily accomplished in adult material. In stained neurons it is possible to make out dendritic branching patterns, the numbers and distribution of dendritic spines, and the course followed by the axon and its branches, including its synaptic boutons. Neurons can be classified on the basis of their Golgi stain morphological structure.

Use of dye and heavy-metal stains. The use of dye stains and of metallic impregnation techniques for demonstrating different portions of cells and for studying different aspects of the anatomy of a nucleus in the brain is illustrated in Fig. I-1. Fig. I-1, *A*, illustrates the cytoarchitectural appearance of a sagittal section through the substantia nigra near the midline of the brain, in which the Nissl substance of the cells is stained with cresyl violet dye (Nissl stain). A globular cluster of neurons of the magnocellular portion of the red nucleus lies in the upper portion of the field. The neurons of the zona compacta of the substantia nigra, which are much smaller than those of the red nucleus, extend horizontally for a distance of 2 mm from the left side of the figure to the level of the exiting fibers of the oculomotor nerve, which are seen as an unstained vertical band. Staining of intrafascicular oligodendroglia nuclei along the course of the fibers outlines the vertical orientation of the exiting axons. Fig. I-1, *B* illustrates the appearance of an adjacent section stained with iron hematoxylin for myelin. Dense-fiber bundles of various thickness and the oculomotor axons are stained. The positions of cell bodies are shown as unstained areas.

The appearance of the large neurons of the zona compacta of the substantia nigra when stained with cresyl violet and examined under higher magnification is illustrated in Fig. I-1, *C*. These cells have prominent clumps of Nissl substance in their cytoplasm. The perikaryon of the neuron is made visible, but only the most proximal portions of the dendrites are seen. The Nissl stain also stains the nuclei of the neurons and glial cells. The cytoplasm of oligodendrocytes is lightly stained, and the cytoplasm of astrocytes is stained only faintly. Darkly stained small nuclei of satellite oligodendrocytes can be seen adjacent to the larger neuron. Lightly stained nuclei of astrocytes that are slightly larger than oligodendrocyte nuclei can be seen scattered in the neuropil, which is stained very faintly.

The appearance of a similar large neuron of the zona compacta when stained with a heavy-metal technique for impregnation of neurofibrils is shown in Fig. I-1, *D*. The perikaryon and all of the cell processes are stained. Fine neurofibrils, which are bundles of neurofilaments, can be seen in the cytoplasm. In addition, many cell processes in the neuropil are stained. The metallic impregnation methods differ in their selectivity, from those such as the Bielschowsky stain that appear to stain all processes, through the Golgi-Cox mercuric impregnation method, which stains a moderate number of cells but not their axons, to the various Golgi silver methods, which stain relatively few cells.

The unselective methods give a picture of the total cell constituents, but it is difficult to follow individual cell processes. The Golgi silver methods allow one to follow dendrites and axons in great detail, but the cells stained may be statistically unrepresentative. Fig. I-1, *E* illustrates the same type of nigral cell impregnated with a rapid Golgi silver method. The axon is stained and can be seen making a characteristic curve as it leaves the axon hillock. In addition, the soma and the voluminous fine processes of an adjacent astrocyte have been impregnated.

Nauta stain. A modified heavy-metal stain was developed by Nauta to demonstrate wallerian degeneration by staining the fragments of the axon. Thus this technique can be used for unmyelinated as well as myelinated fibers, and it shows degeneration as far as the preterminal axon and perhaps as far as the synaptic bouton. The degenerating fibers appear in this stain as a series of droplets of black-colored material; the normal fibers stain lightly and have a continuous structure. The Nauta stain demonstrates degeneration best when the sections are taken so that the degenerating fibers are oriented longitudinally, although heavy degeneration may also be readily observed in sections cut transversely to the pathway undergoing degeneration. A recent modification of the Nauta technique by Fink and Heimer appears to be more successful in demonstrating degenerating synaptic boutons.

Anterograde axoplasmic transport of labelled substances. Another approach to the problem of determining the distribution of the processes of neurons is the use of radioactive labelling of synaptic terminals following axoplasmic transport of radioactive substances. A commonly utilized compound for this purpose is a radiolabelled amino acid, such as tritiated leucine or proline. The tagged substance can be injected intracellularly if the experimental aim is the localization of the processes of a single neuron, or it can be placed in the extracellular space if a group of neurons is to be studied. The amino acid is taken up by the neurons, incorporated into protein, and then transported along the processes. Anterograde axoplasmic flow will convey a radiolabelled substance to the synaptic terminals, which can then be recognized by radioautography. The advantages of this technique to the anterograde degeneration stains are that the process depends on physiological mechanisms rather than on pathological processes; the label does not enter axons in substantial amounts, and so axons passing through a nucleus are not labelled, whereas a lesion would interrupt axons of passage; and the timing of synaptic labelling is predictable from the rate of axoplasmic flow. Disadvantages include the problem of recognizing small amounts of label over background and the time required for photographic exposure to the radioautograms. The scanning of sections with label and the recognition of significant levels above background can be greatly facilitated by use of computer techniques.

Fluorescence histochemistry. A useful tool for the study of pathways in the nervous system that contain monoamines has been developed by the Swedish workers Falck and Hillarp. This is a fluorescence histochemical technique that demonstrates even very fine axons when they contain norepinephrine, dopamine, or serotonin. A great amount of information has already been obtained concerning peripheral autonomic pathways, as well as central monoaminergic pathways. The procedure depends on a reaction between formaldehyde and the monoamines in freeze-dried tissue, and the monoamines fluoresce when examined under ultraviolet light.

Immunofluorescence histochemistry. An alternative way to identify neurons containing specific synaptic transmitters is by the use of an immunofluorescence histochemical procedure. The method depends on the isolation and purification of a specific protein or polypeptide that can be used as an antigen. Antibodies are produced and tagged with a fluorescent compound, such as fluorescein. The antibodies react with tissue sections, and the neurons containing antigen can be identified by the presence of fluorescence. Particular applications include the localization of neurosecretory cells in the hypothalamus and the demonstration of neurons containing choline acetyltransferase (cholinergic neurons), tyrosine hydroxylase or dopamine β-hydroxylase (catecholaminergic neurons), and most recently tryptophan hydroxylase (serotonergic neurons) in the central or peripheral nervous systems. Of current interest is the investigation of possible polypeptide transmitter agents and neurons containing them.

Other light microscopic techniques. Many other techniques using the light microscope have been employed. The polarizing microscope has been used in the study of myelin. Phase contrast microscopy is particularly valuable for the study of neurons and neuroglia in tissue culture. Their long-term behavior can be recorded by time-lapse photography. Radioautography can be employed to follow cell migrations or axoplasmic flow. Dye can be ejected by electrophoresis from microelectrodes to mark the positions of neurons or to demonstrate the morphological structure of a neuron that had previously been studied by electrophysiological methods. A large variety of histochemical procedures may be employed.

An interesting new application of computer techniques to morphology has been the three-dimensional reconstruction of the dendritic patterns of neurons. The neurons of interest are stained with a Golgi technique. The section is scanned using a microscope interfaced with a computer. The coordinates of the cell body are recorded, and then the positions and distances of the branch points of the dendrites with respect to the cell body are entered into the computer memory. Once the entire dendritic tree has been accounted for, which requires scanning the adjacent sections to include dendrites that extend beyond the thickness of a single section, the computer program reconstructs the shape of the neuron. The display can plot in a three-dimensional format the entire dendritic tree, and the display can be changed so that the neuron appears to rotate, allowing it to be viewed from any direction. This technique is useful for cytoarchitectonic studies of nuclear regions within the brain, because it permits a more accurate description and therefore classification of the types of neurons in a particular zone, in contrast to the usual analysis of Golgi material. For instance, this approach has allowed Jones to identify nine different kinds of neurons within the primate visual cortex in addition to the ordinary pyramidal cells.

Electron microscopy. The ultrastructure of nervous tissue has been under intensive investigation for nearly two decades. Peripheral nervous system structures have often been successfully studied by immersion fixation, but in general the central nervous system must be fixed by a perfusion technique. This is often difficult. With suitably fixed material, electron microscopy still has a great deal to demonstrate about normal structure in many areas of the central nervous system. Statistical methods are being developed to help overcome the enormous sampling problems involved in surveys of nervous tissue. Methods are also being developed to enable investigators to be sure of the orientation of blocks of nervous tissue, because the orientation is often crucial for interpretation. An important extension of descriptive electron microscopy is the use of three-dimensional reconstructions from serially sectioned material.

Many experimental procedures are being applied to electron microscopy. For example, it is possible to use Golgi stains and then to observe the relationships of the stained neuron to other structures by cutting thin sections of the Golgi-stained cell. The type of neuron can be determined using the light microscope, and then the arrangement of dendritic branches in the neuropil can be studied at the ultrastructural level. However, with this technique the organization of the cytoplasm is obscured by the electron opaque stain, which completely fills it. This makes it difficult to be sure in all instances that synaptic structures adjacent to the neuron actually connect with it, because the postsynaptic specializations of the synapse cannot be identified.

Degeneration of synaptic endings can be recognized at the ultrastructural level. There appear to be two basic types of degeneration. In one, the amount of neurofilaments increases greatly, accompanied by a swelling of the endings. The more common type of degeneration is characterized by an increased electron density of the cytoplasm and a gradual loss of internal structure. While synaptic vesicles are still visible, however, the degenerating synaptic bouton can be recognized. This technique can be coupled with light microscopy so that preliminary survey with semithin sections allows a region of degeneration to be found, and details can be observed in thin sections with the electron microscope. In this way, the type of synapse can be determined, for example, axosomatic, axodendritic, or axoaxonal. This approach could conceivably be used with a method for identifying the postsynaptic structure to give a certain description of synaptic connections.

A number of other experimental procedures are now being used at the electron microscopic level. Radioautography at an electron microscopic level can provide good resolution, especially if statistical procedures are used to help determine the structures most likely to be associated with the labelled molecule. Electron microscopic histochemistry is just in its infancy as a field of study.

Methods of producing lesions of the nervous system

Ablation of nervous tissue is the oldest method of studying nervous function. Gross ablation of tissue, as of a lobe of the brain, is usually carried out by a combination of sharp excision and removal of the tissue with suction, using fine metal or glass suction tubing. Bleeding is controlled with electrocautery of vessels, which are grasped with a fine forceps through which a very high-frequency current is passed that causes induction heating of the tissue and coagulation of the vessel. Hemostatic agents, such as oxidized cotton and gelfoam, a spongelike form of gelatin derived from collagen, which is soaked in thrombin before application, are also applied to the cut edges of the brain to promote blood clot formation and to stop bleeding from small vessels. Bleeding from large vessels is controlled by the closing of V-shaped metal clips around them.

A number of methods have been devised to make subcortical lesions. The objectives of these methods is to produce a lesion of known size and shape, without causing bleeding at the site of the lesion. The simplest method is the electrolytic lesion, in which a direct current of a few milliamperes is passed through an electrode that is made the anode of a circuit; this produces less gas-bubble formation caused by electrolysis of water and NaCl. Larger and more controlled lesions can be made with induction heating of 70° to 75° C around the tip of an electrode, using radio-frequency current. A thermistor bead or thermocouple in the tip of the electrode is used to monitor and control the brain temperature. This is the most practical way of making lesions at present. Cryosurgical lesions using tubes chilled with liquid nitrogen are also used for making depth lesions.

If a lesion is made slowly, it may be possible to ablate very large areas of the brainstem, which cannot be destroyed abruptly with safety. An excellent method for producing lesions of very precise size over a period of days is to implant small spheres of radioactive isotopes of such metals as yttrium or palladium, which emit beta-radiation and some gamma-radiation.

High-energy beams of sound and of radiation can also be used to produce lesions. Focused ultrasound and beams of high-energy particles have been used to produce lesions within the central nervous system. It is possible to direct a beam of ultrasonic energy or protons to a point deep within the brain, using a modification of the stereotaxic procedure (p. 437), and to destroy small regions of nervous tissue. The advantages of ultrasound and proton beam lesions are that the shape of the lesion can be precisely controlled by making several small lesions, there is no electrode track, the operative morbidity is low, and blood vessels are unharmed. The major disadvantage is the complexity of the equipment required.

Laser beam radiation has also been used as a method of stimulating and damaging single neurons in invertebrate ganglia. Laser radiation applied to the surface of the brain produces a lesion rather like a combination of a heat lesion and one caused by mechanical trauma.

NEUROPHYSIOLOGICAL TECHNIQUES
Stimulation

There are a number of ways in which nervous tissue can be stimulated. The most physiological way is to activate receptor organs by stimuli similar to those that act during the normal life of the organism. A number of special devices have been designed to allow such stimulation to be done relatively quantitatively. For instance, very good control of visual and acoustic stimuli is possible. Mechanical and thermal stimuli are less readily controlled, although an attempt has been made to use these stimuli. The energy applied can be controlled, but it is difficult to overcome the distortion caused by biological tissues separating the stimulus and the receptor organ.

Electrical stimulation is often employed to activate nerve fibers or regions of the central nervous system. The stimuli are generally applied as voltage pulses through low-resistance electrodes. However, sometimes it is more desirable to use current pulses from a high-resistance source of current. This is particularly true if there is a danger that the impedance of the tissue being stimulated would change, thereby altering the amount of current delivered by a voltage pulse. Impedance changes that do not reflect nerve membrane changes could result from such factors as alterations in the extracellular fluid compartment or in blood flow.

Recording

The electrodes commonly employed for recording in neurophysiological experiments include a variety of metal electrodes and glass micropipettes. For recording from peripheral nerve, a frequently used electrode is a platinum wire. For reference purposes, a silver–silver chloride plate is often used. Electrodes to be inserted into the central nervous system may be relatively large metal electrodes (about 0.1 to 1 mm in diameter), metal microelectrodes (1 to 10 μm), or glass microelectrodes filled with electrolyte (0.2 μm outside diameter or larger if broken). The metal electrodes are insulated by some type of enamel. The tip may be sharpened by grinding or electrolysis. Sometimes a metal-filled glass microelectrode is employed. The usual glass microelectrode is filled with a concentration solution of salt, usually 3M KCl. This solution has a minimal junction potential. However, it is sometimes useful to fill the electrodes with other solutions, such as 4M NaCl (good especially for extracellular recording) or 2M potassium acetate or citrate (to prevent the reversal of intracellularly recorded inhibitory postsynaptic potentials caused by leakage of chloride ions). The resistances of metal electrodes are generally below 1 megohm; glass microelectrodes may have resistances of 10 or even 100 megohms.

One of the limitations of glass microelectrodes, particularly those with very fine tips, has been their ability to pass current without changes occurring in the electrode resistance. Electrode polarization may be severe enough to stop current flow altogether, or it may simply interfere with the measurement process by the production of electrical artifacts. A recent improvement in microelectrode technology is the introduction of beveling microelectrode tips by using an abrasive. The amount of beveling can be controlled by simultaneously measuring the resistance of the tip, provided that the microelectrode is filled with electrolyte prior to beveling. The effect of beveling is to increase the surface area of the tip opening without sacrificing a small size; the tip may in fact be sharper.

Special glass microelectrodes have been introduced for selectively measuring the activity of specific ions in solution. These ion-sensitive electrodes are not capable of resolving very rapid changes in ionic concentration, but they are useful for detecting slow changes. Some of the ionic species that can now be measured are hydrogen (pH), sodium, chloride, potassium, and calcium. In some cases, the electrodes can be made small enough for intracellular measurements. One difficulty is that such electrodes may not be completely specific for one ion.

One of the basic principles of recording voltages is that the instrument used as a voltmeter should not draw enough current from the circuit to alter its properties. A measure of this is the relationship between the resistance of the circuit element being studied and the input resistance of the voltmeter. The resistance of the circuit element studied includes the resistance of the electrode employed. For example, when glass microelectrodes are used, the bulk of the circuit resistance is the microelectrode resistance. The microelectrode might have a 10-megohm resistance, and so the input resistance of the amplifier by which potentials are measured, using the microelectrode as a probe, would need to be about 100 megohms for a 10% reduction in the measured potential, or 1,000 megohms for a 1% distortion.

Electrodes, and particularly the electrode–tissue fluid interface, have the electrical properties of resistance, capacitance, and an electromotive potential. A thin silver wire may have a negligible resistance of several ohms, but the interface of a silver wire in saline has a considerable resistance to the flow of direct current. A pair of 1-mm diameter silver ball electrodes in saline will have a resistance to the passage of a small (milliampere) current of about 10,000 ohms. This resistance and the electromotive potential of electrodes are caused by the tendency of the electrode to ionize when placed in a solution. This phenomenon, called polarization, is discussed in greater detail in Appendix II. All electrodes polarize. The degree of polarization is related to the current passing through the interface and, when alternating currents are passed, to the frequency of the current. The degree of polarization can be measured only with respect to another electrode. The hydrogen electrode is used for this purpose, and electrode potentials can be arranged in the so-called electromotive series, with respect to the polarization of the hydrogen electrode. The electromotive potentials are the basis of chemical batteries, and the recording and reference electrodes comprise a battery. Therefore, attempts are made to make the input electrodes of the recording circuit of the same metal so as to reduce the potential between them. Even so, electromotive potentials between electrodes may be much greater than the signal to be recorded. In the case of EEG recording, these potentials are in the millivolt range and the signal is in the microvolt range. Electrode potentials are either balanced out with countervoltages (bucking) or essentially filtered out when resistance-capacitance-coupled (AC-coupled) amplifiers are used. Slight movements of the tissue-electrode interface can change the interface resistance and polarization and produce spurious potentials. To reduce these problems nonpolarizable electrodes are used, although the term is a misnomer. These are electrodes in which the polarization potential is kept highly constant and is reproducible from one electrode to another. This is accomplished by using a metal in contact with a salt of the metal, usually a chloride salt, led by a saline bridge to the tissue. Ag-AgCl-NaCl electrodes are the most commonly used. Pt-Hg-HgCl$_2$-NaCl electrodes may be more stable but cannot be made small as easily as Ag-AgCl electrodes. Voltage differences between these electrodes can be obtained in the microvolt range. A more constant degree of polarization of electrodes can also be obtained by reducing the current drawn by the amplifier through the electrodes by using high-input impedance amplifiers. Nonpolarizable electrodes are particularly used for recording DC-steady or slowly changing potentials. Micropipettes filled with various salt solutions and led to Ag-AgCl electrodes are nonpolarizable electrodes. They usually have an electrode potential of many millivolts with respect to the reference (ground) electrode. Because of their high resistance, the product of their resistance and capacitance can result in a circuit that acts like a filter for high frequencies. Attenuation of high frequencies results in rounded, small spike responses. This is overcome in circuit design of amplifiers used for micropipette recording by an ingenious use of positive feedback.

Recording is done in general by amplifying bioelectrical signals, using a suitable amplifier. For high-input impedance applications, the first stage of amplification is done by one of a variety of devices, such as the cathode follower, the electrometer amplifier, or a field effect transistor amplifier. The input impedance of such instruments may be as high as 10^{13} ohms. Other applications may use amplifiers having a lower input impedance. For instance, for recording from peripheral nerves it is often possible to use an amplifier with a 1-megohm input impedance. Other considerations for the selection of suitable amplifiers include the band-pass filter. For many purposes, an audio amplifier (AC-coupled amplifier) will suffice. However, sometimes it is necessary to have an amplifier that is linear to DC. This is essential when recording membrane potentials. It is also quite important to have an adequate band width for low frequencies in studying extracellular potentials, which usually consist of a mixture of frequencies from about one cycle per second to several hundred cycles per second. If the time constant of an AC–coupled amplifier is much shorter than the slowest frequency to be amplified, the slow-frequency waves will be attenuated and shifted in phase with respect to the faster frequency waves. In addition, when presented with a potential much longer than the time constant, the resistance-capacitance network of the amplifier will first charge

(see Appendix II) and then discharge, producing a voltage of opposite polarity. As an example of this effect, the recording of a prolonged field potential of the type associated with IPSPs, which should be recorded as a slow positive potential, can be recorded as a smaller, faster positive wave followed by a negative wave. Evoked-potential averaging techniques are particularly likely to suffer from this type of artifact, because slow-wave frequencies are often filtered out to produce a more stable baseline for averaging. The upper frequencies of many biological signals do not exceed 10 kc, so it may be possible to reduce noise by filtering out frequencies above this level. For special purposes, operational amplifiers may be used. For example, it is sometimes convenient to integrate or to differentiate signals.

When signals of very small amplitude must be measured against a noisy background, it may be possible to enhance the signal-to-noise ratio through the use of one of the so-called signal averagers. These instruments often are basically analog-to-digital converters. A repeated signal is necessary, and the instrument is triggered by a pulse having a constant timing with reference to the signal. Starting at a fixed time, the instrument digitizes the recorded potential at a chosen rate. Inasmuch as the memory capacity of such an instrument is limited, generally each record is a few hundred to a thousand digital points. The total may represent milliseconds to seconds in time, depending on the sampling rate. With each repetition of the recorded potential, the signal is added in memory in the same digital channels, because the time from onset of digitization is fixed. The noise, which is random, adds in some sweeps, but it will be subtracted in others; so with sufficient repetition it will be averaged to zero.

Techniques for intracellular recording in the central nervous system

The main requirements for intracellular recording in the central nervous system (CNS) are surgical exposure of the area to be studied, reduction of the vascular and respiratory pulsations of the CNS so that the micropipette electrode will remain in an intracellular position, and maintenance of the CNS and the animal in good physiological condition.

With good technique it is possible to record from large neurons such as spinal motoneurons or cortical Betz cells for hours, but in the case of smaller neurons such as spinal interneurons or small basal ganglia neurons, intracellular recordings often can be obtained for only a few minutes. Intracellular recordings in the human brain at the time of craniotomy have been attempted, but the sizable pulsations of the human brain make more than very brief recordings very difficult.

Some of the techniques used in recording in animals are shown in Fig. I-3. The animal, in this case a cat, is shown prepared for a study of responses of brainstem neurons to subcortical stimulation. The skull has been opened in several places for insertion of electrodes. The occipital cortex overlying the upper brainstem has been removed and the recording microelectrode inserted into the brainstem. Warm agar has been poured around the electrode and allowed to harden to protect the brain and to reduce vascular and respiratory pulsations of the brain. In the case of recording from the cortex, a pressor foot, a plastic disc with a central opening for the electrode, may be used. Stimulating electrodes have been placed stereotaxically in the caudate nucleus and in a thalamic nucleus. An electrode has been placed on the sensorimotor cortex to monitor the responses evoked by the stimulating electrodes. The electrocorticogram is recorded with respect to an indifferent electrode on the nose. The indifferent electrode is placed away from the brain, but also away from the heart so as to prevent picking up its electrical activity. The intracellular potentials are recorded with respect to a ground electrode, here placed subcutaneously in the suboccipital area. To further reduce brain pulsations the cisterna magna is opened and drained of CSF. The animal is suspended by the vertebral column, and an artificial pneumo-

thorax is performed. The somatic musculature is relaxed with a neuromuscular blocking agent, gallamine triethiodide. The lungs are inflated as shallowly as possible, with a respirator through a tracheotomy. End-tidal CO_2, and blood gases in some cases, are measured to regulate the respiratory rate. The brain temperature, rectal temperature, and blood pressure are monitored; these physiological functions are maintained at close to normal values by body heating and intravenous fluids.

Stereotaxis. For studies of the brain, it is often desirable to place recording or stimulating electrodes in predetermined regions without seriously disrupting neighboring structures. An instrument designed for this purpose was first developed by Horsley, a British neurosurgeon, and Clarke, a physiologist. This device was popularized by Ranson and his group in the 1930s. The Horsley-Clarke instrument has since become a standard part of the repertory of the neuroanatomist and neurophysiologist. The basic premise is that there is a relatively constant relationship between the parts of the brain and certain skeletal landmarks. In the usual applications of the instrument, the animal is fixed to a frame by tapered bars inserted into the external auditory canals (Fig. I-4). The animal's palate is placed in a horizontal position, with the head held down in position by bars pressing on the inferior orbital ridges. The line between the ear bars is an anteroposterior reference line; for example, points in front

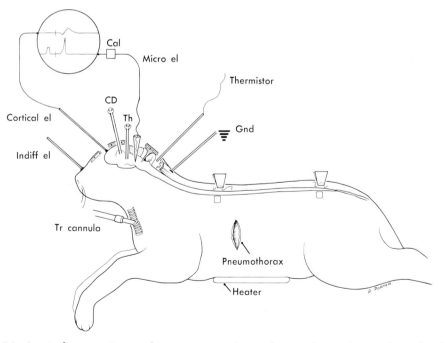

Fig. I-3. Surgical preparation and arrangement of recording and stimulating electrodes for intracellular recording from neurons in the brain in a small animal.

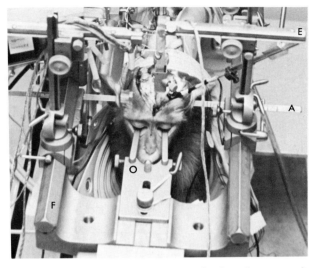

Fig. I-4. Animal stereotaxis. The head of a rhesus monkey is mounted in the main frame, *F*, of a stereotaxic instrument. The basic horizontal plane is determined by the line between bars holding the inferior orbital margins, *O*, and the external acoustic canals, *A*, of the skull. An electrode carrier, *E*, is mounted on the main frame of the instrument.

of this line are so many millimeters anterior, according to the standard terminology. A horizontal reference is provided by an imaginary plane passing 10 mm above the line connecting the ear bars and the inferior orbital margin. The lateral reference can be established by adjusting the ear bars so that the head is centered in the frame; however, this rough adjustment is often corrected by reference to landmarks of the skull or brain. Electrodes are inserted through a hole placed in an appropriate place in the skull until the tip is located at the chosen coordinates. These can be determined by finding the desired structure in a stereotaxic atlas. The initial position of the electrode is found by reading the coordinates of the electrode holder when the tip is positioned between the ear bars, with the animal not yet in the frame. Sometimes another reference point on the frame is provided so that new electrodes can be used without removing the animal's head from the ear bars.

Anesthetics in neurophysiology. Anesthetics are used to abolish consciousness and pain when immobility is required for procedures involving maintaining electrodes in fixed relationships to neurons. Immobility can be produced with neuromuscular blocking agents, but the use of these agents without general or local anesthesia to relieve operative pain cannot be condoned. The barbiturates of short or moderate duration of activity are frequently used as anesthetics, because anesthesia is easily induced by intraperitoneal injection or intravenous (titrated dosage) administra-

tion. The barbiturates also have a good margin of safety between the dosage required for anesthesia and the dosage that produces serious cardiovascular and respiratory depression. When the barbiturates produce surgical anesthesia, they reduce spontaneous neural activity and the amplitude of PSPs, especially if polysynaptic pathways are involved in their generation. In addition, during light barbiturate anesthesia highly synchronized activity of thalamocortical systems (barbiturate spindles) occurs. Although the nervous system is in an abnormal state when an anesthetized animal is studied, the ability of the barbiturates to abolish polysynaptic activity can be useful in studying the properties of monosynaptic and disynaptic pathways in relative isolation without the interference of other pathways.

Hypnotic drugs that do not produce surgical anesthesia but reduce pain and movement have been used in experiments on polysynaptic systems, particularly in sensory physiology. Chloralose, a chloral hydrate derivative, is a drug with effects between those of a hypnotic drug and an anesthetic drug. A number of new hypnoticlike drugs have been introduced into anesthetic practice. Some of these may be useful in neurophysiology.

Inhalation anesthetic has been used on a wider scale in neurophysiology since the introduction into human anesthesia of gaseous agents, such as halothane, which are nonexplosive and have a wider margin of safety than ether or cyclopropane. A mixture of halothane, nitrous oxide, and a muscle relaxant, as often used in human surgery, can provide immobility, pain relief, and comparatively little depression of polysynaptic pathways.

Abolition of pain and immobility can also be produced by transection of the brainstem at the midcollicular level, the so-called cerveau isolé preparation. Surgery is performed while the animal is under a short-acting barbiturate or gas-inhalation anesthetic, and the animal is allowed to recover for several hours before recording is carried out. In these preparations the cortex and thalamus exhibit synchronized activity characteristic of sleep. If the rostral portion of the brain is removed, the preparation is called a decerebrate preparation. Although free of anesthetic effects, the telencephalic and spinal background activity is nevertheless abnormal in the preparations, although as in the case of the use of anesthetics this can be useful for some experimental designs.

Long-term–implanted recording and stimulating electrodes. Recording of electrical activity of the brain in unanesthetized animals in different functional states of activity over long periods of time can be carried out by means of long-term–implanted macroelectrodes

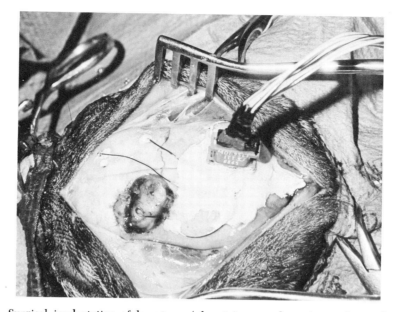

Fig. I-5. Surgical implantation of long-term (chronic) gross electrodes in the epidural space for recording of the electrocorticogram in the cat. The scalp has been opened and retracted laterally. A trephine opening has been made in the left frontal area to expose the dura, and a stainless steel wire electrode can be seen leading to the area. Two other wire electrodes can be seen going to small trephine openings in the right frontal area. The openings are closed with acrylic cement, which holds the electrodes in place. The connector receiving the electrodes is mounted in the midline of the skull in the occipital area and is held in place with acrylic. The male connector with attached cable leads to the first stage of the amplifier.

and microelectrodes. Similar recordings are obtained from the human brain to localize sites of origin of epileptic discharge, particularly in patients with temporal lobe epilepsy.

Three basic types of systems can be used. The simplest method for long-term macroelectrode recording is to implant wires, or wire circuits printed on plastic film, on the dura or on the pia-arachnoid or to implant wire electrodes within the brain, using a stereotaxic machine. The electrodes are led to a female connector, rigidly mounted on the skull to prevent electrode movement and artifactual potentials. A male connector with lead wires to amplifiers is plugged in at the time of recording. The skin site through which the connector is led is prone to infection, which often limits the use of these electrodes, although with meticulous skin care recordings can be obtained for months or years without difficulty. This type of system is illustrated in Fig. I-5.

Another method is to drill and tap the skull and implant a thin metal cannula with a removable cap. At the time of recording, electrodes are inserted through the cannula. This method is suitable for inserting metal microelectrodes for the extracellular recording of the activity of single neurons (units) from the cortex and brainstem. Electrolytically sharpened tungsten or steel wires are generally used because their tips are resistant to breaking, unlike glass pipettes.

Finally, miniaturized radio transmitters and receivers can be implanted on the skull with wires leading to the brain, without the disadvantages of external lead wires. This approach has been used to stimulate the human visual cortex in blind persons. At present the number of functioning stimulation or recording points that have been achieved with transcutaneous or telemetering techniques is small, but with progress in microcircuitry the number will increase.

Data analysis. Recorded information may be kept in a permanent form by photographing the face of an oscilloscope on which it is displayed or by writing it on paper, using a pen recorder. Very rapid activity, such as a nerve impulse, often cannot be recorded directly with a penwriter, because such devices have a limited upper range to their frequency response. Thus, an oscilloscope may be necessary. However, a change in time base may be produced by recording data on a tape recorder and reading the tape out at a different speed than that used for recording. Similarly, the output of a signal averager may be seen by using a penwriter because the contents of the memory can be scanned at a slow rate. The film and paper-strip records can be further analyzed by measurements of the potentials represented on them. A more expensive but more versatile and accurate method of data analysis is to digitize signals and then to analyze them by computer. This can be done "on line" during an experiment or "off line" by storing the information on digital magnetic tape. When the frequency response is not a limiting factor, data can be stored on an analog tape and later analyzed. Many other computer applications, including control by computer of experimental variables, will undoubtedly be common in the near future.

Microiontophoresis. Many drugs will ionize in solution and thus carry a net electrical charge. It is thus possible to enhance their rate of diffusion by applying an electrical field to a solution containing the drug. If a concentrated solution is placed in a microelectrode, it is possible to eject the drug from the tip by means of a small electrical current passed through the electrode. The drug action on nearby neurons could be tested by recording the activity of the neurons through the same microelectrode or through another attached to it. Sometimes it is valuable to make multibarreled microelectrodes so that a number of drugs can be tried on the same neurons. Generally, the recording electrode is extracellular. However, it is possible to manufacture offset microelectrodes, with the leading one capable of intracellular recording while the trailing one(s) ejects a drug extracellularly. This allows a direct analysis of the membrane potential changes in response to the drug, whereas extracellular recording allows indirect inferences based on changes in the rate of firing of the cell. When approaching neurons with electrodes containing very active compounds, a reversed electric field is generally used to restrain the drug from diffusing out of the microelectrode tip.

Optical techniques. It has been shown that nerve impulses are accompanied by changes in the optical properties of nerve fibers. Both light scattering and changes in birefringence have been observed. It is likely that such effects will be helpful in further elucidating the molecular changes that occur in the nerve membrane during activity.

Laboratory values for experimental animals. A great deal of what is known about the central nervous system of humans was first discovered through experimentation on animals. Paradoxically, it is easier to find values in the literature for many physiologically important parameters for humans than it is for animals. Because of this, some baseline values of measurements from the most commonly used experimental animal in neurophysiology, the cat, are given in Table I-1.

Table I-1. Baseline values of measurements in the cat

Normal values of some physiological parameters for the unanesthetized cat	
Temperature	38°-38.5° C
Pulse	110-140/min
Blood pressure	155/100 mm Hg
Respiratory rate	20-30/min
Tidal volume	12-15 ml
Blood volume	5.25% of body weight
Hematocrit level	40% (frequently lower because of disease)
Serum electrolytes and blood gases in arterial blood	
Na	153 ± 5 mEq/l
K	4.3 ± 0.5 mEq/l
Cl	117 ± 4 mEq/l
pCO_2	27 ± 3 mm Hg
pH	7.4 ± 0.4
Glucose	60-100 mg/100 ml (Somogyi)
Cisternal CSF electrolytes	
Na	160 ± 5 mEq/l
K	2.9 ± 0.06 mEq/l
Cl	138 ± 4 mEq/l
Osmolarity	320 mOsm
Brain electrolytes*	
Na	62 ± 5 mEq/l of wet weight
K	98 ± 5 mEq/l of wet weight
Cl	42 ± 2 mEq/l of wet weight
Water content	77%

*Sections of motor cortex taken, largely of gray matter, with some underlying white matter (gray matter 76%, white matter 24%).

BIBLIOGRAPHY

Albrecht, M. H., and Fernstrom, R. C.: A modified Nauta-Gygax method for human brain and spinal cord, Stain Technol. **34**:91-94, 1959.

Alksne, J. F., Blackstad, T. W., Walberg, F., and White, L. E.: Electron microscopy of axon degeneration; a valuable tool in experimental neuroanatomy, Ergebn. Anat. Entwicklungsgesch. **39**:1-31, 1966.

Amatniek, E.: Measurement of bioelectric potentials with microelectrodes and neutralized input capacity amplifiers, Inst. Radio Engrs. Trans. Med. Electron. P.G.M.E. **10**:3-14, 1958.

Barrett, J. N., and Graubard, K.: Fluorescent staining of cat motoneurons in vivo with beveled micropipettes, Brain Res. **18**:565-568, 1970.

Beresford, W. A.: An evaluation of neuroanatomical methods and their relation to neurophysiology, Brain Res. **1**:221-249, 1966.

Berman, A. L.: The brain stem of the cat; a cytoarchitectonic atlas with stereotaxic coordinates, Madison, 1968, University of Wisconsin Press.

Bowsher, D., Brodal, A., and Walberg, F.: The relative values of the Marchi method and some silver impregnation techniques, Brain **83**:150-160, 1960.

Boycott, B. B., Gray, E. G., and Guillery, R. W.: A theory to account for the absence of boutons in silver preparations of the cerebral cortex, based on a study of axon terminals by light and electron microscopy, J. Physiol. (Lond.) **152**:31-35, 1960.

Brodal, A.: Modification of Gudden method for study of cerebral localization, Arch. Neurol. Psychiatry **43:**46-58, 1940.

Brown, P. B., Maxfield, B. W., and Moraff, H.: Electronics for neurobiologists, Cambridge, Mass., 1973, The M.I.T. Press.

Bureš, J., Petráň, M., and Zachar, J.: Electrophysiological methods in biological research, New York, 1967, Academic Press, Inc.

Cowan, W. M., Gottlieb, D. I., Hendrickson, A. E., Price, J. L., and Wollsey, T. A.: The autoradiographic demonstration of axonal connections in the central nervous system, Brain Res. **37:**21-51, 1972.

Fink, R. P., and Heimer, L.: Two methods for selective silver impregnation of degenerating axons and their synaptic endings in the central nervous system, Brain Res. **4:**369-374, 1967.

Fry, W. J.: Intense ultrasound in investigations of the central nervous system. In Lawrence, J. H., and Tobias, C. A., editors: Advances in biological and medical physics, vol. 6, New York, 1958, Academic Press, Inc.

Gergen, J. A., and MacLean, P. D.: A stereotaxic atlas of the squirrel monkey's brain, U. S. Public Health Service Publication No. 933, Washington, D. C., 1962, U. S. Government Printing Office.

Glees, P., and Hasan, M.: The signs of synaptic degeneration; a critical appraisal, Acta Anat. (Basel) **69:**153-167, 1968.

Grant, G., and Aldskogius, H.: Silver impregnation of degenerating dendrites, cells and axons central to axonal transection. I. A Nauta study on the hypoglossal nerve in kittens, Exp. Brain Res. **3:**150-162, 1967.

Heimer, L., and Peters, A.: An electron microscope study of a silver stain for degenerating boutons, Brain Res. **8:**337-346, 1968.

Hillarp, N. A., Fuxe, K., Dahlstrom, A.: Demonstration and mapping of central neurons containing dopamine, noradrenaline, and 5-hydroxytryptamine and their reactions to psychopharmaca, Pharmacol. Rev. **18:**727-743, 1966.

Jones, E. G.: Varieties and distribution of non-pyramidal cells in the somatic sensory cortex of the squirrel monkey, J. Comp. Neurol. **160:**205-268, 1975.

Karlsson, U., and Schultz, R. L.: Fixation of the central nervous system for electron microscopy by aldehyde perfusion. I. Preservation with aldehyde perfusates versus direct perfusion with osmium tetroxide with special reference to membranes and the extracellular space, J. Ultrastruc. Res. **12:**160-186, 1965.

Kater, S. B., and Nicholson, C., editors: Intracellular staining in neurobiology, New York, 1973, Springer-Verlag New York Inc.

Keynes, R. D.: Thermal and optical changes during the nerve impulse. In Proceedings of the International Union of Physiological Science, vol. 6, Washington, D. C., 1968, Federation of American Societies for Experimental Biology, pp. 74-76.

Lasek, R., Joseph, B. S., and Whitlock, D. G.: Evaluation of a radioautographic neuroanatomical tracing method, Brain Res. **8:**319-336, 1968.

LaVail, J. H., and LaVail, M. M.: The retrograde intraaxonal transport of horseradish peroxidase in the chick visual system; a light and electron microscopic study, J. Comp. Neurol. **157:**303-358, 1974.

Lavallée, M., Schanne, O. F., and Hébert, N. C.: Glass microelectrodes, New York, 1969, John Wiley & Sons, Inc.

Lux, H. D., Schubert, P., Kreutzberg, G. W., and Globus, A.: Excitation and axonal flow; autoradiographic study on motoneurons intracellularly injected with a ^{3}H-amino acid, Exp. Brain Res. **10:**197-204, 1970.

Mannen, H.: Contribution to the quantitative study of the nervous tissue, a new method for measurement of the volume and surface area of neurons, J. Comp. Neurol. **126:**75-91, 1966.

Mitchell, H. C., and Thaemert, J. C.: Three dimensions in fine structure, Science **148:**1480-1482, 1965.

Nastuk, W. L., editor: Physical techniques in biological research, vol. 5, Electrophysiological methods, part A; and vol. 6, Electrophysiological methods, part B, New York, 1961, Academic Press, Inc.

Nauta, W. J. H., and Gygax, P. A.: Silver impregnation of degenerating axons in the central nervous system; a modified technique, Stain Technol. **29:**91-93, 1954.

Palay, S. L.: Contributions of electron microscopy to neuroanatomy. In Windle, W. F., editor: New research techniques of neuroanatomy, Springfield, Ill., 1957, Charles C Thomas, Publisher.

Palay, S. L., McGee-Russell, S. M., Gordon, S., and Grillo, M. S.: Fixation of neural tissues for electron microscopy by perfusion with solutions of osmium tetroxide, J. Cell. Biol. **12:**385-410, 1962.

Pease, D. C.: Histological techniques for electron microscopy, New York, 1964, Academic Press, Inc.

Peters, A.: Experiments on the mechanism of silver staining. IV. Electron microscope studies, Q. J. Micr. Sci. **96:**317, 1955.

Ranson, S. W.: On the use of the Horsley-Clarke stereotaxic instrument, Psychiat. Neurol. Bl. **38:**534-543, 1934.

Sabatini, D. D., Bensch, K., and Barrnett, R. J.: Cytochemistry and electron microscopy, J. Cell. Biol. **17:**19-58, 1963.

Salmoiraghi, G. C., and Bloom, F. E.: Pharmacology of individual neurons, Science **144:**493-499, 1964.

Sandlin, R., Lerman, L., Barry, W., and Tasaki, I.: Application of laser interferometry to physiological studies of excitable tissues, Nature (Lond.) **217:**575-576, 1968.

Schaltenbrand, G., and Bailey, P.: Introduction to stereotaxis with an atlas of the human brain, Stuttgart, 1959, Georg Thieme Verlag.

Schoenfeld, R. L., and Milkman, N.: Digital computers in the biological laboratory, Science **146:**190-198, 1964.

Schultz, R. L., and Karlsson, U.: Fixation of the central nervous system for electron microscopy by aldehyde perfusion. II. Effect of osmolarity, pH of perfusate, and fixative concentration, J. Ultrastruct. Res. **12:**187-206, 1965.

Snider, R. S., and Lee, J. C.: A stereotaxic atlas of the monkey brain (Macaca mulatta), Chicago, 1961, University of Chicago Press.

Stretton, A. O. W., and Kravitz, E. A.: Neuronal geometry; determination with a technique of intracellular dye injection, Science **162:**132-134, 1968.

Swank, R. L., and Davenport, H. A.: Chlorate-osmic-formalin methods for staining degenerating myelin, Stain Technol. **10:**87-90, 1935.

Thomas, R. C., and Wilson, V. J.: Marking single neurons by staining with intra-cellular recording microelectrodes, Science **151:**1538-1539, 1966.

Walberg, F.: The early changes in degenerating boutons and the problem of argyrophilia; light and electron microscopic observations, J. Comp. Neurol. **122:**113-137, 1964.

Warwick, R., and Pond, J.: Trackless lesions in nervous tissues produced by high intensity focused ultrasound (high frequency mechanical waves), J. Anat. **102:**387-406, 1968.

Yanof, H. M.: Biomedical electronics, Philadelphia, 1965, F. A. Davis Co.

APPENDIX II

Mathematical concepts

APPLICATIONS OF ELECTRICITY IN NEUROPHYSIOLOGY
Basic electrical concepts

There are a number of mathematical descriptions from the theories of basic electricity that are useful for the understanding of modern neurophysiology; some of these are mentioned here.

Materials may bear a positive or negative charge or they may be electrically neutral. Charged particles attract each other if they are of opposite signs; that is, one is charged positively and the other negatively. Particles of like charge repel each other. The force of attraction or repulsion varies inversely as the square of the distance between the charged objects. The force also depends on the amount of charge on the objects. Coulomb's law relates these quantities:

$$\text{Force} = k \frac{Q_1 Q_2}{d^2} \qquad (1)$$

where k is a proportionality constant, Q_1 and Q_2 are the charges on two objects, and d is the distance between the objects. The unit of charge is the coulomb, which is the charge on 6×10^{18} electrons (one electron has a charge of 1.6×10^{-19} coulombs).

An electric field exists wherever a charged body is acted on by force. This force is a vector quantity. More important for the present discussion is the concept of potential difference. This is the amount of work done in order to move a charged object from one point to another in an electric field. The unit used for the difference in potential between two points is the volt. One volt is equivalent to one joule of work done to move one coulomb of charge.

Charge can be moved readily in some materials, called conductors. Substances that prevent the movement of charge are termed insulators; those that allow a restricted movement of charge are semiconductors.

A device that can store charge is the capacitor. The capacitor consists of two conductors separated by an insulator. A measure of the ability of a capacitor to store charge is its capacitance (C):

$$C = \frac{Q}{V} \qquad (2)$$

where C is in farads, Q is the charge in coulombs on one of the conductive elements, and V is the difference in potential in volts between the two conductors. Usually, capacitors have capacitances in the order of microfarads or less.

The value of capacitance (C) in a capacitor depends on several factors:

$$C = k \frac{K A}{d} \qquad (3)$$

where k is a proportionality constant, K is the dielectric constant (which depends on the material used for the insulator; the dielectric constant of air or of a vacuum is 1), A is the surface area of the conducive elements, and d is the distance between the conductors.

Many electric circuits are designed to move charge through relatively poor conductors known as resistors. The work required to move charge through a resistor is provided by a source of potential difference, such as a battery. The unit of resistance is the ohm. The flow of charge is called a current. The unit of current is the ampere. One ampere is a flow of one coulomb of charge past a given point each second. A potential difference of one volt will move a current of one ampere through a one-ohm resistor. Potential difference, current, and resistance are related in Ohm's law:

$$R = \frac{V}{I} \qquad (4)$$

where R is the resistance in ohms, V the potential difference in volts, and I the current in amperes.

Resistors can be made from a variety of materials. Some materials have a higher resistance for given physical dimensions than do others. The resistance of a standard-sized object made from a given material at a specific temperature is called its resistivity. For material formed into wire, the following equation is used:

$$\text{Resistance} = \frac{\text{resistivity} \times \text{length}}{\text{cross-sectional area}} \qquad (5)$$

When circuits employ a combination of elements, such as capacitors and resistors, it is often possible to replace several such components by a single equivalent element. For example, if several resistors are connected in series, the combination of these resistors can be replaced by a single one whose value equals the sum of the values of the individual ones. Thus, for series resistors:

$$R \text{ total} = R_1 + R_2 + R_3 + \cdots + R_n \qquad (6)$$

For resistors connected in parallel, the total resistance across the combination is related to the individual resistors as follows:

$$\frac{1}{R \text{ total}} = \frac{1}{R_1} + \frac{1}{R_2} + \frac{1}{R} + \cdots + \frac{1}{R_n} \qquad (7)$$

For capacitors connected in parallel, the total capacitance equals the sum of the capacitances of the individual components:

$$C \text{ total} = C_1 + C_2 + C_3 + \cdots + C_n \qquad (8)$$

This is equivalent to increasing the surface area of a single capacitor. For capacitors connected in series, the relationship of total capacitance to the capacitances of the individual elements is:

$$\frac{1}{C \text{ total}} = \frac{1}{C_1} + \frac{1}{C_2} + \frac{1}{C_3} + \cdots + \frac{1}{C_n} \qquad (9)$$

RC networks

Circuits having both resistors and capacitors as components are called RC circuits (Fig. II-1). In this circuit, a resistor *(R)* and a capacitor *(C)* are connected in series with a battery *(E)*. Initially, the circuit is closed at a switch, and the capacitor becomes fully

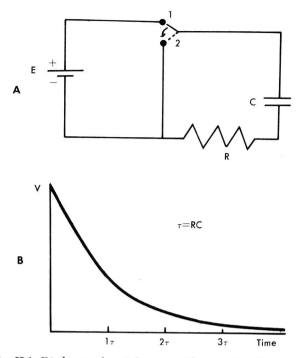

Fig. II-1. Discharge of an RC circuit. The switch in the circuit shown in **A** is initially in position 1. The capacitor, *C*, has been fully charged, so that the battery voltage, *E*, appears across it. When the switch is moved to position 2, current flows through the resistor, *R*, until the voltage, which had been across the capacitor, dissipates. The voltage decreases exponentially, as shown in the curve in **B**. After each period of time, τ *(RC)*, the voltage is reduced to $1/e$ of its former value. This value, τ, is called the time constant.

charged. When the steady state is reached, no current flows because there is by definition an insulator between the two plates of the capacitor. All of the battery voltage appears across the capacitor. If the switch is moved to the other position, as shown by the arrow, the capacitor acts as a source of current. The charge from the capacitor flows through the resistor until there is no longer a difference in potential across the capacitor, as shown in Fig. II-1, *B*. An equation can be developed to describe the potential difference that occurs across the capacitor at each instant in time as its charge is dissipated. Current is the rate of flow of charge:

$$I = \frac{-dQ}{dt} \qquad (10)$$

The negative sign indicates decreasing current with time. The charge on the capacitor can be described by a rearrangement of the equation for capacitance (2):

$$Q = CV \qquad (2a)$$

Substituting for Q in the current equation (10):

$$I = -C \frac{dV}{dt}$$

C is a constant. This relationship gives the current flowing in the series RC circuit during its discharge. At a given instant in time, the current in the resistor can be determined from Ohm's law:

$$I = \frac{V}{R}$$

Because the currents in the two components are the same at a given instant in time,

$$\frac{V}{R} = -C \frac{dV}{dt}$$

The solution of this differential equation is:

$$V = V_o e^{-t/RC} \tag{11}$$

where V_o is the initial voltage to which the capacitor has previously been charged, t is the time elapsed since closing the switch, and R and C are the resistance and capacitance respectively. Note that when $t = RC$, $V = V_o e^{-1}$, or $V = V_o/e$. Thus, the potential difference across the capacitor decreases by a factor of $1/e$ for every unit of elapsed time equal to RC. RC is called the time constant of the circuit, symbolized by τ. It might be surprising that RC would have the dimension of time, but this can be seen from the proper breakdown of the component dimensions:

$$R = \frac{V}{I}; \text{ ohms} = \text{volts/amperes}$$

$$\text{Amperes} = \text{coulombs/seconds}$$

$$C = \frac{Q}{V}; \text{ farads} = \text{coulombs/volt}$$

$$\text{Thus RC} = \text{ohm-farads} = \text{volts-seconds/coulombs}$$

$$\times \frac{\text{coulombs}}{\text{volt}} = \text{seconds}$$

The time constant of a series RC circuit with a resistance of 1 megohm and a capacitance of 1 μF would be:

$$\text{RC} = (10^6 \text{ ohms})(10^{-6} \text{ F}) = 1 \text{ second}$$

It can be shown that the voltage across the capacitor of a series RC circuit is as follows during charging of the capacitor:

$$V = V_o (1 - e^{-t/RC}) \tag{12}$$

The same time constant, RC, is involved in this equation as in the equation for the discharge of the capacitor.

Cable properties

A nerve fiber can be considered analogous to an electric cable. The axoplasm acts as a resistor. The

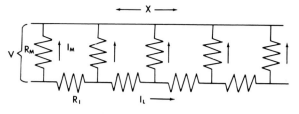

Fig. II-2. Resistance network representing the nerve as a cable. The extracellular fluid is shown as a conductor, the axoplasm as a series of resistors, R_I, and the membrane as a set of parallel resistors, R_M. Distance along the nerve is symbolized by X. Current flowing along the interior of the axon is I_L; current flowing out across the membrane is I_M. Membrane capacitance is ignored in this model because direct currents are being considered.

membrane of a nerve fiber behaves as a sequence of elements having resistance and capacitance. The extracellular fluid is a conductor because its volume is large. The resting potential does not need to be considered in a description of the effects of changes in membrane potential, provided that such changes do not approach threshold.

A series of equations called cable equations have been developed to describe the behavior of a nerve fiber in response to a change in potential at a point along the membrane. The electrical model used is shown in Fig. II-2 (ignoring membrane capacitance, because the relations hold for the steady state). From Ohm's law, the current flowing longitudinally in the axoplasm of such a fiber at a given time would be:

$$i_1 = \frac{-1}{r_i} \frac{dV}{dx} \tag{13}$$

where r_i is the resistance of the axoplasm for a unit length of nerve fiber, V is the drop in potential across the membrane, and x is the distance from the point where an induced change in potential has occurred. The negative sign indicates that the longitudinal current decreases with distance from this point. The reason for this is that some of the current leaks across the membrane. The membrane current, i_m, and the longitudinal current are related by:

$$i_m = \frac{-di_1}{dx} \tag{14}$$

That is, the membrane current at successive points along the nerve fiber is progressively decreased because the longitudinal current is reduced by the outward leakage of membrane current at the preceding points. The membrane current can also be described in terms of the membrane potential drop and the membrane resistance:

$$i_m = \frac{V}{r_m}, \text{ or } V = i_m r_m \tag{15}$$

By combining equations 13 and 14 into 15:

$$V = \frac{r_m d^2 V}{r_i dx^2} \qquad (16)$$

The solution of this equation is:

$$V = A e^{-x/\sqrt{r_m/r_i}} + B e^{+x/\sqrt{r_m/r_i}} \qquad (17)$$

V approaches zero when x approaches infinity, so B must be equal to zero. If $V = V_o$ at $x = 0$, then

$$V = V_o e^{-x/\sqrt{r_m/r_i}} \qquad (18)$$

The term $\sqrt{r_m/r_i}$ is called the length constant, because V falls exponentially to $1/e$ of its value for each such distance.

The length constant obviously increases with r_m and decreases with r_i. Large fibers tend to have large length constants, because r_i is reduced as the diameter of a fiber increases.

When responses to transients must be considered, the cable equation used must take into account the capacitative behavior of the membrane. For the equivalent circuit of nerve, the cable equation would be:

$$i_m = C_m \frac{\delta V}{\delta t} + \frac{V}{r_m} = \frac{1}{r_i + r_e} \frac{\delta^2 V}{\delta x^2} \qquad (19)$$

A further complication arises from the fact that nerve cells may have branching and tapering processes, such as the dendrites of multipolar neurons. Synaptic transmission occurs both on the soma and on dendrites of neurons, and the effects are conveyed across the rest of the cell by its cable properties. A model has been devised by Rall for describing the cable properties of cells with dendrites by dividing the neuron into a series of compartments and considering each compartment to be equivalent to a cylindrical cable. A number of useful features of this model have allowed predictions of the behavior of such neurons that either can or have been tested experimentally.

APPLICATIONS OF PHYSICAL CHEMISTRY IN NEUROPHYSIOLOGY
Electrolytes

Because the electrical currents that are associated with the activity of excitable tissue are carried by ions in solution, some of the properties of electrolytes are considered here briefly.

If electrodes are placed in an aqueous solution containing ions, the negative electrode is called the cathode and the positive one is called the anode. The cathode is a source of electrons, and positive ions or cations migrate toward it. Conversely, the positive electrode is called the anode; it removes electrons and attracts negatively charged ions or anions.

The transfer of current through the electrolyte is accomplished by the addition of electrons to ions at one electrode and the removal of electrons at the other, with the migration of ions through the solution carrying the current between the electrodes. This process is called electrolysis.

Faraday showed that for a given electrolyte the amount of material reacting during electrolysis depends on the amount of current, and that for a given current the amount of electrolyte (or ionized compound) that will move depends on the chemical equivalent weight of the material. Faraday's law is:

96,500 coulombs produces a change in 1 gram-equivalent

The faraday (F) thus equals 96,500 coulombs/gram-equivalent weight. This is an exact law. The faraday is equal to the magnitude of charge on an electron times the number of atoms per gram atomic weight. ($F = 1.60186 \times 10^{-19}$ coulombs times 6.0238×10^{23} atoms/equivalent weight; the latter value is Avogadro's number). Knowing the total amount over time of current used to move a charged compound by electrophoresis allows a computation, using the faraday, of the amount of the compound delivered.

Electrical energy is the product of the voltage and the amount of charge transferred:

$$\text{Electrical energy in joules} = \text{volts} \times \text{coulombs} \qquad (20)$$

A joule is equivalent to one watt-second because:

$$\text{Power (watts)} = \text{volts} \times \text{amperes} = \text{volts} \times \text{coulombs/second} \qquad (21)$$

The conductance of electrolytes is generally used to describe the ease with which currents pass through a solution. The specific conductance is characteristic for a given solution at a particular temperature. It is calculated by:

$$\text{Specific conductance} = 1/\text{specific resistance}$$
$$\text{(see 5)}$$
$$= \text{length/resistance} \times \text{cross-sectional area}$$

In general, salts, such as NaCl and KCl, are strong electrolytes. They produce solutions with high conductances.

The migration of ions of different kinds varies because of differences in size, degree of hydration, and charge. The ability of an ion to migrate in an electric field is measured in terms of its ionic mobility. Conventionally, the direction of current flow in a solution is said to be from positive to negative; this is the direction of net flow of cations. The mobility of an ion can be determined as follows:

$$\text{Mobility } (\mu) = x/tE \qquad (22)$$

where x is the distance the ions move, t is the time elapsed, and E is the electric field strength. The units of μ are cm^2/volt-second. The measurements are done using a moving-boundary apparatus.

The relative mobilities of Na^+, K^+, and Cl^- at 25° C are 52, 76.2, and 79. Thus, K^+ and Cl^- have almost the same mobility, whereas Na^+ has a somewhat smaller mobility. The reason that the smaller Na^+ ion has a lower mobility than K^+, for example, is that it attracts more water molecules because of the intensity of the electric field of its nucleus, and thus it must move a larger shell of water with it. The total electric current through a solution is carried by the various ions in accordance with their relative mobilities. The fraction of the total current carried by a specific ion is given by a quantity called the transference number.

In calculating the expected participation of a given type of ion in solution, one can use the concentration of the ion. This is particularly true if the solution is weak. However, as the concentration increases, the interaction between ions and with the solvent increases, thus decreasing the availability of ions to react. The activity of an ion type is then used for calculations. This is found from the following relationship:

$$\text{Activity} = (\text{concentration})\,(\text{activity coefficient}) \quad (23)$$

Activity coefficients can be found in standard tables for many kinds of ions and a variety of concentrations.

Electrode potentials

When electrodes are placed in a solution of ions, an excess of electrons may develop at one electrode and a deficit of electrons at the other. This results in a difference in potential between the electrodes. The voltaic cell is based on this type of reaction. A battery is constituted of a number of voltaic cells.

The production of a voltaic cell depends on the material selected for the electrodes and the type of solution. If both electrodes were made of the same material, they would each tend to react with the solution in the same fashion, and there would be no difference in potential between them because each would develop an excess or deficiency of electrons to the same degree. However, if one electrode is made from material with a greater tendency to ionize than the other, a difference in potential will develop. The rate of ionization, with loss of material into solution, or the rate of deposition of material at the other electrode, is related to the current that flows according to Faraday's law.

The voltage developed by a voltaic cell can be measured with reference to a standard cell, such as a Weston cadmium cell (which has a voltage of 1.0186 V).

The voltage of a cell is equal to the sum of the voltages at the two electrodes. The potential of an electrode can be determined by comparing it with a reference electrode, which has been given some arbitrary value. It is not possible to measure the potential of a single electrode. The usual reference electrode is a hydrogen electrode, and it has arbitrarily been given the value of 0 V, assuming that certain standard conditions hold. Because of the difficulties in using hydrogen electrodes, it is usually more practical to employ a calomel electrode for a reference, because the potential of the calomel electrode with reference to the hydrogen electrode is well known (−0.2802 V at 25° if 1M KCl is used in making the half cell). Another reference electrode is the silver–silver chloride electrode, commonly used in neurophysiological experiments.

The reactions that occur in voltaic cells are oxidation (release of electrons) at the anode and reduction (uptake of electrons) at the cathode. Equations for these reactions can be predicted from tables of oxidation and reduction potentials, as can the electrode that will be the anode and the one that will be the cathode.

Concentration cell

If two electrodes made from the same material are placed into two identical solutions, no potential difference will develop. However, if the two solutions have different concentrations, a potential difference will develop. The reason for this is that the electrode reactions will differ in rate in the two solutions. The amount of the potential difference will depend on the ratio of the activities (a) of the ions in the two solutions:

$$E = -(RT/nF)\ln(a_1/a_2) \quad (24)$$

If the solutions are dilute, the activities are approximately equal to the concentrations, so:

$$E = -(RT/nF)\ln(c_1/c_2) \quad (25)$$

In these equations, E is the difference in potential between the two electrodes in volts, R is the gas constant (8.3144 joules/degree-mole), T is the absolute temperature, n is the valence, and F is Faraday's constant. This equation is frequently used in neurophysiology, where it is generally referred to as the Nernst equation.

Nernst equation

The Nernst equation can be derived from the consideration that an electrochemical equilibrium is established across a membrane separating solutions of different concentrations. The membrane is considered to be permeable to just one type of ion. The movement of the ion across the membrane in one direction is against an electrical gradient; in the other direction it is against a concentration gradient. The work required to move 1 mole of the ion against the electrical gradient is:

$$\text{Work (joules)} = \text{volts} \times \text{coulombs/mole} = EF \quad (26)$$

The work required for movement of ions against a concentration gradient can be compared with that required to compress gas molecules, because the concentration of ions is similar to the pressure of a gas. Suppose a gram-equivalent of an ideal gas is contained in a cylinder equipped with a piston. The work required to move the piston is given by:

$$\text{Work} = \text{force} \times \text{distance} \quad (27)$$

For a small change in the volume of the gas, the force equals the gas pressure times the cross-sectional area of the cylinder. The increment in work for a small change would be:

$$\Delta W = pA\Delta l = p\Delta v \quad (28)$$

where ΔW is the change in work, p is the pressure, A is the cross-sectional area, Δl is the change in length of the gas column, and Δv is the change in volume of gas. If the pressure is changed slowly, the total work involved in changing the volume from v_1 to v_2 is:

$$W = \int_{v_2}^{v_1} p\,dv \quad (29)$$

However, the ideal gas law shows that:

$$pv = RT \quad (30)$$

Thus,

$$p = RT/v$$

and, substituting,

$$W = RT \int_{v_2}^{v_1} dv/v = RT\,[(ln(v_1) - ln(v_2))] \quad (31)$$
$$= RT\,ln\,v_1/v_2 \quad (32)$$

Similar considerations applied to the work required to move ions against a concentration gradient show this to be:

$$W = RT\,ln\,c_1/c_2 \quad (33)$$

If a membrane separates two solutions of different concentration and if only one type of ion can diffuse across the membrane, the ion will tend to move along the concentration gradient. However, as it does, a potential gradient will develop in the direction that will favor the movement of the ion back across the membrane against the concentration gradient. Eventually, an equilibrium will develop. The work required to move the ion against the electrical gradient will equal that required to move it against the concentration gradient:

$$EF = RT\,ln\,(c_1/c_2)$$

The difference in potential that will exist at the time the equilibrium has been reached is related to the concentration gradient (or activity gradient if the solutions are not dilute) by rearranging the equation:

$$E = RT/F\,ln\,(c_1/c_2) \quad (\text{see 25})$$

The potential calculated by the Nernst equation is known as the equilibrium potential for the ion under consideration. This implies that the potential across a semipermeable membrane would have this value when the ionic concentration gradient is appropriate. The distribution of potassium and chloride ions across the nerve cell membrane is close to that predicted by the Nernst equation, suggesting that these ions are nearly as predicted if the system were passive and in equilibrium. However, the potassium concentration gradient is slightly different from that predicted by the Nernst equation, and the sodium concentration gradient is reversed. This suggests that neither potassium nor sodium are distributed entirely passively.

There is some leakage of small ions across the neuron membrane. This leakage is not great, and the activity of the sodium and potassium pump system prevents any substantial concentration changes in these ions. However, only a very small shift in the concentration of sodium ions within the cytoplasm will reverse the resting potential. The sodium ions are restrained from producing such a change while the neuron is at rest by the fact that the membrane has only a limited permeability to sodium ions. Hodgkin's group has calculated that the permeability of the resting membrane of the squid axon is much higher for potassium ions than for chloride or sodium ions. The ratio of permeabilities for these are $P_K:P_{Na}:P_{Cl} = 1.0:0.04:0.45$. During the initial part of the spike potential, these permeabilities change to $1.0:20.0:0.45$. As the spike potential reverts toward the resting potential level, the permeabilities are $1.8:0:0.45$. Evidently, the membrane potential depends on the permeability to the various small ions, and it is not possible to predict it on the basis of just one ion species.

Goldman-Hodgkin-Katz equation

A useful equation was developed by Hodgkin and Katz from the constant-field theory of Goldman, which relates membrane potential (E), permeability of the membrane to the various ions (P), and the concentration gradients (ion):

$$E = \frac{RT}{F}\,ln\,\frac{P_K\,(K)_o + P_{Na}\,(Na)_o + P_{Cl}\,(Cl)_i}{P_K\,(K)_i + P_{Na}\,(Na)_i + P_{Cl}\,(Cl)_o} \quad (34)$$

The Goldman constant-field equations are based on the assumptions that the ions within the membrane move along concentration gradients by diffusion and along the electric field gradient, similar to the movement of ions in free solution; the electric field across the membrane is constant throughout the membrane; the ionic concentrations at the edges of the membrane are directly proportional to those in solution in the media adjacent to the membrane; and the membrane is homogeneous. Although there is no good evidence that this equation is more than a convenient way of describing these relationships, it has been widely used.

Hodgkin-Huxley equations

Hodgkin and Huxley developed a series of equations to describe the behavior of excited axons in terms of changes in ionic conductances. They used an improved version of the voltage clamp technique, first introduced by Cole's group. The advantages of this approach over previous ones were several. The propagating action potential involves changes at a given point in the membrane potential, membrane conductance, and membrane resistance with time, and the local circuit current flow along the cable structure of the axon results in a progression of these changes from point to point. This behavior can be described by a partial differential equation (the cable equation):

$$i_m = C_m \frac{\delta V}{\delta t} + \frac{V}{r_m} = \frac{1}{r_i + r_e} \frac{\delta^2 V}{\delta x^2} \qquad (19)$$

where i_m is the membrane current, C_m the membrane capacity, V the membrane potential, t the time, r_m the membrane resistance, r_i the internal longitudinal resistance of the axoplasm, r_e the external longitudinal resistance, and x the distance along the axon. By using a feedback control amplifier, the membrane potential along a certain length of axon can be changed uniformly to a predetermined value other than the resting potential. End effects are minimized by guard devices at each end of the clamped region. The current is passed from an electrode placed along the entire clamped region. Current crossing the membrane is measured between two external electrodes. The uniform change in potential along a length of axon eliminates the term $\delta V^2/\delta x^2$ from the cable equation. A simpler differential equation holds:

$$i_m = C_m \frac{dV}{dt} + i_g \ (V,t) \qquad (35)$$

where i_g is the current crossing the membrane through its conductance channels. With the voltage clamp, the capacitative current

$$C_m \frac{dV}{dt}$$

is over rapidly (time constant of 10 μsec), and so only i_g (V,t) needs to be found experimentally.

Furthermore, it was found experimentally that i_g is voltage dependent, making the results of voltage clamping easier to interpret than those of current clamping, for example.

When the membrane is suddenly depolarized beyond threshold by the voltage clamp, an inward and then an outward current flow is observed. The inward current could be shown to be caused by sodium ions, because it reversed at the sodium equilibrium potential and it varied appropriately with changes in external sodium concentration. The later outward current was caused by potassium ions. The two currents could be analyzed separately by recording them in the presence and absence of sodium, and the ionic conductances caused by sodium and potassium could be determined from:

$$g_{Na} = I_{Na}/(V - E_{Na}) \text{ and} \qquad (36)$$
$$g_K = I_K/(V - E_K) \qquad (37)$$

where g is conductance, I is membrane current caused by a particular ion, V is the membrane potential maintained by the voltage clamp, and E is the equilibrium potential for a given ion. A third leakage conductance (other ions) was also found, but this was small. The sodium conductance was transient, even though the membrane potential was held at a constant value for a long time, whereas the potassium conductance increased gradually to a plateau level. The reversal of the sodium conductance was ascribed to a process called inactivation.

In order to provide a quantitative description of their conductance results, Hodgkin and Huxley expressed their results in terms of three parameters, m, h, and n. These varied between 0 and 1, and they had no dimensions. The idea was to describe the increase in sodium conductance in terms of m, the decrease during inactivation in terms of h, and the increase in potassium conductance in terms of n. These parameters could be visualized as charged groups in the membrane, although this is not a necessary connotation. Rate constants were introduced, and it was assumed that these were functions only of the membrane potential. For the simpler case of potassium, the following equation was developed:

$$\frac{dn}{dt} = \alpha_n \ (1 - n) - \beta_n n \qquad (38)$$

where α_n is the rate constant for conversion of the state of the membrane from β to α, and β_n is the rate constant for the reverse reaction. The change in membrane state might be caused by, for example, the movement of charged groups in the membrane structure. This would make it reasonable for α_n and β_n to be voltage dependent. If a step change in voltage is induced and α_n increases while β_n decreases, n will rise exponentially to some plateau level. However, this is not the case experimentally. Instead, the rise in potassium conductance follows a sigmoidal curve. Thus, g_k is proportional to some power of n higher than 2. Hodgkin and Huxley thought that a power of 4 would fit the data satisfactorily, but more recent evidence suggests that a power of 25 would be better. The sigmoidal shape of the potassium conductance curve accounts for the delayed change of potassium permeability in the action potential.

The sodium conductance at first behaves like the potassium conductance, but its increase is much faster. The equation for this is:

$$\frac{dm}{dt} = \alpha_m(1-m) - \beta_m m \qquad (39)$$

where α_m and β_m are larger than α_n and β_n. In this case, g_{Na} is proportional to m^3. However, the increase in g_{Na} is not maintained. Furthermore, the increase in g_{Na} is larger if the initial membrane potential is high than if the axon is depolarized. These facts can be taken into account by considering another process that is voltage dependent but works in the opposite direction to m. This process, called inactivation, is described in terms of h.

$$\frac{dh}{dt} = \alpha_h(1-h) - \beta_h h \qquad (40)$$

where α_h decreases and β_h increases with depolarization. The g_{Na} is proportional to h. When the membrane is at rest, the m groups would tend to be in the β state, whereas the h groups would be in the α state. A depolarization would change the m groups rapidly to the α state, allowing an influx of sodium ions, and the h groups would more slowly change to the β state, preventing the influx of sodium.

The total ionic current, i_g, can be computed from these equations. Once this is found, the action potential in the area affected by the voltage clamp can be computed. The propagated action potential is computed from the cable equation for a constant wave form having a constant conduction velocity, θ. This assumption means that the shape of the curves relating membrane potential to time at a fixed point along the axon and those relating the potential to distance at a fixed time are the same. Because of this, the cable equation can be changed to:

$$\frac{1}{r_i \theta^2} \frac{d^2V}{dt^2} = C_m \frac{dv}{dt} + i_g \qquad (41)$$

This could be solved by using the appropriate value of conduction velocity (determined empirically). The Hodgkin-Huxley equations can be used to test the effects of various experimental procedures using the squid axon. In general, they account for a number of such experimental variables. However, it should be remembered that these equations are not unique; they are empirical descriptions rather than theoretical formulations. However, they have proved to be very useful for predictive purposes, and in altered form they help describe the behavior of excitable membranes other than the squid axon.

CONCEPT OF QUANTAL SYNAPTIC TRANSMISSION
Quantal events in synaptic transmission

Synaptic transmitter appears to be released from nerve terminals in multimolecular packets, rather than molecule by molecule. These packets of transmitter are referred to as quanta. A single quantum of transmitter probably involves several thousand molecules. The synaptic vesicle is considered to be the storage site of transmitter in the chemical synapse, and each vesicle is thought to contain a quantum of transmitter.

In the absence of nerve stimulation, a quantum of transmitter may be released spontaneously from the synaptic terminal from time to time. The effects of a quantum of transmitter may be detected by recording the electrical activity of the postsynaptic element evoked by the transmitter. The best-studied synapse from the standpoint of quantal transmission is the neuromuscular junction. Spontaneously released quanta of transmitter at the neuromuscular junction produce small EPSPs called miniature end-plate potentials. The transmitter agent responsible for the miniature end-plate potentials is acetylcholine. A similar spontaneous release of quanta of transmitter also occurs at other synapses and with other transmitter substances. The quantal release of transmitter appears to be common to chemical synapses, as is the presence of synaptic vesicles.

Nerve stimulation also results in the quantal release of transmitter. The depolarization of the nerve terminal appears to be the initiating event in the release mechanism. As a result of the depolarization, the membrane permeability to calcium increases. An influx of calcium occurs because the electrochemical gradient for calcium is in the inward direction across the membrane. The calcium influx triggers the remaining steps involved in the release mechanism.

In the case of the neuromuscular junction, a nerve impulse normally causes the release of several hundred quanta of transmitter. The end-plate potential is thus the sum of several hundred miniature end-plate potentials. However, if the extracellular concentration of calcium is lowered, fewer quanta of transmitter will be released. Alternatively, raising the extracellular concentration of magnesium will have the same effect.

This suggests that magnesium competes with calcium for some reaction sites but that magnesium cannot trigger the release mechanism.

A statistical description of the events during synaptic transmission has been developed from observations of neuromuscular transmission at end-plates exposed to solutions with a lowered calcium concentration, a raised magnesium concentration, or both.

Poisson distribution

Analysis of the events during quantal synaptic transmission depends on the use of probability theory. The general idea is that there is a population of quanta, tacitly presumed to be associated with synaptic vesicles, within the presynaptic terminal. Each quantum is in either a storage state or in the process of being released. A probability value can be assigned that describes the likelihood that a given quantum will be in the process of release by a given nerve impulse. It is assumed that there is a large population of quanta available for release and that the probability of release for any given quantum is low. For this reason, the statistical distribution that is most applicable is the Poisson distribution. Another distribution that may be applicable is the binominal distribution.

The first relationship used in the analysis of quantal transmission is:

$$m = np \qquad (42)$$

where m is the average number of quanta released by a nerve impulse, n is the number of quanta stored in the nerve terminal and available for release, and p is the average probability of release of the quanta. The Poisson distribution predicts the number of responses containing x quanta from the following relationship:

$$n_x = \frac{Ne^{-m}m^x}{x!} \qquad (43)$$

where n_x is the number of responses with x quanta, x is a small integral number, and N is the number of trials. If no quanta are released, the event is said to be a failure of neuromuscular transmission. In this case, x would be 0. The equation 43 would simplify to:

$$n_0 = Ne^{-m} \qquad (44)$$

This is a very important relationship, because m can be calculated simply from the number of failures of transmission in a known number of trials, using a rearrangement of this equation:

$$m = \ln \frac{N}{n_0} \qquad (44a)$$

A common test of the quantal nature of transmission is a comparison of the value of m, determined in this way, with an estimate of m, m_1, derived from the sizes of the end-plate and miniature end-plate potentials recorded from the same preparation. If the size of a quantum is reflected by the size of a miniature end-plate potential, then the number of quanta that make up the end-plate potential should be approximated by dividing the average amplitude of the end-plate potential, v, by that of the average miniature end-plate potential, v_1:

$$m_1 = \overline{v} / \overline{v_1} \qquad (45)$$

If the end-plate potential is recorded in a preparation not treated with a low calcium-containing or a high magnesium-containing solution, the size of m becomes large. There may be no failures of transmission, so m cannot be calculated from the frequency of failures. Another difficulty is that the estimate of m, m_1, may become inaccurate, because the summation of large numbers of quanta becomes nonlinear as the membrane potential deviates from the resting level toward the equilibrium potential for the synaptic potential. Alternative ways of computing the value of m have been devised, based on the variance of the amplitude of the end-plate potential. Furthermore, it is possible to allow mathematically for the nonlinear summation effect.

The quantal analysis of synaptic transmission has now been applied to a variety of synapses in addition to the neuromuscular junction. It appears to be a generally valid approach to the description of events in chemical synaptic transmission and is a useful technique for determining the mechanism by which various factors, such as drugs, alter transmission.

BIBLIOGRAPHY

Barr, L.: Membrane potential profiles and Goldman equation, J. Theor. Biol. **9**:351-357, 1965.

Cole, K. S.: Membranes, ions and impulses, Berkeley, 1968, University of California Press.

Cole, K. S., Antosiewicz, H. A., and Rabinowitz, P.: Automatic computation of nerve excitation, J. Soc. Indust. Appl. Math. **3**:135-172, 1955.

Cooley, J. W., and Dodge, F. A., Jr.: Digital computer solutions for excitation and propagation of the nerve impulse, Biophys. J. **6**:583-600, 1966.

Cooley, J., Dodge, F., and Cohen, H.: Digital computer solutions for excitable membrane models, J. Cell Physiol. **66**:99-111, 1965.

Daniels, F., and Alberty, R. A.: Physical chemistry, New York, 1955, John Wiley & Sons, Inc.

Fitzhugh, R.: Impulses and physiological states in theoretical models of nerve membrane, Biophys. J. **1**:445-446, 1961.

Fitzhugh, R.: A kinetic model of the conductance changes in nerve membrane, J. Cell. Physiol. **66**:111-119, 1965.

Frankenhaeuser, B.: Computed action potential in nerve from Xenopus Laevis, J. Physiol. (Lond.) **180**:780-788, 1965.

Goldman, D. E.: Potential, impedance and rectification in membranes, J. Gen. Physiol. **27**:37-60, 1943.

Grundfest, H.: Bioelectric potentials, Ann. Rev. Physiol. **2**:213-242, 1940.

Hodgkin, A. L., and Huxley, A. F.: A quantitative description of membrane current and its application to conduction and excitation in nerve, J. Physiol. (Lond.) **117**:500-544, 1952.

Hodgkin, A. L., and Katz, B.: The effect of sodium ions on the electrical activity of the giant axon of the squid, J. Physiol. (Lond.) **108**:37-77, 1949.

Hoyt, R. C.: The squid giant axon; mathematical models, Biophys. J. **3**:399-431, 1963.

Hoyt, R. C.: Non-linear membrane currents with ohmic channels, J. Cell. Physiol. **66**:119-127, 1965.

Katz, B.: Nerve, muscle, and synapse, New York, 1966, McGraw-Hill Book Co.

Lorente de Nó., R.: A study of nerve physiology, New York, 1947, Rockefeller Institute.

Martin, A. R.: Quantal nature of synaptic transmission, Physiol. Rev. **46**:51-66, 1966.

Noble, D.: Applications of Hodgkin-Huxley equation to excitable tissues, Physiol. Rev. **46**:1-51, 1966.

Rall, W.: Distinguishing theoretical synaptic potentials computed for different soma-dendritic distributions of synaptic input, J. Neurophysiol. **30**:1138-1168, 1967.

Atlas of the human brain and spinal cord

The atlas is divided into five sections to illustrate different aspects of the anatomy of the brain and spinal cord. Section A shows gross coronal sections, which are frequently used in the gross neuropathological examination of the brain. In addition, several gross horizontal sections are illustrated. Horizontal views of the brain have become increasingly important since the advent of computer tomography in neurological diagnosis (see Chapter 5). The microphotographs of the thalamus and upper brainstem in sections B and C were cut in stereotaxic coordinates with respect to the AC-PC line. These sections were chosen to illustrate the entry of ascending projection systems into the posterior thalamus and to illustrate the areas in which stereotaxic surgical procedures are carried out for the relief of pain and movement disorders. Section D consists of sections of the brainstem cut in the transverse plane, and section E consists of transverse sections of the spinal cord.

The problem of using consistent neuroanatomical terms, which are also easily usable in verbal communication, remains difficult. Structures have been identified with anglicized names and with names commonly used in clinical practice.

A. HUMAN BRAIN, GROSS CORONAL AND HORIZONTAL SECTIONS

The approximate position of the intercommissural line is indicated by the coordinates along the borders of the plates. Fig. III-1 shows a brain from its right lateral aspect and the locations of a series of coronal sections either anterior to (A), through (O), or posterior to (P) the midpoint of the anterior commissure–posterior commissure line. The coronal sections in Figs. III-2 to III-9 are from another brain, but at approximately the same levels. The brain was stained to enhance the contrast between gray and white matter. The horizontal sections in Figs. III-10 to III-13 are from still another brain, but the tissue was unstained. The coronal and horizontal sections illustrated are life size.

B. POSTERIOR THALAMUS AND UPPER BRAINSTEM OF THE HUMAN BRAIN, CORONAL SECTIONS
Brain of a 66-year-old woman

The cause of death was carcinoma of the stomach. The brain was removed and fixed by perfusion with 10% formalin through the carotid arteries and by subsequent immersion. The brain weight was 1,220 g. The intercommissural distance was 25.5 mm. Markers were placed in the brain in three axes with reference to the intercommissural line. The brainstem and thalamus were sectioned in the coronal plane, perpendicular to the intercommissural line. Frozen-section technique was used, and sections were cut at 30 μm, mounted, and stained with Weil's iron-hematoxylin stain. The shrinkage was less than 5%. Microphotographs of sections are enlarged three times life size.

Fig. III-14 illustrates the brainstem before section-ing. The positions of the sections shown in Figs. III-15 to III-21 are indicated on the lateral view; these sections lie from –2 to –21 mm caudal to the midpoint of the intercommissural line. The position of the inter-commissural line is indicated by the zero coordinates along the borders of the plates.

C. THALAMUS AND UPPER BRAINSTEM OF THE HUMAN BRAIN, SAGITTAL SECTIONS
Brain of a 63-year-old woman

The cause of death was carcinoma of the endome-trium. The weight of the brain was 1,230 g. The inter-commissural distance was 26.5 mm. Markers were placed horizontally through the posterior commissure and foramina of Monro, and the trajectories of these markers can be seen in each section. Fixation, section-ing in the sagittal plane, and staining were done as described in the previous section. Microphotographs of sections are enlarged three times life size.

Fig. III-22 illustrates the midline of the thalamus and upper brainstem before sectioning. The sections shown in Figs. III-23 to III-29 lie from 5.8 to 18.4 mm lateral to the midline of the brain.

There is significant variability in the dimensions of subcortical structures in the human brain. The grid border illustrates only the general dimensions of the structures shown. Atlases of variability and physio-logical localization of targets are required for accurate stereotaxic localization in the human brain.

D. MIDBRAIN, PONS, MEDULLA, AND SPINOMEDULLARY JUNCTION OF THE HUMAN BRAIN, TRANSVERSE SECTIONS
Brain of a 69-year-old woman

The cause of death was acute tubular necrosis. The brain was removed and fixed by immersion in 10% formalin. The weight of the brain after fixation was 1,250 g. The brainstem was sectioned transversely. Frozen-section technique was used, and sections were cut at 30 μm, mounted, and stained with Weil's iron-hematoxylin stain.

Figs. III-30 to III-32 illustrate, on another brain-stem, the approximate levels of the sections in Figs. III-33 to III-42. Sections are enlarged 5.6 times life size.

E. HUMAN SPINAL CORD
Spinal cord of a 69-year-old woman
(see previous section)

Frozen-section technique was used. The cord was sectioned transversely, and the sections were cut at a thickness of 30 μm and stained with Weil's iron-hematoxylin. Microphotographs are enlarged ten times life size in Fig. III-43.

Figs. III-1 to III-43 follow.

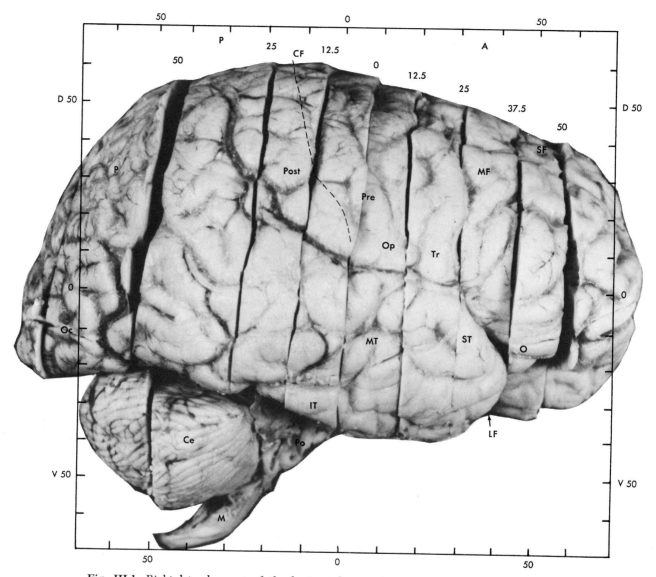

Fig. III-1. Right lateral aspect of the brain, indicating location of sections shown in Figs. III-2 through III-9, in millimeters anterior *(A)* and posterior *(P)* to section 0, which passes through the midpoint of the anterior commissure–posterior commissure line. The horizontal location of the intercommissural line is indicated by the zero marks at the occipital and frontal poles. The anterior commissure lies at A 13, the posterior commissure at P 13. Fissures, sulci: *CF,* central fissure; *LF,* lateral fissure. Lobes, gyri, brain areas: *Ce,* cerebellum; *IT,* inferior temporal gyrus; *M,* medulla; *MF,* middle frontal gyrus; *MT,* middle temporal gyrus; 0, orbital gyri; *Oc,* occipital lobe; *Op,* opercular portion of inferior frontal gyrus; *P,* parietal lobe; *Po,* pons; *Post,* postcentral gyrus; *Pre,* precentral gyrus; *SF,* superior frontal gyrus; *ST,* superior temporal gyrus; *Tr,* triangular portion of inferior frontal gyrus.

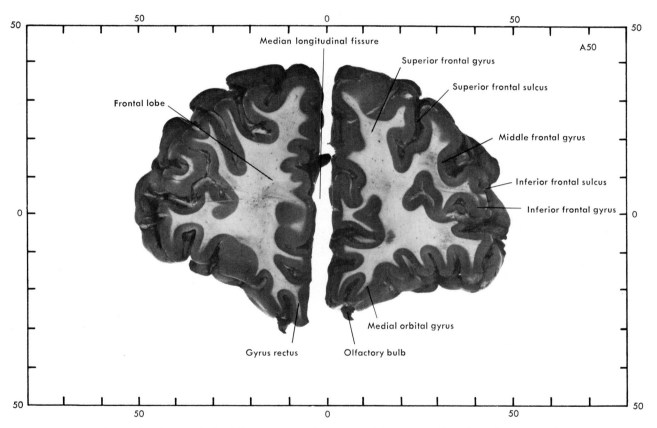

Fig. III-2. These and the following coronal sections of the human brain have been stained to demonstrate the gray matter of the cerebral and cerebellar cortices and of the nuclear areas of the brain. Section shown is through the frontal lobes, rostral to the genu of the corpus callosum.

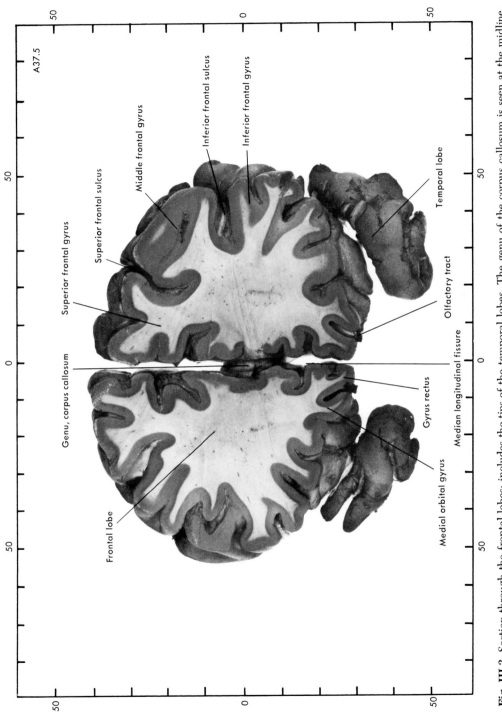

Fig. III-3. Section through the frontal lobes; includes the tips of the temporal lobes. The genu of the corpus callosum is seen at the midline.

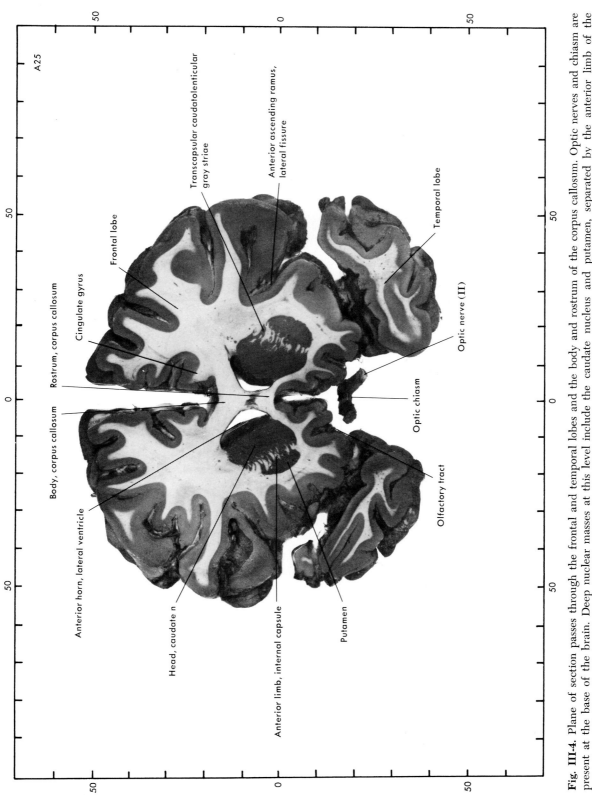

Fig. III-4. Plane of section passes through the frontal and temporal lobes and the body and rostrum of the corpus callosum. Optic nerves and chiasm are present at the base of the brain. Deep nuclear masses at this level include the caudate nucleus and putamen, separated by the anterior limb of the internal capsule.

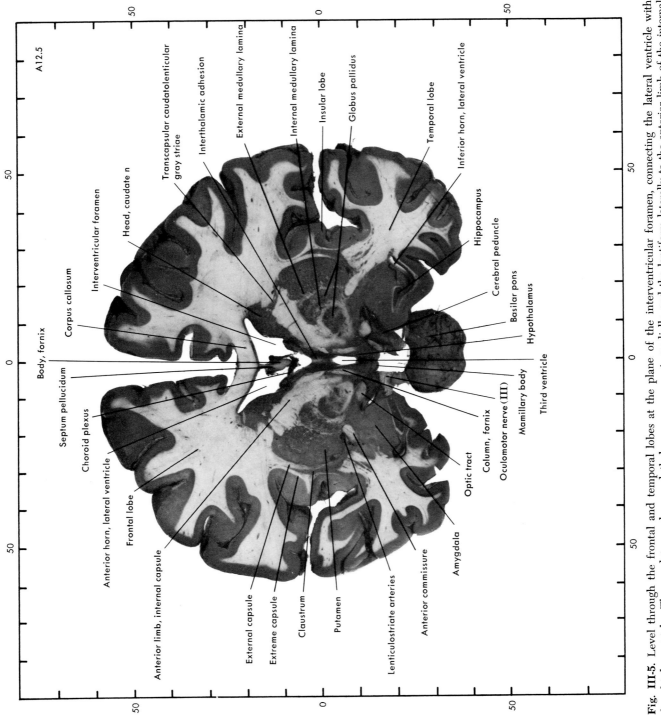

A12.5

Transcapsular caudatolenticular
gray striae

Interthalamic adhesion

External medullary lamina

Internal medullary lamina

Insular lobe

Globus pallidus

Temporal lobe

Inferior horn, lateral ventricle

Hippocampus

Cerebral peduncle

Basilar pons

Hypothalamus

Third ventricle

Mamillary body

Oculomotor nerve (III)

Column, fornix

Optic tract

Anterior commissure

Amygdala

Lenticulostriate arteries

Putamen

Claustrum

Extreme capsule

External capsule

Anterior limb, internal capsule

Frontal lobe

Anterior horn, lateral ventricle

Choroid plexus

Septum pellucidum

Body, fornix

Corpus callosum

Interventricular foramen

Head, caudate n

Fig. III-5. Level through the frontal and temporal lobes at the plane of the interventricular foramen, connecting the lateral ventricle with the third ventricle. The caudate nucleus and thalamus are present medially and the lentiform laterally to the anterior limb of the internal capsule. The amygdaloid nucleus is prominent.

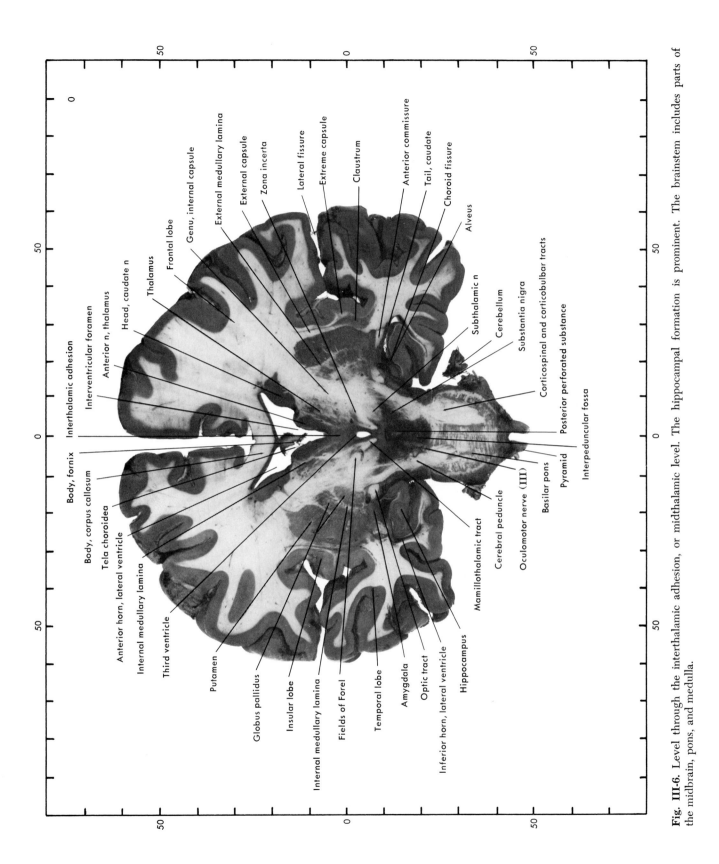

Fig. III-6. Level through the interthalamic adhesion, or midthalamic level. The hippocampal formation is prominent. The brainstem includes parts of the midbrain, pons, and medulla.

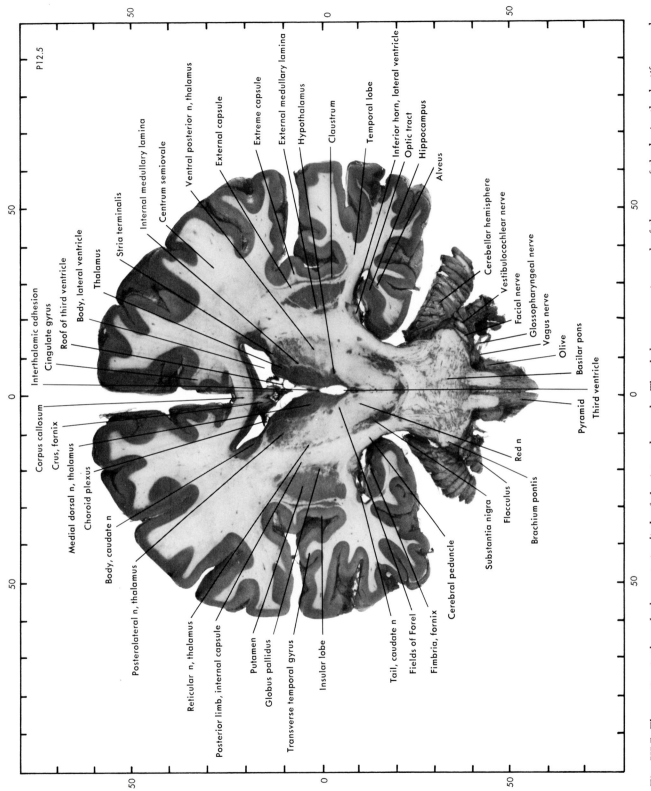

Fig. III-7. The section is through the posterior limb of the internal capsule. The thalamus occupies much of the core of the brain; the lentiform nucleus is near its caudal limit; the cerebellum is appearing.

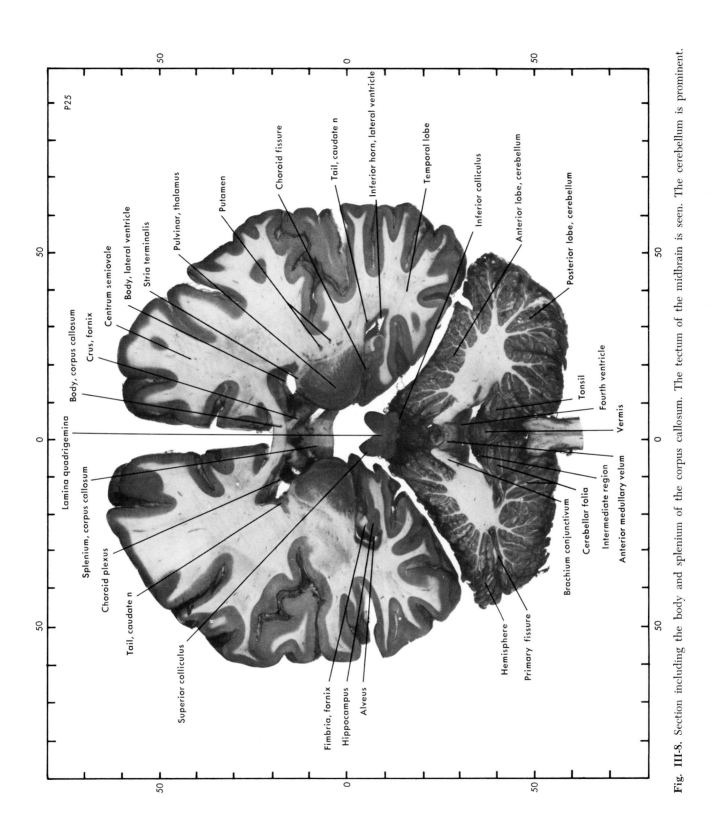

Fig. III-8. Section including the body and splenium of the corpus callosum. The tectum of the midbrain is seen. The cerebellum is prominent.

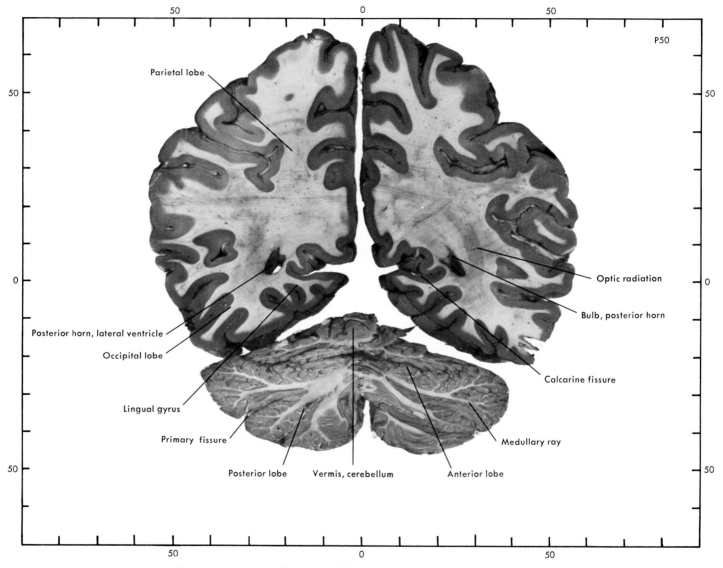

Fig. III-9. Parietal and occipital lobes are shown, as well as the cerebellum.

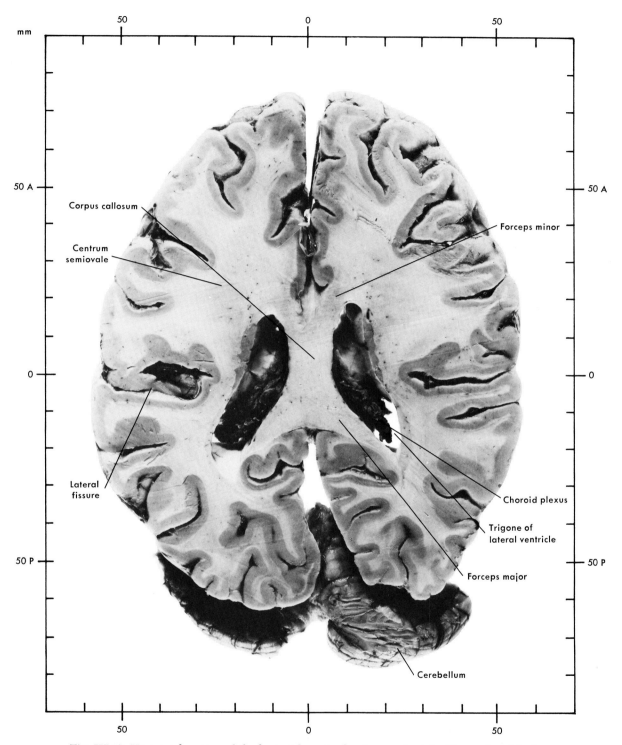

Fig. III-10. Horizontal section of the brain taken at a level approximately 17 mm dorsal to the anterior commissure–posterior commissure line.

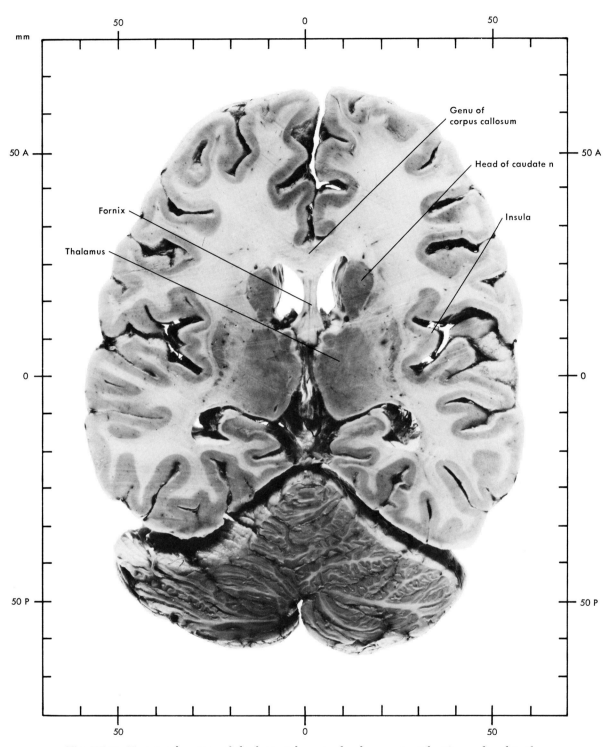

Fig. III-11. Horizontal section of the brain taken at a level approximately 12 mm dorsal to the anterior commissure–posterior commissure line.

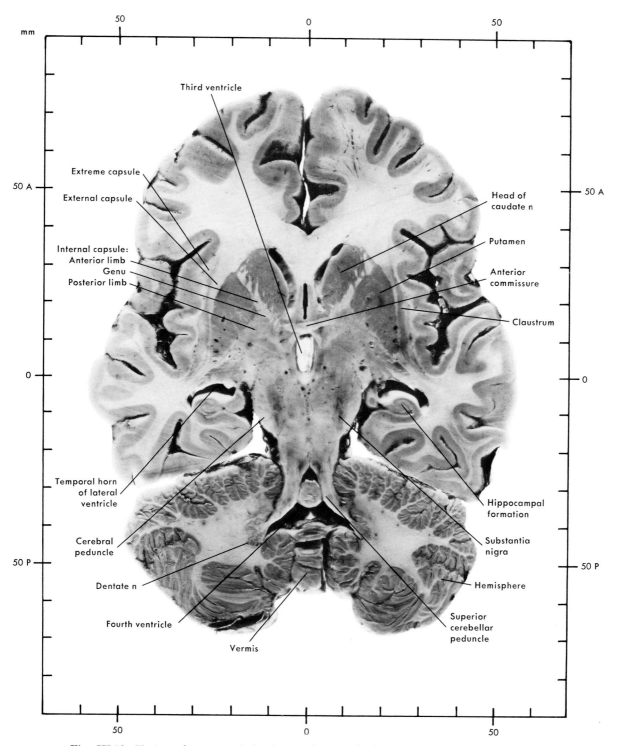

Fig. III-12. Horizontal section of the brain taken at the level of the anterior commissure.

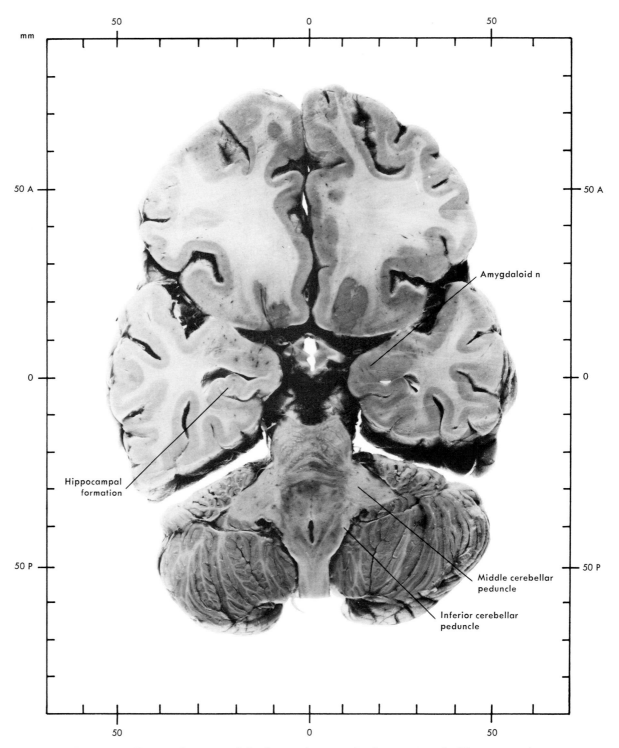

Fig. III-13. Horizontal section of the brain taken at a level approximately 15 mm ventral to the anterior commissure–posterior commissure line.

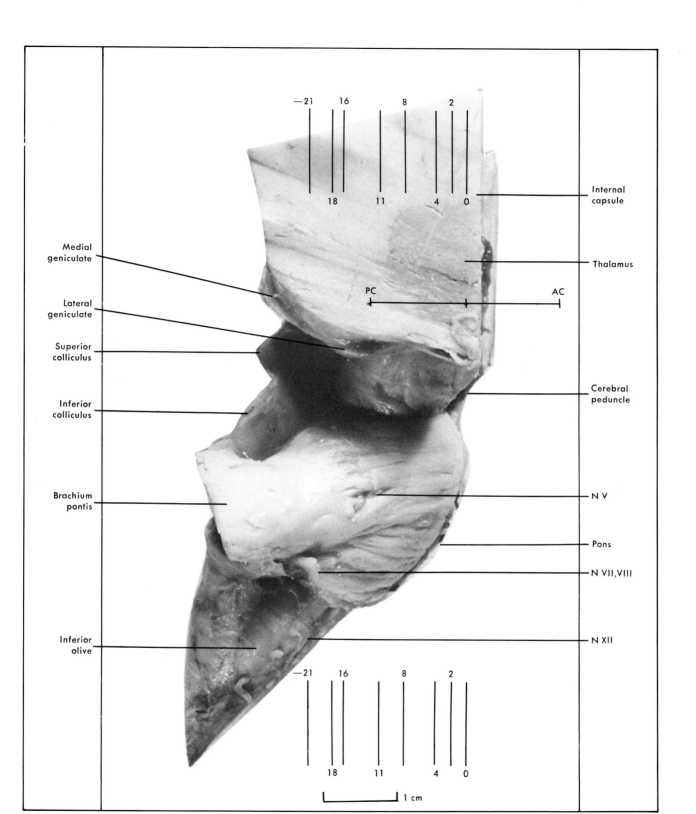

Fig. III-14. Right lateral aspect of the posterior thalamus and upper brainstem, indicating location of sections shown in Figs. III-11 through III-17, with respect to their anterior-posterior (AP) distances from the midpoint of the anterior commissure–posterior commissure *(AC-PC)* line. Abbreviations: *N*, nerve; *n*, nucleus; *Aq*, aqueduct; *V3*, third ventricle.

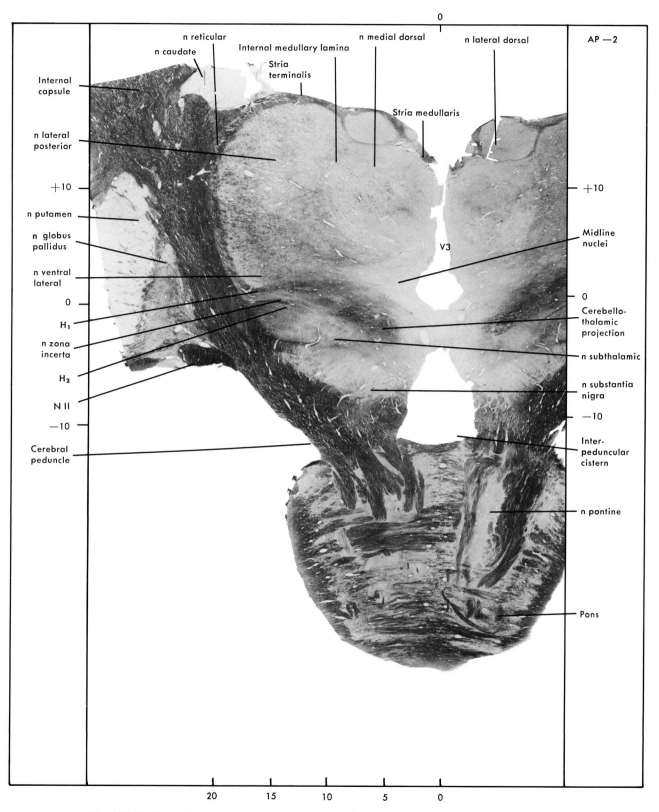

Fig. III-15. Frontal section 2 mm posterior to midpoint of AC-PC line; horizontal level of AC-PC line indicated by 0 markers along the lateral borders of Figs. III-15 through III-21.

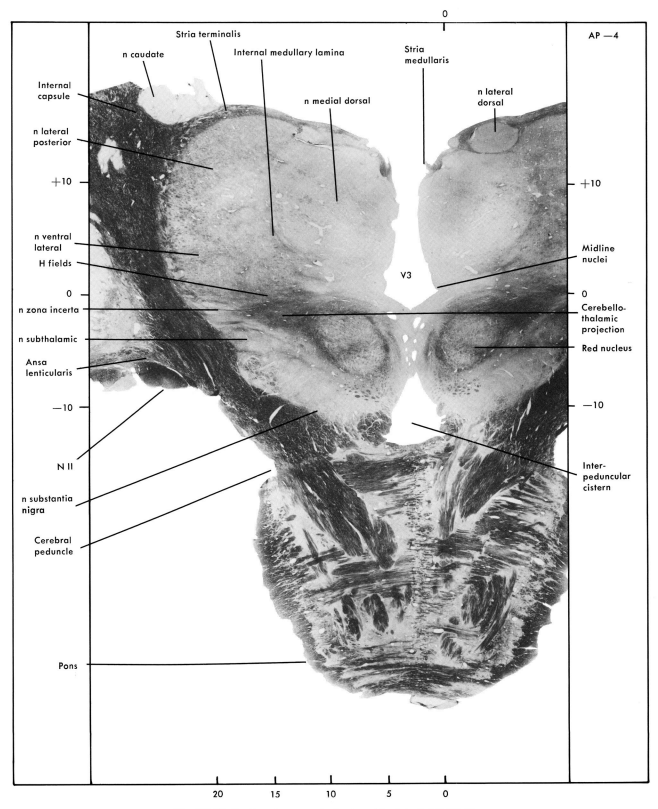

Fig. III-16. Section 4 mm posterior to midpoint of AC-PC line.

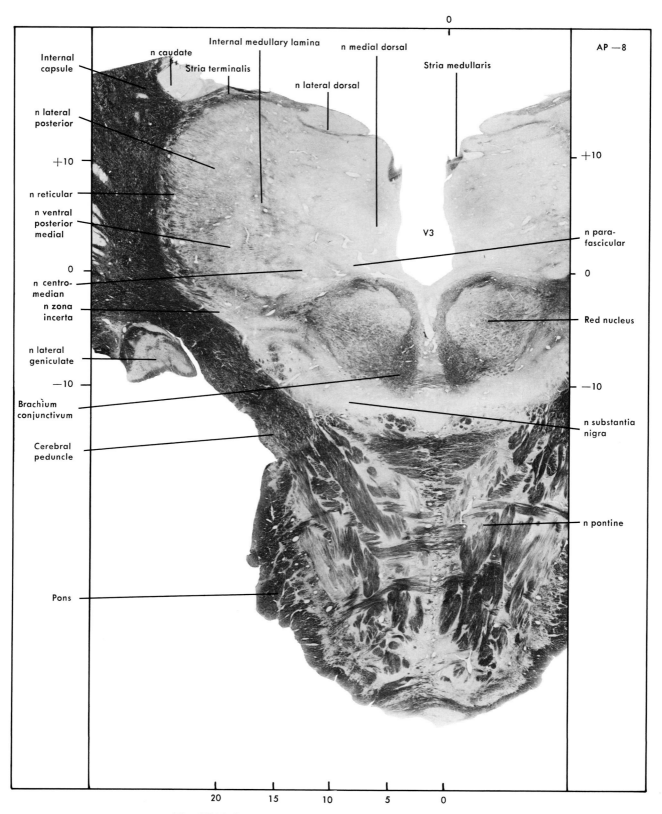

Fig. III-17. Section 8 mm posterior to midpoint of AC-PC line.

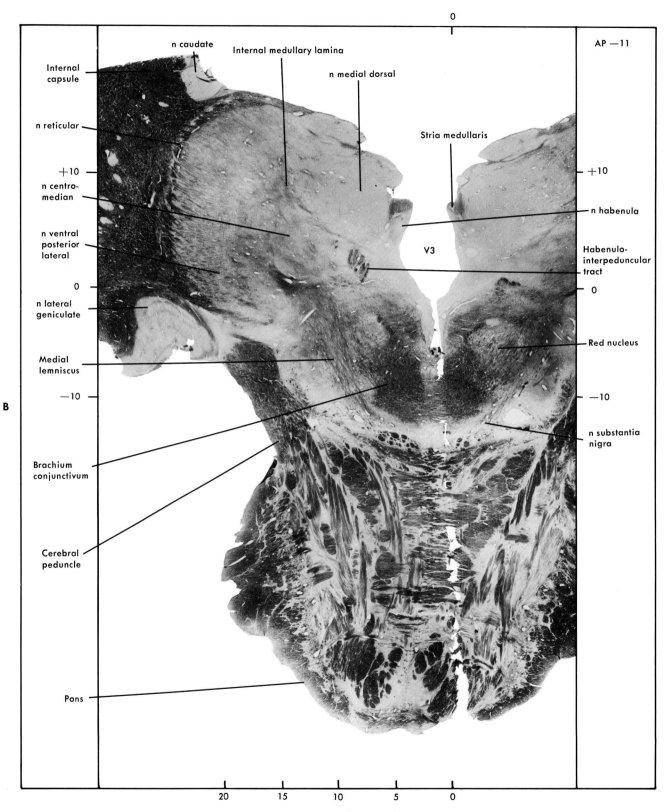

Fig. III-18. Section 11 mm posterior to midpoint of AC-PC line.

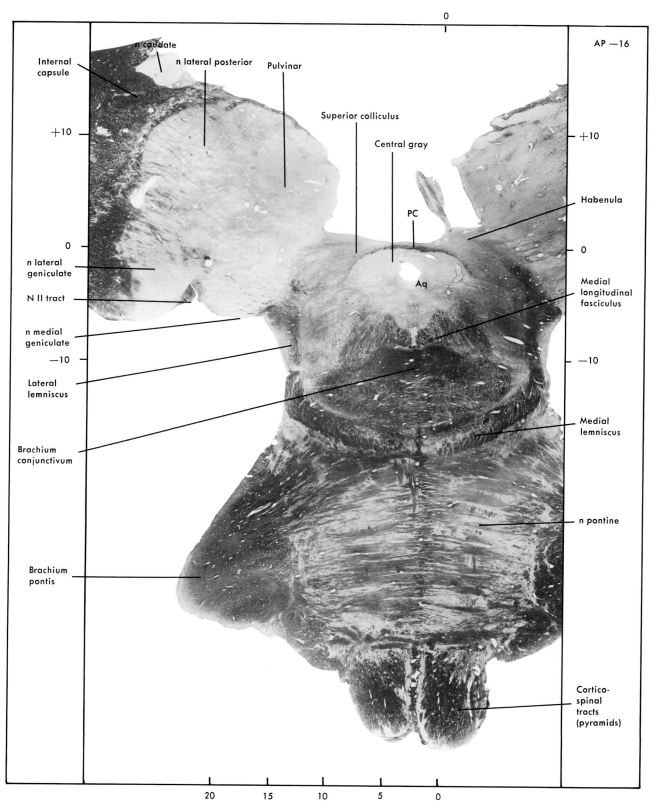

Fig. III-19. Section 16 mm posterior to midpoint of AC-PC line.

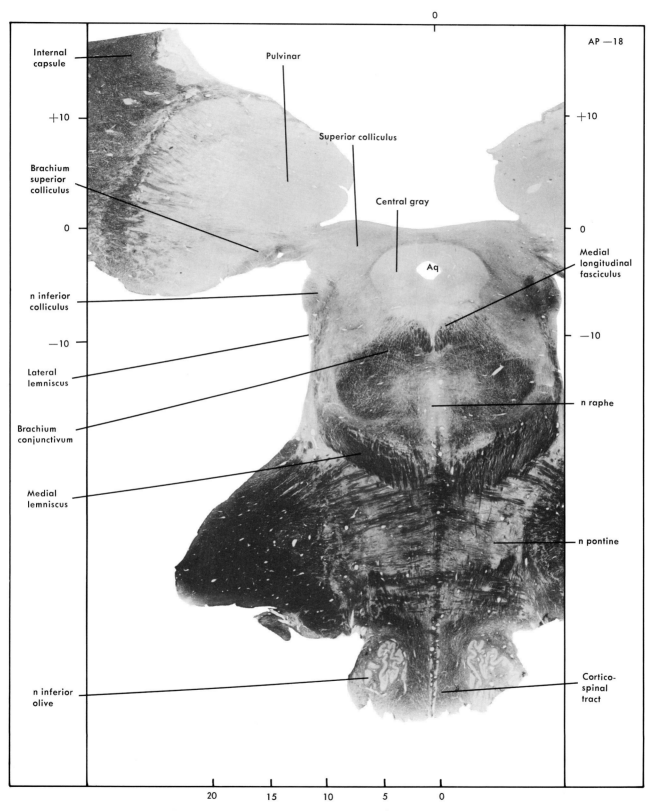

Fig. III-20. Section 18 mm posterior to midpoint of AC-PC line.

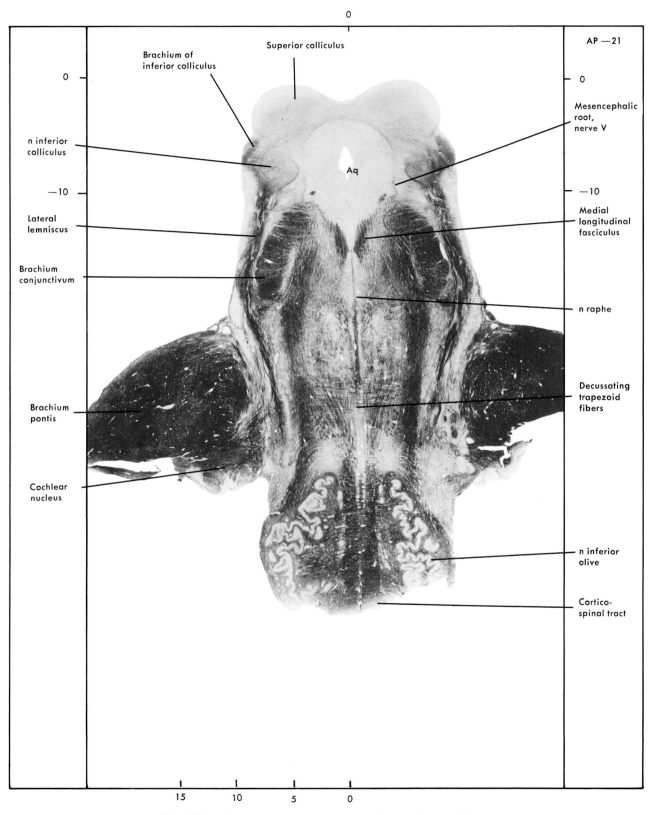

Fig. III-21. Section 21 mm posterior to midpoint of AC-PC line.

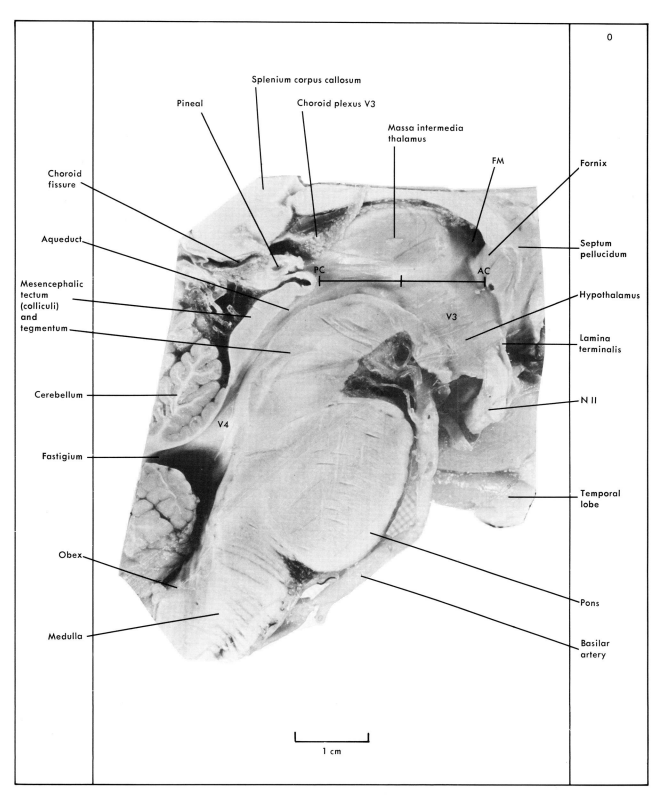

Fig. III-22. Right lateral view of a midsagittal section of the diencephalon and upper brainstem. The sagittal sections shown in Figs. III-23 through III-29 were cut from this block. Abbreviations: *N*, nerve; *n*, nucleus; *AC*, anterior commissure; *PC*, posterior commissure; *V3*, third ventricle; *V4*, fourth ventricle; *VL*, lateral ventricle; *FM*, foramen of Monro. The designation *FM* on the sagittal sections refers to the projection line made by the marker inserted horizontally through the brain at this level, which left a small marking hole in the sections.

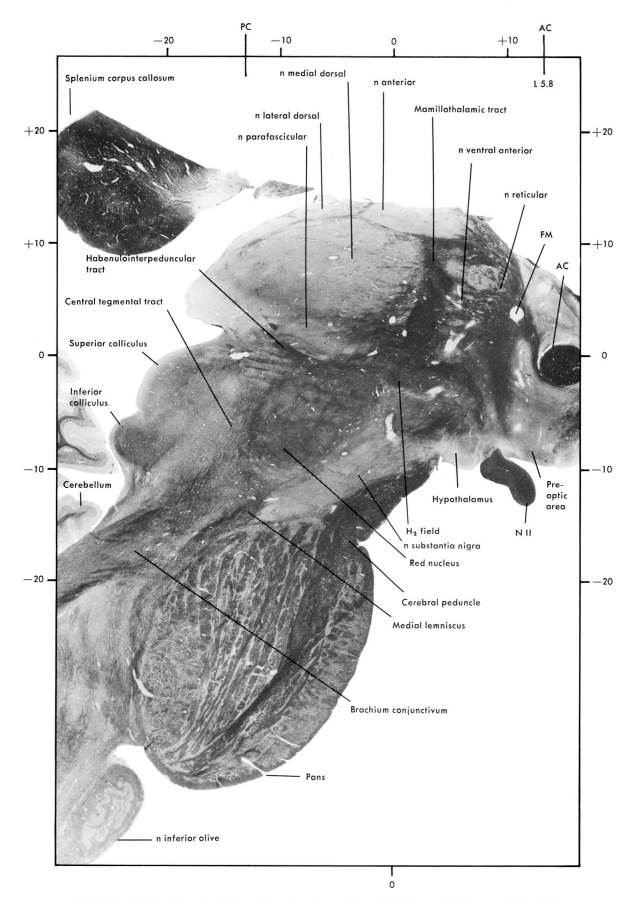

PC   AC
−20   −10   0   +10
L 5.8

Splenium corpus callosum

n medial dorsal

n anterior

n lateral dorsal

Mamillothalamic tract

n parafascicular

n ventral anterior

Habenulointerpeduncular tract

n reticular

FM

AC

Central tegmental tract

Superior colliculus

Inferior colliculus

Cerebellum

Hypothalamus

Pre-optic area

H₂ field

N II

n substantia nigra

Red nucleus

Cerebral peduncle

Medial lemniscus

Brachium conjunctivum

Pons

n inferior olive

0

Fig. III-23. Sagittal section 5.8 mm lateral to the midline of the brain. The horizontal level of the AC-PC line is indicated by the 0 markers along the lateral borders of Figs. III-23 through III-29. The location of the anterior and posterior commissures at the midline of the brain is indicated by the lines labelled *AC* and *PC* along the top border of the figures. The midpoint of the AC-PC line is also indicated along the top and bottom borders of the figures. The line of the projection of the foramen of Monro *(FM)* is also indicated.

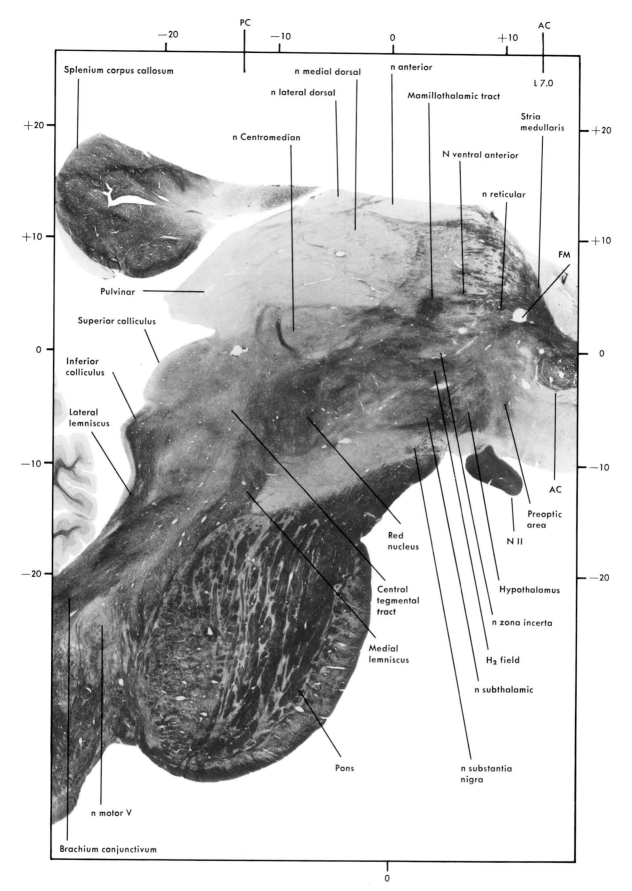

Fig. III-24. Sagittal section 7.0 mm lateral to the midline of the brain.

The following labels appear on the figure:

PC   −20   −10   0   +10   AC

L 7.0

Splenium corpus callosum

n medial dorsal

n lateral dorsal

n anterior

Mamillothalamic tract

n Centromedian

N ventral anterior

Stria medullaris

n reticular

FM

Pulvinar

Superior colliculus

Inferior colliculus

Lateral lemniscus

Red nucleus

Preoptic area

N II

Central tegmental tract

Hypothalamus

Medial lemniscus

n zona incerta

H₂ field

n subthalamic

Pons

n substantia nigra

n motor V

Brachium conjunctivum

AC

+20

+10

0

−10

−20

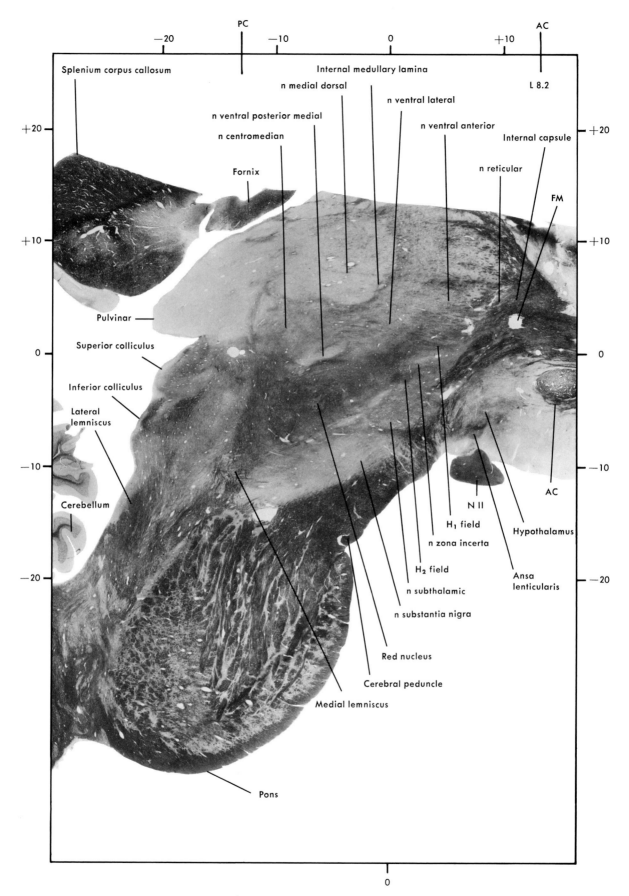

PC   AC

−20   −10   0   +10

L 8.2

Splenium corpus callosum

Internal medullary lamina

n medial dorsal

n ventral posterior medial

n ventral lateral

n centromedian

n ventral anterior

Fornix

Internal capsule

n reticular

FM

+20

+20

+10

+10

Pulvinar

0

0

Superior colliculus

Inferior colliculus

Lateral lemniscus

−10

−10

AC

Cerebellum

N II

H₁ field

Hypothalamus

n zona incerta

Ansa lenticularis

−20

−20

H₂ field

n subthalamic

n substantia nigra

Red nucleus

Cerebral peduncle

Medial lemniscus

Pons

0

Fig. III-25. Sagittal section 8.2 mm lateral to the midline of the brain.

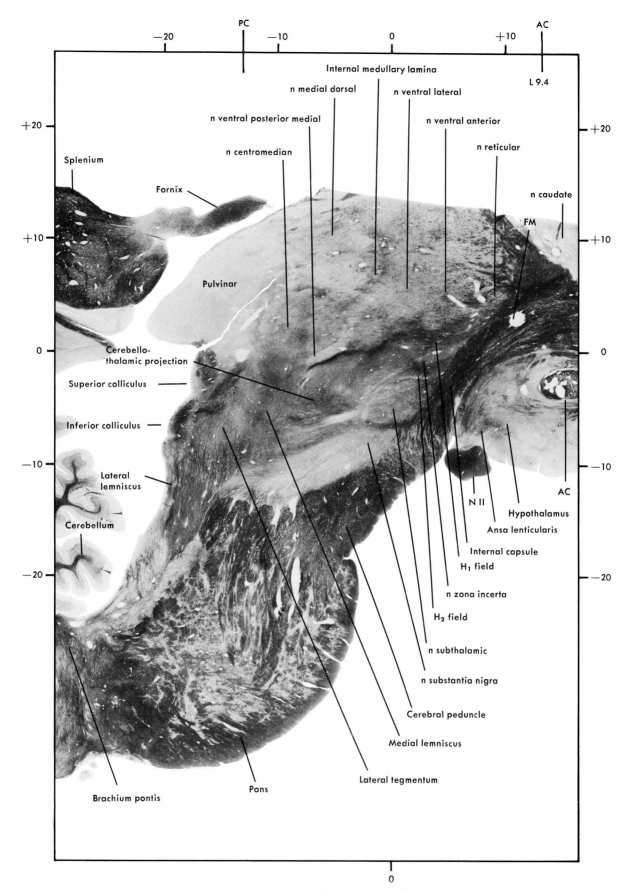

Fig. III-26. Sagittal section 9.4 mm lateral to the midline of the brain.

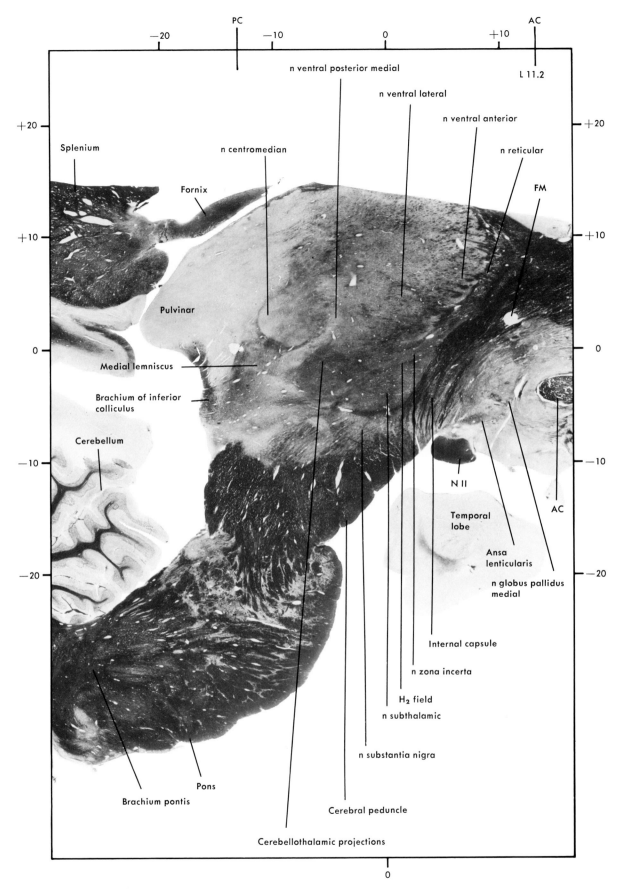

Fig. III-27. Sagittal section 11.2 mm lateral to the midline of the brain.

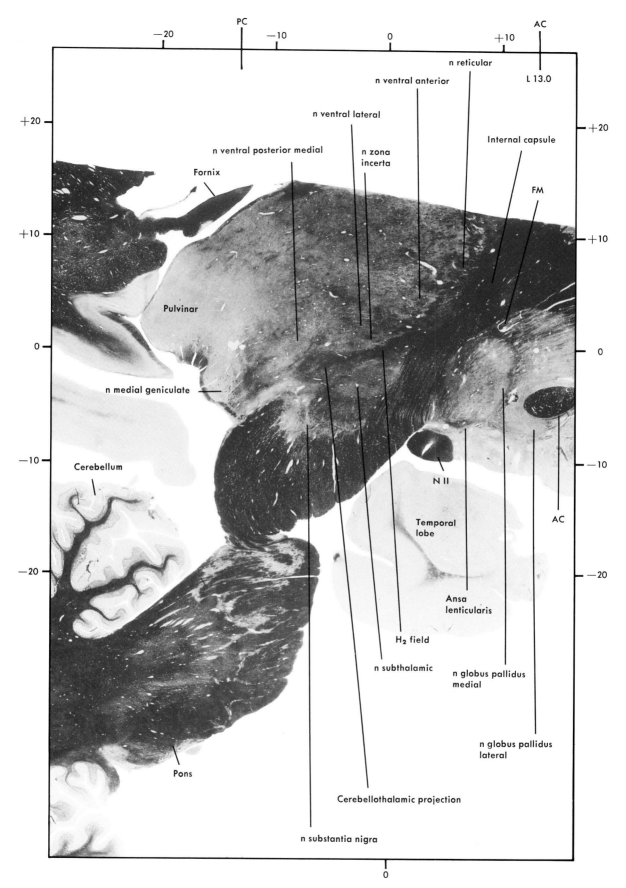

Fig. III-28. Sagittal section 13 mm lateral to the midline of the brain.

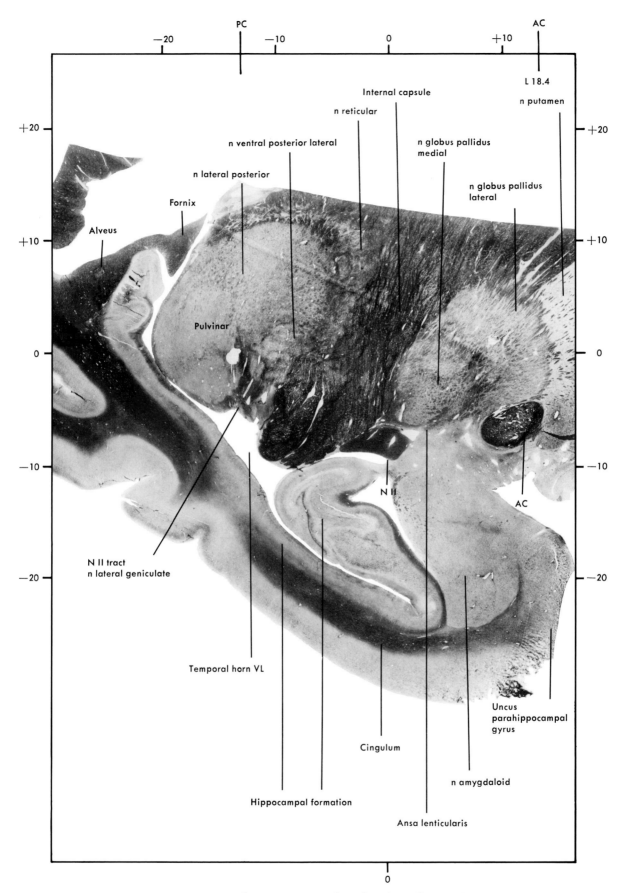

Fig. III-29. Sagittal section 18.4 mm lateral to the midline of the brain.

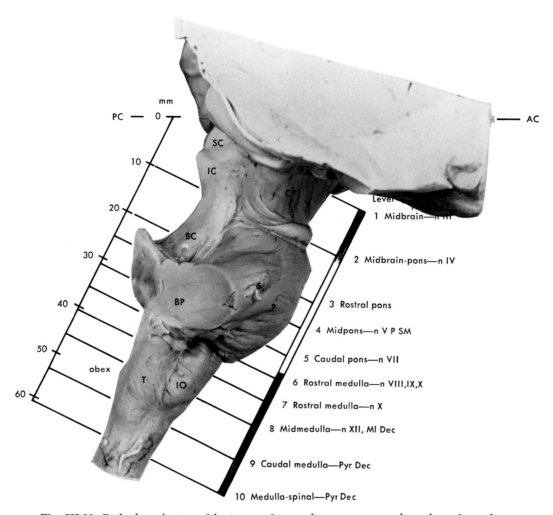

Fig. III-30. Right lateral view of brainstem. Linear dimensions are indicated on the scale on the left, and the locations of the transverse sections shown in Figs. III-33 to III-42 (levels 1 to 10) and the major structures they pass through are indicated on the right. Compare with text, Fig. 5-4. Enlarged 1.4 times life-size. Abbreviations: *AC,* anterior commissure line; *BC,* brachium conjunctivum; *BP,* brachium pontis; *CP,* cerebral peduncle; *IC,* inferior colliculus; *IO,* inferior olive; *Ml Dec,* medial lemniscus decussation; *nVM,* trigeminal nerve motor nucleus; *nVPS,* trigeminal nerve principal sensory nucleus; *nVII,* facial nerve motor nucleus; *nVIII,* statoacoustic (auditory and vestibular) nerve nuclei; *nIX,* glossopharyngeal nerve nuclei; *nX,* vagus nerve nuclei; *nXII,* hypoglossal nerve nucleus; *P,* pons; *PC,* posterior commissure line; *Pyr Dec,* pyramidal decussation; *SC,* superior colliculus; *T,* tuberculum cinereum; *5,* trigeminal nerve roots.

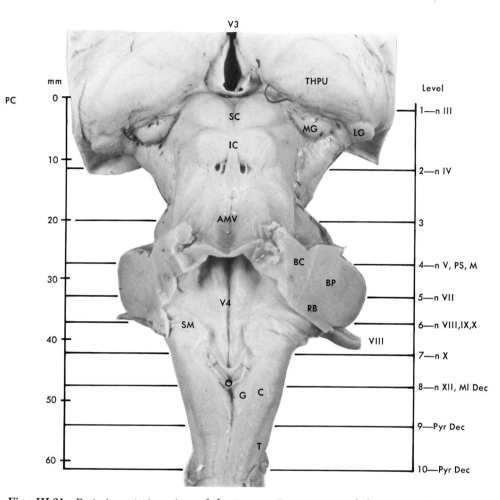

Fig. III-31. Posterior-anterior view of brainstem. Dimensions and locations of transverse sections as in Fig. III-30. Compare with text, Fig. 5-5. Enlarged 1.6 times life-size. Abbreviations: *AMV,* anterior medullary velum; *BC,* brachium conjunctivum; *BP,* brachium pontis; *C,* cuneate tubercle; *G,* gracile tubercle; *IC,* inferior colliculus; *LG,* lateral geniculate; *MG,* medial geniculate; *ML Dec,* medial lemniscus decussation; *nVM,* trigeminal nerve motor nucleus; *nVPS,* trigeminal nerve principal sensory nucleus; *nVII,* facial nerve motor nucleus; *nVIII,* statoacoustic (auditory and vestibular) nerve nuclei; *nIX,* glossopharyngeal nerve nuclei; *nX,* vagus nerve nuclei; *nXII,* hypoglossal nerve nucleus; *O,* obex; *PC,* posterior commissure line; *Pyr Dec,* pyramidal decussation; *RB,* restiform body; *SM,* stria medullaris; *T,* tuberculum cinereum; *THPU,* pulvinar of thalamus; *SC,* superior colliculus; *V3,* third ventricle; *V4,* floor of fourth ventricle; *VIII,* statoacoustic nerve roots.

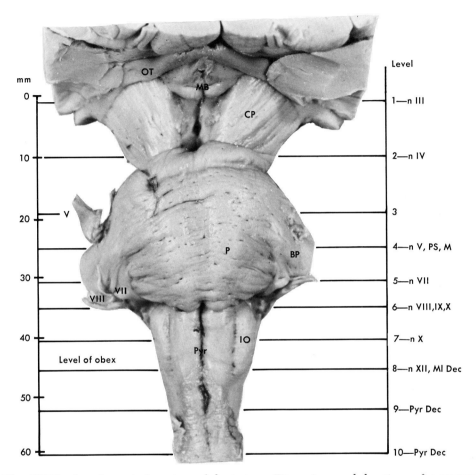

Fig. III-32. Anterior-posterior view of brainstem. Dimensions and locations of transverse sections as in Fig. III-30. Compare with text, Fig. 5-3. Enlarged 1.6 times life-size. Abbreviations: *BP*, brachium pontis; *CP*, cerebral peduncle; *IO*, inferior olive; *MB*, mamillary bodies; *MI Dec*, medial lemniscus decussation; *nVM*, trigeminal nerve motor nucleus; *nVPS*, trigeminal nerve principal sensory nucleus; *nVII*, facial nerve motor nucleus; *nVIII*, statoacoustic (vestibular and auditory) nerve nuclei; *nIX* glossopharyngeal nerve niuclei; *nX* vagus nerve nuclei; *nXII*, hypoglossal nerve nucleus; *OT*, optic tract; *P*, pons; *Pyr*, pyramids; *Pyr Dec*, level of the pyramidal decussation; *V*, trigeminal nerve roots; *VII*, facial nerve root; *VIII*, statoacoustic nerve roots.

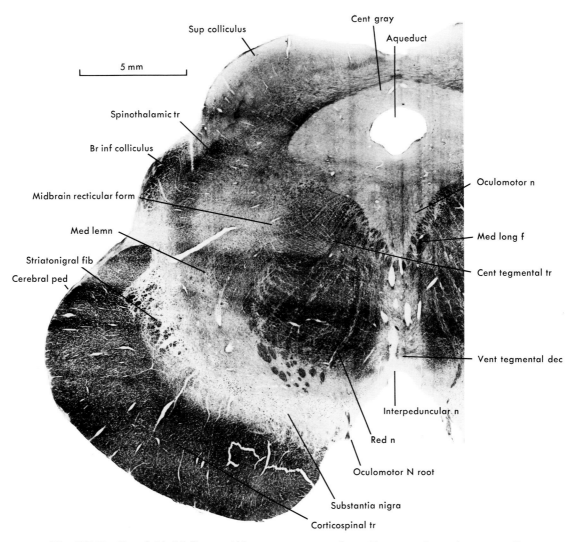

Fig. III-33. (Level 1) Midbrain. Abbreviations: *n*, nucleus; *N*, nerve; *form*, formation; *Br*, brachium; *dec*, decussation; *f*, fasciculus; *fib*, fibers; *lemn*, lemniscus; *ped*, peduncle; *tr*, tract; *Ant*, anterior; *Cent*, central; *Dors*, dorsal; *Inf*, inferior; *Lat*, lateral; *long*, longitudinal; *Med*, medial; *Sup*, superior; *Vent*, ventral.

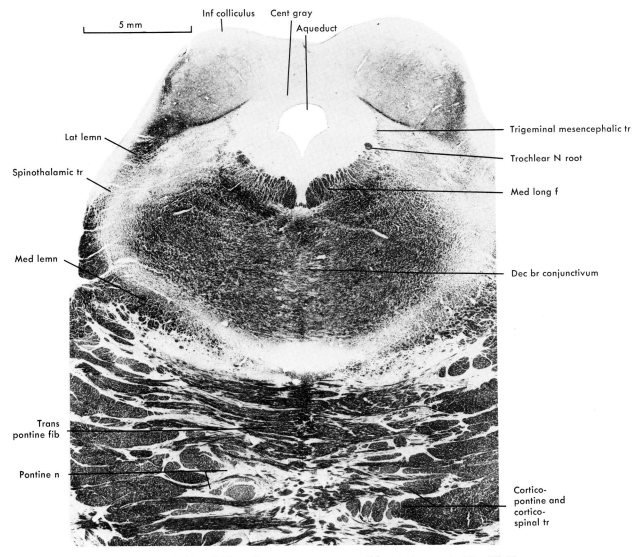

Fig. III-34. (Level 2) Midbrain-pons junction. Abbreviations as in Fig. III-33.

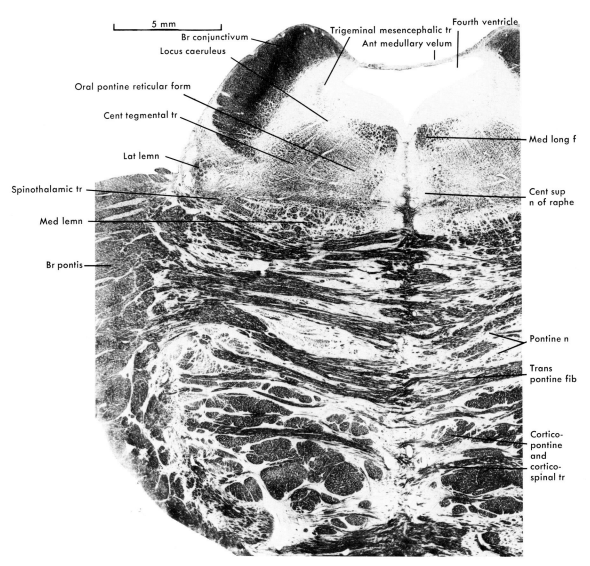

5 mm

Br conjunctivum

Locus caeruleus

Oral pontine reticular form

Cent tegmental tr

Lat lemn

Spinothalamic tr

Med lemn

Br pontis

Trigeminal mesencephalic tr

Ant medullary velum

Fourth ventricle

Med long f

Cent sup n of raphe

Pontine n

Trans pontine fib

Cortico-pontine and cortico-spinal tr

Fig. III-35. (Level 3) Rostral pons. Abbreviations as in Fig. III-33.

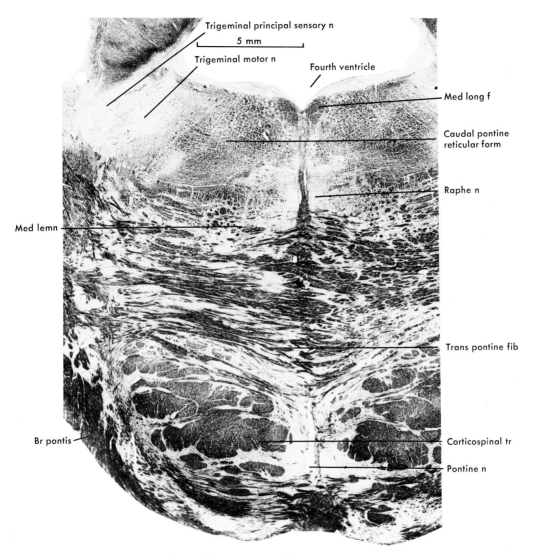

Fig. III-36. (Level 4) Midpons. Abbreviations as in Fig. III-33.

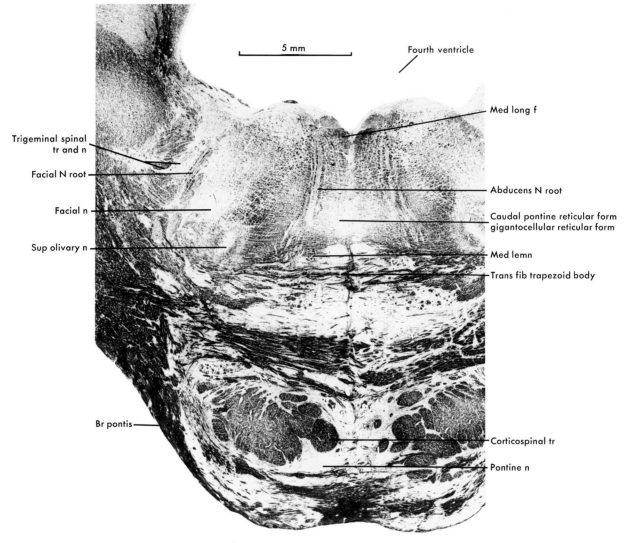

Fig. III-37. (Level 5) Caudal pons. Abbreviations as in Fig. III-33.

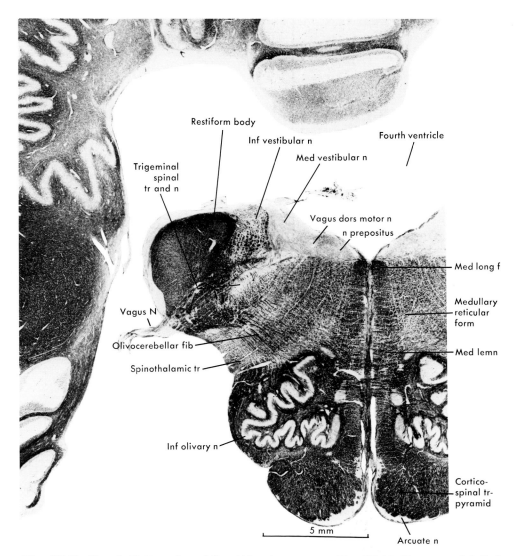

Fig. III-38. (Level 6) Rostral medulla. Abbreviations as in Fig. III-33. Nerve root labelled vagus is part of most rostral rootlets of glossopharyngeal-vagal complex.

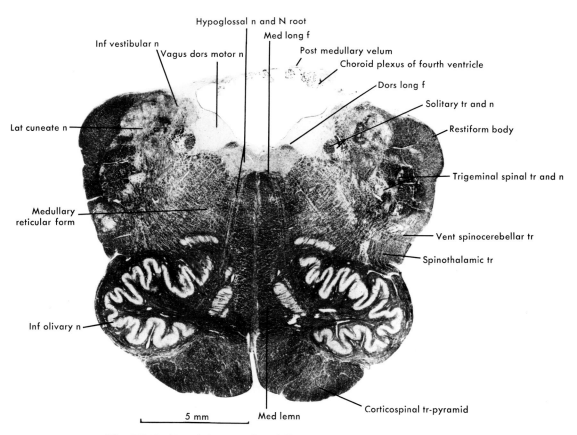

Fig. III-39. (Level 7) Rostral medulla. Abbreviations as in Fig. III-33.

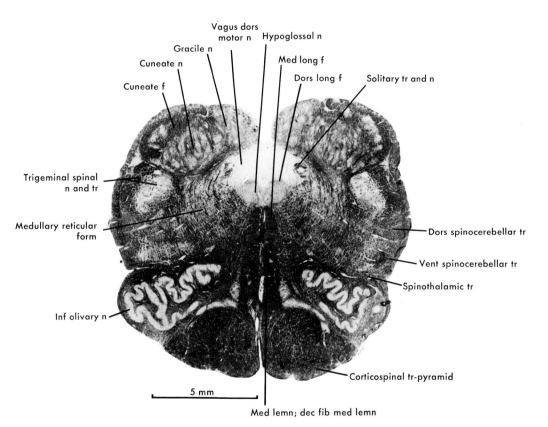

Fig. III-40. (Level 8) Midmedulla. Abbreviations as in Fig. III-33.

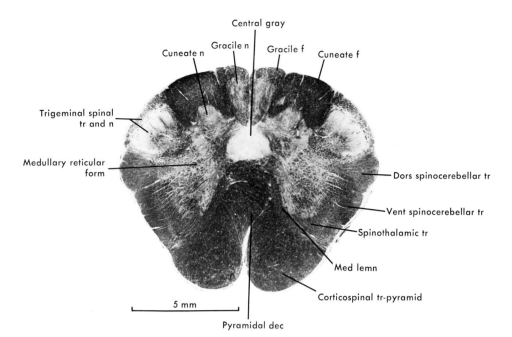

Fig. III-41. (Level 9) Caudal medulla. Abbreviations as in Fig. III-33.

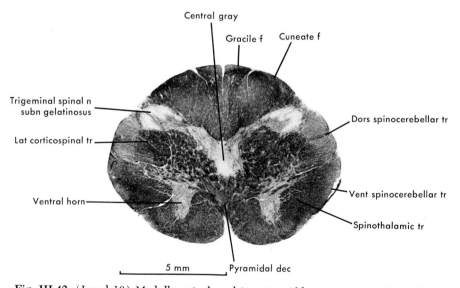

Fig. III-42. (Level 10) Medulla–spinal cord junction. Abbreviations as in Fig. III-33.

Fig. III-43. Human spinal cord. Transverse sections. Sulci, fissures: *DM sul,* dorsal median sulcus; *DI sul,* dorsal intermediate sulcus; *DL sul,* dorsal lateral sulcus; *VM fiss,* ventral median fissure. Areas of gray matter: *D horn,* dorsal horn; *D and V G comm,* dorsal and ventral gray commissures; *V horn,* ventral horn; *n dors,* nucleus dorsalis (Clarke's column); *IML c col,* intermediolateral cell column; *Subs gel,* substantia gelatinosa; *n prop,* nucleus propruis; *Int n,* intermediate nucleus; *Motor n,* motor nucleus; *Comm n,* commissural nucleus; *Laminae I-X,* Rexed's laminae I through X. Areas of white matter: *D fun,* dorsal funiculus; *L fun,* lateral funiculus; *V fun,* ventral funiculus; *Fas gr,* fasciculus gracilis; *Fas cun,* fasciculus cuneatus; *DL fas,* dorsolateral fasciculus; *DCS tr,* dorsal spinocerebellar tract; *VSC tr,* ventral spinocerebellar tract; *CS tr, Rubs tr,* corticospinal tract, rubrospinal tract; *Rets tr,* reticulospinal tracts; *Vests tr,* vestibulospinal tract; *Sthal tr,* spinothalamic tract.

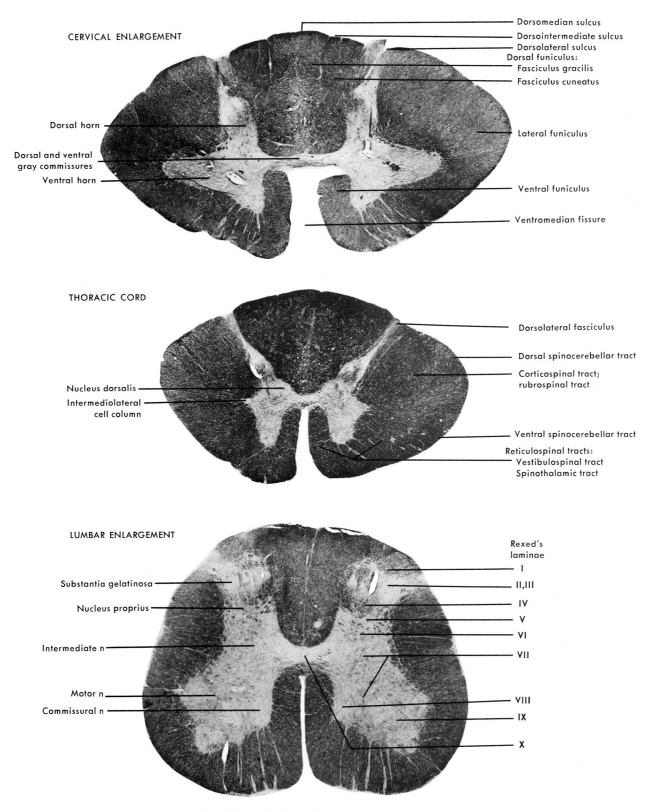

CERVICAL ENLARGEMENT

Dorsomedian sulcus
Dorsointermediate sulcus
Dorsolateral sulcus
Dorsal funiculus:
Fasciculus gracilis
Fasciculus cuneatus

Dorsal horn

Lateral funiculus

Dorsal and ventral
gray commissures
Ventral horn

Ventral funiculus

Ventromedian fissure

THORACIC CORD

Dorsolateral fasciculus

Dorsal spinocerebellar tract

Corticospinal tract;
rubrospinal tract

Nucleus dorsalis
Intermediolateral
cell column

Ventral spinocerebellar tract

Reticulospinal tracts:
Vestibulospinal tract
Spinothalamic tract

LUMBAR ENLARGEMENT

Rexed's
laminae

I

Substantia gelatinosa

II,III

Nucleus proprius

IV

V

VI

Intermediate n

VII

Motor n

VIII

Commissural n

IX

X

Fig. III-43. For legend see opposite page.

Index